Decoding the Pandemic

This comprehensive analysis of COVID-19 draws on the Iceberg Framework—a modified systems thinking model—to examine the deeper forces that shaped the pandemic's trajectory, from structural inequities and institutional fragility to shifting mental models and global behavioral patterns.

Authored by a former Taiwanese Minister of Health and an experienced health system leader, the book combines personal insight with international perspective, offering historical context, contemporary data, and strategic foresight. It situates COVID-19 among history's deadliest pandemics while critically exploring the events, systemic structures, and cultural responses that influenced the crisis. Structured in four parts, the book journeys from echoes of past pandemics and variant-driven disruptions to the hidden foundations of public health responses, culminating in a forward-looking reflection on how COVID-19 has reshaped our understanding of pandemic risk and resilience, while also offering readers a framework for enhanced preparedness in an era of converging global threats.

Timely, accessible, and analytically rigorous, *Decoding the Pandemic* is essential reading for students, researchers, and practitioners in public health, epidemiology, global health policy, and systems science—anyone seeking to understand not just what happened, but why, and what must change before the next pandemic arrives.

Wen-Ta Chiu serves as Co-CEO of AHMC Health System and is the former Taiwan Health Minister and President of Taipei Medical University. A Stanford Fellow with a DrPH from the University of Pittsburgh, he led COVID-19 response efforts across ten hospitals. From 2011 to 2014, he represented Taiwan at the World Health Assembly for four consecutive years, delivering speeches on global health priorities. His leadership has been recognized with 25 awards, including the American Public Health Association's David P. Rall Award.

Jonathan Wu is a prominent medical leader in the United States and founder of AHMC Health System, a network of ten hospitals in California. Under his leadership, AHMC has expanded to include a cancer center, a health insurance company, and long-term care facilities. Dr. Wu also founded Alhambra Medical University and has supported the development of California Northstate University. During the COVID-19 pandemic, he was recognized by a U.S. Congress member as a "Hometown Hero of the Pandemic" for his contributions to public health and community support.

"A comprehensive and insightful analysis of the COVID-19 pandemic's first five years."

—**Dr. Matthew Lin,** *Former Deputy Assistant Secretary and Director of Minority Health, U.S. Department of Health and Human Services*

"A great contribution to physicians, offering clarity and perspective on protecting the communities they serve during a pandemic."

—**Dr. Kenneth Sim,** *Co-Founder and Executive Chairman of Astrana Health*

"A well-researched, systems-level perspective on pandemic resilience, offering practical value for healthcare leaders managing operational and strategic response."

—**Ms. Linda Marsh,** *Senior Executive Vice President, AHMC Healthcare*

"A thoughtful and globally relevant guide for healthcare leaders navigating the complexities of pandemic planning, communication, and clinical coordination."

—**Dr. Alex Chiu,** *Former President, North America Taiwanese Medical Association*

"An invaluable resource for ER physicians and hospital administrators facing pandemic-related challenges."

—**Dr. Stanley Toy,** *CEO, Greater El Monte Community Hospital; Emergency Physician*

"An in-depth exploration of future pandemic risks and the critical lessons learned from COVID-19."

—**Dr. Mike Ly**, *Surveyor for The Joint Commission; Infectious Disease Specialist*

"An essential synthesis of frontline knowledge and public health insight, reflecting lessons drawn from over 130 COVID-related CME sessions and clinical discussions."

—**Dr. Basil Vassantachart,** *CME Program Director, Alhambra Hospital Medical Center; Family Physician*

"Offers clear, experience-based insights into the evolving challenges of critical care during the pandemic—especially valuable for ICU clinicians and hospital planners."

—**Dr. Joseph Kuei,** *Director of Critical Care; Pulmonologist*

"An essential guide for family physicians navigating the challenges of pandemic management."

—**Dr. Josephine Chen,** *Former CMO, Garfield Medical Center; President of Taipei Medical University Alumni Association; Family Physician*

"An informative and engaging narrative that skillfully weaves together history, science, and policy to offer lasting insights into the pandemic and future preparedness."

—**Professor Fu-Tong Liu,** *Academician and Research Fellow, Academia Sinica; Dermatologist*

"A timely and deeply informed contribution that distills five years of pandemic experience into clear, actionable insights for the global health community."

—**Dr. Yun Yen,** *Former Research Director, City of Hope; Former President, Taipei Medical University; Oncologist*

Decoding the Pandemic

Unveiling the Hidden Depths of the COVID-19 Iceberg

Wen-Ta Chiu and Jonathan Wu

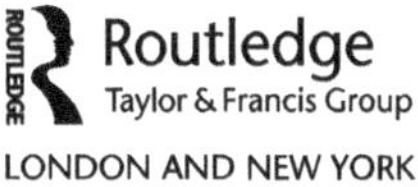

LONDON AND NEW YORK

Designed cover image: Getty Images

First published 2026
by Routledge
4 Park Square, Milton Park, Abingdon, Oxon OX14 4RN

and by Routledge
605 Third Avenue, New York, NY 10158

Routledge is an imprint of the Taylor & Francis Group, an informa business

British Library Cataloguing-in-Publication Data
A catalogue record for this book is available from the British Library

ISBN: 978-1-032-98385-1 (hbk)
ISBN: 978-1-032-98380-6 (pbk)
ISBN: 978-1-003-59556-4 (ebk)

DOI: 10.4324/9781003595564

Typeset in Times New Roman
by KnowledgeWorks Global Ltd.

Contents

List of Figures *ix*
List of Tables *x*
Acknowledgments *xiv*

Introduction: An Overview of the COVID-19 Pandemic Five Years Later 1

PART I
Echoes of the Past: COVID-19's Place in the History of Pandemics 9

1 The Pantheon of Plagues: A Historical Overview 11

2 The Black Death Revisited: Parallels and Contrasts with COVID-19 17

3 A Tale of Two Pandemics: The 1918 Influenza and COVID-19 24

4 The Smallpox Legacy: Eradication Lessons for COVID-19 34

5 Viral Cousins: Comparing Other Coronaviruses to COVID-19 41

6 Pandemic Wisdom: Historical and Contemporary Lessons for COVID-19 49

PART II
The Pandemic Iceberg: Uncovering COVID-19's Hidden Depths 57

7 The Iceberg Ahead: A Framework for Pandemic Analysis 59

8 The Visible Peak: How Global Pandemic Events Triggered Immediate Disruption 65

9 Beneath the Surface: How Underlying Trends Shaped the Evolution of the Pandemic's Trajectory 81

10 Structural Foundations: How Systems and Institutions Shaped the Pandemic Response 128

11 Into the Abyss: How Core Mental Models Influenced Global Pandemic Thinking 173

PART III
Pandemic-Proofing the World: Current Best Practices for Prevention 235

12 Non-Pharmaceutical Interventions: The First Line of Defense 237

13 Vaccines and Treatments: Core Pillars of Pandemic Control 257

14 High-Risk Factors: Understanding Vulnerable Groups in the Pandemic 269

15 Lifestyle as a Shield: Health Behaviors and Pandemic Resilience 278

PART IV
Beyond the Horizon: How COVID-19 Shapes the Next Pandemic Era 301

16 The Long Shadow: Six Enduring Impacts of the Pandemic 303

17 The Long COVID Conundrum: From Medical Mystery to Public Health Priority 326

18 Converging Disease Outbreaks: A Harbinger of Future Pandemics 355

19 A Gathering Storm: The Rise of New Zoonotic Threats 363

20 From Iceberg to Lighthouse: A Final Reflection 375

Index *382*

Figures

0.1	Global COVID-19 Confirmed Cases from 2020 to 2025	1
0.2	Global COVID-19 Reported Deaths from 2020 to 2025	2
0.3	Variant Timeline with Dominant Lineages in the United States from 2020 to 2024	3
0.4	COVID-19 Global Vaccination Coverage from 2020 to 2024	4
0.5	COVID-19 Hospitalizations in the United States (2020–2025)	6
0.6	Flu Hospitalizations in the United States (2019–2025)	6
0.7	RSV Hospitalizations in the United States (2019–2025)	7
3.1	Visualization of First Three Mortality Wave Patterns for 1918 Influenza and COVID-19 Pandemics	25
7.1	Photographic Images of the Titanic (Left) and the Infamous Iceberg That Sank It (Right)	60
7.2	The Systems Thinking Iceberg Model for Pandemic Analysis	63
8.1	Iceberg Model—Events	65
9.1	Iceberg Model—Trends	81
10.1	Iceberg Model—Structures	128
11.1	Iceberg Model—Mental Models	173
14.1	U.S. COVID-19 Deaths by Age Group (01/01/2020–09/27/2023)	274
14.2	Europe COVID-19 Deaths by Age Group (2020–2022)	274
18.1	Resurgence of Multiple Infectious Diseases During the COVID-19 Period (2020–2025). Flu and RSV Saw Significant Resurgence from 2022 to 2025, Mpox from 2022 to 2024, and Norovirus from 2024 to 2025	355
18.2	Test Positivity Rates for COVID-19, Influenza, and RSV in the United States (2022–2025). Flu and RSV Peaked During the Winters of 2022, 2023, and 2024	356
20.1	Lighthouse	380

Tables

1.1	Major Historical Pandemics Comparison	12
2.1	Timeline to Scientific Milestones Between Black Death and COVID-19	21
3.1	Comparative Mortality Statistics Between 1918 Influenza and COVID-19	25
3.2	Comparison of Public Health Interventions Between 1918 Influenza and COVID-19	27
3.3	Comparison of Scientific Understanding and Response Between 1918 Influenza and COVID-19	28
4.1	Key Differences Between Smallpox and COVID-19	36
5.1	Comparison of SARS, MERS, and COVID-19	42
6.1	Historical and Contemporary Pandemic Lessons and Their Relevance to COVID-19	51
8.1	Timeline of COVID-19's Global Spread (December 2019 to March 2020)	66
8.2	ICU System Strain During Early COVID-19 Pandemic (March to April 2020)	68
8.3	Comparative Analysis of Early Lockdown Measures (January to April 2020)	70
8.4	Economic Shock Indicators During Initial COVID-19 Wave (Q1–Q2 2020)	73
9.1	Major SARS-CoV-2 Variants Identified from December 2019 to Early 2025	85
9.2	Epidemiological Trends by Major Global SARS-CoV-2 Variant (2019–2025)	87
9.3	Regional and Seasonal Transmission Patterns of SARS-CoV-2	90
9.4	Comprehensive Analysis of Vaccine Effectiveness Against SARS-CoV-2 Variants (2019–2025)	94
9.5	Comparison of COVID-19 Vaccine Platforms	96
9.6	Global COVID-19 Vaccination and Outcomes by Region	98
9.7	Comparison of COVID-19 Testing Technologies	102
9.8	Comparison of COVID-19 Surveillance Methods	104

9.9 SARS-CoV-2 Genomic Surveillance Capacity by Country Income Level 105
9.10 Antiviral Therapies for COVID-19 108
9.11 Hospital-Based Immune Therapies and Passive Antibody Treatments for COVID-19 110
10.1 Regional Pandemic Strategies, Strengths, and Challenges During COVID-19 129
10.2 Global Health Security Index Rankings of Theoretical Health System Preparedness, Pre-Pandemic (2019) vs. Pandemic (2021) 133
10.3 Global Burnout Rates Among Healthcare Workers During the COVID-19 Pandemic 134
10.4 Factors Associated with Increased Burnout Risk Among Healthcare Workers 136
10.5 Cold Chain Requirements by COVID-19 Vaccine Technology 142
10.6 Initial COVID-19 Vaccine Procurement by Selected High-Income Countries 146
10.7 Cumulative COVID-19 Vaccination Coverage by Country Income Level (2021 vs. 2025) 147
10.8 Initial Pandemic Economic Response by Country (2020–2021) 149
10.9 Initial Pandemic Household and Business Support Measures (2020–2021) 151
10.10 Pandemic Economic Response Implementation Gaps and Access Barriers by Region 152
10.11 Common Misinformation and Conspiracies Spread Throughout the COVID-19 Pandemic, with Corresponding Explanations 160
11.1 Cognitive Biases and Their Underlying Mental Models in COVID-19 Response 175
11.2 Cognitive Cultural Variations in COVID-19 Mental Models 183
11.3 Cultural Mental Models in Pandemic Response 192
11.4 Key Domains of Institutional Mental Models in Pandemic Response 195
11.5 Institutional Mental Models—Rigid vs. Adaptive Models 201
11.6 Temporal Mental Models and Responses Across the COVID-19 Pandemic 203
11.7 Information Processing Models During Public Health Emergencies 213
12.1 Masking Approaches of Select Regions (2020–2025) 239
12.2 Social Distancing Strategies of Select Regions (2020–2025) 241
12.3 Hand Hygiene Policies of Select Regions (2020–2025) 243
12.4 School and Business Closures of Select Regions (2020–2025) 245
12.5 Lockdown Policies of Select Regions (2020–2025) 247
12.6 Travel Restrictions of Select Regions (2020–2025) 249

12.7 Contact Tracing and Quarantining Policies of Select Regions (2020–2025) 251
13.1 Manufacturer, Origin, Type, and Initial Efficacy of COVID-19 Vaccines 258
13.2 Vaccination of Rates by Continent with Select Regions 262
15.1 Impact of Diet on COVID-19 Outcomes 279
15.2 The Role of Vitamins and Trace Elements in Immunity and COVID-19 Outcomes 280
15.3 Key Findings of Physical Activity and Inactivity on COVID-19 Outcomes 284
15.4 Table Summary: Key Findings of Sleep on COVID-19 Outcomes 287
15.5 Pre-Pandemic vs. Pandemic Trends: Alcohol, Opioid, Cannabis, Prescription Drug, and Illicit Drug 293
15.6 Health Impacts and COVID-19 Outcomes of Substance Use 295
16.1 Selected Global Indicators Pre-Pandemic vs. During Pandemic and Beyond 304
16.2 Global and Regional Life Expectancy Changes During the COVID-19 Pandemic (2019–2023) 305
16.3 Global Indirect Health Impacts of COVID-19 306
16.4 Global Mental Health Impacts of the COVID-19 Pandemic (2019–2024) 309
16.5 Global Unemployment Trends by Income Group and Gender, 2019–2024 312
16.6 Global Remote Work Adoption by Income Group and Gender (2020–2024) 313
16.7 Educational Disruption and Learning Loss During COVID-19 (by Region) 315
16.8 Educational Recovery and Response Trends (2024–2025) 316
16.9 Shifts in Public Trust Across Key Institutions During and After COVID-19 317
17.1 Primary Long COVID Symptom Clusters and Estimated Prevalence 327
17.2 Possible Pathophysiological Mechanisms of Long COVID 329
17.3 Organ System Manifestations in Long COVID 331
17.4 Risk Factors for Long COVID Development 335
17.5 Global Long COVID Prevalence by Region 340
17.6 Time Frames for Long COVID Diagnosis Across Major Health Organizations 342
17.7 Current Treatment Approaches for Long COVID by Symptom Category 345
19.1 Major Zoonotic Disease Spillovers of the 21st Century 364
19.2 Expanding Disease Vector Ranges due to Climate Change 365

19.3 Zoonotic Risk Factors in Agricultural and Wildlife Trade Practices 367
19.4 WHO's 2024 Priority Pathogen Watchlist 368
19.5 Core Pillars of One Health for Pandemic Prevention 370
19.6 Cross-Cutting Strategies to Operationalize One Health 371
20.1 The COVID-19 Iceberg: A Framework for Understanding the Pandemic 376

Acknowledgments

Over the past five years, COVID-19 has had a profound impact on California and the United States. Within the AHMC Health System, the ten affiliated hospitals collectively treated over 25,000 COVID-19 cases. In response to this unprecedented challenge, nearly 100 continuing education sessions were organized to support clinical preparedness and professional development.

All healthcare professionals and administrative units across AHMC were fully dedicated to prevention and control efforts. Their strategic recommendations, collaborative spirit, and technical expertise were instrumental in helping the organization navigate some of the most difficult moments in its history—and in shaping the insights presented in this book.

As a result of these collective efforts, AHMC was honored in 2023 with the "Hometown Hero of the Pandemic" award, presented by members of Congress.

The authors would like to extend their appreciation to the following individuals: Dr. Johnson Wu, Dr. Matthew Lin, Mr. Chris Liang, Mr. Tony Yeh, Ms. Linda Marsh, Dr. Kenneth Sim, Dr. Thomas Lam, Dr. Stanley Toy, Ms. Iris Lai, Ms. Evelyn Ku, Mr. Herbert Villafuerte, Mr. Phillip Cohen, Mr. Anthony Nguyen, Ms. Lisa Hahn, Mr. David Batista, Dr. Steve Giordano, Mr. Richard Castro, Ms. Mary Anne Monje, Mr. Sarkis Vartanian, Ms. Judy Saito, Mr. Ash Shehata, Ms. Vivian Yang, Ms. Ariel Qi, Dr. Sonny Wong, Ms. Maan-Huei Hung, Ms. Tarinder Khatkar, Dr. Kevin Chen, Mr. David Allen, Mr. David Huang, Dr. Ahmed El-Bershawi, Dr. Harmohinder Gogia, Dr. Jayakumar Vidhun, Dr. Felix Yip, Dr. Wei Wang, Dr. Raymond Cheung, Dr. Hy Ngo, Dr. Jose Regullano, Dr. Su Kin Lee, Mr. Francis Largoza, Ms. Barbara Tenneson, Ms. Christina Land, Ms. Julie Curtis, Ms. Claudette Caronan, Mr. Michael McGinty, Mr. Jesse Lopez, Ms. Eilyn Caballero, Ms. Kerianne Caligiure, Ms. Jennifer Flores, Dr. William Huang, Mr. Bill Alvarenga, Ms. Nancy Wilson, Mr. Terri Chu, Mr. John Zhuo, Mr. Steven Schulman, Mr. Steve Maekawa, Mr. Jose Ortega, Ms. Rose Tisuthiwongse, Ms. Ericka Smith, Mr. Andrew Grim, Dr. Victor Lange, Dr. Chad Clark, Dr. Stephen Carney, Dr. Josh Child, Dr. Sam McMillan, Dr. Jorge Perez, Dr. Randall Johnson, Dr. Alison Stewart, Dr. Jim Pagano, Dr. John Chon, Dr. Phong Ngo, Dr. Nick Kwan, Dr. Jeremy Williams, Dr. Andrew Shen, Dr. Mike Ly, Dr. Thida Win, Dr. Jamie Lin, Dr. Jessica Mantilla, Dr. Joseph Kuei, Dr. Basil Vassantachart, Dr. Hsiao-Fen Chen, Dr. En-Ming Lai, Mr. Adam Darvish, Ms. Kerri Lee, Ms. Rio Cordova, Ms. Juliette Zhou, Mr. Trevor Roberts,

Dr. Scott Changchien, Dr. Eing-Min Chang, Dr. David Chen, Dr. Joanna Yu, Dr. William Huang, Mr. Ken Lo, Mr. Eugene Chen, Ms. Nicole Chorvat, Ms. Erin Hancock, Ms. Suyen Wu, Ms. Claire Haung, Dr. Ketty Chiu, Mr. Cory Teng, Ms. Cathy Jiang, Ms. Aoife Lin, Ms. Nicole Liu, and Mr. Oscar Yeh.

We also extend our heartfelt thanks to the dedicated physicians, nurses, and technicians across AHMC hospitals and affiliated institutions. Their tireless work across emergency departments, intensive care units, and medical-surgical units formed the foundation for many of the insights shared in this volume.

We are especially grateful to the team at Routledge for their support, editorial guidance, and commitment to bringing this work to publication. Their partnership has helped shape this manuscript into its final form.

The authors would also like to recognize the invaluable support of their editorial team: **Kaveh Aflakian**, **Jessica Toy**, **Naomi Lin**, and **Peggy Pan**. From drafting and translating content to coordinating research, refining language, and organizing and editing the manuscript, their behind-the-scenes efforts were essential throughout the development process. Without their contributions, this book would not have been possible.

Finally, to the readers: thank you for joining us on this journey of reflection, inquiry, and shared responsibility. We hope this work offers not only analysis but also clarity and resolve for the challenges ahead.

Introduction

An Overview of the COVID-19 Pandemic Five Years Later

In March 2020, the world watched as an unfamiliar virus transformed from a distant concern into a global emergency. Within weeks, borders closed, hospitals reached capacity, and societies worldwide found themselves navigating the chaos and disruption of lockdowns, uncertainty, and loss. The virus—SARS-CoV-2—would go on to infect hundreds of millions, claim millions of lives, and leave an enduring legacy of health, economic, and emotional burdens across every continent (Figure 0.1). Excess mortality studies suggest the true global death toll may be two to three times higher than officially reported figures (Figure 0.2).

Now, five years later, we inhabit a transformed landscape. Digital health solutions that might have taken a decade to implement materialized within months. Public awareness of epidemiology, viral transmission, and public health measures also reached levels previously unimaginable. Yet alongside these advances,

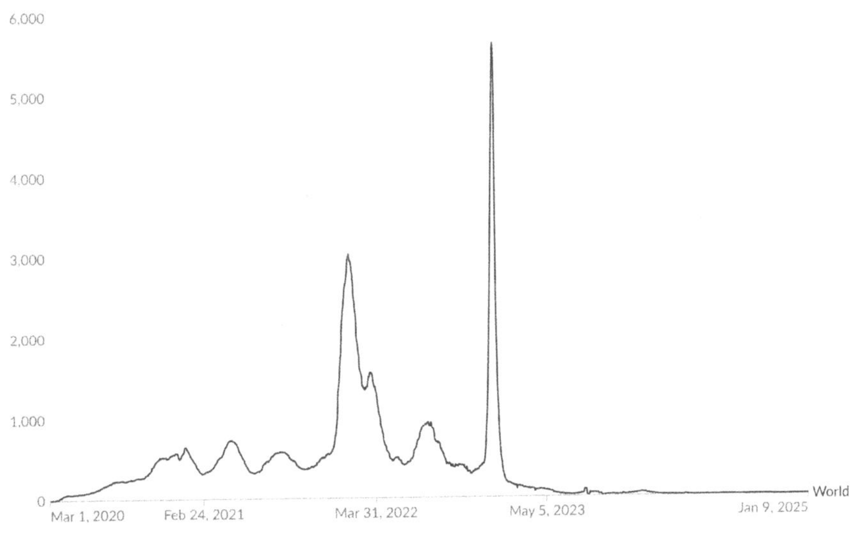

Figure 0.1 Global COVID-19 Confirmed Cases from 2020 to 2025.

Source: Our World in Data (2025); Mathieu et al. (2020).

DOI: 10.4324/9781003595564-1

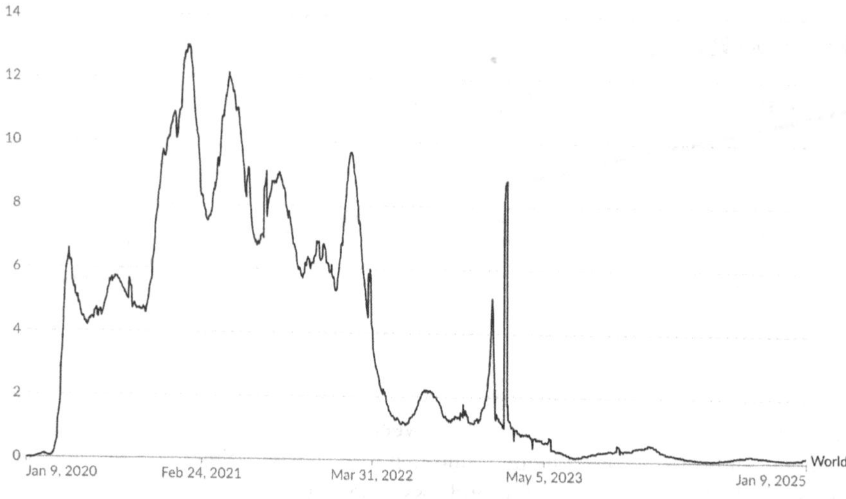

Figure 0.2 Global COVID-19 Reported Deaths from 2020 to 2025.
Source: Our World in Data (2025); Mathieu et al. (2020).

troubling constants remain: misinformation continues to flourish, health systems struggle with chronic fragility, and global cooperation remains inconsistent at best.

Most significantly, we still struggle with fundamental questions about the virus itself—its origins, its true impact, and its long-term consequences for both individuals and societies. These persistent unknowns form not just gaps in our knowledge, but windows into deeper systemic patterns that shaped our collective response.

This five-year period constitutes one of the most consequential chapters in modern global health history. We witnessed COVID-19's evolution from a localized outbreak to a devastating pandemic and finally to an endemic virus with evolving risks. Throughout this journey, case trends surged and receded in multiple distinct waves: the first wave in 2020 exposed unprepared health systems driven by the ancestral strain; the second and third waves in 2021 and early 2022, driven by the Delta and Omicron variants respectively, brought record-breaking case numbers. Death tolls mounted with tragic geographic and demographic variation, with Delta associated with the highest global excess mortality. Meanwhile, the virus itself underwent remarkable genetic evolution, producing variants from Alpha and Delta to Omicron and its sublineages like XBB, JN.1, and XEC, each bringing greater transmissibility and more immune escape (Figure 0.3).

The global response, while unprecedented in its speed and scale, revealed profound disparities. The rapid development of mRNA vaccines represents one of humanity's greatest scientific achievements, with initial rollouts beginning in late 2020 and expanding globally through 2021. Vaccine development initiatives

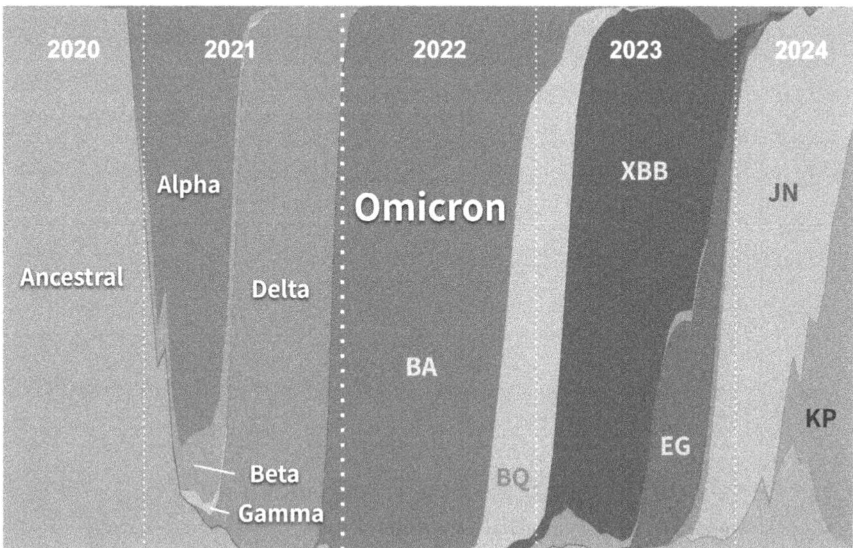

Figure 0.3 Variant Timeline with Dominant Lineages in the United States from 2020 to 2024.

Source: Our World in Data (2025); via GISAID/CoVariants.org (2024).

worldwide compressed typical development timelines from years to months. By mid-2022, over 70% of the world's population had received at least one dose, even despite wide-scale distribution inequity that limited access of vaccines to high-income countries first, while low-income countries were left waiting (Figure 0.4). Over time, waning immunity necessitated regular booster doses, while mounting vaccine hesitancy slowed uptake in various communities. Eventually, this would lead to "booster fatigue," and the shifting variant landscape made public health messaging increasingly complex. Despite these challenges, vaccines were proven to have dramatically reduced severe illness and death even as the virus continued to evolve.

Public health measures saved countless lives while simultaneously exposing social fractures. Digital surveillance tools enabled new forms of containment while raising troubling questions about privacy and power. The economic impact varied dramatically across sectors and populations, with the most vulnerable often bearing the heaviest burdens.

This book adopts a systems thinking framework—specifically, the Iceberg Model—to examine what lies beneath the pandemic's surface events. Like an iceberg, where only a small portion is visible above water, the pandemic's most observable aspects—case counts, policy decisions, and scientific breakthroughs—represent merely the tip of a much deeper structure. Below this visible realm lie recurring patterns, systemic structures, and fundamental mental models that truly determined our collective experience.

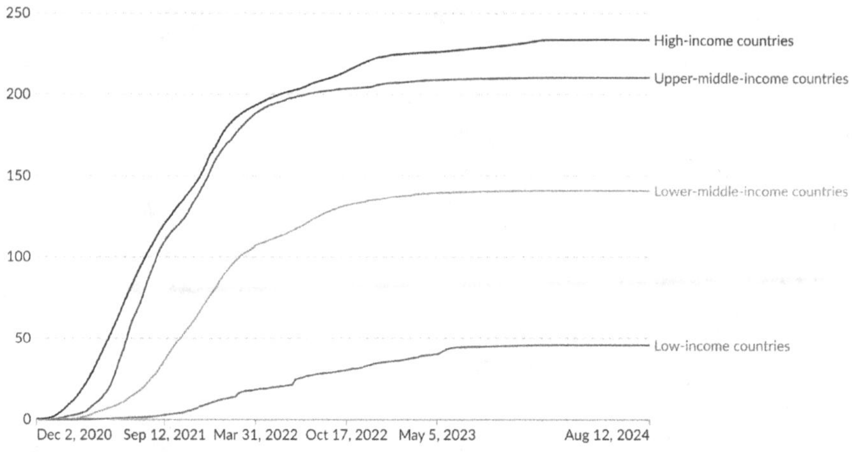

Figure 0.4 COVID-19 Global Vaccination Coverage from 2020 to 2024.

Source: Our World in Data (2025); Mathieu et al. (2020).

As we navigate this exploration, seven critical unknowns serve as our entry points:

1 **What is the true origin of SARS-CoV-2, and why does this question remain unresolved?**

The debate between natural spillover from wildlife and accidental laboratory release continues, complicated by early transparency issues that transformed scientific inquiry into geopolitical controversy. We learned that uncertainty of virus origin undermines public trust and delays critical responses. To better prepare for future pandemics, a global, transparent, and science-based pathogen tracing system is essential, incorporating strict biosafety measures and efficient information-sharing protocols.

2 **How many people truly died from COVID-19, beyond official statistics?**

Official tallies reflect confirmed deaths, but excess mortality studies suggest millions more may have died than reported, highlighting fundamental gaps in our global health surveillance systems. We learned that without accurate data, resources cannot be properly allocated and mistakes cannot be rectified. Public health systems must adopt standardized mortality tracking protocols and be transparent with data during pandemic outbreaks.

3 **What drives the virus's remarkable capacity for mutation and adaptation?**

Each successive variant wave demonstrated SARS-CoV-2's extraordinary adaptability under evolutionary pressure, challenging our vaccine development and public health strategies. We learned that the virus is not a static pathogen. Thus, a broad-spectrum and adaptable vaccine along with the support of genomic surveillance in real time is essential to provide protection against evolving viruses.

4 **How durable is vaccine-induced immunity, and what does this tell us about future protection?**
We now know that antibody immunity wanes within three to four months, while T-cells and memory B-cells provide longer-lasting protection against severe disease, with significant implications for vaccination strategies. We learned that one dose or fixed schedule vaccine programs may not be enough for rapidly mutating viruses. A dynamic, immunity-informed vaccination strategy that incorporates regular immune response monitoring and personalized boosters is crucial for enhanced future protection.

5 **What exactly constitutes long COVID, and what will its long-term societal impact be?**
This persistent syndrome affects millions worldwide, even following mild infections, possibly involving viral remnants, immune dysregulation, or microvascular damage—showing that a virus need not kill to cause devastation. We learned that during pandemics, chronic conditions can become a significant burden. Long-term follow-ups and support systems for post-viral syndromes are essential for comprehensive pandemic response and care.

6 **What was the actual global infection rate, given the limitations of testing and surveillance?**
Estimates suggest that true infections may have been 10–20 times higher than confirmed cases, especially during Omicron surges when widely available at-home testing shrouded true infection counts. This mass level of undetected cases undermines our ability to model future waves and understand herd immunity thresholds. We learned that a robust surveillance strategy, including wastewater monitoring, seroprevalence studies, and digital tracking, is needed to capture the true extent of pandemic outbreaks.

7 **Why did influenza and RSV virtually disappear early in the pandemic only to return with unusual severity?**
In 2020 and 2021, influenza and RSV seasonal infections nearly vanished worldwide, but RSV and influenza returned with concerning strength in 2022–2025, often off-season and with greater severity. Pandemics do not only affect one virus but disrupt entire viral ecosystems (Figures 0.5-0.7). Non-pharmaceutical interventions, including masking and lockdowns, suppressed multiple pathogens and SARS-CoV-2 may have interfered biologically with other viruses. We learned that viral ecosystem disruption can have profound, protracted effects, and that future planning must encompass comprehensive respiratory virus surveillance, extending beyond dominant viruses to monitor the full spectrum of existing, emerging, and reemerging viral threats.

These questions are not merely academic puzzles awaiting resolution. They represent portals through which we can access deeper understandings of our vulnerabilities, capacities, and interdependence. They reveal not just what happened, but why it happened—and what might happen next if we fail to learn and heed the lessons from recent memory.

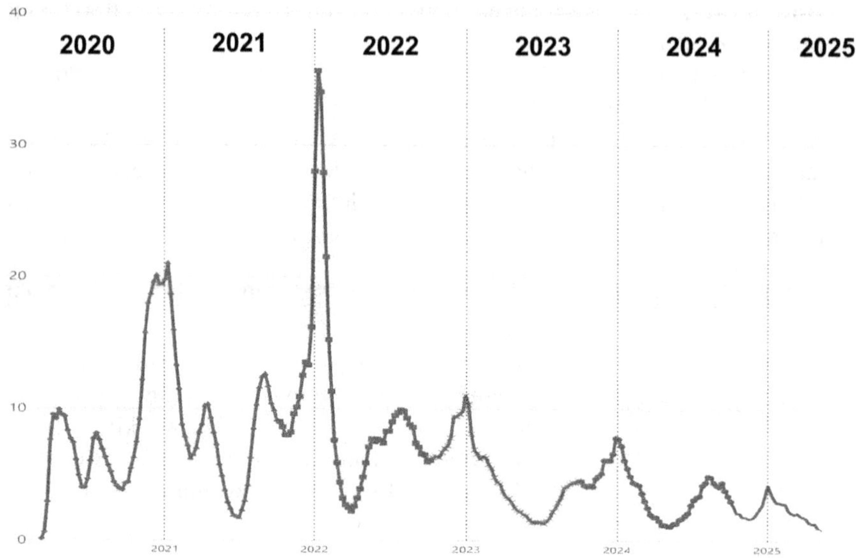

Figure 0.5 COVID-19 Hospitalizations in the United States (2020–2025).
Source: CDC (2025).

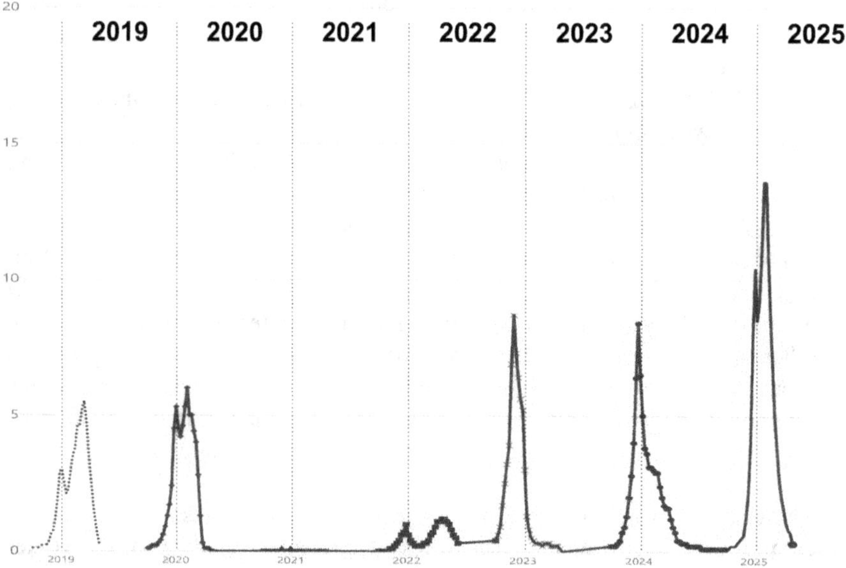

Figure 0.6 Flu Hospitalizations in the United States (2019–2025).
Source: CDC (2025).

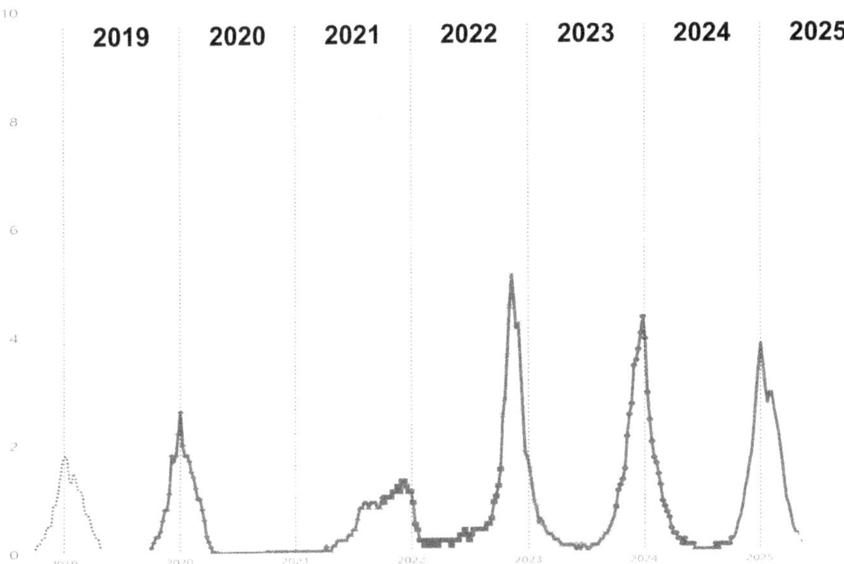

Figure 0.7 RSV Hospitalizations in the United States (2019–2025).

Source: CDC (2025).

This five-year milestone offers a critical moment for reflection. We stand at the threshold between reactive crisis management and proactive, globally coordinated health resilience. The next pandemic may take a different form, from a pathogen that we may possibly have no awareness of, but if we focus only on the specific manifestations of this pandemic rather than the underlying layers that drove its trajectory, we risk repeating history with merely different details.

In the chapters that follow, we will journey through historical pandemics—from the Black Death to the 1918 influenza and beyond—seeking echoes and divergences in our COVID-19 experience. Yet we will not stop at historical comparison. Through systems thinking, we will dive beneath pandemic headline events to explore the patterns they reinforced, the structures they revealed, and the mental models that shaped our collective response.

This layered approach allows us not merely to understand the crisis we endured, but to imagine and construct a world better prepared for what inevitably lies ahead. Five years after COVID-19 emerged, we are no longer left roaming in the dark—but that clarity must not give way to complacency. The insights gained through suffering must now be transformed into wisdom that guides us toward greater resilience, equity, and foresight. This is the journey we now undertake together.

Part I

Echoes of the Past

COVID-19's Place in the History of Pandemics

1 The Pantheon of Plagues

A Historical Overview

The COVID-19 global pandemic has claimed over 7 million officially reported deaths to date, though excess mortality estimates from the World Health Organization suggest the actual figure may be closer to 15–20 million deaths globally. While various rankings of historical pandemics exist using different methodologies, COVID-19 undeniably belongs among major historical diseases such as the Black Death, the 1918 Spanish Influenza, and smallpox in its widespread disruption of global health. This section positions COVID-19 in historical context, comparing mortality rates, societal impacts, and unique challenges to establish the foundation for a more comprehensive exploration of the pandemic's full impact—as well as the lessons that can be derived from this significant chapter in human history.

On March 11, 2020, the World Health Organization (WHO) officially declared COVID-19 a global pandemic. While official figures report approximately 7 million deaths, the actual toll is likely substantially higher due to limitations in testing, reporting inconsistencies, and varying case definitions across countries (Ritchie et al., 2022). Throughout history, major infectious diseases have profoundly disrupted human societies, leaving lasting social, economic, and epidemiological impacts. To understand COVID-19's significance, evolution, and potential trajectory, we must first examine its historical context within the broader landscape of global pandemics.

The Gavi Global Vaccine Alliance has identified the seven deadliest pandemics in recorded history (Table 1.1), with COVID-19 ranking sixth (Gavi, 2025). The following examines these devastating pandemics and their societal impacts:

1. **Black Death (1347–1351):** Caused by the bacterium *Yersinia pestis* and transmitted by fleas on rats, the Black Death originated in Asia and spread to Europe via trade routes. While the main European outbreak occurred between 1347 and 1351, plague outbreaks continued periodically for centuries. Symptoms included fever, chills, weakness, and swollen, painful lymph nodes called buboes. The mortality rate was extremely high, with some estimates suggesting that up to 60% of infected individuals died (Benedictow, 2021). The pandemic had

DOI: 10.4324/9781003595564-3

Table 1.1 Major Historical Pandemics Comparison

Pandemic	*Time Period*	*Pathogen*	*Estimated Deaths*	*Mortality Rate (%)*
Black Death	1347–1351	*Yersinia pestis* (bacterium)	75–200 million	30–60% of infected
1918 Influenza	1918–1920	H1N1 (virus)	50–100 million	Approx. 2.5% average; higher in young adults
Smallpox	Historical–1980	Variola (virus)	>300 million (20th century)	20–45% (variola major); 1–2% (variola minor)
Justinian Plague	541–549	*Yersinia pestis* (bacterium)	15–100 million	50–60% during severe outbreaks
AIDS	1981–present	HIV (virus)	42.3 million (as of 2023)	>99.9% fatal untreated; chronic with treatment
COVID-19	2019–present	SARS-CoV-2 (virus)	>7 million (official), 15–20 million (excess)	0.1–5% varying by age, variant, and vaccination
Third Plague	1855–1960s	*Yersinia pestis* (bacterium)	12–15 million	30–60% without antibiotics

Sources: Benedictow (2021); Centers for Disease Control and Prevention (2025); Christakos et al. (2005, 2007); Gavi (2025); Johnson and Mueller (2002); Karlinsky and Kobak (2021); Morens and Fauci (2020); Ritchie et al. (2022); Roser et al. (2023); Taubenberger and Morens (2006); UNAIDS (2024); Wang et al. (2022); World Health Organization (2022a, 2022b, 2022c, 2025); Yarmol-Matusiak et al. (2021).

profound social, economic, and cultural impacts, leading to widespread labor shortages, the breakdown of feudal systems, and persecution of minority groups erroneously blamed for the disease. Most historical demographic analyses suggest it claimed between 75 and 200 million lives, decimating approximately 30–60% of Europe's population over a relatively short period—though these figures remain subject to ongoing scholarly debate (Christakos et al., 2007).

2 **1918 Spanish Influenza (1918–1920):** The 1918 influenza pandemic, caused by the H1N1 virus, spread rapidly due to troop movements during World War I. Unlike typical influenza outbreaks, which primarily affect the very young and elderly, this pandemic disproportionately affected young adults (Taubenberger & Morens, 2006). Beyond its initial high mortality rate, the pandemic caused widespread social and economic disruption, with schools and businesses closed and healthcare systems overwhelmed. An estimated 50–100 million people died, primarily those aged between 20 and 30 (Johnson & Mueller, 2002).

3 **Smallpox (Historical–1980):** Smallpox, caused by the variola virus, was a devastating disease that affected humanity for thousands of years before its eradication in 1980—the only human disease successfully eradicated to date. While

smallpox has ancient origins, its introduction to the Americas in the 1520s by European colonizers was particularly catastrophic, as indigenous populations had no prior exposure or immunity. Smallpox causes fever and a distinctive, progressive skin rash, potentially leading to encephalitis, blindness, and scarring. The high mortality rate among Native Americans (estimated at 30–90% in different communities) profoundly disrupted their societies and facilitated European colonization (Yarmol-Matusiak et al., 2021). Throughout its entire history, smallpox is estimated to have killed hundreds of millions of people worldwide with conservative estimates suggesting at least 300 million deaths in the 20th century alone before eradication efforts succeeded.

4 **Justinian Plague (541–549):** Like the Black Death, the Justinian Plague was caused by *Y. pestis*, though recent genomic studies indicate it was a different strain. It originated in Africa and spread to Europe and Asia. Named after Byzantine Emperor Justinian I, who contracted but survived the disease, this pandemic contributed to the decline of the Byzantine Empire and had significant economic consequences, disrupting trade and leading to food shortages (Christakos et al., 2005). Contemporary scholarly estimates suggest it claimed between 15 and 100 million lives—with most current research supporting the lower end of this range. Claims about the percentage of world population affected (sometimes cited as 13–26%) should be approached with caution, as demographic data from the 6th century contains significant uncertainties. Recent scholarship tends to favor more conservative mortality estimates than earlier historical analyses.

5 **AIDS (1981–present):** AIDS (acquired immunodeficiency syndrome) is caused by the human immunodeficiency virus (HIV). Transmitted through sexual contact, blood-to-blood contact, and mother-to-child transmission during pregnancy, childbirth, or breastfeeding, HIV weakens the immune system over time, making individuals susceptible to life-threatening opportunistic infections and cancers. The development of antiretroviral therapy has transformed HIV from a typically fatal condition to a manageable chronic disease. According to UNAIDS (2024), approximately 42.3 million people have died from AIDS-related illnesses since the beginning of the epidemic through 2023. While annual AIDS-related deaths have significantly decreased from their peak of 2 million in 2004 to approximately 630,000 in 2023, the pandemic continues to pose significant challenges, particularly in regions with limited healthcare access.

6 **COVID-19 (2019–present):** COVID-19, caused by the SARS-CoV-2 virus, first emerged in Wuhan, China, in late 2019 and spread rapidly worldwide. This respiratory illness can cause fever, cough, breathing difficulties, and in severe cases, pneumonia and organ failure. The pandemic led to unprecedented global lockdown measures, border closures, and economic disruption. The rapid development and distribution of effective vaccines was crucial in controlling the pandemic's overall severity, though access and distribution inequities posed a significant challenge (Morens & Fauci, 2020). As of early 2025, officially reported deaths have reached over 7 million, but excess mortality models from WHO estimate the actual global death toll to be significantly higher—somewhere between 15 and 20 million deaths (Wang et al., 2022).

7 **Third Plague Pandemic (1855–1960s):** The Third Plague Pandemic, again caused by *Y. pestis*, originated in Yunnan, China. While 1959 is often cited as an end date because that's when worldwide cases dropped below 200 per year, isolated outbreaks continued well into the 1960s in some regions (Centers for Disease Control and Prevention, 2025). This pandemic spread worldwide, with major outbreaks in China and India, leading to significant advances in understanding the disease, including Alexandre Yersin's identification of the causative bacterium in 1894 and Paul-Louis Simond's discovery of the rat-flea transmission mechanism in 1898. These scientific breakthroughs improved public health measures such as rat control and quarantine. Contemporary scholarship estimates approximately 12–15 million deaths occurred during this pandemic, with India suffering nearly half of these casualties (Gavi, 2025).

Rankings of historical pandemics by mortality vary considerably depending on methodology, time period considered, and data sources. When accounting for excess mortality estimates rather than just officially reported figures, COVID-19 may rank anywhere from the third to seventh deadliest pandemic in recorded history (Roser et al., 2023). With confirmed cases exceeding 777 million globally, the pandemic's true reach is likely even broader due to limited testing capacity in many regions. The underreporting of deaths is particularly pronounced in low- and middle-income countries, where fragile health systems and limited surveillance infrastructure may obscure the pandemic's full impact (Karlinsky & Kobak, 2021). Moreover, the long-term health consequences of COVID-19 are still being uncovered, suggesting the pandemic's ultimate burden on global health and healthcare systems may not be fully understood for decades to come.

The COVID-19 Landscape: A Future Unresolved

With the acute phase of the COVID-19 pandemic now behind us, the world has entered a complex aftermath phase characterized by different challenges. The declaration by the WHO in May 2023 that COVID-19 no longer constitutes a global public health emergency marked a significant transition point. However, the pandemic's legacy continues to unfold through multiple dimensions: persistent long COVID cases affecting millions globally, healthcare systems still recovering from lingering strain, economic repercussions that have reshaped labor markets and supply chains, and significant public mental health impacts that will require long-term attention (Mathieu et al., 2021).

The post-pandemic landscape also reveals substantial inequities in recovery trajectories. High-income countries with robust vaccination programs and healthcare infrastructure have largely returned to pre-pandemic activities, while many low- and middle-income nations continue to struggle with limited vaccine access, fragile health systems, and economic instability (Yarmol-Matusiak et al., 2021). These disparities are clarion calls to the importance of strengthening global health governance and addressing fundamental inequities in healthcare access.

By understanding COVID-19's place within the historical pantheon of pandemics, we gain valuable context for addressing its long-tail effects and preparing for future public health threats. The subsequent chapters will explore these various dimensions in greater detail, examining both the immediate consequences and long-term implications of what has proven to be one of the most significant global health events of the 21st century.

References

Benedictow, O. J. (2021). *The Black Death 1346-1353: The complete history*. Boydell & Brewer.

Centers for Disease Control and Prevention. (2025, March 25). *Maps and statistics: Plague*. https://www.cdc.gov/plague/maps-statistics/index.html

Christakos, G., Olea, R. A., Serre, M. L., Yu, H. L., & Wang, L. L. (2005). *Interdisciplinary public health reasoning and epidemic modelling: The case of Black Death*. Springer.

Christakos, G., Olea, R. A., & Yu, H. L. (2007). Recent results on the spatiotemporal modelling and comparative analysis of Black Death and bubonic plague epidemics. *Public Health*, *121*(9), 700–720. https://doi.org/10.1016/j.puhe.2006.12.011

Gavi. (2025, February 6). *History's seven deadliest plagues*. https://www.gavi.org/vaccineswork/historys-seven-deadliest-plagues

Johnson, N. P., & Mueller, J. (2002). Updating the accounts: Global mortality of the 1918-1920 "Spanish" influenza pandemic. *Bulletin of the History of Medicine*, *76*(1), 105–115. https://doi.org/10.1353/bhm.2002.0022

Karlinsky, A., & Kobak, D. (2021). Tracking excess mortality across countries during the COVID-19 pandemic with the World Mortality Dataset. *eLife*, *10*, e69336. https://doi.org/10.7554/eLife.69336

Mathieu, E., Ritchie, H., Rodés-Guirao, L., Appel, C., Giattino, C., Hasell, J., Macdonald, B., Dattani, S., Beltekian, D., Ortiz-Ospina, E., & Roser, M. (2021). Coronavirus pandemic (COVID-19). *Our World in Data*. https://ourworldindata.org/coronavirus

Morens, D. M., & Fauci, A. S. (2020). Emerging pandemic diseases: How we got to COVID-19. *Cell*, *182*(5), 1077–1092. https://doi.org/10.1016/j.cell.2020.08.021

Ritchie, H., Mathieu, E., Rodés-Guirao, L., Appel, C., Giattino, C., Ortiz-Ospina, E., Hasell, J., Macdonald, B., Beltekian, D., & Roser, M. (2022). Excess mortality during the coronavirus pandemic (COVID-19). *Our World in Data*. https://ourworldindata.org/excess-mortality-covid

Roser, M., Ritchie, H., & Ortiz-Ospina, E. (2023). What were the death tolls from pandemics in history? *Our World in Data*. https://ourworldindata.org/historical-pandemics

Taubenberger, J. K., & Morens, D. M. (2006). 1918 Influenza: The mother of all pandemics. *Emerging Infectious Diseases*, *12*(1), 15–22. https://doi.org/10.3201/eid1201.050979

UNAIDS. (2024). *2024 global AIDS report. The urgency of now: AIDS at a crossroads*. https://www.unaids.org/en/resources/documents/2024/global-aids-update-2024

Wang, H., Paulson, K. R., Pease, S. A., Watson, S., Comfort, H., Zheng, P., Aravkin, A. Y., Bisignano, C., Barber, R. M., Alam, T., Fuller, J. E., May, E. A., Jones, D. P., Frisch, M. E., Abbafati, C., Adolph, C., Allorant, A., Amlag, J. O., Bang, J. B., … Murray, C. J. L. (2022). Estimating excess mortality due to the COVID-19 pandemic: A systematic analysis of COVID-19-related mortality, 2020–21. *The Lancet*, *399*(10334), 1513–1536. https://doi.org/10.1016/S0140-6736(21)02796-3

World Health Organization. (2022a). *Global excess deaths associated with COVID-19 (modelled estimates)*. https://www.who.int/data/sets/global-excess-deaths-associated-with-covid-19-modelled-estimates

World Health Organization. (2022b). *The true death toll of COVID-19: Estimating global excess mortality.* https://www.who.int/data/stories/the-true-death-toll-of-covid-19-estimating-global-excess-mortality

World Health Organization. (2022c). The WHO estimates of excess mortality associated with the COVID-19 pandemic. *Nature*, *415*, 543–553. https://doi.org/10.1038/s41586-022-05522-2

World Health Organization. (2025). *WHO coronavirus (COVID-19) Dashboard.* https://covid19.who.int/

Yarmol-Matusiak, E. A., Cipriano, L. E., & Stranges, S. (2021). Societal impacts of pandemics: Comparing COVID-19 with history to focus our response. *Frontiers in Public Health*, *9*, 630449. https://www.ncbi.nlm.nih.gov/pmc/articles/PMC8072022/

2 The Black Death Revisited

Parallels and Contrasts with COVID-19

The Black Death, the devastating bubonic plague outbreak of the 14th century, ranks among history's deadliest pandemics, with mortality estimates ranging from 75 to 200 million lives. Understanding of its etiology and transmission route developed gradually, with definitive scientific breakthroughs only emerging in the late 19th century. These advances eventually led to the development of vaccines and, by the mid-20th century, effective antibiotic treatments. This scientific progress resulted from the contributions of key figures including Alexandre Yersin, Paul-Louis Simond, Waldemar Haffkine, and Selman Waksman. In contrast, the scientific response to COVID-19 unfolded at unprecedented speed. Within months rather than centuries, scientists identified the SARS-CoV-2 virus and, within the first two years, had tracked its variants, developed effective vaccines, created therapeutic agents, and implemented preventative measures that significantly reduced mortality.

The Black Death: A Catalyst for Scientific and Social Transformation

The Black Death marked a pivotal moment in human history. Beyond its staggering mortality toll, it fundamentally reshaped societies, triggering social and technological advancements born from desperate bids for survival (Cantor, 2001; McNeill, 1976).

Initially, the plague engendered a sense of helplessness, with many interpreting it as divine retribution. However, as the death toll escalated, a paradigm shift emerged. Desperation compelled Europeans to seek solutions beyond supplication, becoming a catalyst for rational thinking. Society gradually progressed beyond fear and fatalism, embracing a more proactive approach to combating disease. Some historians view this shift as contributing to the Renaissance, with its emphasis on reason and scientific inquiry (Snowden, 2019).

Historical evidence suggests that pandemics often precipitate periods of innovation. The Black Death was no exception, inspiring groundbreaking advances in the understanding and treatment of infectious diseases. By the 17th century, British and Spanish scientists began uncovering associations between microorganisms and infectious diseases. While still uncertain about plague's precise etiology, this discovery facilitated understanding that isolation could impede transmission (Byrne, 2012).

DOI: 10.4324/9781003595564-4

Scientific Breakthroughs in the Study of the Black Death

Several key historical figures made pivotal discoveries that transformed our understanding and treatment of plague:

Alexandre Yersin (1863–1943): Alexandre Yersin, a Swiss-French physician and bacteriologist, made a groundbreaking discovery in 1894 when he identified *Yersinia pestis* as the bacterium responsible for the Black Death (Butler, 2014; Steensma, 2019). During a Hong Kong outbreak, Yersin risked his life to collect and study samples from afflicted patients. His meticulous research allowed him to isolate and identify the bacterial agent. This discovery revolutionized scientific understanding of plague, providing crucial insights into its transmission and potential medical interventions. Yersin's work laid the foundation for subsequent advancements in plague prevention and treatment, including diagnostic tests, antibiotics, and vaccines (Mayo Clinic Proceedings, 2020).

Paul-Louis Simond (1858–1947): French physician and epidemiologist Paul-Louis Simond made a critical discovery in 1898 that transformed understanding of plague transmission. Through careful observation and experimentation, Simond identified that plague was transmitted from infected rats to humans via fleas (Mollaret, 1999; Simond et al., 1998). This breakthrough challenged the prevailing belief that plague spread through direct contact or contaminated air. While Simond's rat-flea-human transmission theory informed public health measures for decades, recent scholarship suggests his experiments were not as conclusive as traditionally portrayed, and he maintained a more complex view of plague transmission that included multiple pathways beyond fleas (Cambau & Drancourt, 2020). Nevertheless, his contributions have had a lasting impact on infectious disease control and prevention.

Waldemar Haffkine (1860–1930): Russian-Jewish bacteriologist Waldemar Haffkine developed one of the first plague vaccines in the late 19th century using heat-killed plague bacteria (Liang, 2020). First tested during an 1897 India outbreak, the vaccine demonstrated remarkable efficacy in preventing infection (T-invariant, 2025). Despite initial skepticism and opposition, the undeniable success of Haffkine's vaccine led to widespread acceptance and implementation. His pioneering efforts in vaccine development laid groundwork for future advancements in immunology and vaccines for other deadly diseases (Hawgood, 2007b; Wilkof, 2017).

Selman Waksman (1888–1973): American microbiologist Selman Waksman was credited with the discovery of streptomycin in 1943, though it was his graduate student Albert Schatz who isolated the compound in Waksman's laboratory (Pringle, 2012; White, 2014). This significant contribution by Schatz led to subsequent controversy and legal proceedings, with Schatz eventually receiving financial compensation and acknowledgment as co-discoverer of streptomycin following a lawsuit in 1950 (Costa, 2024). Streptomycin became the first effective antibiotic against gram-negative bacteria, including *Yersinia pestis*. This discovery came several years after Alexander Fleming's identification of penicillin, as research into antibiotics was accelerating. Streptomycin provided a powerful new tool against plague and tuberculosis, dramatically reducing mortality rates for both diseases. Waksman received the 1952 Nobel Prize in Physiology or Medicine for this discovery, and his methodical research approach to screening soil microbes for antibiotic compounds significantly advanced the field of antimicrobial drug development (Rutgers University, 2024; Woodruff, 2014).

The groundbreaking work of these scientists deepened our understanding of the Black Death and had far-reaching implications for infectious disease management. Their discoveries and innovations established the foundation for modern public health strategies and medical treatments that have saved countless lives to date. The devastating impact of the Black Death ultimately propelled scientific progress that continues to benefit humanity today.

From Plague Doctors to DNA: Tracing Pandemic Management Through History

The Plague Doctor: Precursor to Modern Personal Protective Equipment

The iconic plague doctor, with his beaked mask and full-body covering, symbolizes the medical response to bubonic plague epidemics that ravaged Europe from the 14th to 17th centuries. First designed by French physician Charles de Lorme in 1619, the suit marked a significant advancement in personal protective equipment (Byrne, 2012).

De Lorme's design aimed to protect doctors from miasma, or "bad air," then believed to cause plague. The beaked mask contained aromatic herbs, spices, or vinegar sponges, theorized to purify air and ward off disease. Glass eyes prevented direct contact with infectious fluids, while waxed fabric kept bodily fluids from touching the skin.

The plague doctor's stick served a practical purpose: examining patients while maintaining safe distance from infection. Though primitive by modern standards, this iconic ensemble represents an early attempt at comprehensive disease prevention, combining available medical knowledge with practical design. The image remains a powerful symbol of historical challenges faced by medical professionals and their innovative protective measures against deadly outbreaks (Cantor, 2001).

Confronting Fear: The Role of Religious Communities During Early Pandemics

Historical accounts from the Antonine (165–180 CE) and Cyprian (249–262 CE) plagues that significantly impacted the Roman Empire suggest that early Christian communities developed distinctive responses to epidemic disease. According to historian William McNeill in his work "Plagues and Peoples" and other scholars, these communities often provided care for the sick when others fled (McNeill, 1976; Snowden, 2019).

This period saw multiple outbreaks, including the Antonine Plague and Cyprian Plague, which severely tested Roman society's resilience. While fear and despair were common responses, Christians frequently responded with communal spirit, caring not only for their own but also for pagan neighbors. This practice, rooted in Christian teachings of charity and mercy, distinguished them in a society where many were left to fend for themselves.

Their compassionate care during pandemics enhanced Christianity's reputation when the religion was still gaining a foothold in Roman society. While it's an oversimplification to claim these actions directly led to Christianity becoming the state religion under Constantine, they demonstrated the faith's commitment to principles of love and service, exemplifying how faith-based communities can respond to public health crises with compassion and resilience.

Early Quarantine Measures: Venice and Eyam

As the Black Death swept through Europe in the 14th century, different regions adopted varying strategies to combat disease spread. Venice, a bustling trade hub, implemented organized quarantine measures early. In 1348, Venetian authorities established the world's first lazaretto on Santa Maria di Nazareth island, where incoming ships, cargoes, and crews were isolated for up to forty days—a practice giving rise to the term "quarantine" from Italian "quaranta giorni" (forty days). These measures attempted to control plague spread, protect the city-state's economic interests, and set public health precedents (Benedictow, 2004).

Similarly, the English village of Eyam made a remarkable sacrifice in 1665 when it self-imposed quarantine after plague arrived through contaminated cloth from London. Led by Reverend William Mompesson and his predecessor Thomas Stanley, villagers made the altruistic decision to isolate themselves, preventing contagion from reaching nearby towns. Residents marked village boundaries, and food was left at designated points where coins soaked in vinegar (a rudimentary disinfectant) were left as payment. This self-quarantine resulted in substantial village mortality but successfully halted disease spread beyond Eyam's boundaries (Ziegler, 2013).

Both instances demonstrate early understanding and implementation of quarantine as a public health tool. Venice's approach reflected systematic, government-implemented strategy to safeguard an entire community, while Eyam's story highlighted communal sacrifice and local leadership in crisis management. These historical episodes illuminate the evolution of societal responses to pandemics and quarantine's enduring importance in managing infectious diseases.

21st-Century DNA Studies Confirm Medieval Black Death as Plague

Recent advancements in genetic research have provided profound insights into historical pandemics. 21st-century DNA analysis has conclusively identified *Yersinia pestis* as the causative agent of the medieval Black Death. By extracting and analyzing ancient DNA from dental and skeletal remains of victims buried in mass graves across Europe, scientists have confirmed the bacterial etiology of the 14th-century pandemics (Barbieri et al., 2020).

This breakthrough was achieved through meticulous isolation and sequencing of DNA preserved in dental pulp, where bloodborne pathogens can persist for centuries. The results not only confirmed the bacterial origin but also elucidated its genetic lineage. Subsequent studies have mapped a global phylogenetic tree of plague strains, suggesting the pathogen likely originated in or near China before spreading along the Silk Road and other trade routes to the Crimea and, via maritime trade, throughout Europe (Bramanti et al., 2019).

These findings provide a more comprehensive understanding of plague's historical spread while enhancing our knowledge of pathogen evolution over time—insights crucial for modern epidemiology and understanding how human migration and trade influence infectious disease transmission.

Is COVID-19 a Microcosm of the Black Death? From Centuries to Months and Years

The COVID-19 pandemic demonstrates how modern scientific capabilities have compressed the timeline of pandemic response from centuries to months (Table 2.1). While scientific understanding of the Black Death evolved over many hundreds of years, with definitive identification of its cause only occurring in the 1890s, the SARS-CoV-2 virus was sequenced within weeks of the first reported cases in December 2019. By December 2020, less than a year after the virus's identification, the first mRNA vaccines received emergency use authorization—a process that historically would have taken decades (Williamson et al., 2024).

Table 2.1 Timeline to Scientific Milestones Between Black Death and COVID-19

Milestone	*Black Death (14th century)*	*COVID-19 (2019–2021)*
Pathogen identification	547 years *(1894, by Alexandre Yersin)*	<2 weeks *(January 2020)*
Understanding transmission	551 years *(1898, by Paul-Louis Simond)*	<1–2 months
Vaccine development	550 years *(1897, by Waldemar Haffkine)*	<11 months *(mRNA)*
Treatment development	596 years *(1943, by Selman Waksman & Albert Schatz)*	<1–2 years *(antivirals)*

Sources: Barbieri et al. (2020); Butler (2014); Cambau and Drancourt (2020); Callaway (2020); Costa (2024); Hawgood (2007a, 2007b); Krammer (2020); Li et al. (2020); Liang (2020); Mayo Clinic Proceedings (2020); National Institutes of Health (2020); Pringle (2012); Simond et al. (1998); Steensma (2019); White (2014); Williamson et al. (2024); Woodruff (2014); Zhu et al. (2020).

This accelerated timeline reflects not only technological advances but also the evolution of global scientific collaboration. International research networks, data sharing platforms, and advanced computational models allowed scientists to rapidly characterize the virus, develop diagnostic tests, and design targeted therapeutics. The introduction of antivirals within two years of the pandemic's onset further exemplifies this compressed timeline of scientific response.

Despite these remarkable achievements, both pandemics revealed similar societal vulnerabilities. The Black Death exposed medieval Europe's inadequate sanitation systems and limited medical knowledge, while COVID-19 revealed modern challenges: health system capacity limitations, global supply chain fragilities, and the impact of misinformation in a deeply connected world.

This comparative perspective offers valuable insights for future pandemic preparedness. While scientific capabilities have advanced dramatically, certain fundamental challenges in pandemic response persist across historical contexts. The institutional frameworks, social trust, and public health infrastructures that support scientific innovation remain as crucial today as they were during past pandemics.

References

Barbieri, R., Signoli, M., Chevé, D., Costedoat, C., Tzortzis, S., Aboudharam, G., Raoult, D., & Drancourt, M. (2020). *Yersinia pestis*: The natural history of plague. *Clinical Microbiology Reviews, 34*(1), e00044–19. https://doi.org/10.1128/CMR.00044-19

Benedictow, O. J. (2004). *The Black Death, 1346-1353: The complete history*. Boydell & Brewer.

Bramanti, B., Dean, K. R., Walløe, L., & Stenseth, N. C. (2019). The third plague pandemic in Europe. *Proceedings of the Royal Society B, 286*(1901), 20182429. https://doi.org/10.1098/rspb.2018.2429

Butler, T. (2014). Plague history: Yersin's discovery of the causative bacterium in 1894 enabled, in the subsequent century, scientific progress in understanding the disease and the development of treatments and vaccines. *Clinical Microbiology and Infection, 20*(3), 202–209. https://doi.org/10.1111/1469-0691.12540

Byrne, J. P. (2012). *Encyclopedia of the Black Death*. ABC-CLIO.

Callaway, E. (2020). The race for coronavirus vaccines: A graphical guide. *Nature, 580*(7805), 576–577. https://doi.org/10.1038/d41586-020-01221-y

Cambau, E., & Drancourt, M. (2020). In search of lost fleas: Reconsidering Paul-Louis Simond's contribution to the study of the propagation of plague. *Medical History, 64*(1), 29–51. https://doi.org/10.1017/mdh.2019.74

Cantor, N. F. (2001). *In the wake of the plague: The Black Death and the world it made*. Free Press.

Costa, A. B. (2024). *Waksman discovers the antibiotic streptomycin*. EBSCO Research Starters. https://www.ebsco.com/research-starters/history/waksman-discovers-antibiotic-streptomycin

Hawgood, B. J. (2007a). Alexandre Yersin (1863–1943): Discoverer of the plague bacillus, explorer and agronomist. *Journal of Medical Biography, 15*(1), 9–19. https://doi.org/10.1258/j.jmb.2007.05-59

Hawgood, B. J. (2007b). Waldemar Mordecai Haffkine, CIE (1860-1930): Prophylactic vaccination against cholera and bubonic plague in British India. *Journal of Medical Biography, 15*(1), 9–19. https://doi.org/10.1258/j.jmb.2007.05-59

Krammer, F. (2020). SARS-CoV-2 vaccines in development. *Nature, 586*(7830), 516–527. https://doi.org/10.1038/s41586-020-2798-3

Li, Q., Guan, X., Wu, P., Wang, X., Zhou, L., Tong, Y., Ren, R., Leung, K. S. M., Lau, E. H. Y., Wong, J. Y., Xing, X., Xiang, N., Wu, Y., Li, C., Chen, Q., Li, D., Liu, T., Zhao, J., Liu, M., … & Feng, Z. (2020). Early transmission dynamics in Wuhan, China, of novel coronavirus—Infected pneumonia. *New England Journal of Medicine*, *382*(13), 1199–1207. https://doi.org/10.1056/NEJMoa2001316

Liang, Y. (2020). The pioneer of cholera vaccine and plague vaccine-Haffkine. *Zhonghua Yi Shi Za Zhi*, *50*(2), 103–106. https://doi.org/10.3760/cma.j.issn.0255-7053.2020.02.007

Mayo Clinic Proceedings. (2020). Alexandre Yersin: Discoverer of the plague bacillus. *Mayo Clinic Proceedings*, *95*(1), e5–e6. https://doi.org/10.1016/j.mayocp.2019.10.029

McNeill, W. H. (1976). *Plagues and peoples*. Anchor Books.

Mollaret, H. H. (1999). The discovery by Paul-Louis Simond of the role of the flea in the transmission of the plague. *Bulletin de la Société de Pathologie Exotique*, *92*(5 Pt 2), 383–387.

National Institutes of Health. (2020, December 18). *NIH-Moderna COVID-19 vaccine demonstrates 94.5% efficacy in clinical trials*. U.S. Department of Health and Human Services.https://www.nih.gov/news-events/news-releases/nih-moderna-covid-19-vaccine-demonstrates-94-5-efficacy-clinical-trials

Pringle, P. (2012). The disputed discovery of streptomycin. *The Lancet*, *380*(9838), 194. https://doi.org/10.1016/S0140-6736(12)61202-1

Rutgers University. (2024). Streptomycin & the legacy of Dr. Selman Waksman. School of Environmental and Biological Sciences. https://sebs.rutgers.edu/waksman-museum/streptomycin

Simond, M., Godley, M. L., & Mouriquand, P. D. (1998). Paul-Louis Simond and his discovery of plague transmission by rat fleas: A centenary. *Journal of the Royal Society of Medicine*, *91*(2), 101–104. https://doi.org/10.1177/014107689809100219

Snowden, F. M. (2019). *Epidemics and society: From the Black Death to the present*. Yale University Press.

Steensma, D. P. (2019). Alexandre Yersin: Discoverer of the plague bacillus. *Mayo Clinic Proceedings*, *94*(12), e139–e140. https://doi.org/10.1016/j.mayocp.2019.10.003

T-invariant. (2025, February 20). How a scientist from Odessa saved the 20th century from plague and cholera. Essay on the biography and scientific activities of Vladimir Haffkine. https://t-invariant.org/2023/12/how-a-scientist-from-odessa-saved-the-20th-century-from-plague-and-cholera-essay-on-the-biography-and-scientific-activities-of-vladimir-haffkine/

White, A. (2014). Selman Abraham Waksman. *The Lancet Respiratory Medicine*, *2*(12), 965. https://doi.org/10.1016/S2213-2600(14)70210-3

Wilkof, N. (2017, October 22). Waldemar Haffkine: Pioneer of plague vaccine and the “Little Dreyfus Affair”. The IPKat. https://ipkitten.blogspot.com/2017/10/waldemar-haffkine-pioneer-of-plague.html

Williamson, E. D., Kilgore, P. B., Hendrix, E. K., Neil, B. H., Sha, J., & Chopra, A. K. (2024). Progress on the research and development of plague vaccines with a call to action. *NPJ Vaccines*, *9*(1), 162. https://doi.org/10.1038/s41541-024-00958-1

Woodruff, H. B. (2014). Selman A. Waksman, winner of the 1952 Nobel Prize for Physiology or Medicine. *Applied and Environmental Microbiology*, *80*(1), 2–8. https://doi.org/10.1128/AEM.01143-13

Zhu, N., Zhang, D., Wang, W., Li, X., Yang, B., Song, J., Zhao, X., Huang, B., Shi, W., Lu, R., Niu, P., Zhan, F., Ma, X., Wang, D., Xu, W., Wu, G., Gao, G. F., & Tan, W. (2020). A novel coronavirus from patients with pneumonia in China, 2019. *New England Journal of Medicine*, *382*(8), 727–733. https://doi.org/10.1056/NEJMoa2001017

Ziegler, P. (2013). *The Black Death*. Faber & Faber.

3 A Tale of Two Pandemics

The 1918 Influenza and COVID-19

The 1918 influenza pandemic and COVID-19, separated by a century yet linked by many parallels, demonstrate both scientific advancement and enduring public health challenges. The 1918 H1N1 virus, definitively identified only in 1997, caused 50–100 million deaths with unusual mortality among young adults, while COVID-19 has primarily affected older populations. Both pandemics progressed in waves and prompted similar non-pharmaceutical interventions, though with vastly different scientific responses—from the rudimentary vaccines of 1918 to COVID-19's rapid genomic sequencing and effective immunization development. Public health leaders in both eras faced comparable communication challenges despite radically different information ecosystems. The evolutionary path of the 1918 virus into endemic seasonal influenza suggests SARS-CoV-2 may follow a similar trajectory.

Parallel Pandemics Across a Century

Despite occurring more than a century apart, the 1918 influenza pandemic and COVID-19 exhibit remarkable parallels in their progression and impact. The 1918 pandemic, often characterized as the "progenitor of modern pandemics," infected approximately one-third of the world's population, spreading rapidly around the globe facilitated by World War I troop movements and the absence of effective public health interventions (Crosby, 2003; Taubenberger & Morens, 2006). Comparing these two major pandemics yields valuable insights, despite significant differences in medical knowledge, technology, globalization patterns, and information dissemination capabilities between the eras.

Mortality Patterns and Demographic Impact

Both pandemics progressed in distinct waves (Figure 3.1). The 1918 influenza pandemic unfolded in three major waves: the first began in March 1918, followed by a more lethal second wave in the fall of 1918, and a third wave in the winter and spring of 1919 (Jester et al., 2020). Collectively, these waves resulted in approximately 675,000 American fatalities. COVID-19 followed a similar wave-like pattern, with the initial wave emerging in early 2020. Although its early trajectory resembled that of the 1918 pandemic with regard to the larger waves, subsequent

DOI: 10.4324/9781003595564-5

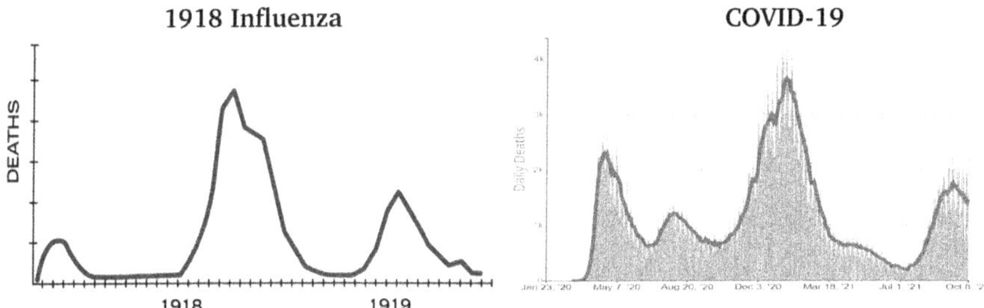

Figure 3.1 Visualization of First Three Mortality Wave Patterns for 1918 Influenza and COVID-19 Pandemics.

Sources: CDC (2018); CDC (2025).

COVID-19 waves were shaped by the emergence of new viral variants and seasonal dynamics (Johns Hopkins University & Medicine, 2025).

A key distinction between these pandemics lies in their demographic impact. The 1918 influenza pandemic disproportionately affected young adults, with peak mortality rates observed in the 20–40 year age cohort (Gagnon et al., 2013; Viboud et al., 2013). This pattern contrasts sharply with typical seasonal influenza, where mortality is highest among the elderly and very young. The mechanisms underlying this atypical mortality distribution are not fully understood, but research suggests it may relate to the virus's capacity to induce cytokine storms—excessive immune responses resulting in severe inflammation and multi-organ dysfunction (Shanks & Brundage, 2012).

In contrast, COVID-19 has predominantly affected older adults, with the highest mortality rates occurring among those aged 65 and above (Centers for Disease Control and Prevention (CDC), 2021). However, certain variants, particularly the Delta variant during its 2021 dominance period, exhibited increased severity among younger age groups compared to the original strain (Centers for Disease Control and Prevention (CDC), 2025). Table 3.1 compares broad mortality statistics between the two.

Table 3.1 Comparative Mortality Statistics Between 1918 Influenza and COVID-19

Metric	*1918 Influenza*	*COVID-19*
Global mortality	50–100 million (2.5–5% of world population)	>7 million confirmed (likely >15–20 million excess deaths)
Primary demographic	Young adults (20–40 years)	Older adults (>65 years)
Case fatality rate	Approximately 2.5%	0.5–5% (depending on region/variant)
Wave pattern	Three distinct waves	Multiple waves (variant-influenced)
Mortality mechanism	Secondary bacterial pneumonia and immune overreaction in young adults	Respiratory failure, hyperinflammation, and vascular complications

Sources: Centers for Disease Control and Prevention (2021, 2025); Crosby (2003); Gagnon et al. (2013); Johns Hopkins University & Medicine (2025); Shanks and Brundage (2012); Taubenberger and Morens (2006); Viboud et al. (2013); Woolf et al. (2020); World Health Organization (WHO) (2023).

Both pandemics resulted in significant excess mortality beyond reported fatalities and showed geographic variations in mortality rates, with certain urban centers, regions, and countries experiencing disproportionate impacts (Woolf et al., 2020; World Health Organization (WHO), 2023). Factors influencing these variations include the timing and nature of public health responses, socioeconomic conditions, population density, age demographics, and healthcare accessibility.

Public Health Interventions: Enduring Strategies

Non-Pharmaceutical Interventions

Despite the century-long interval between pandemics, public health authorities implemented remarkably similar non-pharmaceutical interventions to control viral spread (Markel et al., 2007). Social distancing measures were widely implemented during both crises. During the 1918 pandemic, cities and towns enacted various interventions, including closing schools, churches, theaters, and other public gathering places. Historical analyses have demonstrated that communities implementing these measures early and maintaining them consistently, such as St. Louis, Missouri, experienced lower mortality rates compared to cities that delayed implementation, such as Philadelphia, Pennsylvania (Bootsma & Ferguson, 2007; Hatchett et al., 2007).

During COVID-19, health authorities recommended maintaining physical distance between individuals based on improved understanding of respiratory virus transmission mechanisms (Centers for Disease Control and Prevention (CDC), 2020). Contemporary research distinguishes between respiratory droplets (>5 microns in diameter) that typically fall to surfaces within 6 feet, and aerosols (<5 microns) that can remain suspended longer and travel further. Studies examining SARS-CoV-2 aerosol dynamics found that infectious aerosols can remain suspended for extended periods—up to 16 hours under certain conditions—informing more sophisticated recommendations regarding indoor gathering restrictions, ventilation improvements, and context-specific distancing protocols (National Institutes of Health (NIH), 2021). These interventions are summarized comparatively in Table 3.2.

The Evolution of Respiratory Protection

Respiratory protective devices have evolved significantly between the two pandemics. During the 1918 influenza pandemic, rudimentary cloth masks served as the primary defense against viral transmission (UC Berkeley Library, 2023). These masks, typically constructed from gauze or cotton layers, had limited efficacy but still contributed to reducing transmission rates when properly used and combined with other interventions.

The COVID-19 pandemic witnessed significant advancement in mask technology. The N95 respirator represents a substantial improvement over historical masks, offering enhanced filtration efficiency against airborne pathogens (World Health Organization (WHO), 2020). These respirators comprise multiple layers of synthetic materials, including a critical layer of melt-blown polypropylene functioning as a particulate filter. The electrostatic charge enables N95 respirators to achieve filtration efficiency between 95 and 99.6% against viruses and other airborne particulates—a substantial improvement over cloth masks, which typically demonstrate filtration efficiency of approximately 50–60%.

Personal Hygiene as Enduring Prevention

Both pandemics emphasized handwashing and personal hygiene as key prevention strategies. Modern scientific research has elucidated why handwashing with soap and alcohol-based sanitizers effectively inactivate enveloped viruses like SARS-CoV-2. Soap molecules disrupt the virus's lipid membrane through viral envelope disruption, rendering it non-infectious. Similarly, alcohol-based hand sanitizers denature viral proteins and disrupt lipid membranes, leading to viral inactivation (Hon et al., 2021).

Contemporary public health messaging has emphasized both frequency and duration of handwashing, addressing research findings that many people inadequately wash their hands, failing to reach the recommended minimum of 20 seconds threshold necessary for effective pathogen removal.

Table 3.2 Comparison of Public Health Interventions Between 1918 Influenza and COVID-19

Intervention	*1918 Influenza*	*COVID-19*
Social distancing	School/business closures, bans on public gatherings	6-foot distancing guidelines, capacity restrictions, remote work/learning
Respiratory protection	Gauze/cotton masks (50–60% filtration)	N95 respirators (95%+ filtration), surgical masks, cloth masks
Isolation practices	Home quarantine, temporary influenza wards	Dedicated COVID units, contact tracing, isolation and quarantine protocols
Communication strategies	Newspapers, posters, public announcements	Digital media, daily briefings, real-time dashboards, mobile alerts
Enforcement mechanisms	Local ordinances, voluntary compliance	Stay-at-home orders, business operation restrictions, international travel bans
Personal hygiene	Basic handwashing guidance, general cleanliness	20-second handwashing, 70%+ alcohol hand sanitizers, surface disinfection

Sources: Bootsma and Ferguson (2007); Centers for Disease Control and Prevention (CDC) (2020); Hatchett et al. (2007); Hon et al. (2021); Jester et al. (2020); Markel et al. (2007); National Institutes of Health (NIH) (2021); Taubenberger and Morens (2006); UC Berkeley Library (2023); U.S. National Archives.

Scientific Response: From Limited Understanding to Rapid Innovation

Pathogen Identification and Characterization

The scientific journey between these pandemics is dramatically illustrated in our ability to identify and characterize the causative pathogens. The 1918 influenza virus was only definitively identified as the H1N1 influenza virus in 1997, when researchers recovered and analyzed viral RNA from preserved tissue samples (Taubenberger & Morens, 2006). The complete genetic sequencing of the 1918 H1N1 virus finally revealed the molecular identity of a pathogen that had claimed millions of lives decades earlier.

In contrast, the SARS-CoV-2 genome was sequenced and published within weeks of the first identified cases in Wuhan, China—a testament to modern genomic technologies and international scientific collaboration (Zhu et al., 2020). This rapid identification enabled an unprecedented acceleration of diagnostic testing, viral characterization studies, and targeted vaccine development that would have seemed impossible to physicians struggling against the 1918 pandemic. The contrast in scientific capabilities is detailed in Table 3.3.

Vaccine Development: From Desperate Measures to Scientific Triumph

The 1918 influenza pandemic occurred when vaccine development was in its infancy. Experimental vaccines were rushed to distribution without adequate

Table 3.3 Comparison of Scientific Understanding and Response Between 1918 Influenza and COVID-19

Scientific Element	*1918 Influenza*	*COVID-19*
Pathogen	Initially misidentified as bacterial; H1N1 virus confirmed only in 1997	SARS-CoV-2 genome sequenced within weeks of first cases
Transmission	Limited knowledge of viral spread; focus on droplet transmission	Evolving understanding of droplet, aerosol, and fomite transmission
Diagnostics	Symptom-based diagnosis only; no specific tests	PCR, rapid antigen, antibody tests; genome sequencing
Vaccines	Bacterial vaccines with uncertain efficacy; no effective viral vaccines	Multiple effective vaccines (mRNA, vector, protein) within one year
Treatments	Supportive care, aspirin, unproven “snake oil” remedies	Antivirals, steroids, monoclonals, advanced respiratory support
Research	Minimal global coordination	Significant international collaboration, data sharing, preprints

Sources: Centers for Disease Control and Prevention (CDC) (2022); Ciotti et al. (2023); Fiolet et al. (2022); Kilbourne (2006); Krammer (2020); National Institutes of Health (NIH) (2021); Taubenberger and Morens (2006); Zhu et al. (2020).

testing or evaluation (Ciotti et al., 2023). These products were based on various theories about the pandemic's cause—many later proven incorrect. The effectiveness of these early vaccines was highly questionable, with minimal evidence supporting their efficacy or safety. Despite limited scientific support, a desperate public sought these experimental vaccines, potentially providing false security and leading people to neglect other important public health measures.

In contrast, the COVID-19 pandemic showcases the remarkable advancement of vaccine science. Within one year of the pandemic's onset, multiple highly effective vaccines were developed, rigorously tested through clinical trials, and distributed globally (Krammer, 2020). These vaccines, based on technologies including messenger RNA (mRNA) and viral vector platforms, underwent comprehensive evaluation to ensure safety and efficacy before receiving regulatory authorization.

The overall impact of COVID-19 vaccines on the pandemic's trajectory has been substantial. A study published in June 2022 estimated that COVID-19 vaccines prevented between 14.4 and 19.8 million additional deaths worldwide during their first year of implementation (December 2020 to December 2021) (Fiolet et al., 2022).

Public Health Leadership and Communication

Leadership Under Pressure

Notable parallels exist between the public health leaders who guided response efforts in each era. Dr. Thomas Tuttle, who served as Washington state's Health Commissioner during the 1918 pandemic, strongly endorsed public health interventions including closure of educational institutions, entertainment venues, and other public gatherings (Navarro, 2022). Similarly, Dr. Anthony Fauci, Director of the National Institute of Allergy and Infectious Diseases (NIAID) and Chief Medical Advisor during the COVID-19 pandemic, consistently advocated for face masks, physical distancing, hand hygiene protocols, and isolation to reduce viral transmission (Morens & Fauci, 2021).

Both health leaders faced significant challenges in their efforts to combat their respective pandemics. Dr. Tuttle contended with limited scientific understanding of influenza virology and minimal effective medical interventions beyond supportive care. Dr. Fauci encountered similar challenges during COVID-19, including the rapid dissemination of misinformation and public resistance to health measures. The leadership similarities demonstrate how fundamental principles of epidemiology and public health practice remain consistent across different eras, even as medical knowledge and technology evolve.

Information Ecosystems and Public Response

Both pandemics unfolded in information environments that shaped public understanding and response, though the mechanisms differed dramatically. In 1918, information traveled primarily through newspapers, public announcements, and word of mouth. Wartime censorship in many countries initially suppressed reporting on the pandemic's severity (leading to its "Spanish Flu" misnomer, as Spain's neutral status allowed more open reporting) (Crosby, 2003).

COVID-19 emerged in a hyperconnected world where information—both accurate and inaccurate—spreads globally within seconds. Digital platforms simultaneously enabled a greater degree of scientific collaboration and amplified misconceptions, creating communication challenges for public health authorities (Kupferschmidt, 2020). Both pandemics demonstrate how information ecosystems fundamentally shape societal responses to health crises, with the accelerated pace of modern communication presenting both opportunities and challenges for public health action.

Lessons and Legacy: Institutional Memory and Future Preparedness

Recurring Patterns in Pandemic Impact

Both pandemics revealed how existing social inequities shape health outcomes. Disadvantaged communities experienced disproportionate impacts in both eras. Social determinants of health—including housing conditions, occupational exposure risks, and healthcare access—significantly influenced overall pandemic vulnerability. COVID-19 mortality rates showed substantial disparities by race, ethnicity, and socioeconomic status, a pattern that, while less thoroughly documented, was also observed during the 1918 pandemic (Spreeuwenberg et al., 2018).

Healthcare system capacity to respond to surge demands has been a critical factor in both pandemics. In 1918, healthcare facilities were quickly overwhelmed, with limited options for treating severely ill patients beyond supportive care. During COVID-19, despite significant advances in critical care medicine, many healthcare systems still faced severe capacity constraints during peak surges, necessitating difficult triage decisions (Del Valle et al., 2020).

Viral Evolution and Endemic Transition

The evolutionary trajectories of these pandemic viruses offer a final parallel with important implications for our future. The 1918 H1N1 virus did not disappear after its devastating initial waves. Instead, it became the genetic ancestor of most subsequent influenza A viruses, including seasonal strains that continue to circulate today and the virus responsible for the 2009 H1N1 pandemic (Dowdle, 2018). Over generations, the virus adapted to maintain transmission while generally reducing its virulence.

Virologists anticipate that SARS-CoV-2 will likely follow a similar pattern, establishing itself as an endemic human pathogen and continuing to evolve with varying levels of severity and immune evasion capability. The emergence of increasingly transmissible variants demonstrates this evolutionary process in action (Tregoning et al., 2021). Because our relationship with these pathogens extends far beyond the acute crisis phase of a pandemic, understanding these long-term viral trajectories is essential for sustainable public health planning.

Preparing for Future Pandemics

The lessons from both pandemics highlight the importance of preserving institutional knowledge and maintaining robust public health infrastructure during interpandemic periods. Many of the hard-won insights from 1918 required rediscovery during the COVID-19 pandemic, particularly regarding the effectiveness of early, sustained non-pharmaceutical interventions (Barro, 2020).

The COVID-19 experience demonstrated clearly that scientific knowledge alone is insufficient; despite remarkable advancements, effective public health practice also requires robust implementation systems, clear communication strategies, and sustained political support for optimal preparedness (Jha & Gupta, 2023). By understanding both the parallels and differences between these two watershed pandemic events, we gain valuable perspective for addressing future infectious disease threats. The scientific and technological advances of the past century have dramatically expanded our response capabilities, yet systemic and social challenges of pandemic management remain remarkably persistent across historical contexts.

References

Barro, R. J. (2020). *Non-pharmaceutical interventions and mortality in US cities during the Great Influenza Pandemic, 1918–19*. National Bureau of Economic Research. https://www.nber.org/papers/w27049

Bootsma, M. C., & Ferguson, N. M. (2007). The effect of public health measures on the 1918 influenza pandemic in U.S. cities. *Proceedings of the National Academy of Sciences*, *104*(18), 7588–7593. https://www.pnas.org/doi/10.1073/pnas.0611071104

Centers for Disease Control and Prevention (CDC). (2021). *COVID-19 mortality in adults aged 65 and over*. NCHS Data Brief. https://www.cdc.gov/nchs/products/databriefs/db446.htm

Centers for Disease Control and Prevention (CDC). (2022). *COVID-19 vaccine basics*. https://www.cdc.gov/covid/vaccines/how-they-work.html

Centers for Disease Control and Prevention (CDC). (2018, May 11). *1918 pandemic influenza: Three waves*. U.S. Department of Health & Human Services. https://archive.cdc.gov/#/details?url=https://www.cdc.gov/flu/pandemic-resources/1918-commemoration/three-waves.htm

Centers for Disease Control and Prevention (CDC). (2020). *Coronavirus Disease 2019 (COVID-19): How to protect yourself & others*. https://www.cdc.gov/coronavirus/2019-ncov/prevent-getting-sick/prevention.html

Centers for Disease Control and Prevention (CDC). (2025). *COVID data tracker: Demographics and trends*. https://covid.cdc.gov/covid-data-tracker

Ciotti, M., Ciccozzi, M., Pieri, M., Bernardini, S., Suter, F., & Astorino, R. (2023). Have diagnostics, therapies, and vaccines made the difference in the pandemic evolution of COVID-19 in comparison with "Spanish Flu"? *International Journal of Molecular Sciences*, *24*(16), 12838. https://www.ncbi.nlm.nih.gov/pmc/articles/PMC10384375/

Crosby, A. W. (2003). *America's forgotten pandemic: The influenza of 1918* (2nd ed.). Cambridge University Press.

Del Valle, D. M., Kim-Schulze, S., Huang, H. H., Beckmann, N. D., Nirenberg, S., Wang, B., Lavin, Y., Swartz, T. H., Madduri, D., Stock, A., Marron, T. U., Xie, H., Patel, M., Tuballes, K., Van Oekelen, O., Rahman, A., Kovatch, P., Aberg, J. A., Schadt, E., … & Gnjatic, S. (2020). An inflammatory cytokine signature predicts

COVID-19 severity and survival. *Nature Medicine*, *26*(10), 1636–1643. https://doi.org/10.1038/s41591-020-1051-9

Dowdle, W. R. (2018). Influenza pandemic periodicity, virus recycling, and the art of risk assessment. *Emerging Infectious Diseases*, *12*(1), 34–39. https://www.ncbi.nlm.nih.gov/pmc/articles/PMC3291415/

Fiolet, T., Kherabi, Y., MacDonald, C. J., Ghosn, J., & Peiffer-Smadja, N. (2022). Comparing COVID-19 vaccines for their characteristics, efficacy and effectiveness against SARS-CoV-2 and variants of concern: A narrative review. *Clinical Microbiology and Infection*, *28*(2), 202–221. https://www.ncbi.nlm.nih.gov/pmc/articles/PMC8148145/

Gagnon, A., Miller, M. S., Hallman, S. A., Bourbeau, R., Herring, D. A., Earn, D. J., & Madrenas, J. (2013). Age-specific mortality during the 1918 influenza pandemic: Unravelling the mystery of high young adult mortality. *PLoS One*, *8*(8), e69586. https://www.ncbi.nlm.nih.gov/pmc/articles/PMC3734171/

Hatchett, R. J., Mecher, C. E., & Lipsitch, M. (2007). Public health interventions and epidemic intensity during the 1918 influenza pandemic. *Proceedings of the National Academy of Sciences*, *104*(18), 7582–7587. https://www.pnas.org/doi/10.1073/pnas.0610941104

Hon, K. L., Leung, K. K. Y., Hui, W. F., & Ng, D. K. K. (2021). Applying lessons from influenza pandemics to the COVID-19 pandemic. *Pediatric Pulmonology*, *56*(9), 3071–3074. https://doi.org/10.1002/ppul.25571

Jester, B., Uyeki, T., & Jernigan, D. (2020). Fifty years of influenza A (H3N2) following the pandemic of 1968. *American Journal of Public Health*, *110*(5), 669–676. https://www.ncbi.nlm.nih.gov/pmc/articles/PMC7144439/

Jester, B. J., Uyeki, T. M., & Jernigan, D. B. (2020). Historical and clinical aspects of the 1918 H1N1 pandemic in the United States. *Virology*, *527*, 32–37. https://doi.org/10.1016/j.virol.2018.11.015

Jha, A. K., & Gupta, R. (2023). COVID-19: A comparison to the 1918 influenza and how we can defeat it. *Postgraduate Medical Journal*, *99*(1168), 199–202. https://www.ncbi.nlm.nih.gov/pmc/articles/PMC8108277/

Johns Hopkins University & Medicine. (2025). Coronavirus Resource Center. https://coronavirus.jhu.edu

Kilbourne, E. D. (2006). Influenza pandemics of the 20th century. *Emerging Infectious Diseases*, *12*(1), 9–14. https://doi.org/10.3201/eid1201.051254

Krammer, F. (2020). SARS-CoV-2 vaccines in development. *Nature*, *586*(7830), 516–527. https://doi.org/10.1038/s41586-020-2798-3

Kupferschmidt, K. (2020). Preprints bring 'firehose' of outbreak data. *Science*, *367*(6481), 963–964. https://doi.org/10.1126/science.367.6481.963

Markel, H., Lipman, H. B., Navarro, J. A., Sloan, A., Michalsen, J. R., Stern, A. M., & Cetron, M. S. (2007). Nonpharmaceutical interventions implemented by US cities during the 1918-1919 influenza pandemic. *JAMA*, *298*(6), 644–654. https://www.ncbi.nlm.nih.gov/pmc/articles/PMC7115757/

Morens, D. M., & Fauci, A. S. (2021). A centenary tale of two pandemics: The 1918 influenza pandemic and COVID-19, Part II. *American Journal of Public Health*, *111*(7), 1267–1272. https://www.ncbi.nlm.nih.gov/pmc/articles/PMC8493155/

National Institutes of Health (NIH). (2021). *COVID-19 treatment guidelines – Infection control*. https://www.covid19treatmentguidelines.nih.gov/overview/prevention-of-sars-cov-2/

Navarro, J. A. (2022). Politics, pushback, and pandemics: Challenges to public health orders in the 1918 influenza pandemic. *American Journal of Public Health*, *112*(3), 418–422. https://www.ncbi.nlm.nih.gov/pmc/articles/PMC7893336/

Shanks, G. D., & Brundage, J. F. (2012). Pathogenic responses among young adults during the 1918 influenza pandemic. *Emerging Infectious Diseases*, *18*(2), 201–207. https://www.ncbi.nlm.nih.gov/pmc/articles/PMC3310443/

Spreeuwenberg, P., Kroneman, M., & Paget, J. (2018). Reassessing the 1918 Spanish flu: The role of demographic factors and case fatality. *Influenza and Other Respiratory Viruses*, *12*(5), 507–515. https://doi.org/10.1111/irv.12538

Taubenberger, J. K., & Morens, D. M. (2006). 1918 influenza: The mother of all pandemics. *Emerging Infectious Diseases*, *12*(1), 15–22. https://www.ncbi.nlm.nih.gov/pmc/articles/PMC3291398/

Tregoning, J. S., Flight, K. E., Higham, S. L., Wang, Z., & Pierce, B. F. (2021). Progress of the COVID-19 vaccine effort: Viruses, vaccines and variants versus efficacy, effectiveness and escape. *Nature Reviews Immunology*, *21*(10), 626–636. https://www.nature.com/articles/s41577-021-00592-1

UC Berkeley Library. (2023). *Did masks work?—The 1918 flu pandemic and the meaning of layered interventions*. https://update.lib.berkeley.edu/2020/05/23/did-masks-work-the-1918-flu-pandemic-and-the-meaning-of-layered-interventions/

Viboud, C., Eisenstein, J., Reid, A. H., Janczewski, T. A., Morens, D. M., & Taubenberger, J. K. (2013). Age-specific mortality during the 1918 influenza pandemic: Unravelling the mystery of high young adult mortality. *PLoS One*, *8*(8), e69586. https://www.ncbi.nlm.nih.gov/pmc/articles/PMC3734171/

Woolf, S. H., Chapman, D. A., Sabo, R. T., Weinberger, D. M., & Hill, L. (2020). Excess deaths from COVID-19 and other causes, March-April 2020. *JAMA*, *324*(5), 510–513. https://jamanetwork.com/journals/jama/fullarticle/2768086

World Health Organization (WHO). (2020). *Advice on the use of masks in the context of COVID-19*. https://www.who.int/publications/i/item/advice-on-the-use-of-masks-in-the-community-during-home-care-and-in-healthcare-settings-in-the-context-of-the-novel-coronavirus-(2019-ncov)-outbreak

World Health Organization (WHO). (2023). *Global excess deaths associated with COVID-19*. https://www.who.int/data/stories/global-excess-deaths-associated-with-covid-19

Zhu, N., Zhang, D., Wang, W., Li, X., Yang, B., Song, J., Zhao, X., Huang, B., Shi, W., Lu, R., Niu, P., Zhan, F., Ma, X., Wang, D., Xu, W., Wu, G., Gao, G. F., & Tan, W. (2020). A novel coronavirus from patients with pneumonia in China, 2019. *New England Journal of Medicine*, *382*(8), 727–733. https://doi.org/10.1056/NEJMoa2001017

4 The Smallpox Legacy

Eradication Lessons for COVID-19

Smallpox stands as a singular achievement in the history of public health—the first and only human disease successfully eradicated through deliberate intervention. This devastating airborne disease plagued humanity for over 3,000 years before the World Health Organization certified its global eradication in 1980. This triumph resulted from a coordinated global campaign of vaccination, surveillance, and containment. Given this remarkable precedent, it is natural to ask whether COVID-19 might become the second human disease eliminated from history. While smallpox eradication offers valuable insights for pandemic management, fundamental differences between these pathogens necessitate a nuanced assessment of potential eradication strategies for SARS-CoV-2.

Smallpox: A Historical Perspective

Smallpox, caused by the variola virus, was a highly contagious disease that spread primarily through direct contact with infected individuals and their contaminated belongings, as well as via respiratory droplets during prolonged face-to-face contact (Breman & Henderson, 2002). Although a member of the same Orthopoxvirus genus as monkeypox, smallpox was exclusively a human disease with no known animal reservoir (Tucker, 2001). Its clinical presentation included fever, body aches, and a distinctive rash that progressed to fluid-filled pustules. The disease was frequently severe, with case fatality rates of 20–30% and potential long-term complications including disfigurement, blindness, and infertility among survivors (Barquet & Domingo, 1997).

Smallpox's characteristic progression from fever to its telltale pustular rash allowed for visual recognition of cases—an important factor in the ultimate success of surveillance and containment efforts (Moss, 2011). Death often resulted from overwhelming viremia, secondary bacterial infections, or severe dehydration, with survivors left with distinctive scarring.

The precise origins of smallpox remain uncertain, though archaeological evidence suggests an ancient emergence. The most compelling early evidence comes from Egypt, where researchers have identified pustule marks on the mummy of Pharaoh Ramses V, who died approximately 3,000 years ago (Riedel, 2005). Historical records document smallpox-like symptoms in China during the 4th century,

DOI: 10.4324/9781003595564-6

India in the 7th century, and Turkey in the 10th century, indicating the disease's gradual spread across Eurasia. The disease's impact extended to influencing political succession in imperial China, with historical accounts suggesting that Emperor Kangxi's selection as ruler of the Qing Dynasty at age 8 may have been partially influenced by his survival of smallpox, which gave him lifelong immunity (Hopkins, 1983).

International trade, warfare, and European colonization facilitated smallpox's global transmission, with a particularly catastrophic impact on indigenous American populations following European contact in the 16th century, causing mortality rates estimated between 30 and 90% in affected communities (Bhattacharya, 2008).

Smallpox Eradication Declared in 1980: How Did We Get There?

The journey toward smallpox eradication began when English physician Edward Jenner demonstrated in 1796 that inoculation with cowpox could provide protection against smallpox (Riedel, 2005; Smith, 2011). Observing that milkmaids who had contracted cowpox appeared immune to smallpox, Jenner tested this theory by inoculating a young boy with cowpox material and demonstrating his subsequent immunity to smallpox—the first scientifically documented immunization technique, which he termed "vaccination" (from "vacca," Latin for cow) (Jenner, 1798; Morgan & Parker, 2007).

The Spanish monarchy launched the remarkable Royal Philanthropic Vaccine Expedition (1803–1806), led by physician Francisco Javier Balmis, which brought smallpox vaccination to Spanish colonies across Central and South America and Asia (Franco-Paredes et al., 2005). This early global health initiative employed an innovative technique for preserving the vaccine during long sea voyages by conducting sequential arm-to-arm inoculations among 22 orphan boys who served as living carriers (Mark & Rigau-Pérez, 2009). Isabel Zendal Gómez, the expedition's head nurse, cared for the children and oversaw the vaccination process. The expedition established vaccination programs throughout Latin America, the Philippines, and Macau, delivering millions of vaccinations across three continents—one of history's most ambitious public health initiatives (Franco-Paredes et al., 2005).

By the 1950s, advances in vaccine technology produced a more effective freeze-dried smallpox vaccine that stimulated robust immunity while offering improved stability in tropical climates, though still requiring careful storage management (Fenner et al., 1988). North America and Europe achieved regional smallpox elimination by the early 1950s through systematic vaccination programs.

In 1959, the World Health Assembly adopted a formal resolution to eradicate smallpox globally, though initial efforts achieved limited success (World Health Organization, 1980). Learning from these challenges, the WHO launched the Intensified Smallpox Eradication Program in 1967, with enhanced resources and strategic adjustments (Fenner et al., 1988). The revised campaign employed a comprehensive approach combining mass vaccination in endemic regions with robust surveillance systems for rapid case detection. When outbreaks occurred, health workers implemented targeted ring vaccination to immunize contacts of infected

Table 4.1 Key Differences Between Smallpox and COVID-19

Factor	*Smallpox*	*COVID-19*
Pathogen	Stable virus with limited genetic variation	Rapidly evolving virus with multiple variants
Symptoms	Distinctive visible rash; easy to identify	Often asymptomatic or mild; difficult to visually identify
Animal Reservoirs	None; exclusively human disease	Multiple potential animal hosts (mink, deer, cats, etc.)
Vaccines	Single dose; long-lasting immunity	Multiple doses plus boosters; waning immunity
Vaccine Storage	Thermally stable; minimal cold chain needed	Requires cold or ultra-cold storage chains for mRNA
Transmission	Primarily symptomatic transmission	Significant pre-symptomatic and asymptomatic transmission
Global Coordination	Unified WHO-led campaign	Fragmented national approaches
Eradication Potential	High (achieved)	Low due to biological and socio-political factors

Sources: Breman and Henderson (2002); Centers for Disease Control and Prevention (2021); Crommelin et al. (2021); Dhama et al. (2020); Fenner et al. (1988); Henderson (2009); Huang et al. (2022); Jackson et al. (2020); Kaur and Gupta (2020); Nature (2022); Oreshkova et al. (2020); Palmer et al. (2021); Plotkin and Plotkin (2011); Polack et al. (2020); Sharun et al. (2021); Tarantola and Foster (2011); Tucker (2001); World Health Organization (2022).

individuals, effectively creating barriers to transmission—a strategy particularly effective for smallpox due to its visible symptoms and transmission patterns (Henderson, 2009). These local containment efforts were supported by coordinated international efforts that addressed cross-border transmission through standardized protocols and resource sharing.

These coordinated efforts progressively eliminated smallpox from successive regions: South America was certified smallpox-free in 1971, followed by Asia in 1975 and Africa in 1977 (Fenner et al., 1988). After extensive verification protocols, the World Health Assembly officially declared smallpox eradicated on May 8, 1980—a monumental moment in public health history (World Health Organization, 1980).

Smallpox and COVID-19: Comparative Analysis

The eradication of smallpox offers instructive parallels and contrasts for the management of COVID-19, with several key factors influencing their respective trajectories (Table 4.1). Smallpox presented biological and epidemiological characteristics favorable for eradication. It caused visibly identifiable symptoms, facilitating case identification and contact tracing (Breman & Henderson, 2002). The virus maintained relative genetic stability, allowing vaccines to remain effective without requiring frequent reformulation. Critically, smallpox was exclusively a human disease with no animal reservoir that could reintroduce the virus into human populations (Tucker, 2001).

SARS-CoV-2 presents a more complex eradication challenge from a biological perspective. The virus demonstrates significant genetic variability, with multiple variants emerging that exhibit enhanced transmissibility and partial immune evasion (Huang et al., 2022). A substantial proportion of infections are asymptomatic or mildly symptomatic, complicating case detection (Kaur & Gupta, 2020). The virus has been documented in multiple animal species, including mink, deer, and domestic cats, raising concerns about potential animal reservoirs (Sharun et al., 2021).

Studies have confirmed SARS-CoV-2 infections in white-tailed deer populations with transmission among the deer, suggesting this species could maintain the virus independently (Palmer et al., 2021). Similarly, outbreaks in mink farms have demonstrated not only mink-to-mink transmission but also mink-to-human transmission of variant strains (Oreshkova et al., 2020; Sharun et al., 2021). These findings raise significant concerns about the possibility of wildlife serving as long-term reservoirs for SARS-CoV-2, which could periodically reintroduce the virus into human populations (World Health Organization, 2022). Regardless, these biological characteristics create substantial obstacles to complete eradication.

Vaccination strategies also differ significantly between these pandemics. Smallpox eradication relied on a highly effective vaccine that provided long-lasting immunity with a single dose (Plotkin & Plotkin, 2011). The vaccine's thermal stability facilitated distribution in resource-limited settings without cold chain requirements. Strategic deployment through mass vaccination followed by targeted "ring vaccination" around detected cases proved highly effective at interrupting transmission chains (Henderson, 2009).

In contrast, COVID-19 vaccines have demonstrated impressive efficacy in preventing severe disease and death, but their impact on transmission is more limited, particularly against newer variants (Jackson et al., 2020; Polack et al., 2020). Current vaccines require cold or ultra-cold storage, creating logistical challenges for global distribution. The original mRNA vaccine formulations required storage at temperatures between −90°C and −60°C, though requirements have since been relaxed somewhat as stability data have accumulated (Crommelin et al., 2021). Most formulations require multiple doses to achieve optimal protection, and immunity appears to wane over time, necessitating booster doses (Dhama et al., 2020).

Global coordination represents another area of significant difference. Smallpox eradication succeeded through international cooperation. The WHO coordinated a genuinely global campaign that transcended Cold War politics and regional conflicts (Tarantola & Foster, 2011). The COVID-19 response, while demonstrating remarkable scientific collaboration in vaccine development, has been characterized by fragmented national approaches, vaccine nationalism, and inconsistent implementation of public health measures (Huang et al., 2022). These coordination challenges have impeded effective pandemic management and would present significant obstacles to any eradication effort.

Public health infrastructure played a crucial role in both contexts, though with different levels of development and equity. The smallpox campaign invested in developing public health capacity in participating countries, training healthcare workers, establishing surveillance systems, and creating logistics networks for vaccine distribution (Henderson, 2009). COVID-19 has similarly highlighted the critical importance of robust public health systems. Countries with stronger existing infrastructure generally demonstrated more effective pandemic responses. However, significant global disparities in these capacities have undermined coordinated management efforts and created inequitable outcomes both within and between nations (Gee & Khan, 2021).

Lessons from Smallpox for COVID-19 Management

Despite the biological and structural obstacles that make SARS-CoV-2 eradication unlikely, the smallpox campaign offers valuable tactical and strategic lessons for COVID-19 management.

The smallpox campaign demonstrated the effectiveness of strategically prioritizing vaccination in high-transmission settings and implementing robust surveillance systems (Nature, 2022). For COVID-19, these approaches translate to targeting high-risk populations and enhancing testing, genomic monitoring, and case investigation. Community engagement proved essential in smallpox eradication and remains critical for the COVID-19 response, recognizing that technical solutions require public participation through culturally appropriate communication and collaboration with community leaders (Tarantola & Foster, 2011).

Looking beyond immediate interventions, smallpox eradication reminds us that success against infectious diseases requires sustained effort and methodical region-by-region progress (Fenner et al., 1988). COVID-19 management is evolving toward an endemic approach with focused control efforts in specific geographic areas that can gradually expand, acknowledging uneven progress across regions with varying resources and infrastructure. By combining continued scientific advancement with international coordination that transcends political differences, the global community can substantially reduce COVID-19's ongoing impact while building preparedness for future threats (Gee & Khan, 2021).

References

Barquet, N., & Domingo, P. (1997). Smallpox: The triumph over the most terrible of the ministers of death. *Annals of Internal Medicine*, *127*(8 Pt 1), 635–642. https://doi.org/10.7326/0003-4819-127-8_part_1-199710150-00010

Bhattacharya, S. (2008). *Expunging variola: The control and eradication of smallpox in India, 1947–1977*. Orient Longman.

Breman, J. G., & Henderson, D. A. (2002). Diagnosis and management of smallpox. *New England Journal of Medicine*, *346*(17), 1300–1308. https://doi.org/10.1056/NEJMra020025

Centers for Disease Control and Prevention. (2021). *Smallpox*. https://www.cdc.gov/smallpox/index.html

Crommelin, D. J. A., Anchordoquy, T. J., Volkin, D. B., Jiskoot, W., & Mastrobattista, E. (2021). Addressing the cold reality of mRNA vaccine stability. *Journal of Pharmaceutical Sciences*, *110*(3), 997–1001. https://doi.org/10.1016/j.xphs.2020.12.006

Dhama, K., Sharun, K., Tiwari, R., Dadar, M., Malik, Y. S., Singh, K. P., & Chaicumpa, W. (2020). COVID-19, an emerging coronavirus infection: Advances and prospects in designing and developing vaccines, immunotherapeutics, and therapeutics. *Human Vaccines & Immunotherapeutics*, *16*(6), 1232–1238. https://doi.org/10.1080/21645515.2020.1735227

Nature. (2022, January 24). COVID is here to stay: Countries must decide how to adapt. *Nature*, 601, 481. https://doi.org/10.1038/d41586-022-00057-y

Fenner, F., Henderson, D. A., Arita, I., Jezek, Z., & Ladnyi, I. D. (1988). *Smallpox and its eradication*. World Health Organization.

Franco-Paredes, C., Lammoglia, L., & Santos-Preciado, J. I. (2005). The Spanish Royal Philanthropic Expedition to bring smallpox vaccination to the New World and Asia in the 19th century. *Clinical Infectious Diseases*, *41*(9), 1285–1289. https://doi.org/10.1086/496930

Gee, R. E., & Khan, A. S. (2021). Leading the world again: Creating a 21st century public health agency. *American Journal of Public Health*, *111*(4), 594–596. https://doi.org/10.2105/AJPH.2021.306187

Henderson, D. A. (2009). *Smallpox: The death of a disease*. Prometheus Books.

Hopkins, D. R. (1983). *Princes and peasants: Smallpox in history*. University of Chicago Press.

Huang, S. S. Y., Rifkin-Graboi, A., & Cheon, B. K. (2022). Comparison of COVID-19 and smallpox vaccination hesitancy: Historical and policy lessons. *Health Policy*, *126*(1), 58–66. https://doi.org/10.1016/j.healthpol.2021.11.007

Jackson, L. A., Anderson, E. J., Rouphael, N. G., Roberts, P. C., Makhene, M., Coler, R. N., McCullough, M. P., Chappell, J. D., Denison, M. R., Stevens, L. J., Pruijssers, A. J., McDermott, A., Flach, B., Doria-Rose, N. A., Corbett, K. S., Morabito, K. M., O'Dell, S., Schmidt, S. D., Swanson, P. A., … Beigel, J. H. (2020). An mRNA vaccine against SARS-CoV-2—Preliminary report. *New England Journal of Medicine*, *383*(20), 1920–1931. https://doi.org/10.1056/NEJMoa2022483

Jenner, E. (1798). *An inquiry into the causes and effects of the variolae vaccinae, a disease discovered in some of the western counties of England, particularly Gloucestershire, and known by the name of the cow pox*. Sampson Low.

Kaur, S. P., & Gupta, V. (2020). COVID-19 vaccine: A comprehensive status report. *Virus Research*, *288*, 198114. https://doi.org/10.1016/j.virusres.2020.198114

Mark, C., & Rigau-Pérez, J. G. (2009). The world's first immunization campaign: The Spanish smallpox vaccine expedition, 1803-1813. *Bulletin of the History of Medicine*, *83*(1), 63–94. https://doi.org/10.1353/bhm.0.0173

Morgan, A. J., & Parker, S. (2007). Translational mini-review series on vaccines: The Edward Jenner Museum and the history of vaccination. *Clinical and Experimental Immunology*, *147*(3), 389–394. https://doi.org/10.1111/j.1365-2249.2006.03304.x

Moss, B. (2011). Smallpox vaccines: Targets of protective immunity. *Immunological Reviews*, *239*(1), 8–26. https://doi.org/10.1111/j.1600-065X.2010.00975.x

Oreshkova, N., Molenaar, R. J., Vreman, S., Harders, F., Oude Munnink, B. B., Hakze-van der Honing, R. W., Gerhards, N., Tolsma, P., Bouwstra, R., Sikkema, R. S., Tacken, M. G., de Rooij, M. M., Weesendorp, E., Engelsma, M. Y., Bruschke, C. J., Smit, L. A., Koopmans, M., van der Poel, W. H., & Stegeman, A. (2020). SARS-CoV-2 infection in farmed minks, the Netherlands, April and May 2020. *Euro Surveillance*, *25*(23), 2001005. https://doi.org/10.2807/1560-7917.ES.2020.25.23.2001005

Palmer, M. V., Martins, M., Falkenberg, S., Buckley, A., Caserta, L. C., Mitchell, P. K., Cassmann, E. D., Rollins, A., Zylich, N. C., Renshaw, R. W., Guarino, C., Wagner, B., Lager, K., & Diel, D. G. (2021). Susceptibility of white-tailed deer (*Odocoileus virginianus*) to SARS-CoV-2. *Journal of Virology*, *95*(11), e00083–21. https://doi.org/10.1128/JVI.00083-21

Plotkin, S. A., & Plotkin, S. L. (2011). The development of vaccines: How the past led to the future. *Nature Reviews Microbiology*, *9*(12), 889–893. https://doi.org/10.1038/nrmicro2668

Polack, F. P., Thomas, S. J., Kitchin, N., Absalon, J., Gurtman, A., Lockhart, S., Perez, J. L., Pérez Marc, G., Moreira, E. D., Zerbini, C., Bailey, R., Swanson, K. A., Roychoudhury, S., Koury, K., Li, P., Kalina, W. V., Cooper, D., Frenck, R. W., Hammitt, L. L., … Gruber, W. C. (2020). Safety and efficacy of the BNT162b2 mRNA Covid-19 vaccine. *New England Journal of Medicine*, *383*(27), 2603–2615. https://doi.org/10.1056/NEJMoa2034577

Riedel, S. (2005). Edward Jenner and the history of smallpox and vaccination. *Proceedings (Baylor University. Medical Center)*, *18*(1), 21–25. https://doi.org/10.1080/08998280.2005.11928028

Sharun, K., Dhama, K., Patel, S. K., Pathak, M., Tiwari, R., Singh, B. R., Sah, R., Bonilla-Aldana, D. K., Rodriguez-Morales, A. J., & Leblebicioglu, H. (2021). SARS-CoV-2 in animals: Potential for unknown reservoir hosts and public health implications. *Veterinary Quarterly*, *41*(1), 181–201. https://doi.org/10.1080/01652176.2021.1921311

Smith, K. A. (2011). Edward Jenner and the small pox vaccine. *Frontiers in Immunology*, *2*, 21. https://doi.org/10.3389/fimmu.2011.00021

Tarantola, D., & Foster, S. O. (2011). From smallpox eradication to contemporary global health initiatives: Enhancing human capacity towards a global public health goal. *Vaccine*, *29*(4), D135-D140. https://doi.org/10.1016/j.vaccine.2011.07.027

Tucker, J. B. (2001). *Scourge: The once and future threat of smallpox*. Grove Press.

World Health Organization. (1980). *The global eradication of smallpox: Final report of the global commission for the certification of smallpox eradication*. World Health Organization.

World Health Organization. (2022). *Joint statement on the prioritization of monitoring SARS-CoV-2 infection in wildlife and preventing the formation of animal reservoirs*. https://www.who.int/news/item/07-03-2022-joint-statement-on-the-prioritization-of-monitoring-sars-cov-2-infection-in-wildlife-and-preventing-the-formation-of-animal-reservoirs

5 Viral Cousins

Comparing Other Coronaviruses to COVID-19

Seven distinct coronaviruses are known to infect humans, divided into two categories based on their pathogenicity. The highly pathogenic coronaviruses—SARS-CoV (2003), MERS-CoV (2012), and SARS-CoV-2 (2019)—have caused outbreaks of severe respiratory illnesses: SARS, MERS, and COVID-19, respectively, each with significant mortality rates. Meanwhile, the low pathogenic coronaviruses (HKU1, NL63, 229E, and OC43) typically cause mild to moderate upper-respiratory tract illnesses similar to the common cold. This section focuses specifically on comparing the three highly pathogenic coronaviruses, examining their transmission patterns, clinical presentations, and the valuable lessons they offer for pandemic management.

The Coronavirus Family

Coronaviruses belong to the Coronaviridae family, sharing fundamental characteristics visible under an electron microscope. These viruses have a roughly spherical shape with a diameter of approximately 100–160 nanometers and possess a fatty envelope surrounding their internal components. This envelope, when viewed under electron microscopy, resembles a crown (or corona), which explains the origin of their name (Chen et al., 2020).

SARS-CoV emerged in Guangdong Province, China in late 2002 and spread to 29 countries, infecting 8,096 people and causing 774 deaths. With a mortality rate of approximately 9.6%, it was considered highly lethal. However, strict containment measures effectively controlled the outbreak within seven months, and no cases have been reported worldwide since 2004.

MERS-CoV was first reported in Saudi Arabia in 2012 and has primarily affected countries in the Middle East. It maintains the highest mortality rate among human coronaviruses at approximately 35.9% but demonstrates relatively low transmissibility. Dromedary camels serve as a major reservoir host, with most human infections linked to direct or indirect contact with infected animals. As of early 2025, 2,618 laboratory-confirmed cases and 945 deaths have been reported globally.

SARS-CoV-2, first identified in Wuhan, China in December 2019, quickly achieved global spread, leading to the COVID-19 pandemic. By April 2025,

DOI: 10.4324/9781003595564-7

over 777 million confirmed COVID-19 cases and more than 7 million deaths had been reported worldwide. Despite SARS-CoV-2 having a lower mortality rate compared to SARS-CoV and MERS-CoV, its high transmissibility and capacity for asymptomatic spread have resulted in the COVID-19 pandemic having a far greater total impact worldwide (Petersen et al., 2020). Table 5.1 compares all three comprehensively.

Table 5.1 Comparison of SARS, MERS, and COVID-19

Feature	*SARS-CoV-1 (2002–2004)*	*MERS-CoV (2012–Present)*	*SARS-CoV-2 (2019–present)*
Initial emergence	Guangdong, China	Saudi Arabia	Wuhan, China
Zoonotic source	Bats → civet cats → humans	Bats → camels → humans	Likely bats → intermediate host (TBD) → humans
Global spread	29 countries	Primarily Middle East	Worldwide *(global pandemic)*
Total confirmed cases	Approx. 8,096	Approx. 2,618	≥777,720,205
Total confirmed deaths	Approx. 774	Approx. 945	≥7,094,447
Case fatality rate (CFR)	Approx. 9.6%	Approx. 35.9%	Approx. 0.1–5% *(varies by age, healthcare access, vaccination status, etc.)*
Basic reproduction number (R_0)	Approx. 2–3	Less than 1	Approx. 2.5–5+ *(varies by region/variant)*
Transmission mode	Primarily post-symptomatic	Zoonotic and nosocomial	Asymptomatic, presymptomatic, and symptomatic
Asymptomatic transmission	Rare	Rare	Common *(approx. 40.5% of asymptomatic)*
Clinical onset	Rapid, severe symptoms	Severe symptoms	Wide spectrum *(asymptomatic to severe)*
Containment	Contained by mid-2004 *(no cases since)*	Limited regional outbreaks	Ongoing global circulation
Vaccine availability	No approved vaccine	No approved vaccine	Multiple vaccines *(mRNA, viral vector, protein subunit, etc.)*
Variants of concern	None developed	Minimal genetic drift	Multiple variants *(e.g., Alpha, Delta, and Omicron)*

Sources: World Health Organization (WHO) (2020, 2023a, 2023b, 2024a, 2024b); Centers for Disease Control and Prevention (CDC) (2023, 2024a, 2024b); Buitrago-Garcia et al. (2020); Cevik et al. (2021); Delamater et al. (2019); Fereidouni et al. (2021); He et al. (2020); Hu et al. (2021); Johansson et al. (2021); Lan et al. (2020); Li et al. (2020a); Oran and Topol (2020, 2021); Petersen et al. (2020); Pormohammad et al. (2020); Shang et al. (2020); Toyoshima et al. (2020); Wang et al. (2020); Winkler et al. (2021); Wrapp et al. (2020); Zhu et al. (2020).

Key Similarities and Differences

While these three coronaviruses share a common family, they differ significantly in their transmission dynamics, clinical presentation, and epidemiological impact. Understanding these differences has been crucial for developing effective containment strategies for each virus.

SARS-CoV-2 spreads much faster than either SARS-CoV or MERS-CoV, partially due to its longer incubation period during which individuals may transmit the virus while asymptomatic or experiencing only mild symptoms. A comprehensive analysis of 95 studies, including nearly 30 million cases, indicated that approximately 40.5% of SARS-CoV-2 infections remain asymptomatic (Buitrago-Garcia et al., 2020). Other studies have found estimates ranging from 15 to 25% (Methi & Madslien, 2022) to as high as 40–45% of infections being asymptomatic (Oran & Topol, 2020). More recent systematic reviews have confirmed that approximately 20% of infected individuals remain asymptomatic throughout the course of infection, with higher percentages in certain defined populations (Oran & Topol, 2021). The U.S. CDC found that approximately 59% of SARS-CoV-2 transmission stemmed from asymptomatic cases, with 35% from purely asymptomatic individuals and 24% from presymptomatic individuals (Johansson et al., 2021). This characteristic has greatly complicated COVID-19 containment efforts.

SARS-CoV demonstrated intermediate transmissibility—more efficient than MERS-CoV but less than SARS-CoV-2. Importantly, SARS-CoV transmission typically occurred after symptom onset, making case identification and isolation more straightforward. This characteristic proved crucial to successful containment of the 2003 SARS outbreak.

MERS-CoV exhibits the lowest transmission rate among the three, spreading primarily through contact with infected camels and showing limited human-to-human transmission, typically in healthcare settings or among close household contacts.

The inverse relationship between transmissibility and case fatality among these coronaviruses is notable. MERS-CoV, with its 35–40% mortality rate for MERS, spreads with difficulty between humans. SARS-CoV, with an approximate 10% mortality rate for SARS, demonstrates moderate transmissibility. SARS-CoV-2, with COVID-19's lower mortality rate (0.1–5%, varying significantly by age group, presence of comorbidities, and access to healthcare), shows the highest transmission efficiency—an evolutionary trade-off that has significantly shaped each virus's global impact (Li et al., 2020a).

Structural differences between these viruses partially explain their varying transmission patterns. All three use spike proteins to enter human cells by binding to cell surface receptors, but SARS-CoV-2's spike proteins demonstrate enhanced binding affinity to the ACE2 receptor compared to SARS-CoV (Lan et al., 2020; Winkler et al., 2021). Studies have shown that SARS-CoV-2 spike protein binds to ACE2 with higher affinity than SARS-CoV, which likely contributes to SARS-CoV-2's increased transmissibility (Shang et al., 2020;

Wang et al., 2020; Wrapp et al., 2020). Additionally, variations in accessory proteins across these viruses influence viral replication efficiency and immune evasion capabilities.

Clinical presentations also differ meaningfully among the diseases caused by these coronaviruses. While SARS, MERS, and COVID-19 all cause respiratory symptoms such as fever, cough, and shortness of breath, their typical disease courses vary. SARS and MERS patients frequently developed severe symptoms early in infection, which paradoxically assisted containment efforts by making cases easier to identify. In contrast, COVID-19 presents a spectrum from completely asymptomatic to severe respiratory failure, with many mild cases potentially going undetected and facilitating community spread.

The basic reproduction number (R_0) also varies among these coronaviruses. Studies indicate that SARS-CoV-2 has an estimated R_0 of 2.5 (ranging from 1.8 to 3.6), compared with 2.0–3.0 for SARS-CoV and less than 1 for MERS-CoV (Delamater et al., 2019). This difference in transmissibility partly explains why COVID-19 developed into a global pandemic while SARS and MERS remained more regionally contained (He et al., 2020).

Lessons from Previous Coronavirus Outbreaks

Experience with SARS and MERS provided valuable lessons that informed the COVID-19 response, though implementation of these lessons varied considerably across different regions and time frames.

Rapid identification and isolation of cases proved critical to containing the SARS outbreak in 2003. This insight led to the emphasis on widespread testing and contact tracing during the COVID-19 pandemic, though testing capacity limitations initially hampered these efforts in many countries. The importance of personal protective equipment (PPE) for healthcare workers during both previous coronavirus outbreaks informed protocols that many countries adopted during the COVID-19 pandemic that helped reduce nosocomial transmission.

The MERS outbreak contributed to advances in rapid diagnostic tools, with technologies like polymerase chain reaction (PCR) becoming standard for coronavirus detection. This prior development facilitated the swift creation and deployment of diagnostic tests for SARS-CoV-2, though supply chain challenges and implementation issues created bottlenecks in many regions.

Research into the zoonotic origins of SARS-CoV and MERS-CoV—both traced to bat coronaviruses that likely passed through intermediate animal hosts—informed similar investigations for SARS-CoV-2. This shared evolutionary pattern among highly pathogenic coronaviruses has reinforced the importance of monitoring coronaviruses in wildlife populations and understanding transmission at the human-animal interface.

While neither SARS-CoV nor MERS-CoV resulted in approved vaccines for clinical use due to the limited duration of those outbreaks, the research conducted provided valuable insights into coronavirus immunology and potential vaccine platforms. This groundwork contributed to the unprecedented speed of COVID-19 vaccine development, which benefited from pre-existing knowledge about coronavirus spike proteins as vaccine targets.

Temporal dynamics in viral shedding also differ significantly among the three coronaviruses. Studies have shown that viral shedding of SARS-CoV and MERS-CoV typically begins around the time of symptom onset and peaks during the second week of illness. In contrast, SARS-CoV-2 viral shedding begins during the incubation period and often peaks around or slightly before symptom onset, enabling presymptomatic transmission (Cevik et al., 2021). This distinction has profound implications for containment strategies.

Perhaps most importantly, prior coronavirus outbreaks highlighted the critical value of early implementation of non-pharmaceutical interventions. Countries with direct experience of SARS, particularly in East Asia, generally implemented quarantine, isolation, and social distancing measures more promptly during the COVID-19 pandemic, often achieving better early containment as a result. The effectiveness of these measures for SARS, along with their delayed or inconsistent implementation for COVID-19 in many regions, is a testament to their importance in controlling coronavirus transmission.

Previous outbreaks also demonstrated the crucial role of transparent communication during health emergencies. Initial delays in reporting SARS cases in 2003 contributed to its international spread, a lesson that informed emphasis on more rapid reporting during subsequent outbreaks. Despite this historical precedent, similar challenges with transparency emerged during the early stages of the COVID-19 pandemic, highlighting the persistent difficulty of balancing timely communication with the need for accurate information during emerging outbreaks.

The Unique Challenges of COVID-19 Among Coronavirus Diseases

COVID-19 presented a distinctive set of challenges compared to previous coronavirus outbreaks. Unlike SARS and MERS, where transmission primarily occurred after symptom onset, COVID-19's high rate of asymptomatic transmission made traditional containment measures like temperature checks and symptom monitoring insufficient. Furthermore, SARS-CoV-2's greater transmissibility and capacity for immune evasion have enabled its persistent circulation despite global interventions.

Seasonal patterns also differentiate these coronaviruses. While common human coronaviruses typically exhibit winter seasonality in temperate regions, the global circulation of SARS-CoV-2 has shown more complex patterns influenced by both environmental factors and human interventions (Li et al., 2020b). Understanding these seasonal dynamics may help predict future outbreak patterns and guide ongoing control strategies.

The ongoing evolution of SARS-CoV-2 variants has further complicated response efforts. While SARS-CoV was contained before significant variants could emerge, and MERS-CoV has shown limited genetic diversity over time, SARS-CoV-2 has generated multiple variants of concern with enhanced transmissibility, partial immune evasion, or altered clinical presentations. This evolutionary capacity necessitates continuous monitoring and adaptation of control strategies.

Understanding the similarities and differences between SARS-CoV-2 and its coronavirus relatives has proven essential for developing appropriate public health responses. While we can draw important lessons from previous coronavirus outbreaks, COVID-19's unique epidemiological profile requires tailored approaches to surveillance, containment, and mitigation that account for its distinctive transmission characteristics. The experience with these three highly pathogenic coronaviruses and the diseases they cause collectively highlights the need for flexible, evidence-based strategies and pandemic preparedness systems that can rapidly adapt to the specific challenges posed by emerging viral threats.

References

Buitrago-Garcia, D., Egli-Gany, D., Counotte, M. J., Hossmann, S., Imeri, H., Ipekci, A. M., Salanti, G., & Low, N. (2020). Occurrence and transmission potential of asymptomatic and presymptomatic SARS-CoV-2 infections: A living systematic review and meta-analysis. *PLOS Medicine*, *17*(9), e1003346. https://doi.org/10.1371/journal.pmed.1003346

Centers for Disease Control and Prevention. (CDC). (2023). *SARS basics fact sheet*. Retrieved March 29, 2025, from https://www.cdc.gov/sars/about/fs-sars.html

Centers for Disease Control and Prevention. (CDC). (2024a). *COVID-19 data tracker*. Retrieved March 29, 2025, from https://covid.cdc.gov/covid-data-tracker

Centers for Disease Control and Prevention. (CDC). (2024b). *Middle East respiratory syndrome (MERS)*. Retrieved March 29, 2025, from https://www.cdc.gov/coronavirus/mers/index.html

Cevik, M., Tate, M., Lloyd, O., Maraolo, A. E., Schafers, J., & Ho, A. (2021). SARS-CoV-2, SARS-CoV, and MERS-CoV viral load dynamics, duration of viral shedding, and infectiousness: A systematic review and meta-analysis. *The Lancet Microbe*, *2*(1), e13–e22. https://doi.org/10.1016/S2666-5247(20)30172-5

Chen, Y., Liu, Q., & Guo, D. (2020). Emerging coronaviruses: Genome structure, replication, and pathogenesis. *Journal of Medical Virology*, *92*(4), 418–423. https://doi.org/10.1002/jmv.25681

Delamater, P. L., Street, E. J., Leslie, T. F., Yang, Y. T., & Jacobsen, K. H. (2019). Complexity of the basic reproduction number (R0). *Emerging Infectious Diseases*, *25*(1), 1–4. https://doi.org/10.3201/eid2501.171901

Fereidouni, S. R., Miandehi, N., Fathizadeh, H., Parikhani, A., Khodadadi, E., Mahmoudi, T., Abdoli, A., & Shahbazi, S. (2021). Comparison of the COVID-2019 (SARS-CoV-2) pathogenesis with SARS-CoV and MERS-CoV infections. *Future Virology*, *16*(4), 253–264. https://doi.org/10.2217/fvl-2020-0312

He, X., Lau, E. H., Wu, P., Deng, X., Wang, J., Hao, X., Lau, Y. C., Wong, J. Y., Guan, Y., Tan, X., Mo, X., Chen, Y., Liao, B., Chen, W., Hu, F., Zhang, Q., Zhong, M., Wu, Y., Zhao, L., … & Leung, G. M. (2020). Temporal dynamics in viral shedding and transmissibility of COVID-19. *Nature Medicine*, *26*(5), 672–675. https://doi.org/10.1038/s41591-020-0869-5

Hu, B., Guo, H., Zhou, P., & Shi, Z. L. (2021). Characteristics of SARS-CoV-2 and COVID-19. *Nature Reviews Microbiology*, *19*(3), 141–154. https://doi.org/10.1038/s41579-020-00459-7

Johansson, M. A., Quandelacy, T. M., Kada, S., Prasad, P. V., Steele, M., Brooks, J. T., Slayton, R. B., Biggerstaff, M., & Butler, J. C. (2021). SARS-CoV-2 transmission from people without COVID-19 symptoms. *JAMA Network Open*, *4*(1), e2035057. https://doi.org/10.1001/jamanetworkopen.2020.35057

Lan, J., Ge, J., Yu, J., Shan, S., Zhou, H., Fan, S., Zhang, Q., Shi, X., Wang, Q., Zhang, L., & Wang, X. (2020). Structure of the SARS-CoV-2 spike receptor-binding domain bound to the ACE2 receptor. *Nature*, *581*(7807), 215–220. https://doi.org/10.1038/s41586-020-2180-5

Li, Q., Guan, X., Wu, P., Wang, X., Zhou, L., Tong, Y., Ren, R., Leung, K. S. M., Lau, E. H. Y., Wong, J. Y., Xing, X., Xiang, N., Wu, Y., Li, C., Chen, Q., Li, D., Liu, T., Zhao, J., Liu, M., … & Feng, Z. (2020a). Early transmission dynamics in Wuhan, China, of novel coronavirus-infected pneumonia. *New England Journal of Medicine*, *382*(13), 1199–1207. https://doi.org/10.1056/NEJMoa2001316

Li, Y., Wang, X., & Nair, H. (2020b). Global seasonality of human seasonal coronaviruses: A clue for post-pandemic circulating season of SARS-CoV-2 virus? *The Journal of Infectious Diseases*, *222*(7), 1090–1092. https://doi.org/10.1093/infdis/jiaa436

Methi, F., & Madslien, E.H. (2022). Lower transmissibility of SARS-CoV-2 among asymptomatic cases: Evidence from contact tracing data in Oslo, Norway. *BMC Medicine*, *20*, 427. https://doi.org/10.1186/s12916-022-02642-4

Oran, D. P., & Topol, E. J. (2020). Prevalence of asymptomatic SARS-CoV-2 infection: A narrative review. *Annals of Internal Medicine*, *173*(5), 362–367. https://doi.org/10.7326/M20-3012

Oran, D. P., & Topol, E. J. (2021). The proportion of SARS-CoV-2 infections that are asymptomatic: A systematic review. *Annals of Internal Medicine*, *174*(5), 655–662. https://doi.org/10.7326/M20-6976

Petersen, E., Koopmans, M., Go, U., Hamer, D. H., Petrosillo, N., Castelli, F., Storgaard, M., Al Khalili, S., & Simonsen, L. (2020). Comparing SARS-CoV-2 with SARS-CoV and influenza pandemics. *The Lancet Infectious Diseases*, *20*(9), e238–e244. https://doi.org/10.1016/S1473-3099(20)30484-9

Pormohammad, A., Ghorbani, S., Khatami, A., Razizadeh, M. H., Alborzi, E., Zarei, M., Idrovo, J. P., & Turner, R. J. (2020). Comparison of confirmed COVID-19 with SARS and MERS cases - Clinical characteristics, laboratory findings, radiographic signs and outcomes: A systematic review and meta-analysis. *Reviews in Medical Virology*, *30*(4), e2112. https://doi.org/10.1002/rmv.2112

Shang, J., Ye, G., Shi, K., Wan, Y., Luo, C., Aihara, H., Geng, Q., Auerbach, A., & Li, F. (2020). Structural basis of receptor recognition by SARS-CoV-2. *Nature*, *581*(7807), 221–224. https://doi.org/10.1038/s41586-020-2179-y

Toyoshima, Y., Nemoto, K., Matsumoto, S., Nakamura, Y., & Kiyotani, K. (2020). SARS-CoV-2 genomic variations associated with mortality rate of COVID-19. *Journal of Human Genetics*, *65*(12), 1075–1082. https://doi.org/10.1038/s10038-020-0808-9

Wang, Y., Liu, M., & Gao, J. (2020). Enhanced receptor binding of SARS-CoV-2 through networks of hydrogen-bonding and hydrophobic interactions. *Proceedings of the National Academy of Sciences*, *117*(25), 13967–13974. https://doi.org/10.1073/pnas.2008209117

Winkler, D. A., Piplani, S., Singh, P. K., & Petrovsky, N. (2021). In silico comparison of SARS-CoV-2 spike protein-ACE2 binding affinities across species and implications for virus origin. *Scientific Reports*, *11*(1), 13063. https://doi.org/10.1038/s41598-021-92388-5

World Health Organization. (WHO). (2020). *Report of the WHO-China joint mission on Coronavirus Disease 2019 (COVID-19)*. https://www.who.int/publications/i/item/report-of-the-who-china-joint-mission-on-coronavirus-disease-2019-(covid-19)

World Health Organization. (WHO). (2023a). *Severe acute respiratory syndrome (SARS)*. Retrieved March 29, 2025, from https://www.who.int/health-topics/severe-acute-respiratory-syndrome

World Health Organization. (WHO). (2023b). *Tracking SARS-CoV-2 variants*. Retrieved March 29, 2025, from https://www.who.int/activities/tracking-SARS-CoV-2-variants

World Health Organization. (WHO). (2024a). *Coronavirus disease (COVID-19) pandemic*. Retrieved March 29, 2025, from https://www.who.int/emergencies/diseases/novel-coronavirus-2019

World Health Organization. (WHO). (2024b). *Middle East respiratory syndrome coronavirus (MERS-CoV)*. Retrieved March 29, 2025, from https://www.who.int/health-topics/middle-east-respiratory-syndrome-coronavirus-mers

Wrapp, D., Wang, N., Corbett, K. S., Goldsmith, J. A., Hsieh, C. L., Abiona, O., Graham, B. S., & McLellan, J. S. (2020). Cryo-EM structure of the 2019-nCoV spike in the prefusion conformation. *Science*, *367*(6483), 1260–1263. https://doi.org/10.1126/science.abb2507

Zhu, Z., Lian, X., Su, X., Wu, W., Marraro, G. A., & Zeng, Y. (2020). From SARS and MERS to COVID-19: A brief summary and comparison of severe acute respiratory infections caused by three highly pathogenic human coronaviruses. *Respiratory Research*, *21*(1), 224. https://doi.org/10.1186/s12931-020-01479-w

6 Pandemic Wisdom

Historical and Contemporary Lessons for COVID-19

Throughout history, pandemics have profoundly shaped human societies, each leaving behind valuable insights into effective public health responses and societal adaptation. This section synthesizes the lessons from major historical pandemics—the Black Death, the 1918 Spanish Flu, and Smallpox—alongside more recent outbreaks like SARS, MERS, and others. By examining both historical precedents and contemporary experiences, we can distill critical principles for pandemic management and apply them to our ongoing response to COVID-19.

Enduring Lessons from Historical Pandemics

The Black Death (1347–1351), which devastated medieval European societies, established the value of basic sanitation and isolation practices during disease outbreaks, even before the germ theory of disease was established. Quarantine measures first implemented in 14th-century Venice during this pandemic created a precedent that remains fundamental to modern infectious disease control, with Venice's maritime quarantine becoming a model for other parts of Italy and the world (Conti, 2008; Crawshaw, 2021). The Black Death also revealed how pandemics can drive profound social transformations, restructuring labor relations and accelerating technological innovation as societies adapted to population decline (Benedictow, 2004).

The history of quarantine—how it began, how it was used in the past, and how it is used in the modern era—remains a fascinating topic in the history of public health and sanitation, with its applications evolving from the time of the Black Death to the present day (Gensini et al., 2004; Tognotti, 2013). These early practices demonstrate that public health has always encompassed more than just medicine—it also involves politics, economics, and creating social trust (Crawshaw, 2021).

The 1918 Spanish Influenza pandemic occurred during a period of nascent scientific understanding of viruses and highlighted the critical role of non-pharmaceutical interventions when medical countermeasures are limited. Historical analyses of city-level responses during this pandemic have shown that locations implementing early, sustained social distancing measures experienced significantly lower mortality rates (Bootsma & Ferguson, 2007; Crosby, 2003). As mentioned

DOI: 10.4324/9781003595564-8

in Chapter 3 one prominent historical example is the contrast between St. Louis, which had excess deaths of 347 per 100,000 people, and Philadelphia, which recorded 748 per 100,000 (Hatchett et al., 2007). This dramatic difference resulted from Philadelphia's decision to proceed with a large parade despite warnings, while St. Louis swiftly implemented restrictions within days of detecting cases (Markel et al., 2007).

The public health response in Philadelphia and St. Louis differed dramatically during the 1918 pandemic; Philadelphia downplayed the significance of early cases and allowed a city-wide parade to continue, while St. Louis acted quickly to ban public gatherings and close schools (Barry, 2004). This pandemic further revealed the necessity for transparent public communication during health crises, as wartime censorship and misinformation hampered effective public health responses in many countries.

Smallpox eradication represents humanity's greatest triumph over infectious disease and offers invaluable insights for contemporary pandemic management. This achievement exemplified the power of global coordination and political commitment in confronting pathogens that transcend national boundaries (Foege, 2011; Henderson, 2009). The successful ring vaccination strategy employed during the campaign illustrated the effectiveness of targeted approaches when universal coverage is not immediately achievable, while also affirming the value of community engagement and cultural sensitivity in implementing public health measures across diverse settings with varying healthcare resources (Henderson, 2009).

Insights from Contemporary Outbreaks

Recent infectious disease outbreaks have yielded additional lessons applicable to pandemic management (Table 6.1). The 2003 SARS outbreak demonstrated the effectiveness of rapid case identification and isolation in containing novel coronaviruses, particularly when transmission occurs primarily after symptom onset. Healthcare settings became significant amplification points for SARS, highlighting the need for robust infection control protocols. The international response to SARS led to improvements in global health governance for novel pathogens, including revisions to the International Health Regulations that enhanced reporting requirements (Fidler, 2004; Heymann & Rodier, 2004).

The 2009 H1N1 influenza pandemic, though less severe than initially feared, provided valuable experience in accelerated vaccine development and global distribution mechanisms. It exposed weaknesses in equitable vaccine access, as high-income countries secured supplies before others—a pattern subsequently repeated during COVID-19. This pandemic also revealed the challenges of risk communication when disease severity remains uncertain during early stages (Fineberg, 2014).

The 2014–2016 Ebola outbreak in West Africa illustrated the crucial role of trust in public health interventions. Research conducted during the Ebola epidemic in Liberia found that respondents who expressed low trust in government were much less likely to take precautions against Ebola in their homes or to abide by government-mandated social distancing mechanisms (Blair et al., 2017). Initial resistance to contact tracing and safe burial practices hampered containment efforts.

Trust was fostered through open, transparent, and adaptive communication that was accountable to community-led response efforts, with responders engaging "technologies of trust"—including reflexivity, openness, and accountability—to facilitate relations of trust (Viergever & Hendriks, 2016). When authorities began

Table 6.1 Historical and Contemporary Pandemic Lessons and Their Relevance to COVID-19

Pandemic	*Time Period*	*Key Lessons Learned*	*Relevance to COVID-19*
Black Death	1347–1351	Introduced quarantine and isolation; revealed pandemics reshape society	Reinforced isolation as a core response; showed long-term societal impacts
1918 Influenza	1918–1920	Demonstrated effectiveness of NPIs; highlighted harm of censorship	Validated timely interventions and transparent communication
Smallpox	Historical–1980	Achieved through global coordination, ring vaccination, and trust-building	Informed global vaccine campaigns and the importance of public trust
SARS-CoV-1	2002–2004	Showed value of early detection, isolation, and health system readiness	Strengthened surveillance and international reporting standards
H1N1 Influenza	2009	Exposed vaccine access inequities; challenged risk communication	Foreshadowed unequal distribution and messaging difficulties
Ebola *(West Africa)*	2014–2016	Emphasized local engagement and culturally sensitive responses	Highlighted that trust and cooperation are critical to success
MERS-CoV	2012–present	Advanced zoonotic surveillance and hospital infection control	Reinforced One Health approaches and healthcare preparedness
Zika Virus	2015–2016	Revealed need for agile surveillance and rapid research	Emphasized adaptability to unexpected disease outcomes
COVID-19	2019–present	Integrated past lessons; exposed gaps in equity, trust, and systems	Stress-tested preparedness and need for inclusive, digital-era responses

Sources: Barry (2004); Bedford et al. (2019); Blair et al. (2017); Bootsma and Ferguson (2007); Crawshaw (2021); Crosby (2003); Fidler (2004); Foege (2011); Gensini et al. (2004); Graham et al. (2018); Hatchett et al. (2007); Henderson (2009); Heymann and Rodier (2004); Larson (2020); Lee et al. (2020); Markel et al. (2007); Moon et al. (2015); Oppenheim et al. (2019); Petersen et al. (2016); Tangcharoensathien et al. (2020); Tognotti (2013); Vinck et al. (2019); Vraga and Bode (2020); Whitelaw et al. (2020); Zumla et al. (2016).

collaborating with community leaders and addressing local concerns, compliance with control measures improved substantially (Vinck et al., 2019).

The MERS outbreak, ongoing since 2012 but primarily contained within the Arabian Peninsula, has advanced understanding of zoonotic disease transmission at the human-animal interface. Identifying dromedary camels as the primary reservoir for MERS-CoV shaped surveillance strategies and interventions to reduce spillover events. This experience reinforced the value of interdisciplinary collaboration between human and veterinary health sectors using a One Health approach for emerging infectious diseases (Zumla et al., 2016).

The Zika virus outbreak in the Americas (2015–2016) revealed the challenges of responding to pathogens with unexpected clinical manifestations. The association between Zika infection during pregnancy and congenital abnormalities showed how novel pathogens can produce unanticipated consequences beyond their immediate symptoms. This outbreak emphasized the necessity for comprehensive surveillance systems capable of detecting unusual disease patterns and the importance of research agility during emerging infectious disease events (Petersen et al., 2016).

Applying Pandemic Wisdom to COVID-19 and Future Threats

The COVID-19 pandemic validated historical lessons while revealing new dimensions of pandemic management. The rapid development of vaccines within one year represents a scientific achievement built on decades of research. While global collaboration through genomic sequencing and data sharing reached unprecedented levels, inequitable vaccine distribution confirmed that technological solutions also require effective implementation systems.

Non-pharmaceutical interventions proved essential in mitigating transmission, reinforcing lessons from the 1918 influenza pandemic. Their effectiveness depended primarily on implementation quality and societal adherence rather than policy adoption alone, highlighting the need for context-appropriate interventions (Bootsma & Ferguson, 2007).

Critical areas requiring attention for future pandemic preparedness span multiple dimensions. Early warning systems must pair with governance structures that incentivize timely reporting and response rather than penalizing transparency. COVID-19 demonstrated that countries detecting and responding quickly generally achieved better outcomes, though political and economic factors often delayed crucial public health measures (Bedford et al., 2019; Moon et al., 2015; Oppenheim et al., 2019).

Research platforms capable of pivoting to emerging threats require sustained investment during interpandemic periods. The remarkable success of mRNA vaccines built upon decades of previously under-recognized research, suggesting that similar long-term investments across multiple technological platforms could benefit responses to future outbreaks (Graham et al., 2018).

Public health infrastructure must maintain adequate capacity between crises rather than expanding and contracting with each threat. The pandemic revealed that countries with robust testing, contact tracing, and isolation facilities already in place due to prior experiences with SARS or MERS responded most effectively in the crucial early stages of COVID-19 (Lee et al., 2020).

Digital transformation created unprecedented possibilities for disease surveillance and healthcare delivery during COVID-19, though success varied dramatically across settings. These experiences reinforce the importance of adapting digital solutions to local infrastructure, privacy considerations, and user acceptance, meaning that technological solutions must be contextually appropriate to achieve their full potential (Whitelaw et al., 2020).

Misinformation management emerged as another critical component of effective pandemic response, as the rapid spread of false information complicated public health messaging and undermined trust. Future preparedness must include proactive communication strategies that address misinformation while building trust in scientific institutions and governmental authorities (Larson, 2020; Tangcharoensathien et al., 2020; Vraga & Bode, 2020).

Equity considerations must be addressed proactively to ensure resources reach vulnerable populations both within and between countries. The disproportionate impact of COVID-19 on disadvantaged communities highlighted persistent structural inequities in global health systems that require deliberate, sustained attention to correct (Ahmed et al., 2020; Bambra et al., 2020; Patel et al., 2020).

The Historical Context of COVID-19 vs. Past Pandemics

Placing COVID-19 within the broader historical context of pandemics reveals both unique aspects of this outbreak and recurring patterns connecting it to previous infectious disease crises. What distinguishes our current era is not the fundamental nature of pandemic threats, which have remained constant throughout human history, but rather our enhanced capacity to respond through scientific knowledge, technological tools, and global coordination mechanisms. Yet the COVID-19 experience demonstrates that these advanced capabilities must be paired with political will, social cooperation, and equitable implementation to effectively control pandemic spread.

As we navigate the transition from pandemic response to preparedness for future threats, the integrated historical perspective presented in this chapter provides a foundation for more effective and equitable approaches. By synthesizing lessons from past pandemic management—from medieval plague outbreaks to 21st-century coronavirus epidemics—we can build more resilient health systems and societies capable of mitigating the impact of inevitable future pandemic events.

To fully harness these lessons, however, we must go beyond historical parallels and adopt a structured framework for understanding the deeper dynamics of pandemic crises. Just as past outbreaks exposed multiple layers of societal vulnerability and resilience, COVID-19 demands analysis that reaches beneath surface-level events. Part II introduces the Iceberg Theory—a systems thinking approach that helps uncover not only the visible consequences of the pandemic (cases, deaths, disruptions), but also the hidden patterns, structures, and mental models that shaped its trajectory.

References

Ahmed, F., Ahmed, N., Pissarides, C., & Stiglitz, J. (2020). Why inequality could spread COVID-19. *The Lancet Public Health*, *5*(5), e240. https://doi.org/10.1016/S2468-2667(20)30085-2

Bambra, C., Riordan, R., Ford, J., & Matthews, F. (2020). The COVID-19 pandemic and health inequalities. *Journal of Epidemiology and Community Health*, *74*(11), 964–968. https://doi.org/10.1136/jech-2020-214401

Barry, J. M. (2004). *The great influenza: The story of the deadliest pandemic in history*. Viking.

Bedford, J., Farrar, J., Ihekweazu, C., Kang, G., Koopmans, M., & Nkengasong, J. (2019). A new twenty-first century science for effective epidemic response. *Nature*, *575*(7781), 130–136. https://doi.org/10.1038/s41586-019-1717-y

Benedictow, O. J. (2004). *The Black Death, 1346-1353: The complete history*. Boydell & Brewer.

Blair, R. A., Morse, B. S., & Tsai, L. L. (2017). Public health and public trust: Survey evidence from the Ebola Virus Disease epidemic in Liberia. *Social Science & Medicine*, *172*, 89–97. https://doi.org/10.1016/j.socscimed.2016.11.016

Bootsma, M. C., & Ferguson, N. M. (2007). The effect of public health measures on the 1918 influenza pandemic in U.S. cities. *Proceedings of the National Academy of Sciences*, *104*(18), 7588–7593. https://doi.org/10.1073/pnas.0611071104

Conti, A. A. (2008). Quarantine through history. In *International encyclopedia of public health* (pp. 454–462). Academic Press. https://doi.org/10.1016/B978-012373960-5.00380-4

Crawshaw, J. L. S. (2021). *Plague hospitals: Public health for the city in early modern Venice*. Routledge.

Crosby, A. W. (2003). *America's forgotten pandemic: The influenza of 1918*. Cambridge University Press.

Fidler, D. P. (2004). *SARS, governance and the globalization of disease*. Palgrave Macmillan.

Fineberg, H. V. (2014). Pandemic preparedness and response—Lessons from the H1N1 influenza of 2009. *New England Journal of Medicine*, *370*(14), 1335–1342. https://doi.org/10.1056/NEJMra1208802

Foege, W. H. (2011). *House on fire: The fight to eradicate smallpox*. University of California Press.

Gensini, G. F., Yacoub, M. H., & Conti, A. A. (2004). The concept of quarantine in history: From plague to SARS. *Journal of Infection*, *49*(4), 257–261. https://doi.org/10.1016/j.jinf.2004.03.002

Graham, B. S., Mascola, J. R., & Fauci, A. S. (2018). Novel vaccine technologies: Essential components of an adequate response to emerging viral diseases. *JAMA*, *319*(14), 1431–1432. https://doi.org/10.1001/jama.2018.0345

Hatchett, R. J., Mecher, C. E., & Lipsitch, M. (2007). Public health interventions and epidemic intensity during the 1918 influenza pandemic. *Proceedings of the National Academy of Sciences*, *104*(18), 7582–7587. https://doi.org/10.1073/pnas.0610941104

Henderson, D. A. (2009). *Smallpox: The death of a disease*. Prometheus Books.

Heymann, D. L., & Rodier, G. (2004). SARS: A global response to an international threat. *Brown Journal of World Affairs*, *10*(2), 185–197.

Larson, H. J. (2020). Blocking information on COVID-19 can fuel the spread of misinformation. *Nature*, *580*(7803), 306. https://doi.org/10.1038/d41586-020-00920-w

Lee, V. J., Chiew, C. J., & Khong, W. X. (2020). Interrupting transmission of COVID-19: Lessons from containment efforts in Singapore. *Journal of Travel Medicine*, *27*(3), taaa039. https://doi.org/10.1093/jtm/taaa039

Markel, H., Lipman, H. B., Navarro, J. A., Sloan, A., Michalsen, J. R., Stern, A. M., & Cetron, M. S. (2007). Nonpharmaceutical interventions implemented by US cities during the 1918-1919 influenza pandemic. *JAMA*, *298*(6), 644–654. https://doi.org/10.1001/jama.298.6.644

Moon, S., Sridhar, D., Pate, M. A., Jha, A. K., Clinton, C., Delaunay, S., Edwin, V., Fallah, M., Fidler, D. P., Garrett, L., Goosby, E., Gostin, L. O., Heymann, D. L., Lee, K., Leung, G. M., Morrison, J. S., Saavedra, J., Tanner, M., Leigh, J. A., … & Piot, P. (2015). Will Ebola change the game? Ten essential reforms before the next pandemic. The report of the Harvard-LSHTM Independent Panel on the Global Response to Ebola. *The Lancet*, *386*(10009), 2204–2221. https://doi.org/10.1016/S0140-6736(15)00946-0

Oppenheim, B., Gallivan, M., Madhav, N. K., Brown, N., Serhiyenko, V., Wolfe, N. D., & Ayscue, P. (2019). Assessing global preparedness for the next pandemic: Development and application of an Epidemic Preparedness Index. *BMJ Global Health*, *4*(1), e001157. https://doi.org/10.1136/bmjgh-2018-001157

Patel, J. A., Nielsen, F., Badiani, A. A., Assi, S., Unadkat, V. A., Patel, B., Ravindrane, R., & Wardle, H. (2020). Poverty, inequality and COVID-19: The forgotten vulnerable. *Public Health*, *183*, 110–111. https://doi.org/10.1016/j.puhe.2020.05.006

Petersen, L. R., Jamieson, D. J., Powers, A. M., & Honein, M. A. (2016). Zika virus. *New England Journal of Medicine*, *374*(16), 1552–1563. https://doi.org/10.1056/NEJMra1602113

Tangcharoensathien, V., Calleja, N., Nguyen, T., Purnat, T., D'Agostino, M., Garcia-Saiso, S., Landry, M., Rashidian, A., Hamilton, C., AbdAllah, A., Ghiga, I., Hill, A., Hougendobler, D., van Andel, J., Nunn, M., Brooks, I., Sacco, P. L., De Domenico, M., Mai, P., … & Briand, S. (2020). Framework for managing the COVID-19 infodemic: Methods and results of an online, crowdsourced WHO technical consultation. *Journal of Medical Internet Research*, *22*(6), e19659. https://doi.org/10.2196/19659

Tognotti, E. (2013). Lessons from the history of quarantine, from plague to influenza A. *Emerging Infectious Diseases*, *19*(2), 254–259. https://doi.org/10.3201/eid1902.120312

Viergever, R. F., & Hendriks, T. C. (2016). The 10 largest public and philanthropic funders of health research in the world: What they fund and how they distribute their funds. *Health Research Policy and Systems*, *14*(1), 12. https://doi.org/10.1186/s12961-015-0074-z

Vinck, P., Pham, P. N., Bindu, K. K., Bedford, J., & Nilles, E. J. (2019). Institutional trust and misinformation in the response to the 2018–19 Ebola outbreak in North Kivu, DR Congo: A population-based survey. *The Lancet Infectious Diseases*, *19*(5), 529–536. https://doi.org/10.1016/S1473-3099(19)30063-5

Vraga, E. K., & Bode, L. (2020). Defining misinformation and understanding its bounded nature: Using expertise and evidence for describing misinformation. *Political Communication*, *37*(1), 136–144. https://doi.org/10.1080/10584609.2020.1716500

Whitelaw, S., Mamas, M. A., Topol, E., & Van Spall, H. G. (2020). Applications of digital technology in COVID-19 pandemic planning and response. *The Lancet Digital Health*, *2*(8), e435–e440. https://doi.org/10.1016/S2589-7500(20)30142-4

Zumla, A., Dar, O., Kock, R., Muturi, M., Ntoumi, F., Kaleebu, P., Eusebio, M., Mfinanga, S., Bates, M., Mwaba, P., Ansumana, R., Khan, M., Alagaili, A. N., Cotten, M., Azhar, E. I., Maeurer, M., Ippolito, G., & Petersen, E. (2016). Taking forward a 'One Health' approach for turning the tide against the Middle East respiratory syndrome coronavirus and other zoonotic pathogens with epidemic potential. *International Journal of Infectious Diseases*, *47*, 5–9. https://doi.org/10.1016/j.ijid.2016.06.012

Part II

The Pandemic Iceberg

Uncovering COVID-19's Hidden Depths

7 The Iceberg Ahead

A Framework for Pandemic Analysis

The COVID-19 pandemic, like the sinking of the Titanic, represents a catastrophic failure to heed critical warnings. To fully understand the pandemic and its wide-ranging impacts, we apply a systems thinking approach using the Iceberg Theory framework. This framework breaks the pandemic into four critical layers: Events (the observable outcomes), Trends (the patterns that reinforced those events), Structures (the systems and institutions that produced those trends), and Mental Models (deeply held beliefs that sustained those structures). These layers reveal both the visible and hidden dimensions of the crisis, offering a comprehensive view that can inform public health policy and future pandemic preparedness.

The Titanic Story

In 1912, the maritime world witnessed the tragic sinking of the Titanic, a symbol of human achievement hailed as unsinkable and the largest luxury liner of its era. This disaster unfolded against the backdrop of a significant natural event: the fracturing of the Greenland ice sheet, which led to the creation of between 15,000 and 30,000 icebergs, drifting into the shipping lanes of the North Atlantic (Bigg & Wilton, 2014). Among these icebergs was a colossal mass of ice weighing approximately 1.5 million tons and standing 30 meters tall, of which a mere 10% was visible above the water's surface. This iceberg had drifted to a location roughly 2,400 kilometers from the open ocean, presenting a hidden danger to maritime navigation (Figure 7.1) (Bassett, 2000).

On April 14, 1912, as the Titanic was on its maiden voyage from Southampton to New York, the ship was surrounded by claims of its invincibility (National Archives, 2012). However, the journey soon turned perilous. Despite receiving six warnings from other ships about the presence of icebergs ahead, the Titanic's crew chose to ignore these advisories, pressing on at a high speed of 20.5 knots (23.6 MPH) (National Museum of American History, 2012). As the ship drew closer to the peril, it received three more urgent warnings, with the final alert being a stark "Iceberg right ahead!" Yet, these cautions were disregarded, leading to a catastrophic collision with a massive iceberg that would ultimately claim over 1,500 lives (Garzke & Brown, 1996).

DOI: 10.4324/9781003595564-10

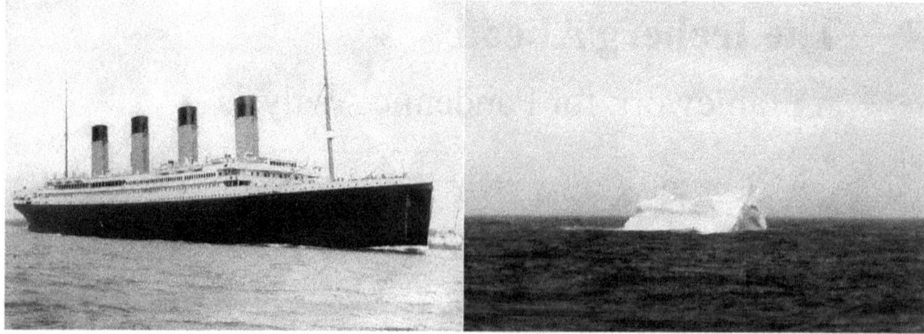

Figure 7.1 Photographic Images of the Titanic (Left) and the Infamous Iceberg That Sank It (Right).

The Iceberg Analogy

This tragic event perfectly illustrates how visible dangers often represent only a fraction of the total threat. Just as only 10% of an iceberg is visible above the waterline while 90% lurks beneath the surface, the Titanic catastrophe stemmed not merely from the collision itself, but from deeper structural and operational failures, such as inadequate safety protocols, insufficient lifeboats, and a culture that prioritized speed and power over safety. This hidden complexity directly parallels our understanding of systemic risks in public health.

The COVID-19 pandemic, much like an iceberg, has visible impacts—cases, hospitalizations, and deaths that dominated public discourse. Yet beneath these observable outcomes lies a complex interplay of hidden factors, such as evolving viral variants, structural weaknesses in healthcare systems, inadequate public health infrastructure, and the social and cultural behaviors that shaped responses. All these factors combined contributed significantly to the crisis's severity and persistence (Leischow & Milstein, 2006).

Human Negligence Leads to a Catastrophic Pandemic of the Century

Human oversight, hubris, and political indecision undoubtedly played a pivotal role in the escalation of COVID-19 into a catastrophic global pandemic, much like the negligence that led to the Titanic's tragic collision with an iceberg. Despite several early warnings about the virus, a collective failure to heed these signs allowed the disease to spread rapidly and uncontrollably across the globe.

The timeline below highlights critical moments when more decisive action might have mitigated the pandemic's impact:

- **December 2019:** Early signs of a novel coronavirus appear in Wuhan, China, with the first reported cases of a "mysterious pneumonia" linked to a seafood market. Despite initial concerns, local authorities downplay the threat. The virus is identified, but it takes until January 11, 2020, for China to share genetic data with the WHO, missing an earlier opportunity for global coordination (WHO, 2020).

- **January 14, 2020:** The WHO publicly reports "no clear evidence of human-to-human transmission," based on incomplete data from Chinese authorities. This statement fosters a false sense of security, delaying efforts to recognize the virus's true airborne nature and potential for global spread. Meanwhile, cases are already emerging in Thailand, Japan, and South Korea (CDC, 2024).
- **January 20, 2020:** China acknowledges human-to-human transmission. However, this realization comes too late for countries like the United States and many in Europe, where early responses are slow. Despite this crucial admission, international travel remains largely unrestricted, facilitating the global spread of the virus (CDC, 2024).
- **January 23, 2020:** The first city-wide lockdown is imposed in Wuhan, China, as cases spike. At this point, the virus is present in at least eight countries. Despite mounting evidence of a global threat, international health bodies deem travel and trade restrictions unnecessary. This failure to act reflects the reluctance to acknowledge the magnitude of the crisis and hampers containment efforts (WHO, 2020).
- **January 30, 2020:** The WHO declares a Public Health Emergency of International Concern (PHEIC) as the virus spreads to 22 countries. However, this declaration comes too late for many regions already experiencing community transmission, and inconsistent messaging leaves many governments uncertain of how to proceed (WHO, 2020).
- **February 5, 2020:** The *Diamond Princess* cruise ship is quarantined off the coast of Japan after an outbreak among passengers. This event serves as another early warning of the virus's rapid spread in enclosed spaces, yet policies for dealing with such outbreaks are still fragmented and inconsistent (Yale Medicine, 2021).
- **February 7, 2020:** Dr. Li Wenliang, the Chinese doctor who first tried to raise alarms about the virus, dies from COVID-19. His tragic death reflects the suppression of early whistleblowers and the consequences of failing to act swiftly on warnings from frontline medical professionals (Yale Medicine, 2021).
- **February 20, 2020:** Despite cases spreading across continents, including widespread transmission in Italy, South Korea, and Iran, the international community hesitates to label COVID-19 a "global pandemic." Many countries continue to believe containment is possible within national borders, leading to patchwork responses that prove ineffective in stopping the spread (WHO, 2020).
- **March 11, 2020:** The WHO officially declares COVID-19 a global pandemic after the virus afflicts 113 countries and regions. By this time, countries like Italy have already entered full-scale crisis mode, with overwhelmed hospitals and mounting death tolls. The delay in pandemic recognition allows the virus to take root in communities worldwide, with fatal consequences (WHO, 2020).
- **Mid-March 2020:** Major Western countries, including the United States and many in Europe, begin implementing large-scale lockdowns and travel restrictions. However, the initial reluctance to take decisive action results in the virus spreading unchecked for months. By now, global supply chains are disrupted, and critical shortages of personal protective equipment and ventilators have emerged in hospitals across the globe (Jack, 2020).

- **April 2020:** Global cases surpass 1 million, with the epicenter shifting to Europe and North America. The delays in coordinated response efforts between nations, as well as conflicting guidance on mask use and social distancing, further exacerbate the uncontrollable spread (WHO, 2020).
- **Summer 2020:** While some countries manage to flatten their infection curves, others, particularly in the Americas, experience spikes in cases due to premature re-openings, poor public health messaging, and politicization of the virus. Countries that took swift action informed by past epidemics demonstrated that timely interventions, such as strict lockdowns and widespread testing, can suppress the virus, but these lessons are not being adopted universally (Jack, 2020).

These milestones represent the progression of a crisis that grew from localized cases to a global emergency, and how early opportunities for containment diminished over time. As we analyze the pandemic's full impact, we must look beyond these visible events to understand the deeper, less obvious consequences. Much like an iceberg, where the visible portion represents only a fraction of its mass, the pandemic's effects extend far beyond immediate health impacts.

The Origins and Applications of the Iceberg Theory

The Iceberg Theory, originally conceptualized by psychoanalyst Sigmund Freud, employs the iceberg as a metaphorical representation of human consciousness. The visible portion above water symbolizes the conscious mind, while the substantially larger submerged mass represents the preconscious and unconscious mind that functions beyond immediate recognition or awareness (McLeod, 2024).

This metaphor has transcended its psychoanalytic origins. In literature, Ernest Hemingway formalized the "Iceberg Principle" as a literary technique wherein minimal narrative elements are explicitly presented while others are hidden away, compelling readers to derive deeper implications and meanings independently.

Within systems thinking, scholars have adapted this metaphor to demonstrate how observable phenomena within systems constitute merely superficial manifestations, while fundamental structures and patterns remain obscured (Meadows, 2008). This analytical approach facilitates the identification of strategic intervention points for implementing sustainable solutions to complex systemic challenges.

Consequently, we have selected the systems thinking framework of the Iceberg Theory as our methodological approach for analyzing the multifaceted complexities of the COVID-19 pandemic.

The Application of the Iceberg Theory in the COVID-19 Pandemic

To gain a deeper understanding of the pandemic, we utilize a four-layered Iceberg framework (Figure 7.2):

i **Events:** The visible, surface-level manifestations of the pandemic, such as infection rates, death tolls, and immediate social and economic impacts (Carey et al., 2015).

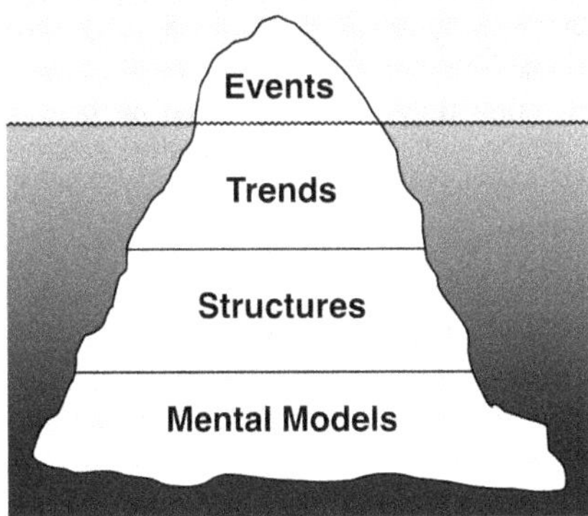

Figure 7.2 The Systems Thinking Iceberg Model for Pandemic Analysis.

ii **Trends/Patterns:** This layer represents underlying patterns, including the mutation and evolution of COVID-19 variants, as well as transmission dynamics. These trends were not always visible in real time but were critical to shaping the trajectory of the pandemic (Leischow & Milstein, 2006).

iii **Systemic Structures:** Beneath the trends lie systemic factors such as healthcare infrastructure, government policies, and global collaboration efforts. These structures influenced the global capacity to respond to the pandemic, from the speed of vaccine development to the effectiveness of public health interventions (Rutter et al., 2017).

iv **Mental Models/Behaviors:** At the deepest level, we examine mental models—individual, collective, institutional, and temporal responses to the crisis. This includes compliance with public health measures, the role of misinformation, and the psychological and cultural factors that shaped how societies managed or failed to manage the pandemic (Knai et al., 2018).

With the Iceberg Theory as our analytical framework, we now begin our descent through the pandemic's layered impacts. In the following section, we explore the most visible tier: the immediate global effects that transformed societies worldwide.

References

Bassett, V. (2000). Causes and effects of the rapid sinking of the Titanic. *Inquiry Journal, University of Pennsylvania*. https://writing.engr.psu.edu/uer/bassett.html

Bigg, G. R., & Wilton, D. J. (2014). Iceberg risk in the Titanic year of 1912: Was it exceptional? *Weather*, *69*(4), 100–104. https://rmets.onlinelibrary.wiley.com/doi/10.1002/wea.2238

Carey, G., Malbon, E., Carey, N., Joyce, A., Crammond, B., & Carey, A. (2015). Systems science and systems thinking for public health: A systematic review of the field. *BMJ Open*, *5*(12), e009002. https://pmc.ncbi.nlm.nih.gov/articles/PMC4710830/

CDC. (2024, July 8). *CDC Museum COVID-19 timeline*. https://www.cdc.gov/museum/timeline/covid19.html

Garzke, W. H., & Brown, D. K. (1996). How did the Titanic really sink? *Naval History Magazine, 10*(5). https://www.usni.org/magazines/naval-history-magazine/1996/october/how-did-titanic-really-sink
Jack, L. (2020). Disseminating timely peer-reviewed content in 2020: COVID-19 and chronic disease, public health and pharmacy, eliminating health disparities, global health, and student research. *Preventing Chronic Disease, 17*, E100. https://www.cdc.gov/pcd/issues/2020/20_0447.htm
Knai, C., Petticrew, M., Mays, N., Capewell, S., Cassidy, R., Cummins, S., Eastmure, E., Fafard, P., Hawkins, B., Jensen, J. D., Katikireddi, S. V., Mwatsama, M., Orford, J., & Weishaar, H. (2018). Systems thinking as a framework for analyzing commercial determinants of health. *The Milbank Quarterly, 96*(3), 472–498.
Leischow, S. J., & Milstein, B. (2006). Systems thinking and modeling for public health practice. *American Journal of Public Health, 96*(3), 403–405. https://pmc.ncbi.nlm.nih.gov/articles/PMC1470500/
McLeod, S. (2024, January 25). *Freud's theory of the unconscious mind.* Simply Psychology. https://www.simplypsychology.org/unconscious-mind.html
Meadows, D. H. (2008). *Thinking in systems: A primer*. Chelsea Green Publishing.
National Archives. (2012). They said it couldn't sink. *Prologue Magazine, 44*(1). https://www.archives.gov/publications/prologue/2012/spring/titanic.html
National Museum of American History. (2012). *The iceberg that sank Titanic*. https://americanhistory.si.edu/collections/object/nmah_1416178
Rutter, H., Savona, N., Glonti, K., Bibby, J., Cummins, S., Finegood, D. T., Greaves, F., Harper, L., Hawe, P., Moore, L., Petticrew, M., Rehfuess, E., Shiell, A., Thomas, J., & White, M. (2017). The need for a complex systems model of evidence for public health. *The Lancet, 390*(10112), 2602–2604.
WHO. (2020). *Timeline of WHO's response to COVID-19*. https://www.who.int/emergencies/diseases/novel-coronavirus-2019/interactive-timeline
Yale Medicine. (2021, March 9). *Our pandemic year—A COVID-19 timeline*. https://www.yalemedicine.org/news/covid-timeline

8 The Visible Peak

How Global Pandemic Events Triggered Immediate Disruption

The COVID-19 pandemic triggered widespread visible disruptions to global society, as nations rushed to contain a virus that would reshape everyday life. From the first cases in Wuhan to the cascade of lockdowns across continents, the immediate impact of SARS-CoV-2 manifested in overwhelmed hospitals, shuttered businesses, empty streets, and radical changes to social behavior. These visible events—the tip of the pandemic iceberg—represent the most immediate and observable manifestations of a crisis that would expose deeper systemic vulnerabilities (Figure 8.1).

The First Wave: From Local Outbreak to Global Pandemic

The emergence of COVID-19 marked a pivotal moment in global health history, as a localized outbreak in central China evolved into the first major pandemic of the fully interconnected modern era (Table 8.1). On December 31, 2019, Chinese officials reported a cluster of pneumonia cases linked to the Huanan Seafood Wholesale Market in Wuhan, Hubei Province (World Health Organization, 2020a). Epidemiological analysis would later establish that human-to-human transmission was already occurring with an estimated reproductive number of 2.2

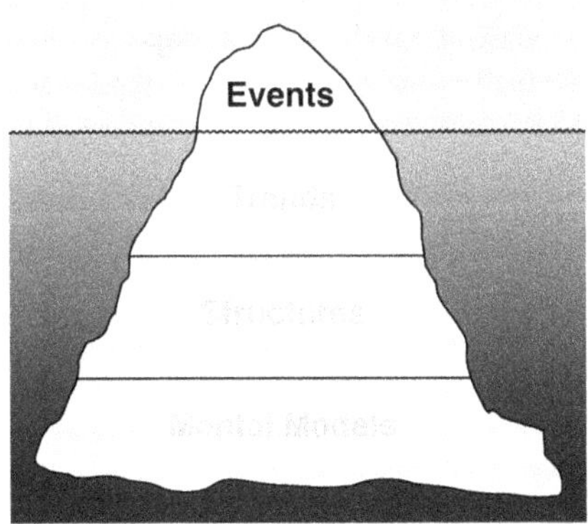

Figure 8.1 Iceberg Model—Events.

DOI: 10.4324/9781003595564-11

(Li et al., 2020). Local authorities closed the market on January 1, 2020, implementing environmental sanitation measures. By January 7, scientists identified a novel coronavirus as the causative agent, initially designated as 2019-nCoV (Zhu et al., 2020).

The early response in Wuhan revealed the inherent challenges of identifying and containing a novel pathogen. Dr. Li Wenliang, an ophthalmologist at Wuhan Central Hospital, attempted to warn colleagues about patients presenting with SARS-like symptoms on December 30, 2019 (Green, 2020). Around the same time, researchers were documenting familial clusters of pneumonia cases, providing early evidence of possible person-to-person transmission (Chan et al., 2020). Yet local authorities responded by reprimanding Dr. Li for "spreading rumors," a decision that would later exemplify the obstacles to early warning and transparent communication. Dr. Li's subsequent death from COVID-19 on February 7, 2020 was an awakening to the growing concerns about information management during the outbreak's crucial early phase (Cheng et al., 2020).

The virus's movement beyond China's borders demonstrated the limitations of traditional border screening measures in the modern era of global mobility. Thailand reported the first international case on January 13, 2020—a Wuhan resident who had arrived in Bangkok (Bastola et al., 2020). Japan and South Korea soon confirmed cases, establishing the pathogen's presence across East Asia and revealing the inadequacy of temperature screening and travel history questionnaires for containing spread.

Table 8.1 Timeline of COVID-19's Global Spread (December 2019 to March 2020)

Date	*Event*	*Significance*
Dec 31, 2019	Pneumonia cluster reported in Wuhan	First official outbreak report
Jan 7, 2020	Novel coronavirus identified (2019-nCoV)	Virus formally identified
Jan 13, 2020	First case outside China (Thailand)	First international transmission
Jan 23, 2020	Wuhan lockdown begins	First major citywide lockdown
Jan 30, 2020	WHO declares global health emergency	PHEIC formally declared
Feb 2, 2020	First death outside China (The Philippines)	Confirms fatal spread abroad
Feb 4, 2020	Diamond Princess outbreak	Rapid spread in confined setting
Feb 21, 2020	Major outbreak in Lombardy, Italy	First large-scale EU transmission
Feb 26, 2020	First case in Brazil	Virus reaches South America
Feb 29, 2020	First COVID-19 death in United States	North American fatalities begin
Mar 11, 2020	WHO declares COVID-19 a pandemic	Global spread formally recognized

Sources: Centers for Disease Control and Prevention (2020); European Centre for Disease Prevention and Control (2020); Ministry of Health Brazil (2020); Reuters (2020); World Health Organization (2020).

Several early clusters illuminated the virus's transmission patterns and foreshadowed challenges that would soon become global. The *Diamond Princess* cruise ship outbreak, beginning February 4, created a closed system for observing viral spread, with 712 of 3,711 passengers and crew ultimately testing positive (Moriarty et al., 2020). In South Korea, an outbreak accelerated when a single individual associated with the Shincheonji Church in Daegu infected over 5,000 others, demonstrating the virus's capacity for rapid transmission in communal settings (Kim et al., 2020). Italy's first major outbreak emerged in the Lombardy region, with the town of Codogno's first case on February 21 preceding a rapid cascade of infections throughout northern Italy. Despite implementing a local lockdown on February 23, existing cases had already seeded widespread community transmission (Remuzzi & Remuzzi, 2020).

The WHO's response evolved as evidence mounted of international spread. WHO Director-General Dr. Tedros Adhanom Ghebreyesus declared a Public Health Emergency of International Concern (PHEIC) on January 30, 2020, after transmission to 22 countries (World Health Organization, 2020). The subsequent pandemic declaration on March 11 came as cases exceeded 118,000 across 114 countries, formally acknowledging the virus's establishment on every inhabited continent.

By mid-March 2020, what began as a cluster of unusual pneumonia cases in one Chinese city had transformed into a worldwide crisis with unprecedented velocity. The virus had established footholds across global networks at a speed that overwhelmed traditional containment strategies, setting the stage for the extraordinary public health measures and healthcare system challenges that would follow.

Healthcare Systems Under Siege: A Global Struggle to Adapt and Endure

The COVID-19 pandemic subjected healthcare systems worldwide to unprecedented strain, creating scenes that seemed unimaginable in modern medical facilities. From makeshift morgues in hospital parking lots to patients treated in corridors, the visible signs of overwhelmed healthcare systems provided some of the pandemic's most dramatic illustrations of what happens when a novel pathogen outpaces medical infrastructure capacity (Ji et al., 2020).

As COVID-19 cases surged, healthcare systems worldwide scrambled to expand capacity beyond normal operational limits (Table 8.2). The first dramatic images of healthcare systems in crisis emerged from Wuhan in January 2020. Footage showed overcrowded emergency rooms, patients sleeping on floors, and hastily constructed field hospitals. The 1,000-bed Huoshenshan Hospital, built in just ten days, as well as the 1,600-bed Leishenshan Hospital that followed shortly after, demonstrated the extraordinary measures required to handle the unprecedented influx of patients (Pan et al., 2020).

Italy's Lombardy region provided the first Western example of a healthcare system in collapse. By early March 2020, hospitals in Bergamo and surrounding areas faced catastrophic overcrowding. Intensive care units operated far beyond capacity, forcing doctors to make impossible triage decisions (Grasselli et al., 2020). Emergency rooms became improvised ICUs, while hospital corridors filled with patients on gurneys. The region's sophisticated healthcare system, typically a source of pride, buckled under the viral onslaught (Armocida et al., 2020).

New York City's crisis in March and April 2020 exemplified urban healthcare systems under extreme pressure. The Javits Convention Center transformed into a 2,500-bed field hospital (O'Brien, 2020). The USNS Comfort, a Navy hospital ship, docked in Manhattan to provide additional capacity (USNI News, 2020). Central Park hosted an emergency field hospital, complete with respiratory care units. These highly visible emergency measures in America's largest city dramatized the pandemic's impact on even the most resourced healthcare systems (Ranney et al., 2020).

Beyond physical space limitations, the pandemic exposed critical vulnerabilities in medical supply chains and resource allocation systems. The global shortage of personal protective equipment (PPE) created immediate, visible crises in

Table 8.2 ICU System Strain During Early COVID-19 Pandemic (March to April 2020)

Region/ Country	*Pre-Pandemic ICU Beds*	*Peak ICU Demand*	*% Over Capacity*	*Emergency Measures*
Wuhan, China	Approx. 600	2,087+ (Jan–Feb 2020)	**248 ↑**	*Built temporary hospitals; rapidly expanded ICU capacity*
New York, U.S.A.	Approx. 1,600	3,500+ (April 2020)	**119 ↑**	*Converted spaces into ICUs; deployed field hospitals*
Lombardy, Italy	Approx. 720	1,200+ (March 2020)	**66 ↑**	*ICU triage; military assistance*
Madrid, Spain	Approx. 700	1,400+ (March 2020)	**100 ↑**	*Temporary ICUs; hospital expansion*
Paris, France	Approx. 5,080	7,148+ (April 2020)	**40 ↑**	*Temporary ICUs; patient transfers*
São Paulo, Brazil	Approx. 1,000	1,800+ (May 2020)	**80 ↑**	*ICU waiting lists; expanded capacity*
Tehran, Iran	Approx. 5,000	7,000+ (Mar–Apr 2020)	**40 ↑**	*ICU expansion; resource reallocation*
London, U.K.	Approx. 4,122	5,702+ (April 2020)	**38 ↑**	*NHS Nightingale Hospitals; ICU capacity growth*

Sources: Bhatraju et al. (2020); Grasselli et al. (2020); Li et al. (2020); NHS England (2020); Pan et al. (2020); Phua et al. (2020); Remuzzi and Remuzzi (2020); Rosenbaum (2020).

healthcare facilities worldwide. Medical staff resorted to wearing garbage bags, reusing single-use masks, and improvising face shields from office supplies (Ranney et al., 2020). Images of healthcare workers with facial bruises from extended mask use became powerful symbols of the pandemic's toll on medical professionals. Ventilator shortages emerged as another critical bottleneck, with doctors facing gut-wrenching decisions about which patients would receive ventilator support (Emanuel et al., 2020). Hospital oxygen systems, never designed for simultaneous use by hundreds of patients, began failing under the strain. Hospitals in Brazil's Manaus region faced catastrophic oxygen shortages in January 2021, with patients suffocating in their beds as supply systems failed (Reuters, 2021). This crisis was compounded by logistical challenges in the Amazon region and political responses that sacrificed lives while advancing unrelated infrastructure agendas (Ferrante & Fearnside, 2023). Similar crises emerged in India during its devastating second wave, with families desperately searching for oxygen cylinders as hospitals depleted their supply under sustained duress (Thadhani, 2021).

The pandemic's toll on healthcare workers became immediately visible and constituted a crisis within the broader crisis. Photos of exhausted staff sleeping on floors or slumped in chairs circulated globally. Deaths among medical professionals mounted, with Italy losing over 100 doctors during the first wave alone (Armocida et al., 2020). Healthcare workers organized protests over PPE shortages, staging demonstrations with signs declaring "We are not expendable" (Spoorthy et al., 2020). The staffing crisis worsened as workers fell ill or required quarantine after exposure. New York called for healthcare worker volunteers from across the country, while Italy graduated medical students early to bolster hospital staffing. Travel nurses commanded extraordinary salaries as hospitals competed for scarce personnel (Adams & Walls, 2020).

Healthcare facilities rapidly reconfigured physical spaces to accommodate the surge of COVID-19 patients while minimizing transmission risk. Elective surgeries ceased worldwide, transforming operating rooms into makeshift ICUs. Parking lots became triage centers and drive-through testing sites, while hospitals erected tents outside emergency departments to screen potential COVID-19 patients. Negative pressure rooms were constructed using plastic sheeting and portable fans. Regular hospital rooms were converted to ICU spaces with temporary monitoring equipment. As the pandemic progressed, hospitals developed new protocols visible to patients and visitors. Temperature screening stations appeared at entrances. Plastic barriers arose at reception desks. Waiting rooms implemented strict distancing measures. These physical changes transformed the familiar landscape of healthcare facilities into something more isolating, forbidding, and fear-inducing (Legido-Quigley et al., 2020).

Initial Public Health Measures and Governance Responses

The implementation of public health measures during COVID-19 marked the most extensive deployment of non-pharmaceutical interventions in modern history.

From city-wide lockdowns to ubiquitous mask wearing, these measures transformed public spaces and daily routines into visible manifestations of pandemic response. Governance approaches varied dramatically across nations and regions, revealing contrasting philosophies about balancing public health imperatives with economic and social considerations (Hale et al., 2020).

The pandemic ushered in a new era of government-mandated movement restrictions, beginning with China's strict interventions in Wuhan. On January 23, 2020, Chinese authorities sealed off a city of 11 million people—a containment measure of historical significance in both scale and scope (Lau et al., 2020). Footage circulated globally showing Wuhan's deserted boulevards and silent intersections, with surveillance drones monitoring compliance and broadcasting instructions to the few visible pedestrians. This extraordinary approach established a model that governments worldwide would adapt to their own contexts in the months ahead (Table 8.3). In the weeks that followed, epidemiological modeling helped validate such measures, suggesting that uncontrolled spread could overwhelm healthcare systems and lead to hundreds of thousands of deaths in countries like the United Kingdom and the United States (Ferguson et al., 2020).

Italy's national lockdown in March 2020 marked the first such action in a Western democracy, requiring citizens to carry permission forms for essential movement. While effective in reducing viral transmission, widespread quarantine

Table 8.3 Comparative Analysis of Early Lockdown Measures (January to April 2020)

Country	*Start Date*	*Mandated Restrictions*	*Enforcement Measures*	*Estimated Mobility Drop (%)*
China (Wuhan)	Jan 23, 2020	Full city lockdown; no travel allowed	Digital tracking; barriers	**90 ↓**
Italy	Mar 9, 2020	National stay-home; non-essentials closed	Police checkpoints; fines	**85 ↓**
Spain	Mar 14, 2020	National lockdown; tight movement limits	Military; drones; fines	**80 ↓**
France	Mar 17, 2020	Stay-home with permit; non-essentials closed	Police deployment; fines	**85 ↓**
India	Mar 24, 2020	Sudden national lockdown	Police; fines; beatings	**75 ↓**
U.K.	Mar 23, 2020	National stay-home order	Police; tiered fines	**75 ↓**
U.S.A. (varied)	Mar–Apr 2020	State-by-state lockdowns; varied responses	Mixed; mostly advisory	**40–80 ↓**
Sweden	No lockdown	Voluntary distancing	Minimal enforcement	**25–30 ↓**

Sources: Apple (2020); Chinazzi et al. (2020); Flaxman et al. (2020); Google (2020); Hale et al. (2020); Hsiang et al. (2020); Lau et al. (2020); Patel et al. (2020).

measures carried psychological costs, including post-traumatic stress symptoms, confusion, and anger (Brooks et al., 2020). The sight of armed police checking documents on Rome's empty streets highlighted the extraordinary nature of these restrictions. France followed with similarly strict measures, requiring signed attestations for any outdoor activity (Flaxman et al., 2020). Meanwhile, India's lockdown announcement, made with just 4 hours' notice, triggered one of the largest internal migrations in modern history as urban workers fled cities for rural villages. The resulting chaos—with thousands walking hundreds of kilometers along highways—demonstrated the challenges of implementing strict containment measures in developing nations with large informal economies and limited social safety nets (Patel et al., 2020).

The implementation of border controls further restricted movement at international scales. Travel bans proliferated worldwide, though they were often implemented after the virus had already entered target countries. Quarantine requirements for international travelers became standard, with some countries establishing dedicated quarantine facilities. These measures represented the most significant restrictions on international travel since World War II, transforming once-bustling airports into near-empty terminals with parked aircraft visible for miles (Chinazzi et al., 2020).

As countries worked to contain the spread, testing infrastructure expanded at exponential rates, reshaping urban landscapes. Drive-through testing sites emerged in parking lots and community spaces, creating scenes reminiscent of disaster response operations. The sight of medical workers in full PPE administering tests through car windows became a defining image of the pandemic response. National approaches to testing revealed marked differences in capacity and strategy. South Korea's early success with mass testing set standards that other nations would struggle to match. Their high-capacity testing centers, capable of processing thousands of samples daily, demonstrated how rapid diagnosis could support containment efforts. By contrast, testing shortages in many Western nations forced strict prioritization of limited resources, undermining early containment efforts (Kucirka et al., 2020).

Contact tracing efforts revealed divergent approaches to technology and privacy across societies. South Korea's comprehensive digital tracking system used credit card records, CCTV footage, and mobile phone data to track potential exposure. This aggressive approach proved effective but raised concerns about surveillance that would be unacceptable in many Western democracies (Park et al., 2020). Singapore's TraceTogether program offered a middle ground, using Bluetooth tokens and mobile applications to track potential exposure while attempting to preserve privacy. The visible presence of these systems—from QR code check-ins at venues to tracking tokens worn by citizens—highlighted how public health measures were reshaping daily life and expectations of privacy.

The pandemic transformed everyday behaviors in public spaces, most visibly through mask requirements and physical distancing practices. Initially discouraged outside healthcare settings, masks became mandatory in many jurisdictions by mid-2020. This shift manifested in striking visual changes—from Tokyo's Shibuya

Crossing to New York's Times Square, masked faces became the norm rather than the exception, creating one of the pandemic's most emblematic symbols (Howard et al., 2021). Simultaneously, physical distancing transformed navigation of public spaces. Floor markers indicating safe distances appeared in stores worldwide, while plastic barriers at checkout counters and reception desks became ubiquitous. These changes created new forms of public choreography as people learned to maintain the newly sacrosanct "six feet of separation" while conducting essential activities.

Throughout these varied responses, the pandemic revealed significant contrasts in crisis governance and public communication strategies worldwide. New Zealand's approach, marked by decisive action and consistent messaging, stood in sharp relief against the fragmented responses seen in Brazil and the United States. Communication styles varied dramatically—from South Korea's transparent daily briefings to the inconsistent and often politicized messaging evident in countries where pandemic response became entangled with partisan politics (Ko et al., 2021). These differences in governance approaches would ultimately influence both the immediate effectiveness of containment measures and the long-term impact of the pandemic on affected societies.

The First Shocks: Societal and Economic Disruption

The COVID-19 pandemic triggered the most severe global economic crisis since the Great Depression while simultaneously transforming daily life in unprecedented ways. From vacant business districts to virtual classrooms, the pandemic fundamentally altered how people worked, learned, worshipped, and connected with one another. These disruptions revealed both the vulnerability of established systems and humanity's remarkable capacity for adaptation under extreme pressure (Baldwin & Weder di Mauro, 2020).

The pandemic's economic impact manifested first in global financial markets before rapidly affecting the real economy (Table 8.4). The U.S. stock market's decline in March 2020 marked the fastest bear market in history, triggering circuit breakers—automatic trading halts—multiple times in a single month (U.S. Securities and Exchange Commission, 2020). The New York Stock Exchange's trading floor stood nearly empty, with the few remaining traders wearing masks and separated by plexiglass barriers. Oil markets provided perhaps the most dramatic illustration of this disruption when U.S. futures plunged below zero for the first time in history on April 20, 2020, reaching negative $37.63 per barrel as sudden demand collapse collided with limited storage capacity (Le et al., 2021).

The employment crisis quickly became visible across societies. Lines at food banks stretched for miles in wealthy nations like the United States, creating scenes reminiscent of Great Depression photographs, while unemployment office websites crashed under extreme demand as state systems struggled to process millions of claims simultaneously (U.S. Bureau of Labor Statistics, 2020). Small businesses were particularly vulnerable, with surveys in April 2020 indicating that 43% of responding U.S. small businesses had temporarily closed, and employment among these businesses had

Table 8.4 Economic Shock Indicators During Initial COVID-19 Wave (Q1–Q2 2020)

Indicator	*Pre-Pandemic Baseline*	*Peak Disruption*	*% Change*	*Significance/ Context*
S&P 500 Index	3,386.15 *(Feb 2020)*	2,237.40 *(Mar 2020)*	**−34**	*Fastest bear market in history; multiple circuit breakers triggered*
WTI Crude Oil Futures	$63.27/barrel *(Jan 2020)*	–$37.63/barrel *(Apr 2020)*	**Negative price**	*First negative price in history due to demand crash/storage issues*
Global Air Travel	4.5B passengers *(2019 total)*	1.8B passengers *(2020 total)*	**−60**	*Largest industry contraction in aviation history*
Jobless Claims (U.S.)	200,000/week	6.87M *(March 2020)*	**+3,335**	*Highest ever recorded; overwhelmed state systems*
Global Supply Chain Pressure Index (GSCPI)	0.0 *(normalized)*	4.3 *(May 2020)*	**+430**	*Major disruptions in global logistics*
Retail Foot Traffic (U.S.)	100 *(baseline)*	17.9 *(April 2020)*	**−82.1**	*Retail collapse during initial lockdowns*
Global Manufacturing Purchasing Index (PMI)	50.1 *(Jan 2020)*	39.6 *(Apr 2020)*	**−21**	*Near all-time low; manufacturing slowed globally*
Remote Work (U.S.)	5% workforce	Approx. 35% *(April 2020)*	**+600**	*Massive workforce shift to telecommuting*

Sources: Barman et al. (2021); Dingel and Neiman (2020); Federal Reserve Bank of New York (2020); Gössling et al. (2020); International Air Transport Association (2020); International Energy Agency (2020); International Monetary Fund (2020); Le et al. (2021); McKibbin and Fernando (2020); S&P Dow Jones Indices (2020); S&P Global (2020); SafeGraph (2020); U.S. Bureau of Labor Statistics (2020); U.S. Department of Labor (2020); U.S. Securities and Exchange Commission (2020).

Note: The Global Supply Chain Pressure Index (GSCPI) is normalized to a pre-pandemic average of zero (1997–2019), with values above zero indicating heightened global logistics strain; a reading of +4.3 in May 2020 marked a historically extreme disruption. The Global Manufacturing PMI (Purchasing Managers' Index) signals contraction when below 50; its April 2020 value of 39.6 reflected severe global manufacturing decline.

fallen by 40% (Bartik et al., 2020). Meanwhile, supply chain disruptions evolved from early shortages of toilet paper and hand sanitizer to widespread manufacturing gaps. Car dealership lots emptied as semiconductor shortages halted production, electronics stores struggled to maintain inventory, and furniture deliveries faced months-long delays. The crisis became physically visible as dozens of container ships anchored off major ports, particularly Los Angeles and Long Beach, created floating traffic jams. Containers stacked in port facilities formed metal mountains, revealing the fragility of just-in-time delivery systems that had previously operated invisibly in the background of global commerce (Barman et al., 2021).

Educational systems experienced a fundamental shift at an unprecedented scale. By April 2020, UNESCO data revealed that school closures affected more than 1.6 billion students globally. The physical infrastructure of education—classrooms, playgrounds, lecture halls—fell silent as learning shifted to digital platforms. Students attended class from dining tables and bedrooms, while teachers adapted to instructing through screens displaying matrices of students' faces. The transformation extended to institutions with centuries of uninterrupted operation; Harvard University conducted its first online commencement in its 384-year history, illustrating how thoroughly the pandemic had altered even the most established academic traditions (UNESCO, 2020).

The emptying of public spaces offered perhaps the most striking visual evidence of societal change. City centers typically teeming with activity stood deserted during lockdown periods—Times Square in New York City appeared abandoned in aerial photographs, Venice's canals ran clear as tourism ceased, and Paris's Champs-Élysées emptied of traffic. Popular tourist destinations that normally hosted thousands daily became ghost towns overnight: Disney closed all its theme parks for the first time in its history, the Las Vegas Strip went dark as casinos shuttered, and the Vatican's St. Peter's Square remained empty during Holy Week, with Pope Francis delivering his Easter blessing to a vacant plaza (Gössling et al., 2020).

Cultural and sporting events halted worldwide in previously unimaginable ways. The Tokyo 2020 Olympics were postponed for the first time in peacetime history, professional sports leagues suspended seasons mid-play, and the NBA's abrupt suspension on March 11, 2020, marked a turning point in American recognition of the crisis. Broadway went dark for the first time since the 1918 Spanish Influenza pandemic, while museums worldwide closed their doors, including the Louvre's first closure since World War II (Heisbourg, 2020).

Religious communities faced profound disruptions to worship practices that had remained consistent for generations. Mecca's Grand Mosque stood empty as Saudi Arabia suspended the Umrah pilgrimage, Jerusalem's Western Wall plaza accommodated only small, distanced groups, and churches worldwide conducted services online or moved to parking lot gatherings with attendees remaining in their cars. Funeral practices underwent particularly painful changes as families couldn't gather to mourn their dead, traditional burial customs were modified or suspended, and video-streamed memorial services became the norm. These changes profoundly affected grieving processes and denied many the comfort of communal mourning that had previously helped societies process collective trauma (Yamin, 2020).

As physical spaces emptied, digital platforms experienced unprecedented growth to fill the void. Video conferencing tools like Zoom became household essentials rather than business utilities, virtual social gatherings attempted to replace in-person connections, and remote work transformed homes into offices. This digital shift manifested visibly in urban landscapes as rush hour traffic disappeared from many cities and delivery vehicles replaced commuter cars on city streets, creating new patterns of movement and commerce (Dingel & Neiman, 2020).

The social response to the pandemic evolved in stages that revealed shifting community dynamics. Early crisis periods saw remarkable displays of solidarity—residents confined to homes staged impromptu balcony concerts that became powerful symbols of unity, while healthcare workers received widespread acclaim through coordinated public applause in major cities worldwide. As the pandemic progressed, this initial unity gave way to more complex social tensions. Anti-lockdown protests emerged in capital cities, and mask wearing evolved from public health measure to political statement, with videos of confrontations in stores and public spaces highlighting growing divisions over pandemic response (Bavel et al., 2020).

Throughout these disruptions, communities developed new ways to acknowledge loss and process collective grief. In Washington, DC, rows of white flags on the National Mall represented lives lost to COVID-19, while similar memorials appeared worldwide—from empty chairs in Prague to painted hearts along London's Thames River. These public expressions of mourning provided visible reminders of the pandemic's human toll while offering spaces for collective grieving despite physical distancing requirements (Honey-Rosés et al., 2020).

The societal and economic disruptions of COVID-19 created enduring images of a world transformed. Empty streets, masked faces, and distance markers on floors became universal symbols of the pandemic era. These visible changes to familiar routines and spaces revealed both society's vulnerability to disruption and its capacity for rapid adaptation to dire circumstances—demonstrating both the fragility of global systems and the remarkable resilience of human communities in the face of crisis. Yet these observable phenomena represent only the surface manifestations of deeper patterns and trends that would ultimately determine the pandemic's full trajectory, which we will explore in the next chapter.

References

Adams, J. G., & Walls, R. M. (2020). Supporting the health care workforce during the COVID-19 global epidemic. *JAMA*, *323*(15), 1439–1440. https://doi.org/10.1001/jama.2020.3972

Apple. (2020). *COVID-19 – Mobility trends reports*. https://covid19.apple.com/mobility

Armocida, B., Formenti, B., Ussai, S., Palestra, F., & Missoni, E. (2020). The Italian health system and the COVID-19 challenge. *The Lancet Public Health*, *5*(5), e253. https://doi.org/10.1016/S2468-2667(20)30074-8

Baldwin, R., & Weder di Mauro, B. (Eds.). (2020). *Economics in the time of COVID-19*. CEPR Press. https://voxeu.org/content/economics-time-covid-19

Barman, A., Das, R., & De, P. K. (2021). Impact of COVID-19 in food supply chain: Disruptions and recovery strategy. *Current Research in Behavioral Sciences*, *2*, 100017. https://doi.org/10.1016/j.crbeha.2021.100017

Bartik, A. W., Bertrand, M., Cullen, Z., Glaeser, E. L., Luca, M., & Stanton, C. (2020). The impact of COVID-19 on small business outcomes and expectations. *Proceedings of the National Academy of Sciences*, *117*(30), 17656–17666. https://doi.org/10.1073/pnas.2006991117

Bastola, A., Sah, R., Rodriguez-Morales, A. J., Lal, B. K., Jha, R., Ojha, H. C., Shrestha, B., Chu, D. K. W., Poon, L. L. M., Costello, A., Morita, K., & Pandey, B. D. (2020). The first 2019 novel coronavirus case in Nepal. *The Lancet Infectious Diseases*, *20*(3), 279–280. https://doi.org/10.1016/S1473-3099(20)30067-0

Bavel, J. J. V., Baicker, K., Boggio, P. S., Capraro, V., Cichocka, A., Cikara, M., Crockett, M. J., Crum, A. J., Douglas, K. M., Druckman, J. N., Drury, J., Dube, O., Ellemers, N., Fiske, S. T., Goya-Tocchetto, D., Hamann, J. L., Hutcherson, C. A., Jetten, J., Keltner, D., … Willer, R. (2020). Using social and behavioural science to support COVID-19 pandemic response. *Nature Human Behaviour*, *4*(5), 460–471. https://doi.org/10.1038/s41562-020-0884-z

Bhatraju, P. K., Ghassemieh, B. J., Nichols, M., Kim, R., Jerome, K. R., Nalla, A. K., Greninger, A. L., Pipavath, S., Wurfel, M. M., Evans, L., Kritek, P. A., West, T. E., Luks, A., Gerbino, A., Dale, C. R., Goldman, J. D., O'Mahony, S., & Mikacenic, C. (2020). Covid-19 in critically ill patients in the Seattle region—Case series. *New England Journal of Medicine*, *382*(21), 2012–2022. https://doi.org/10.1056/NEJMoa2004500

Brooks, S. K., Webster, R. K., Smith, L. E., Woodland, L., Wessely, S., Greenberg, N., & Rubin, G. J. (2020). The psychological impact of quarantine and how to reduce it: Rapid review of the evidence. *The Lancet*, *395*(10227), 912–920. https://doi.org/10.1016/S0140-6736(20)30460-8

Centers for Disease Control and Prevention. (2020). *CDC museum COVID-19 timeline*. https://www.cdc.gov/museum/timeline/covid19.html

Chan, J. F.-W., Yuan, S., Kok, K.-H., To, K. K.-W., Chu, H., Yang, J., Xing, F., Liu, J., Yip, C. C.-Y., Poon, R. W.-S., Tsoi, H.-W., Lo, S. K.-F., Chan, K.-H., Poon, V. K.-M., Chan, W.-M., Ip, J. D., Cai, J.-P., Cheng, V. C.-C., Chen, H., … Yuen, K.-Y. (2020). A familial cluster of pneumonia associated with the 2019 novel coronavirus indicating person-to-person transmission: A study of a family cluster. *The Lancet*, *395*(10223), 514–523. https://doi.org/10.1016/S0140-6736(20)30154-9

Cheng, V. C. C., Wong, S. C., Chen, J. H. K., Yip, C. C. Y., Chuang, V. W. M., Tsang, O. T. Y., Sridhar, S., Chan, J. F. W., Ho, P. L., & Yuen, K. Y. (2020). Escalating infection control response to the rapidly evolving epidemiology of the coronavirus disease 2019 (COVID-19) due to SARS-CoV-2 in Hong Kong. *Infection Control & Hospital Epidemiology*, *41*(5), 493–498. https://doi.org/10.1017/ice.2020.58

Chinazzi, M., Davis, J. T., Ajelli, M., Gioannini, C., Litvinova, M., Merler, S., Pastore y Piontti, A., Mu, K., Rossi, L., Sun, K., Viboud, C., Xiong, X., Yu, H., Halloran, M. E., Longini, I. M., Jr, & Vespignani, A. (2020). The effect of travel restrictions on the spread of the 2019 novel coronavirus (COVID-19) outbreak. *Science*, *368*(6489), 395–400. https://doi.org/10.1126/science.aba9757

Dingel, J. I., & Neiman, B. (2020). How many jobs can be done at home? *Journal of Public Economics*, *189*, 104235. https://doi.org/10.1016/j.jpubeco.2020.104235

Emanuel, E. J., Persad, G., Upshur, R., Thome, B., Parker, M., Glickman, A., Zhang, C., Boyle, C., Smith, M., & Phillips, J. P. (2020). Fair allocation of scarce medical resources in the time of Covid-19. *New England Journal of Medicine*, *382*(21), 2049–2055. https://doi.org/10.1056/NEJMsb2005114

European Centre for Disease Prevention and Control. (2020). *COVID-19 situation update worldwide*. https://www.ecdc.europa.eu/en/geographical-distribution-2019-ncov-cases

Federal Reserve Bank of New York. (2020). *Global Supply Chain Pressure Index*. https://www.newyorkfed.org/research/policy/gscpi

Ferguson, N. M., Laydon, D., Nedjati-Gilani, G., Imai, N., Ainslie, K., Baguelin, M., Bhatia, S., Boonyasiri, A., Cucunubá, Z., Cuomo-Dannenburg, G., Dighe, A., Dorigatti, I., Fu, H., Gaythorpe, K., Green, W., Hamlet, A., Hinsley, W., Okell, L. C., van Elsland, S., … Ghani, A. C. (2020). *Impact of non-pharmaceutical interventions (NPIs) to reduce COVID-19 mortality and healthcare demand*. Imperial College London. https://doi.org/10.25561/77482

Ferrante, L., & Fearnside, P. M. (2023). Brazil's Amazon oxygen crisis: How lives and health were sacrificed during the peak of COVID-19. *Global Health, 19*(1), 39. https://doi.org/10.1186/s12992-023-00935-8

Flaxman, S., Mishra, S., Gandy, A., Unwin, H. J. T., Mellan, T. A., Coupland, H., Whittaker, C., Zhu, H., Berah, T., Eaton, J. W., Monod, M., Imperial College COVID-19 Response Team, Ghani, A. C., Donnelly, C. A., Riley, S., Vollmer, M. A. C., Ferguson, N. M., Okell, L. C., Bhatt, S. (2020). Estimating the effects of non-pharmaceutical interventions on COVID-19 in Europe. *Nature, 584*(7820), 257–261. https://doi.org/10.1038/s41586-020-2405-7

Google. (2020). *COVID-19 community mobility reports*. https://www.google.com/covid19/mobility/

Gössling, S., Scott, D., & Hall, C. M. (2020). Pandemics, tourism and global change: A rapid assessment of COVID-19. *Journal of Sustainable Tourism, 29*(1), 1–20. https://doi.org/10.1080/09669582.2020.1758708

Grasselli, G., Pesenti, A., & Cecconi, M. (2020). Critical care utilization for the COVID-19 outbreak in Lombardy, Italy: Early experience and forecast during an emergency response. *JAMA, 323*(16), 1545–1546. https://doi.org/10.1001/jama.2020.4031

Green, A. (2020). Li Wenliang. *The Lancet, 395*(10225), 682. https://doi.org/10.1016/S0140-6736(20)30382-2

Hale, T., Angrist, N., Kira, B., Petherick, A., Phillips, T., & Webster, S. (2020). *Variation in government responses to COVID-19* [Blavatnik School of Government Working Paper, 31, 2020–11]. https://www.bsg.ox.ac.uk/sites/default/files/2020-05/BSG-WP-2020-032-v6.0.pdf

Heisbourg, F. (2020). From Wuhan to the world: How the pandemic will reshape geopolitics. *Survival, 62*(3), 7–24. https://doi.org/10.1080/00396338.2020.1763608

Honey-Rosés, J., Anguelovski, I., Chireh, V. K., Daher, C., Konijnendijk van den Bosch, C., Litt, J. S., Mawani, V., McCall, M. K., Orellana, A., Oscilowicz, E., Sánchez, U., Senbel, M., Tan, X., Villagomez, E., Zapata, O., & Nieuwenhuijsen, M. J. (2020). The impact of COVID-19 on public space: An early review of the emerging questions – Design, perceptions and inequities. *Cities & Health, 5*(sup1), S263–S279. https://doi.org/10.1080/23748834.2020.1780074

Howard, J., Huang, A., Li, Z., Tufekci, Z., Zdimal, V., van der Westhuizen, H. M., von Delft, A., Price, A., Fridman, L., Tang, L. H., Tang, V., Watson, G. L., Bax, C. E., Shaikh, R., Questier, F., Hernandez, D., Chu, L. F., Ramirez, C. M., & Rimoin, A. W. (2021). An evidence review of face masks against COVID-19. *Proceedings of the National Academy of Sciences, 118*(4), e2014564118. https://doi.org/10.1073/pnas.2014564118

Hsiang, S., Allen, D., Annan-Phan, S., Bell, K., Bolliger, I., Chong, T., Druckenmiller, H., Huang, L. Y., Hultgren, A., Krasovich, E., Lau, P., Lee, J., Rolf, E., Tseng, J., & Wu, T. (2020). The effect of large-scale anti-contagion policies on the COVID-19 pandemic. *Nature, 584*(7820), 262–267. https://doi.org/10.1038/s41586-020-2404-8

Ko, K., Sakuwa, K., Suzuki, K., Poocharoen, O., Nguyen, T., Henderson, S., Withers, M., Ahonen, P., Kuhlmann, S., Franzke, J., Dahlström, C., Lindvall, J., Comfort, L., & Kim, D. Y. (2021). *International Comparative Analysis of COVID19 Responses* (p. 346). KDI School of Public Policy and Management. https://www.kdevelopedia.org/Resources/view/InternationalComparativeAnalysisofCOVID19Responses99202202040168675

International Air Transport Association. (2020). *Annual Review 2020*. https://www.iata.org/contentassets/c81222d96c9a4e0bb4ff6ced0126f0bb/iata-annual-review-2020.pdf

International Energy Agency. (2020). *Oil market report – April 2020*. https://www.iea.org/reports/oil-market-report-april-2020

International Monetary Fund. (2020). *World economic outlook, April 2020: The great lockdown*. https://www.imf.org/en/Publications/WEO/Issues/2020/04/14/weo-april-2020

Ji, Y., Ma, Z., Peppelenbosch, M. P., & Pan, Q. (2020). Potential association between COVID-19 mortality and health-care resource availability. *The Lancet Global Health, 8*(4), e480. https://doi.org/10.1016/S2214-109X(20)30068-1

Kim, S. W., Park, J. W., Jung, H. D., Lee, J. Y., Lee, J. S., Kim, T. H., Hong, K. J., & Jang, Y. S. (2020). Risk factors for transmission of Middle East respiratory syndrome coronavirus infection during the 2015 outbreak in South Korea. *Clinical Infectious Diseases*, *70*(3), 450–457. https://doi.org/10.1093/cid/ciz272

Kucirka, L. M., Lauer, S. A., Laeyendecker, O., Boon, D., & Lessler, J. (2020). Variation in false-negative rate of reverse transcriptase polymerase chain reaction-based SARS-CoV-2 tests by time since exposure. *Annals of Internal Medicine*, *173*(4), 262–267. https://doi.org/10.7326/M20-1495

Lau, H., Khosrawipour, V., Kocbach, P., Mikolajczyk, A., Schubert, J., Bania, J., & Khosrawipour, T. (2020). The positive impact of lockdown in Wuhan on containing the COVID-19 outbreak in China. *Journal of Travel Medicine*, *27*(3), taaa037. https://doi.org/10.1093/jtm/taaa037

Le, T. H., Le, A. T., & Le, H. C. (2021). The historic oil price fluctuation during the Covid19 pandemic: What are the causes? *Research in International Business and Finance*, *58*, 101489. https://doi.org/10.1016/j.ribaf.2021.101489

Legido-Quigley, H., Mateos-García, J. T., Campos, V. R., Gea-Sánchez, M., Muntaner, C., & McKee, M. (2020). The resilience of the Spanish health system against the COVID-19 pandemic. *The Lancet Public Health*, *5*(5), e251–e252. https://doi.org/10.1016/S2468-2667(20)30060-8

Li, Q., Guan, X., Wu, P., Wang, X., Zhou, L., Tong, Y., Ren, R., Leung, K. S. M., Lau, E. H. Y., Wong, J. Y., Xing, X., Xiang, N., Wu, Y., Li, C., Chen, Q., Li, D., Liu, T., Zhao, J., Liu, M., … Feng, Z. (2020). Early transmission dynamics in Wuhan, China, of novel coronavirus-infected pneumonia. *New England Journal of Medicine*, *382*(13), 1199–1207. https://doi.org/10.1056/NEJMoa2001316

Li, R., Rivers, C., Tan, Q., Murray, M. B., Toner, E., & Lipsitch, M. (2020). Estimated demand for US hospital inpatient and intensive care unit beds for patients with COVID-19 based on comparisons with Wuhan and Guangzhou, China. *JAMA Network Open*, *3*(5), e208297. https://doi.org/10.1001/jamanetworkopen.2020.8297

McKibbin, W. J., & Fernando, R. (2020). The global macroeconomic impacts of COVID-19: Seven scenarios. *Asian Economic Papers*, *20*(2), 1–30. https://doi.org/10.1162/asep_a_00796

Ministry of Health Brazil. (2020). *Coronavirus in Brazil*. https://www.gov.br/saude/pt-br/assuntos/saude-de-a-a-z/c/covid-19

Moriarty, L. F., Plucinski, M. M., Marston, B. J., Kurbatova, E. V., Knust, B., Murray, E. L., Pesik, N., Rose, D., Fitter, D., Kobayashi, M., Toda, M., Cantey, P. T., Scheuer, T., Halsey, E. S., Cohen, N. J., Stockman, L., Albrecht, D. R., Bancroft, E. A., Thornburg, N. J., … Richards, J. (2020). Public health responses to COVID-19 outbreaks on cruise ships—Worldwide, February–March, 2020. *MMWR. Morbidity and Mortality Weekly Report*, *69*(12), 347–352. https://doi.org/10.15585/mmwr.mm6912e3

NHS England. (2020). *COVID-19 hospital activity*. https://www.england.nhs.uk/statistics/statistical-work-areas/covid-19-hospital-activity/

O'Brien, J. (2020). Hospital ship comfort ends NYC COVID-19 mission after treating 182 patients. *USNI News*. https://news.usni.org/2020/04/27/hospital-ship-comfort-ends-nyc-covid-19-mission-after-treating-182-patients

Pan, A., Liu, L., Wang, C., Guo, H., Hao, X., Wang, Q., Huang, J., He, N., Yu, H., Lin, X., Wei, S., & Wu, T. (2020). Association of public health interventions with the epidemiology of the COVID-19 outbreak in Wuhan, China. *JAMA*, *323*(19), 1915–1923. https://doi.org/10.1001/jama.2020.6130

Park, S., Choi, G. J., & Ko, H. (2020). Information technology-based tracing strategy in response to COVID-19 in South Korea—privacy controversies. *JAMA*, *323*(21), 2129–2130. https://doi.org/10.1001/jama.2020.6602

Patel, J., Fernandes, G., & Sridhar, D. (2020). How can we improve self-isolation and quarantine for Covid-19? *BMJ*, *372*, n625. https://doi.org/10.1136/bmj.n625

Phua, J., Weng, L., Ling, L., Egi, M., Lim, C. M., Divatia, J. V., Shrestha, B. R., Arabi, Y. M., Ng, J., Gomersall, C. D., Nishimura, M., Koh, Y., & Du, B. (2020). Intensive care management of coronavirus disease 2019 (COVID-19): Challenges and recommendations. *The Lancet Respiratory Medicine*, *8*(5), 506–517. https://doi.org/10.1016/S2213-2600(20)30161-2

Ranney, M. L., Griffeth, V., & Jha, A. K. (2020). Critical supply shortages—The need for ventilators and personal protective equipment during the Covid-19 pandemic. *New England Journal of Medicine*, *382*(18), e41. https://doi.org/10.1056/NEJMp2006141

Remuzzi, A., & Remuzzi, G. (2020). COVID-19 and Italy: What next? *The Lancet*, *395*(10231), 1225–1228. https://doi.org/10.1016/S0140-6736(20)30627-9

Reuters. (2020, February 2). *Philippines reports first coronavirus death outside China*. https://www.reuters.com/article/us-china-health-philippines-idUSKBN1ZW05T

Reuters. (2021, January 14). *Brazil's Amazonas state running out of oxygen as COVID-19 surges*. Reuters. https://www.reuters.com/article/us-health-coronavirus-brazil-amazon/brazils-amazonas-state-running-out-of-oxygen-as-covid-19-surges-idUSKBN29J2SJ/

Rosenbaum, L. (2020). Facing Covid-19 in Italy—Ethics, logistics, and therapeutics on the epidemic's front line. *New England Journal of Medicine*, *382*(20), 1873–1875. https://doi.org/10.1056/NEJMp2005492

S&P Dow Jones Indices. (2020). *S&P 500 Index*. https://www.spglobal.com/spdji/en/indices/equity/sp-500/

S&P Global. (2020, April). *J.P. Morgan Global Manufacturing PMI™*. https://www.pmi.spglobal.com/Public/Home/PressRelease/3854205c66d34b09849f1961ecc7c89d

SafeGraph. (2020). *U.S. consumer activity during COVID-19 pandemic*. https://www.safegraph.com/dashboard/covid19-commerce-patterns

Spoorthy, M. S., Pratapa, S. K., & Mahant, S. (2020). Mental health problems faced by healthcare workers due to the COVID-19 pandemic—A review. *Asian Journal of Psychiatry*, *51*, 102119. https://doi.org/10.1016/j.ajp.2020.102119

Thadhani, A. (2021). *Preventing a repeat of the COVID-19 second-wave oxygen crisis in India* [Observer Research Foundation, Special Report No. 151]. https://www.orfonline.org/research/preventing-a-repeat-of-the-covid-19-second-wave-oxygen-crisis-in-india

U.S. Bureau of Labor Statistics. (2020). *The employment situation—March 2020*. https://www.bls.gov/news.release/archives/empsit_04032020.pdf

U.S. Department of Labor. (2020). *Unemployment insurance weekly claims*. https://www.dol.gov/ui/data.pdf

U.S. Securities and Exchange Commission. (2020). *SEC takes targeted action to assist funds and advisers, allows virtual board meetings and provides conditional relief from certain filing procedures*. https://www.sec.gov/news/press-release/2020-63

UNESCO. (2020). *Education: From disruption to recovery*. UNESCO. https://en.unesco.org/covid19/educationresponse

USNI News. (2020). Hospital ship comfort ends NYC COVID-19 mission after treating 182 patients. *USNI News*. https://news.usni.org/2020/04/27/hospital-ship-comfort-ends-nyc-covid-19-mission-after-treating-182-patients

World Health Organization. (2020a). *Archived: WHO timeline – COVID-19*. https://www.who.int/news/item/27-04-2020-who-timeline---covid-19

World Health Organization. (2020b). *Novel coronavirus (2019-nCoV): Situation report, 1*. https://www.who.int/docs/default-source/coronaviruse/situation-reports/20200121-sitrep-1-2019-ncov.pdf

World Health Organization. (2020c). *WHO coronavirus (COVID-19) dashboard*. https://covid19.who.int/

World Health Organization. (2020d). *WHO Director-General's opening remarks at the media briefing on COVID-19 – 11 March 2020*. https://www.who.int/director-general/

speeches/detail/who-director-general-s-opening-remarks-at-the-media-briefing-on-covid-19---11-march-2020

Yamin, D. (2020). Counting the cost of COVID-19. *International Journal of Infectious Diseases*, *100*, 88–91. https://doi.org/10.1016/j.ijid.2020.07.063

Zhu, N., Zhang, D., Wang, W., Li, X., Yang, B., Song, J., Zhao, X., Huang, B., Shi, W., Lu, R., Niu, P., Zhan, F., Ma, X., Wang, D., Xu, W., Wu, G., Gao, G. F., & Tan, W. (2020). A novel coronavirus from patients with pneumonia in China, 2019. *New England Journal of Medicine*, *382*(8), 727–733. https://doi.org/10.1056/NEJMoa2001017

9 Beneath the Surface

How Underlying Trends Shaped the Evolution of the Pandemic's Trajectory

While the immediate events of COVID-19 commanded global attention, a more complex story was unfolding beneath the surface (Figure 9.1). Like the vast body of an iceberg hidden underwater, the pandemic's deeper patterns and trends shaped its trajectory in ways not immediately visible to observers. The evolution of viral variants, the seasonal waves of infection, and the emergence of long-term health impacts revealed patterns that would prove crucial for understanding both the immediate crisis and the deeper structural issues that would allow it to persist.

This chapter examines the key patterns and trends of viral evolution that shaped changes and adaptations in response:

- ***The Variant Timeline: From Ancestral to Omicron and Beyond***
- ***Transmission Dynamics Across Waves, Regions, and Seasons***
- ***Viral Evolution's Impact on Vaccine Efficacy and Immunity***
- ***Evolving Testing and Surveillance Adaptations***
- ***Treatment Advances and Clinical Understanding***

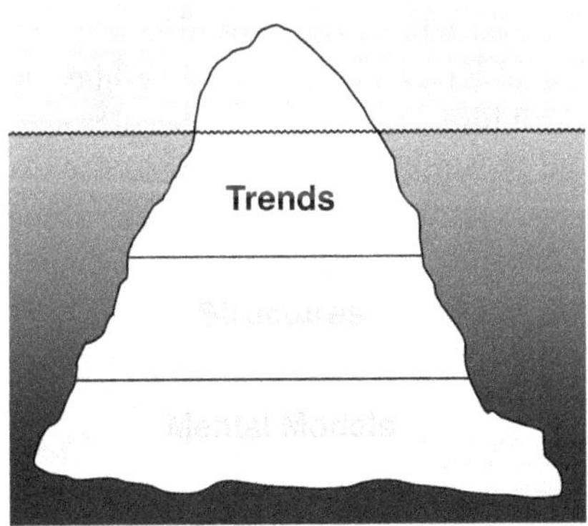

Figure 9.1 Iceberg Model—Trends.

DOI: 10.4324/9781003595564-12

The Variant Timeline: From Ancestral to Omicron and Beyond

The evolution of SARS-CoV-2 has progressed through distinct phases marked by the emergence of variants with increased transmissibility, immune evasion capabilities, or both. This evolutionary trajectory has fundamentally shaped the pandemic's course, with four major variants—Ancestral, Alpha, Delta, and Omicron—driving successive global waves of infection. Understanding this progression provides crucial insights into viral adaptation patterns and their implications for public health response.

Variant Classification Systems

Before examining the evolutionary timeline (Table 9.1), it's important to understand how SARS-CoV-2 variants are classified and named. Three main nomenclature systems are widely used to track SARS-CoV-2 evolution (O'Toole et al., 2021). The Pango lineage system offers a hierarchical, dynamic nomenclature (e.g., B.1.1.7, BA.2) designed to capture the leading edge of pandemic transmission, with each lineage representing an epidemiologically relevant phylogenetic cluster (Rambaut et al., 2020). The Global Initiative on Sharing All Influenza Data (GISAID) classification identifies global clades based on genetic markers and phylogenetic relationships (e.g., S, G, GH, GR, GV). Meanwhile, the Nextstrain system tracks pathogen evolution in real-time using broader clade designations (e.g., 19A, 20A, 21A). To facilitate public communications, the World Health Organization (WHO) introduced a simplified naming system using Greek alphabet letters (Alpha, Beta, etc.) for Variants of Concern (VOCs) and Variants of Interest (VOIs), while scientific nomenclature continues to use the more technical systems for precision (World Health Organization (WHO), 2025a, 2025b).

The Ancestral Period: December 2019–December 2020

The initial phase of the pandemic was dominated by the original SARS-CoV-2 strain first identified in Wuhan, China (Gutierrez et al., 2020). This period established baseline characteristics for viral transmission and pathogenicity, against which subsequent variants would be measured. While the original strain demonstrated high transmissibility compared to other coronaviruses, it had not yet developed the enhanced transmission or immune escape capabilities that would characterize later variants. During this phase, the virus accumulated mutations that would later prove significant for variant emergence. Genomic surveillance, though limited in many regions, began identifying patterns in viral evolution that would help predict and understand variant behavior (Volz et al., 2021). The D614G mutation, which increased viral infectivity, emerged during this period and became globally dominant, providing early evidence of the virus's adaptive capabilities (Plante et al., 2021; Zhang et al., 2020).

The D614G mutation in the spike protein represented the first significant evolutionary adaptation in SARS-CoV-2. Laboratory studies demonstrated that this mutation enhanced viral replication in human lung epithelial cells and primary human airway tissues by increasing the infectivity and stability of virions (Plante et al., 2021). The mutation did not alter the virus's susceptibility to neutralizing antibodies but improved viral transmission efficiency. By May 2020, variants carrying the D614G mutation accounted for approximately 70% of global isolates, demonstrating how rapidly beneficial mutations could achieve dominance (Gutierrez et al., 2020; Zhang et al., 2020).

The Alpha Period: September 2020–June 2021

The emergence of the Alpha variant (B.1.1.7) in the United Kingdom marked the first major evolutionary shift in SARS-CoV-2's capabilities (Volz et al., 2021). This variant demonstrated approximately 50% higher transmissibility than the ancestral strain, attributed to mutations in the spike protein that enhanced receptor binding (Wang et al., 2021). The rapid displacement of previous strains by Alpha revealed how new variants could achieve dominance through enhanced transmission efficiency. Alpha's spread coincided with initial vaccine rollouts, creating a race between immunization efforts and viral evolution. This variant showed modest immune escape capabilities but remained generally susceptible to vaccine-induced immunity (Wang et al., 2021). However, its enhanced transmissibility necessitated more stringent public health measures even as vaccination campaigns began, highlighting the challenge of controlling more efficiently spreading variants.

The Delta Period: October 2020–December 2021

The Delta variant (B.1.617.2) represented another significant evolutionary advancement in viral fitness and adaptability (Kurhade et al., 2023). First identified in India, Delta combined increased transmissibility—estimated at 60% higher than Alpha—with partial immune escape capabilities (Sil et al., 2024). This combination proved particularly effective at driving new infection waves, even in populations with relatively high vaccination rates. Delta's period of dominance coincided with growing population immunity from both vaccination and prior infection. The variant showed an increased ability to cause breakthrough infections in vaccinated individuals, though vaccines remained highly effective at preventing severe disease (Yisimayi et al., 2024). This pattern revealed how viral evolution was being shaped by growing immune pressure, leading to adaptations that could partially circumvent existing immunity while maintaining high transmission rates.

The Omicron Era: November 2021–Present

The emergence of Omicron (B.1.1.529) marked the most dramatic evolutionary shift yet observed in SARS-CoV-2 (WHO, 2021a). This variant family, beginning with BA.1 and continuing through numerous subvariants including BA.2, BA.4/5, XBB, JN.1, KP.2, and XEC, demonstrated unprecedented immune escape capabilities while maintaining high transmissibility (Centers for Disease Control and

Prevention (CDC), 2024b). Omicron's extensive spike protein mutations—over 30 compared to the ancestral strain—enabled it to evade much of the immunity developed against previous variants (WHO, 2021a).

The Omicron lineage has evolved through several distinct phases. The initial Omicron variant (BA.1), first detected in November 2021 in South Africa and Botswana, rapidly spread globally due to its enhanced transmissibility and immune evasion properties (WHO, 2021a). Laboratory studies demonstrated significantly reduced neutralization by antibodies from vaccination or previous infection. By late 2021, the BA.2 subvariant emerged and showed approximately 1.4 times higher transmissibility than BA.1 (Lyngse et al., 2022). By March 2022, BA.2 had become dominant in many regions worldwide. The BA.4 and BA.5 subvariants, first detected in South Africa in early 2022, demonstrated additional mutations that enhanced immune escape (Kurhade et al., 2023). BA.5 became globally dominant by mid-2022.

The evolution of Omicron continued with XBB and other recombinant lineages. XBB, a recombinant of two BA.2 sublineages, emerged in mid-2022 and exhibited enhanced immune evasion capabilities (Sluvkin et al., 2024). Subsequently, XBB.1.5 demonstrated increased ACE2 binding affinity along with immune escape, becoming dominant in early 2023. By late 2023, JN.1, a descendant of BA.2.86, emerged and became dominant by early 2024 (CDC, 2024). The KP lineages (KP.2, KP.3) subsequently emerged with further adaptations in immune evasion. By mid-2024, the XEC variant, a recombinant of JN.1 lineages KS.1.1 and KP.3.3, began increasing in prevalence across multiple regions (CDC, 2024).

This evolutionary pattern has differed from previous variants in several crucial ways. Rather than being displaced by entirely new variants, Omicron has generated a series of increasingly optimized subvariants. Each new subvariant has shown incremental advantages in transmission or immune escape, allowing them to outcompete their predecessors while maintaining the basic Omicron framework (Sluvkin et al., 2024).

SARS-CoV-2 Evolution: Current Dynamics and Future Outlook

By late 2023 through early 2025, SARS-CoV-2 evolution has demonstrated consistent patterns of modest but significant advantages in emerging variants (European Centre for Disease Prevention and Control, 2025). This reflects the virus's adaptation to populations with high immunity levels, requiring more sophisticated immune escape mechanisms while preserving transmission efficiency.

The primary driver of viral evolution appears to be immune pressure, pushing variants to develop increasingly complex evasion strategies (Focosi et al., 2024). Different viral lineages frequently acquire similar beneficial mutations independently, suggesting there may be limited optimal evolutionary pathways available to the virus. This phenomenon of convergent evolution has become particularly evident in the spike protein region, where multiple lineages independently develop similar mutations (Sluvkin et al., 2024). Such convergence indicates constrained

Table 9.1 Major SARS-CoV-2 Variants Identified from December 2019 to Early 2025

Variant Name	*Classification (WHO/Pango)*	*First Identified*	*Region of Origin*	*Key Impact or Significance*
Original Strain	Ancestral (A)	Dec 2019	Wuhan, China	*Caused initial global outbreak and pandemic*
Alpha	VOC (B.1.1.7)	Sep 2020	United Kingdom	*Increased transmissibility; higher severity than original*
Beta	VOC (B.1.351)	May 2020	South Africa	*Immune escape; reduced vaccine efficacy*
Gamma	VOC (P.1)	Nov 2020	Manaus, Brazil	*Immune escape; reinfection concerns*
Delta	VOC (B.1.617.2)	Oct 2020	Maharashtra, India	*Highly transmissible; increased severity*
Omicron BA.1	VOC (B.1.1.529)	Nov 2021	South Africa/ Botswana	*Rapid spread; substantial immune escape*
Omicron BA.2	VOC (BA.2)	Nov-Dec 2021	South Africa/ Global	*Higher transmissibility than BA.1*
Omicron BA.4/ BA.5	VOC (BA.4, BA.5)	Jan-Feb 2022	South Africa	*Increased reinfections; partial immune evasion*
Omicron XBB/ XBB.1.5	VOI (XBB, XBB.1.5)	Aug-Oct 2022	Singapore/ U.S.A.	*Enhanced transmissibility; notable antibody evasion*
Omicron EG.5	VOI (EG.5)	Feb 2023	Multiple countries	*Increased transmissibility; moderate immune escape*
Omicron BA.2.86	VOI (BA.2.86)	July-Aug 2023	Multiple countries	*Initial concern due to high mutations; later lower risk*
Omicron JN.1	VOI (BA.2.86.1.1)	Aug 2023	Luxembourg	*Rapid global spread late 2023*
Omicron KP.2	VUM (KP.2)	Jan 2024	Multiple countries	*Potential immune evasion*
Omicron KP.3	VUM (KP.3)	Feb 2024	Multiple countries	*Additional spike mutations*
Omicron XEC	REC (KS.1.1 + KP.3.3)	Sep 2024	Germany/ Global	*Recombinant lineage; increased transmissibility*

Sources: WHO (2025a, 2025b); GISAID (n.d., 2025); CDC (2024); European Centre for Disease Prevention and Control (2025); Sluvkin et al. (2024); Focosi et al. (2024); Kurhade et al. (2023); Lyngse et al. (2022); Volz et al. (2021).

evolutionary options for the virus as it balances enhanced transmission with immune evasion.

Up to now, the relationship between transmission and severity appears to follow a predictable pattern: variants generally maintain or increase transmissibility without necessarily evolving toward greater severity (Plante et al., 2021).

The tracking of these evolutionary patterns relies heavily on global surveillance networks. Organizations like GISAID have developed platforms enabling rapid sharing of genomic data for near real-time monitoring (GISAID, n.d.; WHO, 2025a, 2025b). However, significant disparities in surveillance capabilities across regions create blind spots in our collective global understanding.

Current evidence suggests SARS-CoV-2 will continue to evolve, though likely at a more gradual pace than during earlier pandemic phases. The virus appears to be optimizing its spread within populations characterized by complex immunity profiles from prior infections and vaccinations (CDC, 2024; European Centre for Disease Prevention and Control, 2025).

In the next section, we'll explore how these viral adaptations combine with geographic and seasonal factors to create distinct transmission dynamics across different regions and time periods.

Transmission Dynamics Across Waves, Regions, and Seasons

The global transmission of SARS-CoV-2 from 2019 to 2025 followed complex patterns shaped by evolving viral variants, changing immunity landscapes, and regional factors. Four distinct variant waves—Ancestral, Alpha, Delta, and Omicron—each brought unique transmission characteristics, with progressive changes in transmissibility and severity. While case numbers increased dramatically with each new variant, severity generally decreased over time, particularly after widespread vaccination began. Regional and seasonal patterns emerged, with temperate regions experiencing predictable winter surges while equatorial areas showed less seasonality. Urban environments, population mobility, and housing patterns significantly influenced local transmission dynamics. These diverse patterns highlight why the pandemic's impact varied so dramatically across regions and why effective response strategies required locally-tailored approaches rather than universal solutions.

Wave-by-Wave Transmission Overview

While Section 2.3.1 defines the timing, characteristics, and classification of global waves, here we focus on their concrete impacts across health system indicators, and the patterns that emerged as the pandemic evolved (Table 9.2).

The Ancestral Wave (Early 2020)

The Ancestral Wave in early 2020 resulted in a significant global spread of the virus. According to data reported to the WHO, by June 2020, there were

Table 9.2 Epidemiological Trends by Major Global SARS-CoV-2 Variant (2019–2025)

Variant	*Time Period*	*Estimated Global Cases*	*Estimated Global Deaths*	*Estimated Global CFR (%)*	*Notable Traits*
Ancestral	Late 2019–Mid 2020	8–12 million	400,000–600,000	2.5–4.0	No prior immunity; limited testing
Alpha	Late 2020–Early 2021	110–130 million	2.3–2.5 million	2.0–3.0	More transmissible; coincided with vaccine rollout
Delta	Mid–Late 2021	200–250 million	1.4–1.6 million	1.5–2.5	Higher severity; unvaccinated most impacted
Omicron	Late 2021–2025	700–900 million (ongoing)	1.3–1.6 million	0.3–1.0	Immune escape; overlapping waves of subvariants

Sources: WHO (2022a, 2025a, 2025b); Mathieu et al. (2020a, 2020b); CDC (2022a); Wang et al. (2022); Wolter et al. (2022); Li et al. (2023); Sheikh et al. (2021, 2023); Twohig et al. (2022); Nyberg et al. (2022); Maslo et al. (2022); Fisman & Tuite (2021).

approximately 10 million confirmed cases globally and around 500,000 deaths (Mathieu et al., 2020a, 2020b). Meta-analyses have estimated the case fatality rate (CFR) during this ancestral strain period at approximately 3.6%, though rates varied significantly by region, with higher rates observed in Europe and the Americas (Baud et al., 2020; Li et al., 2023; WHO, 2022a). Hospitalization data remains incomplete globally for this period, but healthcare systems in Italy, Iran, and New York City experienced severe overwhelm (Grasselli et al., 2020; Zhou et al., 2020). This initial wave was characterized by limited testing capacity, significant underreporting, and extremely high CFRs in countries hit earliest in the pandemic timeline.

The transmissibility of the ancestral strain, while high compared to other human coronaviruses, remained lower than subsequent variants. Research demonstrated a basic reproduction number (R_0) between 2.2 and 3.6 for the original strain, before the emergence of the D614G mutation, which increased transmissibility by approximately 20% (Volz et al., 2021). The virus spread most effectively in crowded indoor environments with poor ventilation and prolonged person-to-person contact, establishing a transmission pattern that would persist throughout the pandemic (Adam et al., 2020; Rader et al., 2020).

The Alpha Wave (Late 2020–Early 2021)

The Alpha Wave spanning late 2020 to early 2021 saw global cases increase dramatically. First identified in the United Kingdom, the Alpha variant demonstrated approximately 50% higher transmissibility than the ancestral strain (Volz et al.,

2021). By March 2021, global confirmed cases had reached approximately 130 million, with the global death toll approaching 2.9 million cumulative fatalities. Studies have estimated the CFR during the Alpha variant period at approximately 2.6%, representing a modest reduction from the ancestral strain (Challen et al., 2021; Wang et al., 2022; Sheikh et al., 2021). Hospitalization trends during this period showed sharp increases across the United Kingdom, United States, and Central Europe, with studies demonstrating that Alpha infections carried a 30–70% higher risk of hospitalization than the ancestral strain (Davies et al., 2021; Twohig et al., 2022; Nyberg et al., 2022).

Alpha's spread notably coincided with the initiation of global vaccination campaigns, creating a race between immunization efforts and viral evolution. Countries with earlier and more robust vaccination programs generally experienced lower mortality during this wave, though vaccine inequity meant this protection was unevenly distributed globally (Petherick et al., 2021). Mathematical modeling demonstrated that the Alpha variant's higher transmissibility necessitated a higher population immunity threshold to achieve herd immunity, estimated at approximately 80% compared to 60–70% for the ancestral strain (Kissler et al., 2020).

The Delta Wave (Mid–Late 2021)

The Delta Wave through mid to late 2021 caused a significant increase in global cases and hospitalizations. Research indicates Delta was approximately 60% more transmissible than Alpha (Fisman & Tuite, 2021) and showed increased severity. Hospitalization surges were particularly pronounced in South and Southeast Asia, with India experiencing a devastating surge that overwhelmed healthcare systems (Tian et al., 2020), while also causing significant stress on intensive care units (ICU) across the southern United States and Eastern Europe. Studies found the Delta variant had a higher risk of hospitalization, ICU admission, and mortality compared to previous variants, with hospitalization risk approximately 2.3 times higher than Alpha (Sheikh et al., 2021; Twohig et al., 2022).

Meta-analyses have estimated the CFR during this period at approximately 2.0%, which, while lower than previous waves, still represented substantial mortality given Delta's increased transmissibility (Wang et al., 2022). Despite growing vaccination coverage globally, Delta's increased transmissibility and partial immune evasion capabilities created disproportionate impacts among unvaccinated populations. Research demonstrated 10–15 times higher hospitalization rates among unvaccinated individuals compared to vaccinated ones during this wave (CDC, 2022a).

Globally, Delta replaced Alpha as the predominant strain in all regions by August 2021, though the timing and severity of resulting epidemic waves varied considerably. Regional resurgences were influenced by population immunity levels, vaccination coverage, and public health measures, creating a complex mosaic of infection peaks (Haldane et al., 2021). Notably, countries with high vaccination coverage but relaxed public health measures experienced substantial transmission, though with significantly lower hospitalization and mortality rates than observed in less-vaccinated regions (Sharma et al., 2021).

The Omicron Wave (Late 2021–2025)

The Omicron Wave, beginning in late 2021 and continuing through various sublineages, caused an explosive surge in global case numbers. First identified in Botswana and South Africa in November 2021, Omicron demonstrated unprecedented transmissibility and immune escape capabilities (Wolter et al., 2022). In January 2022 alone, the WHO reported over 15 million new cases in a single week, the highest number recorded in the pandemic (WHO, 2022a). While studies showed Omicron generally caused less severe disease than Delta (with a 50–70% reduced risk of hospitalization), the sheer volume of infections still led to substantial hospitalization numbers and continued mortality (Maslo et al., 2022; Nyberg et al., 2022).

Multiple meta-analyses have estimated the CFR during the Omicron period at approximately 0.7%, representing a significant reduction compared to previous variants but still resulting in substantial mortality due to the extraordinarily high case numbers (Li et al., 2023; Wang et al., 2022). Hospitalization patterns changed noticeably during this wave. Despite record case numbers, hospital stays were generally shorter, though some regions reported increased pediatric admissions compared to previous waves (CDC, 2022b).

Rather than producing a single global peak, Omicron's sublineages (including BA.1, BA.2, BA.4/5, XBB, and others) created overlapping regional surges that extended the wave's impact for multiple years (Lyngse et al., 2022). Initial BA.1 infections showed high attack rates in both vaccinated and previously infected individuals due to immune escape mutations, with transmission rates three to five times higher than Delta in household studies (Lyngse et al., 2022). The emergence of the BA.2 subvariant approximately 60 days after BA.1 created a "wave within a wave" in many regions, with BA.2 demonstrating approximately 30% higher transmissibility than BA.1 (Lyngse et al., 2022).

Subsequent sublineages followed a similar pattern, with BA.4/5 emerging in mid-2022, XBB lineages in late 2022, and JN.1 and KP variants through 2023–2024, each showing incremental advantages in immune escape that enabled new waves of transmission even in highly exposed populations (WHO, 2025b). This successive pattern of subvariants, each characterized by greater immune evasion rather than increased intrinsic severity, appears to represent SARS-CoV-2's evolutionary stabilization as it optimizes transmission in a highly immune global population (Wang et al., 2022).

Seasonal and Environmental Patterns Across Regions

While scientific consensus indicates that SARS-CoV-2 is not strictly seasonal in the manner of influenza, recurring seasonal patterns (Table 9.3) nevertheless influenced transmission throughout the pandemic (Moriyama et al., 2020; Sajadi et al., 2020).

In the Northern Hemisphere, particularly across North America and Europe, transmission consistently peaked during winter months (November through

Table 9.3 Regional and Seasonal Transmission Patterns of SARS-CoV-2

Region	*Peak Period Transmission*	*Environmental Drivers*	*Social/Cultural Factors*	*Observed Patterns*
Northern Hemisphere (North America, Europe)	Winter (Nov–Feb)	Cold temps, low humidity, indoor air	Holiday gatherings, more indoor activity	Winter surges driven by indoor exposure; less in warmer months
Asia	Variable; often mid-year peaks	Monsoons, humidity, climate diversity	Major festivals, regional mobility	Variant-driven surges by festivals, climate, and containment
Southern Cone (South America)	Winter (Jun–Aug)	Cold seasonal shifts	Travel during winter months	Mirrors Northern Hemisphere with inverted timing
Equatorial Regions (South America, Southeast Asia)	Irregular; not very seasonal	Minor temp variation; some humidity effects	Large gatherings, varying containment efforts	Driven more by new variants and policy shifts than seasonality
Africa	Variable; often during rainy seasons	Rainfall, indoor crowding	Limited indoor infrastructure; festival timing	Data gaps may obscure trends; modest seasonal impact observed
Oceania	Variable; tied to travel waves	Geographic isolation, climate variation	Domestic travel, reopening phases	Early containment; later peaks with reopenings

Sources: Baker et al. (2020); Carlson et al. (2020); Ma et al. (2021); Moriyama et al. (2020); Sajadi et al. (2020); Merow and Urban (2020); Richardson et al. (2023); Sharma et al. (2021).

February), driven by colder temperatures, reduced humidity, and increased indoor gatherings (Merow & Urban, 2020; Moriyama et al., 2020). Studies demonstrated that a 10°C decrease in temperature was associated with a 22.1% increase in SARS-CoV-2 transmission, while a 30% decrease in relative humidity increased transmission by approximately 18.7% (Ma et al., 2021). These environmental factors were further amplified by behavioral changes during winter, with mathematical models attributing approximately 40% of winter transmission increases to indoor gathering behaviors compared to 60% from direct environmental effects (Sharma et al., 2021).

Asian transmission dynamics presented more complex patterns, influenced by environmental shifts, cultural behaviors, and variant introductions (Tian et al., 2020). Many regions experienced distinct mid-year transmission peaks corresponding to monsoon seasons and significant cultural events. Countries such as

India and Bangladesh recorded substantial infection spikes during major festivals and high humidity periods, with movement data showing 20–40% increases in mobility during these events despite ongoing pandemic conditions (Zhou et al., 2020).

South America displayed notable variability between its northern and southern regions. The southern cone nations, including Argentina and Chile, experienced predictable transmission peaks during their winter months (June through August), mirroring the seasonality observed in the Northern Hemisphere but with inverted timing (Mena et al., 2021). Equatorial regions across the continent showed less predictable patterns primarily, driven by variant introductions and changing public health measures rather than seasonal changes. Studies in Brazil demonstrated that temperature effects on transmission were approximately one-third as strong in equatorial regions compared to temperate ones (Ma et al., 2021).

Africa and Oceania, while reporting lower overall transmission rates, still exhibited meaningful seasonal influences. African transmission patterns often corresponded with regional rainfall patterns and humidity, particularly during rainy seasons when indoor crowding increased in sub-Saharan regions (WHO, 2022a, 2025a). Oceania's geographic isolation combined with stringent public health measures helped limit the spread, yet seasonal shifts remained evident, particularly during periods of increased domestic travel and tourism (Haldane et al., 2021).

Environmental conditions influenced viral behavior throughout these regional patterns. Laboratory studies indicated that SARS-CoV-2 may survive more efficiently at cooler temperatures and that humidity levels affect airborne transmission dynamics, with lower humidity potentially enhancing aerosol stability (Moriyama et al., 2020; Richardson et al., 2023). These factors, combined with increased indoor gathering during colder months, likely contributed to the elevated transmission observed during winter in many temperate regions.

Social patterns amplified these environmental effects considerably. Winter months combined both environmental and behavioral risks as indoor gatherings increased during traditional holidays and family events (Petherick et al., 2021). Though transmission typically declined during summer periods, large-scale events and enclosed air-conditioned spaces during extreme heat waves continued providing significant transmission opportunities throughout warmer seasons (Rader et al., 2020).

Regional Variation, Urban Dynamics, and Immunity Landscapes

The movement of variants across regions revealed distinct transmission networks that shaped the timing and impact of successive variant waves. Early pandemic patterns typically showed variants emerging in one region before spreading globally, as observed with Alpha in the United Kingdom and Delta in India (Sheikh et al., 2021; Volz et al., 2021). However, this pattern evolved substantially with Omicron and its subvariants, which demonstrated the ability to emerge and spread through multiple regions almost simultaneously, creating complex overlapping transmission waves that challenged traditional containment approaches (WHO, 2022a).

Vaccination coverage and prior infection created widely varying immunity landscapes across regions. High-income countries generally secured early access to mRNA vaccines, while lower and middle-income regions relied more heavily on inactivated virus or viral vector vaccines with different effectiveness profiles (Haldane et al., 2021). Prior exposure to specific variants further complicated these immunity patterns. South Africa's significant experience with the Beta variant created a distinct immunological backdrop that influenced its experience with subsequent waves differently than regions where Beta had limited circulation (Wolter et al., 2022).

Urbanization patterns played crucial roles in how these dynamics unfolded locally. Megacities with high population density and extensive public transportation networks created persistent environments for close contact transmission (Hamidi et al., 2020; Jay et al., 2020). Research demonstrated that cities with population densities above 5,000 people per square kilometer experienced 1.5–2.1 times higher cumulative incidence of COVID-19 than less dense areas, even after accounting for testing rates and demographic factors (Hamidi et al., 2020; Rader et al., 2020). Studies of mobility patterns revealed that densely populated urban cores acted as persistent transmission hubs throughout successive pandemic waves, with case rates often correlating strongly with public transit usage patterns (Jay et al., 2020).

However, population density alone did not determine outcomes—cities like Hong Kong and Singapore, despite being among the world's most densely populated urban centers, maintained relatively low transmission through exceptional surveillance systems and rapid containment responses (Tian et al., 2020). Comprehensive analysis of metropolitan areas found that connectivity and mobility patterns were often stronger predictors of transmission than raw population density, with areas featuring high intra-urban movement experiencing substantially greater spread regardless of overall density metrics (Rader et al., 2020).

Housing and transportation patterns also influenced transmission. Multi-generational housing arrangements, common across parts of Asia and Mediterranean regions, potentially contributed to intra-household transmission (Mena et al., 2021). Similarly, transportation infrastructure shaped risk exposure, with areas reliant on public transit potentially experiencing different transmission patterns than those with lower population mobility or private transportation predominance (Jay et al., 2020). Spatiotemporal analysis of urban transmission dynamics found disproportionate impacts in lower-income neighborhoods, with studies in major U.S. cities demonstrating two to four times higher positivity rates in zip codes with median household incomes below regional averages, even after controlling for testing accessibility (Yang et al., 2021).

Understanding the Pandemic's Uneven Global Impact

From wave to wave, the pandemic's burden was unevenly distributed—modulated by season, geography, infrastructure, and immunity profiles (Haldane et al., 2021).

These complex patterns reveal why global surges never followed uniform trajectories, and why preparedness and response strategies must always be locally informed rather than universally applied. The distinct characteristics of each major variant wave, combined with geographic and seasonal variations, shaped the highly uneven global experience of the pandemic.

Understanding these transmission dynamics proves essential for interpreting how variant waves unfolded and how public health responses adapted across different regions. These insights provide the necessary foundation for analyzing vaccine performance across diverse settings—a topic explored in the next section. As we continue to refine our understanding of SARS-CoV-2 transmission patterns, our ability to predict and mitigate future respiratory pandemic threats will similarly evolve, incorporating these hard-won lessons from COVID-19's complex global journey.

Viral Evolution's Impact on Vaccine Efficacy and Immunity

COVID-19 vaccines have undergone a remarkable journey from 2020 to 2025, facing the continuous challenge of viral evolution. While initial vaccines showed extraordinary effectiveness against early variants, each new variant—particularly Omicron—required vaccines to adapt. Over time, vaccination strategies shifted from achieving sterilizing immunity to preventing severe outcomes, eventually adopting an annual updating approach similar to influenza vaccines. Different vaccine technologies offered varied benefits, with some excelling in speed of development and others in accessibility or durability. Despite scientific advances, global implementation revealed persistent inequities in vaccine access and coverage. This section explores this evolution of vaccines against a changing virus and the lessons learned for future pandemic preparedness.

Initial Vaccine Effectiveness and the Challenge of Emerging Variants

First-generation COVID-19 vaccines, developed against the ancestral strain, demonstrated exceptional efficacy in both clinical trials and early real-world applications. mRNA vaccines in particular showed efficacy rates exceeding 90% against symptomatic infection with original and Alpha variants. During clinical trials, the Pfizer-BioNTech vaccine achieved 95% efficacy in preventing symptomatic disease (Polack et al., 2020), while Moderna's vaccine showed 94.1% efficacy (Baden et al., 2021). These promising results established high expectations for vaccine performance, though they would soon be challenged by viral evolution.

The emergence of successive variants revealed a pattern of increasing immune evasion. The Delta variant showed the first significant reduction in vaccine effectiveness against infection, though protection against severe disease remained robust. Real-world data demonstrated that two-dose mRNA vaccine effectiveness against Delta infection dropped to approximately 65%, though protection against hospitalization remained between 84 and 90% (Pouwels et al., 2021; Sheikh et al., 2021, 2023).

The arrival of Omicron marked a more dramatic shift. This variant's extensive mutations enabled unprecedented immune escape, with initial two-dose vaccine effectiveness against infection dropping below 40% (Andrews et al., 2022; Kirsebom et al., 2022). Studies across multiple countries showed similar patterns—data from the U.K. Health Security Agency revealed that while protection against severe disease remained significant at 72%, effectiveness against symptomatic infection had declined to 34% four months after the second dose (Kirsebom et al., 2022). This substantial reduction in effectiveness against infection underscored how rapidly the virus was evolving to evade vaccine-induced immunity.

The data in Table 9.4 illustrates the progressive increase in immune escape across variants from 2019 to 2025, with protection against symptomatic infection declining dramatically from 95% against the ancestral strain to less than 10% against recent variants (Lee et al., 2024; Lin et al., 2024). While protection against severe disease has been better preserved, it has still shown concerning decline from over 90% initially to approximately 55–70% against the most recent variants (Link-Gelles, 2024, 2025; Self et al., 2024). This pattern of evolution has fundamentally changed the role of COVID-19 vaccines, which by 2025 primarily function to prevent severe outcomes rather than infection (Krammer & Ellebedy, 2023).

Table 9.4 Comprehensive Analysis of Vaccine Effectiveness Against SARS-CoV-2 Variants (2019–2025)

SARS-CoV-2 Lineage	*Emergence Timeline*	*Antibody Levels Required*	*Efficacy Against Symptomatic Infection (%)*	*Efficacy Against Severe Disease (%)*
Ancestral Strain	Dec 2019	1× (reference)	Approx. 95.00	High (>90)
Alpha (B.1.1.7)	Sep 2020	1–2×	Approx. 90.00 (↓)	High (>90)
Delta (B.1.617.2)	Dec 2020	3–5×	Approx. 65.00 (↓)	Approx. 80–90 (↓)
Omicron (B.1.1.529)	Nov 2021	10–15×	Approx. 25.00 (↓)	Approx. 55–80 (↓)
Omicron BA.4/5	Apr 2022	15–20×	Approx. 15–20 (↓)	Approx. 60–70 (↓)
XBB Variants	Late 2022	20–30×	Approx. 10–15 (↓)	Approx. 65–75
JN Variants	Late 2023	25–35×	<10 (↓)	Approx. 70–80
KP Variants	2024	30–45×	<10 (↓)	Approx. 65–75 (↓)
New 2025 Variants	2025	35–50×	Approx. 5–10 (↓)	Approx. 60–70 (↓)

Sources: Andrews et al. (2022); Baden et al. (2021); CDC (2024, 2025c); Ferdinands et al. (2022); Huiberts et al. (2024); Kirsebom et al. (2022, 2024); Lee et al. (2024); Lin et al. (2024); Link-Gelles et al. (2022, 2024, 2025); Lopez Bernal et al. (2021); Polack et al. (2020); Self et al. (2024); Sheikh et al. (2021, 2023); Tartof et al. (2024); Tenforde et al. (2021); UK Health Security Agency (2023-2024); Wang et al. (2023); Bar-On et al. (2021).

Vaccine Platform Diversity and Strategic Adaptations to Variant Escape

The challenge of waning immunity and variant escape drove the development of booster strategies. Initial boosters using original strain vaccines showed significant benefit—a large-scale study in Israel demonstrated that a third dose restored protection against hospitalization to over 90% during the Delta wave (Bar-On et al., 2021). However, this protection proved less durable against Omicron, leading to the development of bivalent vaccines targeting both ancestral and Omicron strains (Goldberg et al., 2021).

Data from the first bivalent booster campaign in late 2022 showed mixed results. While these updated vaccines generated stronger antibody responses against Omicron variants, real-world effectiveness proved more modest than anticipated. CDC data from September to December 2022 indicated that bivalent boosters provided 43–56% additional protection against symptomatic infection compared to previous vaccination status, with effectiveness varying significantly by age group and time since vaccination (Link-Gelles et al., 2022). More recent data on monovalent XBB.1.5-targeted vaccines introduced in 2023 showed initial effectiveness against symptomatic infection at approximately 54%, declining to about 20% after 20 weeks, while maintaining stronger protection against hospitalization (Kirsebom et al., 2024; Link-Gelles et al., 2024).

Different vaccine platforms have demonstrated varying capabilities for adaptation to new variants. mRNA vaccines showed particular advantages in rapid modification, with new variant-specific versions developed within 100 days (Krause et al., 2021). Their flexibility enabled quick deployment of updated formulations, though manufacturing complexity and cold chain requirements limited global accessibility (Mathieu et al., 2023).

Viral vector vaccines demonstrated more stable but generally lower effectiveness. While they achieved 60–70% efficacy against symptomatic disease from early variants (Voysey et al., 2021), their protection declined more significantly against Omicron. However, their easier storage requirements made them crucial for global vaccination efforts, particularly in regions lacking ultra-cold chain infrastructure (Sandoval et al., 2023).

Protein subunit vaccines emerged later but showed promising results, achieving 90% efficacy against original and Alpha variants during clinical trials (Dunkle et al., 2022). Their traditional technology platform offered potential advantages for production scaling and storage, though development timelines proved longer than mRNA platforms.

The performance characteristics in Table 9.5 reveal important patterns in vaccine platform evolution throughout the pandemic. mRNA platforms demonstrated unparalleled speed and adaptability, with clinical data showing they could be rapidly updated to target new variants while maintaining robust safety profiles (Krammer & Ellebedy, 2023; Thomas et al., 2021). Viral vector vaccines offered a valuable balance of accessibility and effectiveness, though most were discontinued by 2025 in favor of other platforms due to their more limited adaptability to new variants (Sandoval et al., 2023).

Table 9.5 Comparison of COVID-19 Vaccine Platforms

COVID-19 Vaccine Platform	*Speed to Development*	*Adaptability to Variants*	*Effectiveness Duration*	*Safety Profile*
mRNA *(Pfizer-BNT, Moderna)*	Very high (≤100 days)	Very high	Moderate (4–6 months)	High
Viral Vector *(AstraZeneca, J&J, Sputnik)*	Moderate (6–9 months)	Moderate	Moderate (5–7 months)	High[a]
Protein Subunit *(Novavax, Sanofi)*	Slow (9–12 months)	High	Long (6–8 months)	Very High
Inactivated Virus *(Sinovac, Sinopharm)*	Moderate (6–9 months)	Low	Short (3–5 months)	High
Live Attenuated[b] *(Codagenix)*	Slow (12+ months)	Moderate	Long (8+ months)	Moderate
Virus-Like Particles *(Medicago)*	Slow (9–12 months)	Moderate	Moderate (5–7 months)	High
DNA Vaccines[b] *(Inovio, Zydus Cadila)*	High (4–6 months)	High	Unknown to moderate (5–7 months)	High
Self-Amplifying RNA[b] *(Arcturus)*	Very high (≤100 days)	Very high	Long (7–9 months)	High

Sources: Chemaitelly et al. (2022); Dunkle et al. (2022); Heath et al. (2024); Krammer and Ellebedy (2023); Mathieu et al. (2023); Sandoval et al. (2023); Thomas et al. (2021); Voysey et al. (2021); WHO (2023b, 2024); Wu et al. (2024).

Notes

[a] Rareblood-clotting issues affected the perception of safety among the public.

[b] Real-world data still lacking for live attenuated, DNA, and saRNA platforms.

Protein subunit vaccines like Novavax showed excellent safety profiles and stability, with recent data showing comparable protection against severe outcomes to mRNA vaccines (Heath et al., 2024; Wu et al., 2024). A 2024 network meta-analysis comparing all major vaccine platforms found that while initial effectiveness varied, the gap had narrowed for prevention of severe disease, with protein subunit vaccines showing particularly durable protection (Wu et al., 2024). Inactivated virus vaccines enabled widespread vaccination in resource-limited regions despite their modest effectiveness against variants (Mathieu et al., 2023).

Newer technologies such as self-amplifying RNA and DNA vaccines emerged to address limitations of first-generation vaccines, though with more limited deployment (Krammer & Ellebedy, 2023).

Evolution of Real-World Effectiveness and Shift Toward Preventing Severe Disease

Real-world data has revealed complex patterns in vaccine performance across different populations and contexts. A meta-analysis of 23 studies involving over

100 million vaccinated individuals showed that effectiveness varies significantly with age, comorbidities, and time since vaccination (Sandoval et al., 2023). In adults over 65, initial vaccine effectiveness against severe disease started at 85% but declined to approximately 70% after six months, prompting recommendations for earlier booster doses in this age group (UK Health Security Agency, 2023-2024).

The rapid evolution of SARS-CoV-2 has created a continuous challenge for vaccine-induced immunity. Studies tracking neutralizing antibody responses show that each major variant has required progressively higher antibody levels for protection. Laboratory data indicate that neutralization of Omicron subvariants requires 10–40 times higher antibody levels compared to ancestral strains, explaining the increased occurrence of breakthrough infections even in vaccinated populations (Sluvkin et al., 2024; Wang et al., 2023).

A comprehensive analysis of 241,204 breakthrough infections across four continents revealed that while vaccination continues to provide robust protection against severe outcomes, effectiveness against infection follows a relatively predictable decline pattern: 90–100% in first month, 70–80% at three months, 50–60% at six months, and below 50% after six months without boosting (Sandoval et al., 2023; Tenforde et al., 2021).

The evolving nature of SARS-CoV-2 has prompted a shift in vaccination strategy from achieving sterilizing immunity to preventing severe disease. Recent data from the 2023–2024 vaccination campaign showed that the XBB.1.5-targeted monovalent vaccines provided approximately 54% protection against symptomatic infection in the first two months after vaccination, declining to approximately 20% after 20 weeks (Link-Gelles et al., 2024). However, protection against hospitalization remained stronger at about 65% initially, declining to around 50–55% after several months (Self et al., 2024). The effectiveness varied significantly by variant, with notably lower protection seen against the JN.1 lineage that became dominant in early 2024 (Huiberts et al., 2024; Moustsen-Helms et al., 2024).

Specifically, a study from the VISION Network covering 26 hospitals from October 2023 to March 2024 found that the 2023–2024 XBB.1.5 monovalent vaccines provided 57% effectiveness against XBB lineage hospitalizations but only 49% against BA.2.86/JN.1 lineage hospitalizations, highlighting the impact of variant evolution on vaccine performance (Self et al., 2024). A Danish nationwide register-based study similarly found that relative vaccine protection was approximately 15–20% lower against JN.1 compared to earlier XBB variants (Moustsen-Helms et al., 2024).

Global Implementation Disparities and Lessons for Future Pandemic Response

Global disparities in vaccine access have created distinct challenges for variant control, with significant implications for mortality and healthcare system resilience (Mathieu et al., 2023; WHO, 2021b).

Table 9.6 Global COVID-19 Vaccination and Outcomes by Region

	Vaccination Coverage Estimate (%)		*COVID-19 Mortality Rate Estimate per 100,000*	
Region	*2021–2022*	*2023–2025*	*2021–2022*	*2023–2025*
North America	60–75 %	75–85 ↑	45–60	15–30 ↓
Western Europe	70–80 %	80–90 ↑	30–45	10–25 ↓
Eastern Europe	50–65 %	60–75 ↑	60–80	30–45 ↓
East Asia	70–85 %	80–90 ↑	25–35	10–20 ↓
South Asia	40–60 %	60–75 ↑	70–90	35–50 ↓
Middle East	60–80 %	70–85 ↑	40–60	20–35 ↓
North Africa	30–45 %	50–60 ↑	60–80	35–50 ↓
Sub-Saharan Africa	15–30 %	30–40 ↑	60–80	50–75 ↓
South America	60–75 %	75–90 ↑	65–80	30–45 ↓
Oceania	70–85 %	80–90 ↑	20–35	5–20 ↓
Global Average	**55–65 %**	**65–75 ↑**	**55–70**	**25–40 ↓**

Sources: Mathieu et al. (2023); WHO (2024, 2025a); European Centre for Disease Prevention and Control (2024); CDC (2024, 2025c); European Centre for Disease Prevention and Control (2024).

The global vaccination data presented in Table 9.6 highlights several critical findings from the pandemic response. Analysis revealed a strong inverse correlation between vaccination coverage and mortality rates, with countries achieving >80% coverage reporting mortality rates 70-80% lower than those with <40% coverage (Mathieu et al., 2023). Notably, healthcare integration proved more predictive of sustained protection than vaccination rates alone, as regions that effectively incorporated COVID-19 vaccination into existing health systems maintained better outcomes (WHO, 2021b).

While regional disparities narrowed after 2023, significant gaps remained in 2025, particularly in Sub-Saharan Africa, where infrastructure limitations continued to hamper vaccination efforts, with coverage reaching only 25–35% compared to 80–90% in Western Europe and East Asia (Mathieu et al., 2023; WHO, 2024). By 2025, countries with successful healthcare integration maintained moderate protection despite reduced emphasis on mass campaigns. Annual vaccination adoption rates varied significantly by region, with 40–60% uptake in high-income countries compared to just 10–20% in low-income regions, reflecting ongoing challenges in achieving global vaccine equity (WHO, 2024).

In early 2024, WHO data showed substantial differences in vaccine distribution: high-income countries averaged 3.2 doses per person, while low-income countries averaged just 0.3 doses (WHO, 2024). These disparities were reflected in mortality rates, with comprehensively vaccinated populations experiencing one-fifth the death rate of those with limited vaccine access (Mathieu et al., 2023).

Experience from 2021 to 2025 has demonstrated that successful vaccination programs require integration with existing healthcare infrastructure. Countries that incorporated COVID-19 vaccination into routine healthcare delivery achieved 35-45% higher coverage rates compared to those relying solely on mass vaccination campaigns (WHO, 2021b). This insight, combined with the need for ongoing variant surveillance and vaccine adaptation, points toward the critical importance of building sustainable, integrated systems for future pandemic response. However, these comparisons should be interpreted cautiously given variations in testing capacity, death reporting standards, and demographic factors across regions.

Current research focuses on three main approaches to improve vaccine protection: universal coronavirus vaccines targeting conserved viral regions with potential for broader cross-variant protection (Krammer & Ellebedy, 2023), mucosal immunity enhancement through nasal vaccines (which has shown promising effectiveness in preventing upper respiratory tract infection in clinical trials), and novel adjuvant development that has demonstrated increased neutralizing antibody persistence (Krause et al., 2021; Wu et al., 2024).

As of 2025, COVID-19 vaccination has largely transitioned to an annual model similar to influenza, with vaccines updated each year to target the predominant circulating strains from recent months (CDC, 2025c; Yale Medicine, 2024b). For example, the 2024–2025 vaccines were formulated to target JN.1 and KP.2 variants, providing improved protection compared to previous XBB.1.5-targeted vaccines against the variants circulating in 2024–2025 (Link-Gelles, 2024, 2025).

This trajectory reflects both scientific ingenuity and the necessity of adaptation in response to an evolving virus. While early vaccines provided robust protection, the emergence of immune-evasive variants required continual refinement of formulations and strategies. As COVID-19 continues its transition into a managed endemic threat, sustained innovation and integration into routine healthcare remain central to long-term protection. The ongoing pressure from viral evolution also highlights the importance of enhanced testing and surveillance systems, critical for rapidly anticipating and responding to emerging threats—topics we explore in the next section.

Evolving Testing and Surveillance Adaptations

The evolution of SARS-CoV-2 variants required ongoing adaptation in testing and surveillance. These changes reflected both advances in detection technology and deeper insight into variant behavior. This shift—from rudimentary to sophisticated—was key to tracking spread, anticipating new variants, and informing targeted public health responses across pandemic phases.

Early Pandemic Testing Challenges

As SARS-CoV-2 began its initial spread, early 2020 testing data revealed significant disparities in national capacities. South Korea, with a population of about 51 million, had performed 109,591 COVID-19 tests by early March—equivalent to roughly 2,138 tests per million people (Worldometer, 2020). This rapid response capability was largely due to South Korea's previous experience with the 2015 MERS outbreak, which had prompted the development of emergency testing protocols and infrastructure (Choi & Kim, 2024; You, 2020). In contrast, the United

States had conducted only 472 tests through the CDC by late February, amounting to fewer than 1 test per million people despite having a population more than six times larger (Engelberg et al., 2020; Worldometer, 2020). Italy and the United Kingdom also lagged behind, with 23,345 tests (386 per million) and 13,525 tests (199 per million), respectively (Worldometer, 2020).

These discrepancies reflected fundamentally different approaches to pandemic response. South Korea leveraged its existing infrastructure to implement innovative solutions like drive-through testing centers, while the United States initially limited testing to individuals with severe symptoms or known exposures, hampered by restrictive CDC guidelines and technical failures with early test kits (Engelberg et al., 2020). The CDC's first test kits, distributed in early February 2020, contained faulty reagents that produced inconclusive results, leading to significant delays in expanding testing capacity during a critical early window for containment (Choi & Kim, 2024).

By late 2023, global testing capacity had expanded dramatically. The United States, once a testing laggard, had conducted over 1.18 billion cumulative tests—roughly 3.5 million per million people—marking one of the most dramatic diagnostic scale-ups globally (Mathieu et al., 2020a; Worldometer, 2024). The United Kingdom also launched extensive mass testing efforts, ultimately surpassing 522 million tests, or about 7.6 million per million population. Italy and France each conducted over 270 million tests, exceeding 4 million per million. South Korea, which led in early containment through targeted testing, reached approximately 15.8 million tests by 2023, or around 308,000 per million people—favoring precision over volume (Mathieu et al., 2020a; Worldometer, 2024). Brazil and India, despite their large populations, reported lower per capita testing rates at around 296,000 and 665,000 per million, respectively (Worldometer, 2024). These patterns reflected not only resource availability, but deeper strategic differences in how countries opted to confront the evolving demands of the pandemic.

The Evolution of Testing Technologies

While the initial phase of the pandemic revealed critical weaknesses in global testing infrastructure, testing technologies faced their own ongoing challenges and adaptations (Table 9.7). Early polymerase chain reaction (PCR) tests, designed to detect the original Ancestral strain, demonstrated high analytical sensitivity under laboratory conditions, approaching nearly 99.9% in ideal settings (College of American Pathologists (CAP), 2022). However, real-world performance varied significantly, with clinical sensitivity rates ranging from 70 to 80% due to sample collection timing and quality (Wang et al., 2021; Woloshin et al., 2020). Multiple studies reported that PCR sensitivity was highest three to five days after symptom onset, but could drop to as low as 38% if testing occurred very early in infection or late in the recovery phase (Wikramaratna et al., 2020).

The rapid emergence of new variants quickly disrupted existing testing protocols. The Alpha variant's N501Y mutation and H69/V70 deletion initially caused S-gene target failure in some PCR tests, inadvertently providing an early warning system for variant spread (Kirsebom et al., 2022). When Delta emerged, this specific detection mechanism no longer worked, requiring new approaches to variant detection. By late 2020, laboratories had developed multiplexed assays capable of simultaneously screening for multiple variants, though deployment remained costly (Navarro et al., 2021).

Molecular testing capabilities have evolved significantly through multiple technological generations. Loop-mediated isothermal amplification (LAMP) tests emerged as a cost-effective alternative to PCR, offering results in under 30 minutes at a fraction of the cost (Kashir & Yaqinuddin, 2020). By mid-2021, LAMP testing achieved high concordance with PCR while requiring minimal laboratory infrastructure, making it particularly valuable in resource-limited settings (Yoshikawa et al., 2020). RT-LAMP assays demonstrated the ability to detect less than 100 viral genome copies within 30 minutes, with studies showing 99.9% sensitivity and 96.1% specificity for viral loads above 100 copies (Amaral et al., 2021). However, field evaluations sometimes showed more modest performance metrics, with sensitivity ranging from 90 to 95% compared to standard PCR, particularly when viral loads were low (Larremore et al., 2021).

The development of multiplexed PCR assays marked another crucial advance. These tests could simultaneously detect SARS-CoV-2 and distinguish between VOCs, significantly reducing the time between detection and variant identification (Vogels et al., 2021). Some multiplex assays performed comparably to commercial tests but at substantially lower costs, with reagent costs reduced by as much as 60–80% in some implementations (Wang et al., 2023). Multiplexed RT-qPCR approaches proved highly effective for variant surveillance, providing a cost-efficient complement to whole genome sequencing for population-level monitoring (Umunnakwe et al., 2022). These technological innovations enabled both expanded testing access and improved variant tracking, creating critical tools for pandemic response despite resource constraints in many settings.

COVID-19 Surveillance: New Innovations and Challenges

The COVID-19 pandemic drove unprecedented advances in pathogen monitoring through global genomic surveillance networks. The GISAID initiative served as the backbone of this effort, amassing approximately 17.2 million SARS-CoV-2 genetic sequences across 215 countries and territories by 2025 (Global Initiative on Sharing All Influenza Data (GISAID), n.d., 2025). This vast repository enabled researchers to track viral evolution in near real-time, informing critical public health decisions throughout the pandemic.

As the pandemic evolved, public health authorities were forced to transition away from case counts and test positivity rates as the primary metrics for tracking community transmission. In the pandemic's early phases, clinical testing and case reporting provided reasonably accurate estimates of COVID-19 prevalence. However, as the virus became endemic and self-testing became more widespread, reported case counts increasingly underrepresented actual infection rates (Peccia et al., 2020). By late 2021, at-home rapid antigen test use became mainstream, and

Table 9.7 Comparison of COVID-19 Testing Technologies

Testing Method	*Sensitivity (%)*	*Specificity (%)*	*Time*	*Advantages*	*Limitations*
PCR	95–99	>99	4–24 hours	• *High accuracy* • *Gold standard*	• *High cost* • *Lab required*
Rapid Antigen	50–85	97–100	15–30 minutes	• *Fast, inexpensive* • *Widely accessible*	• *Lower sensitivity* • *False negatives*
LAMP (lab/field use)	90–95	98–99	20–45 minutes	• *Portable; field-friendly* • *Faster than PCR*	• *Slightly lower accuracy than PCR*
LAMP (home use)	90–95	98–100	30–45 minutes	• *Fast and convenient* • *Molecular accuracy*	• *High cost* • *Limited supply*
Multiplex PCR	>95	>99	4–24 hours	• *Can detect multiple pathogens concurrently*	• *Very high cost* • *Lab required*
Serology (antibody)	85–95 (post-infection)	>95	1–2 days	• *Can identify prior infection or immunity*	• *Not for acute infection diagnosis*

Sources: CAP (2022); Woloshin et al. (2020); Yoshikawa et al. (2020); Amaral et al. (2021); Vogels et al. (2021); Larremore et al. (2021); Li et al. (2023).

Note: PCR = Polymerase chain reaction; LAMP = Loop-mediated isothermal amplification fewer people sought testing at clinics or local testing sites, with these unreported results creating significant blind spots in surveillance efforts. While hospitalizations and deaths remained reliable indicators of disease severity, the delayed nature of their timing—lagging infections by up to two weeks or more—limited their usefulness for early intervention (Baker et al., 2020).

In this context, wastewater surveillance emerged as a powerful tool for tracking community transmission. Wastewater monitoring provided a non-selective sampling of entire communities regardless of testing behavior or access. It effectively captured both symptomatic and asymptomatic infections, providing a more comprehensive picture of viral circulation (Medema et al., 2020). Studies consistently demonstrated that viral signals in wastewater typically preceded confirmed cases by 10–14 days, with some researchers detecting SARS-CoV-2 in sewage weeks before the first clinical cases were reported in certain regions (WHO, 2023a). This early detection capability allowed communities to implement preventive measures before transmission reached exponential growth (Peccia et al., 2020).

The expansion of wastewater-based epidemiology (WBE) has proven to be a cost-effective and reliable early-warning tool. In 2025, the U.S. CDC's National Wastewater Surveillance System (NWSS) included over 1,500 U.S. sites and monitored additional pathogens like RSV, influenza, and mpox (CDC, 2025a). The European Union mandated wastewater monitoring under its revised Urban Wastewater Treatment Directive, while Canada, Australia, and several EU member states integrated WBE into public health infrastructure. In Uganda, wastewater projects launched in schools, hospitals, and transport hubs enhanced early detection of viral threats in high-risk areas (WHO, 2023a, 2024). Some countries also initiated aircraft wastewater testing to monitor incoming international travelers. The U.S., Canada, and Belgium implemented pilot programs to detect emerging variants through wastewater collected from arriving flights. Collectively, these efforts positioned WBE as a core component of next-generation disease surveillance, offering durable infrastructure for monitoring future outbreaks (CDC, 2025a, 2025b; Naughton et al., 2021).

Overall, the integration of multiple surveillance approaches (Table 9.8) proved especially valuable. Sentinel surveillance networks, strategically positioned in high-risk populations, provided another vital layer of monitoring that helped overcome biases in conventional indicators. In Europe, an artificial intelligence (AI)-based sentinel system using data from networked dialysis clinics successfully predicted local outbreak risks (Bellocchio et al., 2021). These networks, combined with advanced analytics, enabled rapid variant detection, transmission tracking, and impact prediction, with researchers integrating next-generation sequencing and phylogenetic methods to identify potentially concerning variants before widespread transmission could manifest.

Global Genomic Surveillance: Inequities and Progress

The COVID-19 pandemic accelerated the development of pathogen genomic surveillance capabilities worldwide, though with profound geographic disparities in

Table 9.8 Comparison of COVID-19 Surveillance Methods

Surveillance Method	*Advantages*	*Limitations*	*Typical Lead Time for Detection*
Clinical Case Reporting	• Individual-level data • Symptom tracking	• Dependent on testing access • Misses asymptomatic cases	**0 days** *(baseline)*
Wastewater Surveillance	• Global coverage (50+ nations) • Captures asympto-matic cases	• Cannot identify individuals	**10–14 days** *before surge*
Genomic Sequencing	• Detects specific variants • Tracks viral evolution	• Costly • Requires technical expertise	***Variant-dependent***
Sentinel Networks	• Focuses on high-risk populations	• Limited to sentinel groups • Not population-wide	**3–7 days** *before surge*

Sources: CDC (2024); WHO (2025a); GISAID (n.d.); Medema et al. (2020); Peccia et al. (2020); Brito et al. (2022).

implementation, capacity, and timeliness. The most significant disparity existed between high-income and low-income nations. By early 2022, high-income countries had sequenced approximately 3.53% of their COVID-19 cases, while low and middle-income countries averaged just 0.35% (with 78% of high-income countries sequencing above 0.5% of cases vs. only 42% of low and middle-income countries) (Brito et al., 2022). This tenfold difference in sequencing intensity created significant blind spots in global variant tracking, potentially allowing emerging variants to spread undetected in under-resourced regions before being identified elsewhere (Table 9.9).

Despite these disparities, surveillance capacity was shaped by more than just national wealth. A key determinant was whether countries had pre-existing genomic infrastructure. Many nations—especially those without such systems—were compelled to initiate or expand genomic surveillance during the pandemic. For instance, 77% of upper-middle-income and 78% of high-income countries sequencing SARS-CoV-2 had previously established influenza virus sequencing programs. In contrast, only 37.5% of low-income countries had such infrastructure, highlighting how the pandemic served as a catalyst for building new genomic surveillance systems in resource-limited settings (Brito et al., 2022).

While ongoing disparities in genomic surveillance vary by income level, the landscape has shifted significantly since the early phases of the COVID-19 pandemic. In 2025, high-income countries have largely scaled back broad sequencing programs due to reduced funding and shifting priorities, relying instead on more targeted approaches such as representative sampling and wastewater-based surveillance (WHO, 2025b). Conversely, some middle-income countries have expanded their sequencing capacity through international support and regional infrastructure, modestly improving their detection potential. These shifts have narrowed certain gaps while introducing new variability in surveillance strategy and data quality.

Table 9.9 SARS-CoV-2 Genomic Surveillance Capacity by Country Income Level

Country Income Level	*Estimated % of Cases Sequenced*	*Detection Ability (%)*	*Estimated % of Cases Infected Before Detection*	*Surveillance Capabilities*
High Income	0.6–1.2 *(High)*	85–99 *(High)*	1–3 *(Low)*	High-resolution lineage tracking and dynamics
Upper-Middle Income	0.3–0.6 *(Moderate)*	70–90 *(Moderate-High)*	5–8 *(Moderate)*	Track spread and identify emerging patterns
Lower-Middle Income	0.1–0.3 *(Moderate)*	50–70 *(Moderate)*	10–15 *(Moderate-High)*	Estimate prevalence and detect early spread
Low Income	< 0.1 *(Low)*	20–40 *(Low)*	20–30 *(High)*	Detect dominant lineages only

Sources: Synthesized from Brito et al. (2022); CDC (2024); GISAID (n.d., 2025); and WHO Epidemiological Updates (2025a).

Regional initiatives have also played a crucial role in addressing surveillance disparities. By 2022, 40 of 47 African member states (85%) had established in-country genomic sequencing capabilities through efforts coordinated by the Africa CDC's Pathogen Genomics Initiative (Agboli et al., 2025). Similarly, the creation of regional sequencing hubs in South America and Southeast Asia helped build sustainable infrastructure that could be maintained beyond emergency funding cycles (WHO, 2024). Despite these advances, political tensions and data sharing concerns often impeded effective cooperation, as evidenced by delays in sequence submission during critical periods of variant emergence (Nemudryi et al., 2020).

The sequencing turnaround time, which is the period between sample collection and data availability, emerged as another critical metric beyond raw sequencing numbers. Early variant detection requires not just genomic data, but timely genomic data. During the first two years of the pandemic, only about 25% of sequences from high-income countries were submitted within 21 days of sample collection, compared to just 5% from low and middle-income countries (Brito et al., 2022). This disparity in timeliness reduced the utility of sequence data for informing time-sensitive public health decisions in many regions.

Future Directions and Sustainable Models

The landscape of COVID-19 surveillance has been transformed by technological innovation and practical experience. Portable sequencing devices now enable faster analysis with less laboratory infrastructure, and while costs have decreased significantly, they still remain a barrier for widespread adoption in resource-limited settings (Brito et al., 2022). Advanced machine learning approaches have shown impressive capabilities in predicting viral evolution, with some models achieving accuracy rates above 90% in identifying mutations that may lead to immune escape (Ma et al., 2021).

AI applications in surveillance have expanded beyond genomic analysis to include automated wastewater testing, anomaly detection in clinical data, and integrated multi-parameter early warning systems. A study published in 2023 demonstrated that machine learning algorithms could predict the emergence of new SARS-CoV-2 variants 45–60 days before they became dominant by analyzing patterns in existing sequences (Han et al., 2023). These predictive applications show promise for directing targeted surveillance resources more efficiently in future outbreaks.

The integration of surveillance modalities has emerged as a best practice for comprehensive monitoring. Countries that successfully combined clinical testing, wastewater monitoring, genomic surveillance, and sentinel networks demonstrated superior early warning capabilities compared to those relying on any single approach (WHO, 2024). For example, Denmark's integrated surveillance system could detect emerging variants within days of their introduction into the country by cross-correlating signals from wastewater, clinical testing, and genomic analysis (Krogsgaard et al., 2024).

Despite this progress, the economic sustainability of global surveillance systems remains uncertain. Studies suggest that adequate pandemic preparedness in low and middle-income countries requires annual investments of approximately $3–4 billion, a fraction of the economic impact of delayed variant detection (Global Burden of Disease 2021 Health Financing Collaborator Network, 2023). However, securing consistent funding has proven challenging as public attention has largely faded. A World Bank report estimated that in 2024, global funding for pandemic surveillance had declined by 45% from its 2021 peak, raising concerns about diminished capacity for early detection of future threats (World Bank, 2024).

The path forward requires not only continued technological innovation to reduce costs further, but also new frameworks for international cooperation that address both economic disparities and data sharing concerns. The COVID-19 testing and surveillance experience has shown us that technological capability must be paired with sustainable models that overcome systemic barriers to create truly global early warning systems for future pandemic threats. In the next section, we examine how clinical understanding and therapeutic approaches evolved in parallel, marking another critical dimension of the pandemic's trajectory.

Treatment Evolution and Clinical Understanding

The development of COVID-19 treatments followed a rapid but uneven trajectory as clinical understanding of the disease evolved. Initial approaches, often based on repurposed medications, gave way to more targeted therapies as knowledge of viral pathogenesis improved. This evolution in treatment strategies reflected growing insight into both the virus's mechanisms of action and the body's immune response to infection.

Early Approaches and Antiviral Strategies (2020–2021)

The first wave of the pandemic saw widespread experimentation with existing medications, often with limited evidence of efficacy. Hydroxychloroquine emerged as an early candidate following in vitro studies, leading to emergency use authorizations (EUA) in many countries. However, large-scale clinical trials involving 96,000 patients across 671 hospitals eventually demonstrated no benefit and potential harm in the form of cardiac toxicity (RECOVERY Collaborative Group, 2020).

Convalescent plasma also emerged as a possible treatment and was rapidly deployed under EUA in March 2020 as a form of passive antibody therapy. Although it initially showed promise based on theoretical benefit and historical precedent, large randomized trials later demonstrated inconclusive clinical impact, leading to a phase out of hospital protocols and an EUA revocation (Roberts et al., 2022).

By mid-2020, clinical understanding had advanced sufficiently to identify distinct phases of COVID-19 illness—viral replication, inflammatory response, and in severe cases, hypercoagulation. This framework led to more targeted treatment approaches based on disease stage (Wiersinga et al., 2020). Early data from the RECOVERY trial showed that dexamethasone reduced mortality by one-third in ventilated patients, marking the first proven treatment for severe COVID-19 and establishing the role of immunomodulation in late-stage disease (RECOVERY Collaborative Group, 2021a).

Remdesivir became the first antiviral treatment approved for COVID-19, though its impact proved modest. Initial trials showed a reduction in recovery time from 15 to 11 days in hospitalized patients, but no significant effect on mortality (Beigel et al., 2020). Real-world data from 28,855 patients across 41 hospitals revealed that the drug's effectiveness varied significantly based on timing of administration, with early treatment (within seven days of symptom onset) showing a 15% reduction in mortality compared to negligible benefit when started later (Goldman et al., 2020; Wang et al., 2020). More recent meta-analyses from 2023 to 2024 have confirmed this pattern, with pooled data showing remdesivir reduced mortality in patients with severe COVID-19 (RR = 0.57, 95% CI 0.48–0.68) and shortened time to clinical improvement (Chen et al., 2023). A comprehensive individual patient data meta-analysis further demonstrated mortality benefits primarily in patients requiring no or conventional oxygen support, with limited effect for ventilated patients (Amstutz et al., 2023).

The development of oral antivirals marked a more significant advance (Table 9.10). Nirmatrelvir-ritonavir (Paxlovid) initially demonstrated an 89% reduction in hospitalization among high-risk unvaccinated patients when started within three days of symptom onset (Hammond et al., 2022). More recent data from 2024 show somewhat lower but still substantial effectiveness, with the CDC reporting an 87% reduction in hospitalization and death in high-risk patients with early treatment. Real-world effectiveness across broader populations has proven more variable—around 54% overall in preventing hospitalizations and up to 73% in adults over 65 (Yale Medicine, 2024a). The emergence of Paxlovid rebound, occurring in approximately 10–20% of treated patients, highlighted the complexity of

Table 9.10 Antiviral Therapies for COVID-19

Therapy	*Key Dates*	*Primary Mechanism*	*Setting*	*Mortality Reduction*	*Hospitalization Reduction*
Hydroxychloroquine	Mar 2020 (EUA); Jun 2020 (revoke)	Endosomal pH modulator	Outpatient/ Hospitalized	No benefit demonstrated	No benefit demonstrated
Remdesivir	May 2020 (EUA); Oct 2020 (full)	RNA polymerase inhibitor	Hospitalized	0–15% (timing dependent)	N/A
Remdesivir (Outpatient)	Jan 2022 (full)	RNA polymerase inhibitor	Outpatient	Not significant	87% for high-risk patients
Paxlovid	Dec 2021 (EUA); May 2023 (full)	Protease inhibitor	Outpatient	Not assessed directly	89% (unvaccinated), 54–73% (general)
Molnupiravir	Dec 2021 (EUA)	Viral RNA mutagenesis	Outpatient	Not assessed directly	30%
Extended Paxlovid	Jan 2024 (research use)	Persistent viral suppression	Long COVID	N/A	N/A

Sources: RECOVERY Collaborative Group (2020); Beigel et al. (2020); Gottlieb et al. (2022); Hammond et al. (2022); Jayk Bernal et al. (2022); Yale Medicine (2024a); University of California San Francisco (2024).

antiviral treatment administration, though studies have found that rebound symptoms are typically mild and resolve within days without additional treatment (Yale Medicine, 2024a).

Comparative effectiveness studies published in 2024 have offered important insights into antiviral selection. A target trial emulation study in The Lancet Infectious Diseases found no indication that combination therapy with nirmatrelvir-ritonavir and remdesivir provided advantages over nirmatrelvir-ritonavir monotherapy, suggesting that single-agent therapy with Paxlovid may be the most efficient approach for many patients (Choi et al., 2024). However, other research has highlighted that remdesivir maintains an important place in the therapeutic armamentarium, particularly for patients with drug interactions that preclude Paxlovid use (National Institutes of Health, 2025).

Immunomodulation and Evolving Treatment Paradigms (2021–2022)

Clinical understanding of COVID-19's immunopathology led to more sophisticated use of immune-targeting treatments (Table 9.11). By late 2021, evidence supported a staged approach to treatment based on disease progression. For early disease, antivirals and monoclonal antibodies showed the greatest benefit. As the disease progressed, targeted immunomodulation with IL-6 inhibitors became crucial. In severe disease, broad immunosuppression with corticosteroids proved lifesaving (Sweeney et al., 2024).

Baricitinib, a JAK1/2 inhibitor, emerged as a pivotal immunomodulatory therapy. Unlike other immunomodulators, baricitinib demonstrated significant mortality benefits in placebo-controlled trials, with a 38.2% relative reduction and 5 percentage point absolute reduction in 28-day all-cause mortality (Marconi et al., 2021). This treatment works through a dual mechanism, simultaneously inhibiting viral entry into cells and dampening the inflammatory cascade by blocking cytokine signaling. In 2022, the RECOVERY trial confirmed these benefits in a larger population, finding baricitinib reduced mortality by 13% compared to usual care (RR 0.87, 95% CI 0.77–0.98) (RECOVERY Collaborative Group, 2022).

Recent comparative studies from 2024 show that baricitinib may be particularly effective against newer variant strains such as Omicron, with one nationwide cohort study demonstrating lower 30-day mortality rates compared to tocilizumab (53.8% vs. 61.5%) during the Omicron period (You et al., 2025). A systematic review and meta-analysis published in 2022 found a statistically significant reduction in 28-day mortality (OR 0.69, 95% CI 0.50–0.94) in patients receiving baricitinib (Marconi et al., 2021). Direct comparisons between baricitinib and tocilizumab published in 2024 suggest that while both are effective, baricitinib may offer advantages in terms of ease of administration (oral vs. intravenous), shorter half-life, and lower cost of treatment (Sweeney et al., 2024).

Clinical experience revealed distinct patient subgroups with varying treatment needs and outcomes. Analysis of 150,000 hospitalized patients across three continents identified four major phenotypes, each requiring different therapeutic approaches (Marconi et al., 2021; Sweeney et al., 2024). The rapid progressive

Table 9.11 Hospital-Based Immune Therapies and Passive Antibody Treatments for COVID-19

Therapy	*Key Dates*	*Primary Mechanism*	*Setting*	*Mortality Reduction*
Convalescent plasma	Mar 2020 (EUA) Feb 2021 (revoked)	Passive antibody transfer	Hospitalized	Inconclusive
Dexamethasone	June 2020	Broad anti-inflammatory	Hospitalized	17% overall, 33% in ventilated
Baricitinib + Remdesivir	Dec 2020 (EUA)	JAK1/JAK2 inhibitor + antiviral	Hospitalized	30–39%
Tocilizumab	Apr 2021	IL-6 inhibitor	Hospitalized	4–7% relative reduction
Baricitinib (monotherapy)	Jul 2021 (expanded EUA); May 2022 (full)	JAK1/JAK2 inhibitor	Hospitalized	38.2% relative reduction
Dexamethasone + Tocilizumab	Apr 2021	Complementary anti-inflammatory	Hospitalized	30–35%
Vilobelimab	Mar 2024	Complement C5a inhibitor	Critical illness	24% relative reduction
Baricitinib for Long COVID	Jun 2024 (trial initiated)	JAK1/JAK2 inhibitor	Long COVID	Trial ongoing

Sources: RECOVERY Collaborative Group (2021a, 2021b); Kalil et al. (2021); Marconi et al. (2021); Roberts et al. (2022); Sweeney et al. (2024); Vanderbilt University Medical Center (2024).

phenotype, characterized by quick deterioration and high inflammatory markers, showed the best response to early aggressive immunomodulation, with mortality decreasing from 40% to 25% with early intervention. Patients with the hypercoagulable phenotype, marked by elevated D-dimer and thrombotic complications, required intensive anticoagulation, with protocol-driven approaches reducing major thrombotic events by 45%. The hypoxic phenotype with limited inflammation, showing severe hypoxemia but modest inflammatory markers, benefited most from supportive care and prone positioning. Finally, the multisystem inflammatory phenotype, often seen in younger patients with severe organ involvement, responded best to combined immunomodulation strategies (Ferrando et al., 2020; Phua et al., 2020).

Advances in Supportive Care and Specialized Interventions (2021–2023)

Understanding of optimal supportive care evolved significantly as the pandemic progressed. Early aggressive intubation approaches gave way to more nuanced respiratory support strategies as clinicians gained experience. Data from over 89,000 ICU admissions demonstrated that a staged approach to oxygen support—starting with high-flow nasal oxygen and carefully selected progression to mechanical ventilation—reduced mortality by 30% compared to early intubation protocols that characterized the initial pandemic response (Ferrando et al., 2020; Tobin et al., 2020).

The development of specialized interventions reflected a growing understanding of COVID-19's complex pathophysiology. Prone positioning emerged as a crucial intervention for improving oxygenation in severely ill patients. A meta-analysis of 25 studies involving 40,643 patients showed a 26% reduction in mortality when prone positioning was implemented early in severe cases (Guérin et al., 2020). Hospital systems that developed dedicated pruning teams reduced complications by 40% compared to ad hoc approaches, demonstrating the importance of standardized protocols in managing novel clinical challenges.

ECMO utilization similarly evolved through evidence-based patient selection as experience accumulated. Data from the ELSO registry covering 4,812 COVID-19 ECMO cases demonstrated 90-day survival rates of 48% overall, but reaching 65% in carefully selected patients under age 65 without significant comorbidities (Barbaro et al., 2021; Schmidt et al., 2020). These findings led to more precise ECMO protocols, improving resource utilization during surge periods when critical care resources were stretched thin.

The emergence of new variants necessitated continuous adaptation of treatment strategies throughout this period. Monoclonal antibody treatments particularly illustrated this challenge of therapeutic obsolescence in the face of viral evolution. Real-world effectiveness studies demonstrated substantial declines in monoclonal antibody performance, with risk ratios declining from approximately 0.53-0.55 against Alpha and Delta variants to 0.71 against Omicron variants, indicating reduced protection (Kip et al., 2023). Early monoclonal antibody treatments like casirivimab/imdevimab (REGEN-COV) showed strong efficacy against original strains (Weinreich et al., 2021), but subsequently demonstrated complete loss of neutralizing activity against Omicron BA.1 variants. Similarly, sotrovimab, which initially showed promise for early COVID-19 treatment (Gupta et al., 2021), maintained some efficacy against BA.1 but failed against subsequent BA.2 subvariants (Rey et al., 2024). Laboratory studies revealed that nearly all approved monoclonal antibodies demonstrated significant decreases in neutralizing activities against Omicron and its subvariants, with some showing 20-fold or greater reductions in effectiveness (Gruell et al., 2022; Takashita et al., 2022). By 2023, newer combination approaches such as amubarvimab plus romlusevimab emerged as potential treatments (Evering et al., 2023), while select antibodies like bebtelovimab retained activity against certain Omicron sublineages, though even these faced limitations against newer variants like BQ.1 and XBB lineages (Pochtovyi et al., 2023; Wang et al., 2023). This pattern of therapeutic obsolescence reinforced the critical need for continued development of pan-variant treatments and the importance of targeting more conserved viral regions.

Long-Term Complications and Treatment Evolution (2022–2025)

As acute management improved, persistent symptoms following COVID-19 infection emerged as a significant clinical challenge. This condition, termed

Long COVID or Post-Acute Sequelae of SARS-CoV-2 (PASC), represented a new frontier in pandemic response. According to the CDC, approximately 1 in 13 U.S. adults (17.6 million Americans) have experienced Long COVID (CDC, 2025d, 2025e). A 2023 systematic review of 130 publications found prevalence estimates generally ranging from 15 to 30% of COVID-19 survivors experiencing symptoms persisting at least six months post-infection (Woodrow et al., 2023). Global estimates from the Global Burden of Disease study suggest similar patterns, with substantial proportions of individuals experiencing persistent fatigue, cognitive, and respiratory symptoms following symptomatic COVID-19 (Global Burden of Disease Long COVID Collaborators et al., 2022)

Long COVID manifestations cross multiple organ systems, with cardiopulmonary (32%), neurological (25%), psychiatric (20%), and musculoskeletal (15%) symptoms being most common (Deer et al., 2021). The pathophysiology appears complex, involving persistent viral reservoirs, dysregulated immune responses, microthrombi, and autonomic dysfunction (Mehandru & Merad, 2022). Research from 2024 suggests Long COVID risk may be declining with successive variants and increasing vaccination rates, though it remains a significant public health concern (Davis et al., 2023). A deeper exploration of Long COVID epidemiology, pathophysiology, and management will be presented in Chapter 17.

By early 2024, the therapeutic landscape for both acute COVID-19 and its long-term sequelae had become increasingly sophisticated. AI-driven predictive models achieved 80% accuracy in treatment response prediction, enabling more personalized therapeutic approaches (Evashwick et al., 2023). Healthcare systems worldwide developed more resilient treatment infrastructures, with standardized protocols showing significant improvements in outcomes. However, access disparities persisted, particularly in resource-limited settings. The cost of advanced therapeutics remained substantial, ranging from $500 to $5,000 per patient, creating significant barriers to global implementation (WHO, 2023b; Infectious Disease Society of America (IDSA), 2025).

The evolution of COVID-19 treatment approaches has demonstrated both the remarkable adaptability of medical science and the persistent challenges of ensuring equitable access to effective therapies. As viral evolution continues and immunization strategies adapt, therapeutic approaches will likely require ongoing refinement to address both acute COVID-19 and its long-term sequelae.

The emergence of these treatment patterns revealed deeper systemic vulnerabilities. The difficulty in scaling innovations and ensuring consistent care across regions was not just a matter of resources, but of structural preparedness. Collectively, these interlinked trends in viral evolution, transmission dynamics, immunity, surveillance, and clinical care reveal the complexity beneath the surface of the pandemic. Understanding these connections sets the stage for analyzing broader structural factors that further define global responses and outcomes.

References

Adam, D. C., Wu, P., Wong, J. Y., Lau, E. H., Tsang, T. K., Cauchemez, S., Leung, G. M., & Cowling, B. J. (2020). Clustering and superspreading potential of SARS-CoV-2 infections in Hong Kong. *Nature Medicine*, *26*(11), 1714–1719. https://doi.org/10.1038/s41591-020-1092-0

Agboli, E., Bitew, M., Malaka, C. N., Kallon, T. M. P. S., Jalloh, A. M. S., Yankonde, B., Shempela, D. M., Sikalima, J. F. M., Joseph, M., Kasonde, M., Demeke, F. M., Valdese, A. F. I., Grace, L. B., Célestin, G., Papkiauri, A., Berlange, S. Y. F., Majanja, J., Omwenga, V. K., Wambugu, E. N., … Moir, M. (2025). Building pathogen genomic sequencing capacity in Africa: Centre for epidemic response and innovation fellowship. *Tropical Medicine and Infectious Disease*, *10*(4), 90. https://doi.org/10.3390/tropicalmed10040090

Amaral, C., Antunes, W., Moe, E., Duarte, A. G., Lima, L. M. P., Santos, C., Gomes, I. L., Afonso, G. S., Vieira, R., Teles, H. S. S., Reis, M. S., Ramalho da Silva, M. A., Henriques, A. M., Fevereiro, M., Ventura, M. R., Serrano, M., & Pimentel, C. (2021). A molecular test based on RT-LAMP for rapid, sensitive and inexpensive colorimetric detection of SARS-CoV-2 in clinical samples. *Scientific Reports*, *11*, Article 16430. https://doi.org/10.1038/s41598-021-95799-6

Amstutz, A., Speich, B., Mentré, F., Rueegg, C. S., Belhadi, D., Assoumou, L., Burdet, C., Murthy, S., Dodd, L. E., Wang, Y., Malvy, D., Kaiser, L., Nasraway, S. A., Järvisalo, M. J., Zwahlen, M., Sadeghipour, P., Peto, T. J., Schlegel, M., Siegfried, N., … Tikkinen, K. A. O. (2023). Effects of remdesivir in patients hospitalised with COVID-19: A systematic review and individual patient data meta-analysis of randomised controlled trials. *The Lancet Respiratory Medicine*, *11*(8), 746–757. https://doi.org/10.1016/S2213-2600(22)00528-8

Andrews, N., Stowe, J., Kirsebom, F., Toffa, S., Rickeard, T., Gallagher, E., Gower, C., Kall, M., Groves, N., O'Connell, A. M., Simons, D., Blomquist, P. B., Zaidi, A., Nash, S., Iwani Binti Abdul Aziz, N., Thelwall, S., Dabrera, G., Myers, R., Amirthalingam, G., ... Lopez Bernal, J. (2022). COVID-19 vaccine effectiveness against the Omicron (B.1.1.529) variant. *New England Journal of Medicine*, *386*(16), 1532–1546. https://doi.org/10.1056/NEJMoa2119451

Baden, L. R., El Sahly, H. M., Essink, B., Kotloff, K., Frey, S., Novak, R., Diemert, D., Spector, S. A., Rouphael, N., Creech, C. B., McGettigan, J., Khetan, S., Segall, N., Solis, J., Brosz, A., Fierro, C., Schwartz, H., Neuzil, K., Corey, L., … COVE Study Group. (2021). Efficacy and safety of the mRNA-1273 SARS-CoV-2 vaccine. *New England Journal of Medicine*, *384*(5), 403–416. https://doi.org/10.1056/NEJMoa2035389

Baker, R. E., Yang, W., Vecchi, G. A., Metcalf, C. J. E., & Grenfell, B. T. (2020). Susceptible supply limits the role of climate in the early SARS-CoV-2 pandemic. *Science*, *369*(6501), 315–319. https://doi.org/10.1126/science.abc2535

Barbaro, R. P., MacLaren, G., Boonstra, P. S., Iwashyna, T. J., Slutsky, A. S., Fan, E., & Brodie, D. (2021). Extracorporeal membrane oxygenation support in COVID-19: An international cohort study of the extracorporeal life support organization registry. *The Lancet*, *398*(10307), 1230–1240. https://doi.org/10.1016/S0140-6736(21)01960-7

Bar-On, Y. M., Goldberg, Y., Mandel, M., Bodenheimer, O., Freedman, L., Kalkstein, N., Mizrahi, B., Alroy-Preis, S., Ash, N., Milo, R., & Huppert, A. (2021). Protection of BNT162b2 vaccine booster against Covid-19 in Israel. *New England Journal of Medicine*, *385*(15), 1393–1400. https://doi.org/10.1056/NEJMoa2114255

Baud, D., Qi, X., Nielsen-Saines, K., Musso, D., Pomar, L., & Favre, G. (2020). Real estimates of mortality following COVID-19 infection. *The Lancet Infectious Diseases*, 20(7), 773. https://doi.org/10.1016/S1473-3099(20)30195-X

Beigel, J. H., Tomashek, K. M., Dodd, L. E., Mehta, A. K., Zingman, B. S., Kalil, A. C., Hohmann, E., Chu, H. Y., Luetkemeyer, A., Kline, S., Lopez de Castilla, D., Finberg, R. W., Dierberg, K., Tapson, V., Hsieh, L., Patterson, T. F., Paredes, R., Sweeney, D. A., Short, W. R., … Lane, H. C. (2020). Remdesivir for the treatment of COVID-19 – Final report. *New England Journal of Medicine, 383*(19), 1813–1826. https://doi.org/10.1056/NEJMoa2007764

Bellocchio, F., Carioni, P., Lonati, C., Garbelli, M., Martínez-Martínez, F., Stuard, S., & Neri, L. (2021). Enhanced sentinel surveillance system for COVID-19 outbreak prediction in a large European dialysis clinics network. *International Journal of Environmental Research and Public Health, 18*(18), 9739. https://doi.org/10.3390/ijerph18189739

Brito, A. F., Semenova, E., Dudas, G., Hassler, G. W., Kalinich, C. C., Kraemer, M. U. G., Ho, J., Tegally, H., Githinji, G., Agoti, C. N., Khaemba, E., Otieno, E., Davis, M., Goldstein, E., Pybus, O. G., de Oliveira, T., Khan, K., Scarpino, S. V., Sabino, E. C., … Faria, N. R. (2022). Global disparities in SARS-CoV-2 genomic surveillance. *Nature Communications, 13*(1), Article 7003. https://doi.org/10.1038/s41467-022-33713-y

Carlson, C. J., Gomez, A. C., Bansal, S., & Ryan, S. J. (2020). Misconceptions about weather and seasonality must not misguide COVID-19 response. *Nature Communications, 11*(1), 4312. https://doi.org/10.1038/s41467-020-18150-z

Centers for Disease Control and Prevention (CDC). (2022a). COVID-19–Associated hospitalizations among adults during SARS-CoV-2 Delta and Omicron variant predominance, by race/ethnicity and vaccination status—COVID-NET, 14 States, July 2021–January 2022. *Morbidity and Mortality Weekly Report, 71*(12), 466–473. https://doi.org/10.15585/mmwr.mm7112e2

Centers for Disease Control and Prevention (CDC). (2022b). Genomic surveillance for SARS-CoV-2 variants: Predominance of the Delta (B.1.617.2) and Omicron (B.1.1.529) variants—United States, June 2021–January 2022. *Morbidity and Mortality Weekly Report, 71*(6), 206–211. https://doi.org/10.15585/mmwr.mm7106a4

Centers for Disease Control and Prevention (CDC). (2024). Genomic surveillance for SARS-CoV-2 variants: Circulation of Omicron XBB and JN.1 lineages—United States, May 2023–September 2024. *Morbidity and Mortality Weekly Report, 73*(42), 1–7. https://www.cdc.gov/mmwr/volumes/73/wr/mm7342a1.htm

Centers for Disease Control and Prevention (CDC). (2025a). *COVID-19 National Wastewater Data*. National Wastewater Surveillance System (NWSS). https://www.cdc.gov/nwss/rv/COVID19-national-data.html

Centers for Disease Control and Prevention (CDC). (2025b). *COVID-19 Variants in the Wastewater*. https://www.cdc.gov/nwss/rv/COVID19-variants.html

Centers for Disease Control and Prevention (CDC). (2025c). *COVID-19 Variant Proportions*. https://www.cdc.gov/covid/long-term-effects/index.html

Centers for Disease Control and Prevention (CDC). (2025d). *Long COVID basics*. https://www.cdc.gov/covid/long-term-effects/index.html

Centers for Disease Control and Prevention (CDC). (2025e). *CDC Science and the Public Health Approach to Long COVID*. https://www.cdc.gov/long-covid/php/scientific-approach/index.html

Challen, R., Brooks-Pollock, E., Read, J. M., Dyson, L., Tsaneva-Atanasova, K., & Danon, L. (2021). Risk of mortality in patients infected with SARS-CoV-2 variant of concern 202012/1: Matched cohort study. *BMJ, 372*, n579. https://doi.org/10.1136/bmj.n579

Chemaitelly, H., Yassine, H. M., Benslimane, F. M., Al Khatib, H. A., Tang, P., Hasan, M. R., Malek, J. A., Coyle, P., Ayoub, H. H., Al Kanaani, Z., Al Kuwari, E., Jeremijenko, A., Mohamoud, Y. A., Goodman, A. L., Thomas, A. G., Kaleeckal, A. H., Latif, A. N., Bertollini, R., & Abu-Raddad, L. J. (2022). mRNA-1273 COVID-19 vaccine effectiveness against the B.1.1.7 and B.1.351 variants and severe COVID-19 disease in Qatar. *Nature Medicine, 27*(9), 1614–1621. https://doi.org/10.1038/s41591-021-01446-y

Chen, C., Fang, J., Chen, S., Rajaofera, M. J. N., Li, X., Wang, B., & Xia, Q. (2023). The efficacy and safety of remdesivir alone and in combination with other drugs for the treatment of COVID-19: A systematic review and meta-analysis. *BMC Infectious Diseases, 23*(1), 672. https://doi.org/10.1186/s12879-023-08525-0

Choi, O., & Kim, S. (2024). Comparison of the efficacy of COVID-19 responses in South Korea and the United States. *Global Health Action*, *17*(1). https://doi.org/10.1080/16549716.2024.2370611

Choi, M. H., Wan, E. Y. F., Wong, I. C. K., Chan, E. W. Y., Chu, W. M., Tam, A. R., Yuen, K. Y., & Hung, I. F. N. (2024). Comparative effectiveness of combination therapy with nirmatrelvir–ritonavir and remdesivir versus monotherapy with remdesivir or nirmatrelvir–ritonavir in patients hospitalised with COVID-19: A target trial emulation study. *The Lancet Infectious Diseases*, *24*(11), 1213–1224. https://doi.org/10.1016/S1473-3099(24)00353-0

College of American Pathologists (CAP). (2022). *How good are COVID-19 (SARS-CoV-2) diagnostic PCR tests?* https://www.cap.org/member-resources/podcasts/how-good-are-covid-19-diagnostic-pcr-tests

Davies, N. G., Jarvis, C. I., CMMID COVID-19 Working Group, Edmunds, W. J., Jewell, N. P., Diaz-Ordaz, K., & Keogh, R. H. (2021). Increased mortality in community-tested cases of SARS-CoV-2 lineage B.1.1.7. *Nature*, *593*(7858), 270–274. https://doi.org/10.1038/s41586-021-03426-1

Davis, H. E., Assaf, G. S., McCorkell, L., Wei, H., Low, R. J., Re'em, Y., Redfield, S., Austin, J. P., & Akrami, A. (2023). Characterizing long COVID in an international cohort: 7 months of symptoms and their impact. *EClinicalMedicine*, *38*, 101019. https://doi.org/10.1016/j.eclinm.2021.101019

Deer, R. R., Rock, M. A., Vasilevsky, N., Carmody, L., Rando, H., Anzalone, A. J., Basson, M. D., Bennett, T. D., Bergquist, T., Boudreau, E. A., Bramante, C. T., Byrd, J. B., Callahan, T. J., Chan, L. E., Chu, H., Chute, C. G., Coleman, B. D., Davis, H. E., Gagnier, J., … Robinson, P. N. (2021). Characterizing long COVID: Deep phenotype of a complex condition. *EBioMedicine*, *74*, 103722. https://doi.org/10.1016/j.ebiom.2021.103722

Dunkle, L. M., Kotloff, K. L., Gay, C. L., Áñez, G., Adelglass, J. M., Barrat Hernández, A. Q., Harper, W. L., Duncanson, D. M., McArthur, M. A., Florescu, D. F., McClelland, R. S., Garcia-Fragoso, V., Riesenberg, R. A., Musante, D. B., Fried, D. L., Clarke, D. K., Medina, F. A., Cho, I., Glenn, G. M., … Dubovsky, F. (2022). Efficacy and safety of NVX-CoV2373 in adults in the United States and Mexico. *New England Journal of Medicine*, *386*(6), 531–543. https://doi.org/10.1056/NEJMoa2116185

Engelberg, S., Song, L., & DePillis, L. (2020, March 17). *How South Korea scaled coronavirus testing while the U.S. fell dangerously behind*. ProPublica. https://www.propublica.org/article/how-south-korea-scaled-coronavirus-testing-while-the-us-fell-dangerously-behind

European Centre for Disease Prevention and Control. (2024). *COVID-19 vaccine effectiveness against hospitalisation and death using electronic health records in eight European countries in the VEBIS monitoring network – October 2023 to April 2024* [Technical Report]. https://www.ecdc.europa.eu/en/publications-data/covid-19-vaccine-effectiveness-hospitalisation--death-health-records

European Centre for Disease Prevention and Control. (2025). *SARS-CoV-2 variants of concern as of 25 April 2025*. https://www.ecdc.europa.eu/en/covid-19/variants-concern

Evashwick, J. D., Van Hauser, K. M., Kennedy, J. N., Rolfes, M. A., Patel, M. M., Gaglani, M., Ginde, A. A., Douin, D. J., Talbot, H. K., Casey, J. D., Mohr, N. M., Johnson, N. J., Shapiro, N. I., Gibbs, K. W., Files, D. C., Hager, D. N., Shehu, A., Prekker, M. E., Erickson, H. L., & Zaccaro, D. J. (2023). Development of data-driven COVID-19 outcome prediction models comparing monotherapy with combination therapy approaches. *JAMA Network Open*, *6*(11), e2342098. https://doi.org/10.1001/jamanetworkopen.2023.2342098

Evering, T. H., Chew, K. W., Giganti, M. J., Moser, C., Pinilla, M., Wohl, D. A., Currier, J. S., Eron, J. J., Javan, A. C., Bender Ignacio, R., Margolis, D., Zhu, Q., Ma, J., Zhong, L., Yan, L., D'Andrea Nores, U., Hoover, K., Mocherla, B., Choudhary, M. C., Deo, R., Ritz, J., Fischer, W. A., Fletcher, C. V., Li, J. Z., Hughes, M. D., Smith, D., & Daar, E. S., for the ACTIV-2/A5401 Study Team. (2023). Safety and efficacy of combination SARS-CoV-2 neutralizing monoclonal antibodies amubarvimab plus romlusevimab in nonhospitalized patients with COVID-19. *Annals of Internal Medicine*, *176*(5), 658–666. https://doi.org/10.7326/M22-3428

Ferdinands, J. M., Rao, S., Dixon, B. E., Mitchell, P. K., DeSilva, M. B., Irving, S. A., Lewis, N., Natarajan, K., Stenehjem, E., Grannis, S. J., Han, J., Adams, K., Crane, B., Reese, S. E., Embi, P., Dascomb, K., Klein, N. P., DeSilva, M., Vazquez-Benitez, G., … Patel, M. (2022). Waning of vaccine effectiveness against moderate and severe COVID-19 among adults in the US from the VISION network: Test negative case-control study. *BMJ*, *379*, e072141. https://doi.org/10.1136/bmj-2022-072141

Ferrando, C., Suarez-Sipmann, F., Mellado-Artigas, R., Hernández, M., Gea, A., Arruti, E., Aldecoa, C., Martínez-Pallí, G., Martínez-González, M. A., Slutsky, A. S., & Villar, J. (2020). Clinical features, ventilatory management, and outcome of ARDS caused by COVID-19 are similar to other causes of ARDS. *Intensive Care Medicine*, *46*(12), 2200–2211. https://doi.org/10.1007/s00134-020-06192-2

Fisman, D. N., & Tuite, A. R. (2021). Evaluation of the relative virulence of novel SARS-CoV-2 variants: A retrospective cohort study in Ontario, Canada. *CMAJ: Canadian Medical Association Journal*, *193*(42), E1619–E1625. https://doi.org/10.1503/cmaj.211248

Focosi, D., Franchini, M., Joyner, M. J., & Casadevall, A. (2024). Neutralization of SARS-CoV-2 Omicron XBB.1.5 and JN.1 variants after COVID-19 booster-vaccination and infection. *Journal of General Virology*, *105*(1), 001886. https://doi.org/10.1099/jgv.0.001886

Global Burden of Disease 2021 Health Financing Collaborator Network. (2023). Global investments in pandemic preparedness and COVID-19: Development assistance and domestic spending on health between 1990 and 2026. *The Lancet Global Health*, *11*(3), e385–e413. https://doi.org/10.1016/S2214-109X(23)00007-4

Global Burden of Disease Long COVID Collaborators, Wulf Hanson, S., Abbafati, C., Aerts, J. G., Al-Aly, Z., Ashbaugh, C., Ballouz, T., Blyuss, O., Bobkova, P., Bonsel, G., Borzakova, S., Buonsenso, D., Butnaru, D., Carter, A., Chu, H., De Rose, C., Diab, M. M., Ekbom, E., El Tantawi, M., Fomin, V., … Vos, T. (2022). Estimated global proportions of individuals with persistent fatigue, cognitive, and respiratory symptom clusters following symptomatic COVID-19 in 2020 and 2021. *JAMA*, *328*(16), 1604–1615. https://doi.org/10.1001/jama.2022.18931

Global Initiative on Sharing All Influenza Data (GISAID). (n.d.). *hCoV-19 variants*. https://gisaid.org/hcov19-variants/

Global Initiative on Sharing All Influenza Data (GISAID). (2025, April 30). *hCoV-19 data sharing: 215 countries and territories*. https://gisaid.org/fileadmin/c/gisaid/files/pdfs/215_Countries_hCoV_data_sharing.pdf

Goldberg, Y., Mandel, M., Bar-On, Y. M., Bodenheimer, O., Freedman, L., Haas, E. J., Milo, R., Alroy-Preis, S., Ash, N., & Huppert, A. (2021). Waning immunity after the BNT162b2 vaccine in Israel. *New England Journal of Medicine*, *385*(24), e85. https://doi.org/10.1056/NEJMoa2114228

Goldman, J. D., Lye, D. C. B., Hui, D. S., Marks, K. M., Bruno, R., Montejano, R., Spinner, C. D., Galli, M., Ahn, M. Y., Nahass, R. G., Chen, Y. S., SenGupta, D., Hyland, R. H., Osinusi, A. O., Cao, H., Blair, C., Wei, X., Gaggar, A., Brainard, D. M., … Subramanian, A. (2020). Remdesivir for 5 or 10 days in patients with severe COVID-19. *New England Journal of Medicine*, *383*(19), 1827–1837. https://doi.org/10.1056/NEJMoa2015301

Gottlieb, R. L., Vaca, C. E., Paredes, R., Mera, J., Webb, B. J., Perez, G., Oguchi, G., Ryan, P., Nielsen, B. U., Brown, M., Hidalgo, A., Sachdeva, Y., Mittal, S., Osiyemi, O., Skarbinski, J., Juneja, K., Hyland, R. H., Osinusi, A., Chen, S., … Sealfon, R. S. (2022). Early remdesivir to prevent progression to severe COVID-19 in outpatients. *New England Journal of Medicine*, *386*(4), 305–315. https://doi.org/10.1056/NEJMoa2116846

Grasselli, G., Pesenti, A., & Cecconi, M. (2020). Critical care utilization for the COVID-19 outbreak in Lombardy, Italy: Early experience and forecast during an emergency response. *JAMA*, *323*(16), 1545–1546. https://doi.org/10.1001/jama.2020.4031

Gruell, H., Vanshylla, K., Tober-Lau, P., Hillus, D., Schommers, P., Lehmann, C., Kurth, F., Sander, L. E., & Klein, F. (2022). mRNA booster immunization elicits potent neutralizing serum activity against the SARS-CoV-2 Omicron variant. *Nature Medicine, 28*(3), 477–480. https://doi.org/10.1038/s41591-021-01676-0

Guérin, C., Albert, R. K., Beitler, J., Gattinoni, L., Jaber, S., Marini, J. J., Munshi, L., Papazian, L., Pesenti, A., Vieillard-Baron, A., & Mancebo, J. (2020). Prone position in ARDS patients: Why, when, how and for whom. *Intensive Care Medicine, 46*(12), 2385–2396. https://doi.org/10.1007/s00134-020-06306-w

Gupta, A., Gonzalez-Rojas, Y., Juarez, E., Crespo Casal, M., Moya, J., Falci, D. R., Sarkis, E., Solis, J., Zheng, H., Scott, N., Cathcart, A. L., Hebner, C. M., Sager, J., Mogalian, E., Tipple, C., Peppercorn, A., Alexander, E., Pang, P. S., Free, A., … Shapiro, A. E. (2021). Early treatment for COVID-19 with SARS-CoV-2 neutralizing antibody sotrovimab. *New England Journal of Medicine, 385*(21), 1941–1950. https://doi.org/10.1056/NEJMoa2107934

Gutierrez, J. M., Groves, H. E., Isabel, M. R., Patel, S. N., Gubbay, J. B., Guttman, D. S., & Poutanen, S. M. (2020). Evolutionary and structural analyses of SARS-CoV-2 D614G spike protein mutation now documented worldwide. *Scientific Reports, 10*, 14031. https://doi.org/10.1038/s41598-020-70827-z

Haldane, V., De Foo, C., Abdalla, S. M., Jung, A. S., Tan, M., Wu, S., Chua, A., Verma, M., Shrestha, P., Singh, S., Perez, T., Tan, S. M., Bartos, M., Mabuchi, S., Bonk, M., McNab, C., Werner, G. K., Panjabi, R., Nordström, A., … Legido-Quigley, H. (2021). Health systems resilience in managing the COVID-19 pandemic: Lessons from 28 countries. *Nature Medicine, 27*(6), 964–980. https://doi.org/10.1038/s41591-021-01381-y

Hamidi, S., Sabouri, S., & Ewing, R. (2020). Does density aggravate the COVID-19 pandemic? Early findings and lessons for planners. *Journal of the American Planning Association, 86*(4), 495–509. https://doi.org/10.1080/01944363.2020.1777891

Hammond, J., Leister-Tebbe, H., Gardner, A., Abreu, P., Bao, W., Wisemandle, W., Baniecki, M., Hendrick, V. M., Damle, B., Simón-Campos, A., Pypstra, R., & Rusnak, J. M. (2022). Oral nirmatrelvir for high-risk, nonhospitalized adults with COVID-19. *New England Journal of Medicine, 386*(15), 1397–1408. https://doi.org/10.1056/NEJMoa2118542

Han, W., Chen, N., Xu, X., Sahil, A., Zhou, J., Li, Z., Zhong, H., Gao, E., Zhang, R., Wang, Y., Sun, S., Cheung, P. P.-H., & Gao, X. (2023). Predicting the antigenic evolution of SARS-CoV-2 with deep learning. *Nature Communications, 14*, 3478. https://doi.org/10.1038/s41467-023-39199-6

Heath, P. T., Galiza, E. P., Baxter, D. N., Boffito, M., Browne, D., Burns, F., Chadwick, D. R., Clark, R., Cosgrove, C. A., Galloway, J., Goodman, A. L., Heer, A., Higham, A., Iyengar, S., Jeanes, C., Kalra, P. A., Kyriakidou, C., Bradley, J. M., Munthali, C., Minassian, A. M., … Toback, S. (2023). Safety and efficacy of the NVX-CoV2373 coronavirus disease 2019 vaccine at completion of the placebo-controlled phase of a randomized controlled trial. *Clinical Infectious Diseases, 76*(3), 398–407. https://doi.org/10.1093/cid/ciac803

Huiberts, A. J., Hoeve, C. E., de Gier, B., Cremer, J., van der Veer, B., de Melker, H. E., van de Wijgert, J. H. H. M., van den Hof, S., Eggink, D., & Knol, M. J. (2024). Effectiveness of Omicron XBB.1.5 vaccine against infection with SARS-CoV-2 Omicron XBB and JN.1 variants, prospective cohort study, the Netherlands, October 2023 to January 2024. *Eurosurveillance, 29*(10), 2400109. https://doi.org/10.2807/1560-7917.ES.2024.29.10.2400109

Infectious Disease Society of America (IDSA). (2025). *IDSA guidelines on the treatment and management of patients with COVID-19*. Infectious Diseases Society of America Guidelines. https://www.idsociety.org/practice-guideline/covid-19-guideline-treatment-and-management/

Jay, J., Bor, J., Nsoesie, E. O., Lipson, S. K., Jones, D. K., Galea, S., & Raifman, J. (2020). Neighbourhood income and physical distancing during the COVID-19 pandemic in the United States. *Nature Human Behaviour, 4*(12), 1294–1302. https://doi.org/10.1038/s41562-020-00998-2

Jayk Bernal, A., Gomes da Silva, M. M., Musungaie, D. B., Kovalchuk, E., Gonzalez, A., Delos Reyes, V., Martín-Quirós, A., Caraco, Y., Williams-Diaz, A., Brown, M. L., Du, J., Pedley, A., Assaid, C., Strizki, J., Grobler, J. A., Shamsuddin, H. H., Tipping, R., Wan, H., Paschke, A., … De Anda, C. (2022). Molnupiravir for oral treatment of COVID-19 in nonhospitalized patients. *New England Journal of Medicine*, *386*(6), 509–520. https://doi.org/10.1056/NEJMoa2116044

Kalil, A. C., Patterson, T. F., Mehta, A. K., Tomashek, K. M., Wolfe, C. R., Ghazaryan, V., Marconi, V. C., Ruiz-Palacios, G. M., Hsieh, L., Kline, S., Tapson, V., Iovine, N. M., Jain, M. K., Sweeney, D. A., El Sahly, H. M., Branche, A. R., Regalado Pineda, J., Lye, D. C., Sandkovsky, U., … Doernberg, S. B. (2021). Baricitinib plus remdesivir for hospitalized adults with COVID-19. *New England Journal of Medicine*, *384*(9), 795–807. https://doi.org/10.1056/NEJMoa2031994

Kashir, J., & Yaqinuddin, A. (2020). Loop mediated isothermal amplification (LAMP) assays as a rapid diagnostic for COVID-19. *Medical Hypotheses*, *141*, 109786. https://doi.org/10.1016/j.mehy.2020.109786

Kip, K. E., McCreary, E. K., Collins, K., Minnier, T. E., Snyder, G. M., Garrard, W., McKibben, J. C., Yealy, D. M., Seymour, C. W., Huang, D. T., Bariola, J. R., Schmidhofer, M., Wadas, R. J., Angus, D. C., Kip, P. L., & Marroquin, O. C. (2023). Evolving real-world effectiveness of monoclonal antibodies for treatment of COVID-19: A cohort study. *Annals of Internal Medicine*, *176*(4), 496–504. https://doi.org/10.7326/M22-1286

Kirsebom, F. C. M., Andrews, N., Stowe, J., Toffa, S., Sachdeva, R., Gallagher, E., Simmons, R., Lopez Bernal, J., Ramsay, M., Dabrera, G., Amirthalingam, G., & Brown, K. (2022). COVID-19 vaccine effectiveness against the Omicron (BA.2) variant in England. *The Lancet Infectious Diseases*, *22*(7), 931–933. https://doi.org/10.1016/S1473-3099(22)00309-7

Kirsebom, F. C. M., Stowe, J., Lopez Bernal, J., Hall, V., Andrews, N., Simpson, C., Mathieu, E., Coughlan, L., Cole, R., & Amirthalingam, G. (2024). Effectiveness of autumn 2023 COVID-19 vaccination and residual protection of prior doses against hospitalisation in England. *Journal of Infection*, *89*(1), 106177. https://doi.org/10.1016/j.jinf.2024.02.017

Kissler, S. M., Tedijanto, C., Goldstein, E., Grad, Y. H., & Lipsitch, M. (2020). Projecting the transmission dynamics of SARS-CoV-2 through the postpandemic period. *Science*, *368*(6493), 860–868. https://doi.org/10.1126/science.abb5793

Krammer, F., & Ellebedy, A. H. (2023). Variant-adapted COVID-19 booster vaccines. *Science (New York, N.Y.)*, *382*(6667), 157–159. https://doi.org/10.1126/science.adh2712

Krause, P. R., Fleming, T. R., Longini, I. M., Peto, R., Briand, S., Heymann, D. L., Beral, V., Snape, M. D., Rees, H., Ropero, A. M., Balicer, R. D., Cramer, J. P., Muñoz-Fontela, C., Gruber, M., Gaspar, R., Singh, J. A., Subbarao, K., Van Kerkhove, M. D., Swaminathan, S., … Henao-Restrepo, A. M. (2021). SARS-CoV-2 variants and vaccines. *New England Journal of Medicine*, *385*(2), 179–186. https://doi.org/10.1056/NEJMsr2105280

Krogsgaard, L. W., Benedetti, G., Gudde, A., Richter, S. R., Rasmussen, L. D., Midgley, S. E., Qvesel, A. G., Nauta, M., Bahrenscheer, N. S., von Kappelgaard, L., McManus, O., Hansen, N. C., Pedersen, J. B., Haimes, D., Gamst, J., Nørgaard, L. S., Jørgensen, A. C. U., Ejegod, D. M., Møller, S. S., Clauson-Kaas, J., Knudsen, I. M., Franck, K. T., & Ethelberg, S. (2024). Results from the SARS-CoV-2 wastewater-based surveillance system in Denmark, July 2021 to June 2022. *Water Research*, *252*, 121223. https://doi.org/10.1016/j.watres.2024.121223

Kurhade, C., Zou, J., Xia, H., Liu, M., Chang, H. C., Ren, P., Xie, X., & Shi, P. Y. (2023). Low neutralization of SARS-CoV-2 Omicron BA.2.75.2, BQ.1.1, and XBB.1 by parental mRNA vaccine or a BA.5 bivalent booster. *Nature Medicine*, *29*(2), 344–347. https://doi.org/10.1038/s41591-022-02162-x

Larremore, D. B., Wilder, B., Lester, E., Shehata, S., Burke, J. M., Hay, J. A., Tambe, M., Mina, M. J., & Parker, R. (2021). Test sensitivity is secondary to frequency and turnaround time for COVID-19 screening. *Science Advances*, *7*(1), eabd5393. https://doi.org/10.1126/sciadv.abd5393

Lee, C. Y., Kuo, H. W., Liu, Y. L., Chuang, J. H., & Chou, J. H. (2024). Population-Based Evaluation of Vaccine Effectiveness against SARS-CoV-2 Infection, Severe Illness, and Death, Taiwan. *Emerging Infectious Diseases*, *30*(3), 478–489. https://doi.org/10.3201/eid3003.230893

Li, B., Deng, A., Li, K., Hu, Y., Li, Z., Shi, Y., Xiong, Q., Liu, Z., Guo, Q., Zou, L., Zhang, H., Zhang, M., Ouyang, F., Su, J., Su, W., Xu, J., Lin, H., Sun, J., … Lu, J. (2022). Viral infection and transmission in a large, well-traced outbreak caused by the SARS-CoV-2 Delta variant. *Nature Communications*, *13*, 460. https://doi.org/10.1038/s41467-022-28089-y

Li, J. X., Liao, P. L., Wei, J. C., Hsu, S. B., & Yeh, C. J. (2023). A chronological review of COVID-19 case fatality rate and its secular trend and investigation of all-cause mortality and hospitalization during the Delta and Omicron waves in the United States: A retrospective cohort study. *Frontiers in Public Health*, *11*, 1143650. https://doi.org/10.3389/fpubh.2023.1143650

Lin, D. Y., Xu, Y., Gu, Y., Zeng, D., Wheeler, B., Young, H., Sunny, S. K., & Moore, Z. (2024). Study shows effectiveness of updated COVID-19 vaccines wanes moderately over time, is lower against currently circulating variants. *New England Journal of Medicine*, *390*(22), 2079–2082. https://doi.org/10.1056/NEJMc2402779

Link-Gelles, R., Ciesla, A. A., Fleming-Dutra, K. E., Smith, Z. R., Britton, A., Wiegand, R. E., Ilang, C. N., Miller, J. D., Accorsi, E. K., Schrag, S. J., Verani, J. R., MacNeil, A., & Patel, M. M. (2022). Effectiveness of bivalent mRNA vaccines in preventing symptomatic SARS-CoV-2 infection—Increasing Community Access to Testing program, United States, September–November 2022. *Morbidity and Mortality Weekly Report*, *71*(48), 1526–1530. https://doi.org/10.15585/mmwr.mm7148e1

Link-Gelles, R., Ciesla, A. A., Mak, J., Roper, L. E., Iuliano, A. D., Britton, A., Fleming-Dutra, K. E., Smith, Z. R., Miller, J. D., Accorsi, E. K., Schrag, S. J., MacNeil, A., & Patel, M. M. (2024). Early estimates of updated 2023–2024 (monovalent XBB.1.5) COVID-19 vaccine effectiveness against symptomatic SARS-CoV-2 infection attributable to co-circulating Omicron variants among immunocompetent adults. *Morbidity and Mortality Weekly Report*, *73*(4), 102–107. https://doi.org/10.15585/mmwr.mm7304a2

Link-Gelles, R., Chickery, S., Webber, A., Ong, T. C., Rowley, E. A. K., DeSilva, M. B., Dascomb, K., Irving, S. A., Klein, N. P., Grannis, S. J., Barron, M. A., Reese, S. E., McEvoy, C., Sheffield, T., Naleway, A. L., Zerbo, O., Rogerson, C., Self, W. H., Zhu, Y., … CDC COVID-19 Vaccine Effectiveness Collaborators. (2025). Interim estimates of 2024–2025 COVID-19 vaccine effectiveness among adults aged ≥18 years—VISION and IVY Networks, September 2024–January 2025. *MMWR. Morbidity and Mortality Weekly Report*, *74*(6), 74–82.

Lopez Bernal, J., Andrews, N., Gower, C., Gallagher, E., Simmons, R., Thelwall, S., Stowe, J., Tessier, E., Groves, N., Dabrera, G., Myers, R., Campbell, C. N. J., Amirthalingam, G., Edmunds, M., Zambon, M., Brown, K. E., Hopkins, S., Chand, M., & Ramsay, M. (2021). Effectiveness of the Pfizer-BioNTech and Oxford-AstraZeneca vaccines on COVID-19 related symptoms, hospital admissions, and mortality in older adults in England: Test negative case-control study. *BMJ*, *373*, n1088. https://doi.org/10.1136/bmj.n1088

Lyngse, F. P., Kirkeby, C. T., Denwood, M., Christiansen, L. E., Mølbak, K., Møller, C. H., Skov, R. L., Krause, T. G., Rasmussen, M., Sieber, R. N., Johannesen, T. B., Lillebaek, T., Fonager, J., Fomsgaard, A., Møller, F. T., Stegger, M., Overvad, M., Spiess, K., & Mortensen, L. H. (2022). Household transmission of SARS-CoV-2 Omicron variant of concern subvariants BA.1 and BA.2 in Denmark. *Nature Communications*, *13*, 5760. https://doi.org/10.1038/s41467-022-33498-0

Ma, Y., Pei, S., Shaman, J., Dubrow, R., & Chen, K. (2021). Role of meteorological factors in the transmission of SARS-CoV-2 in the United States. *Nature Communications*, *12*(1), 3602. https://doi.org/10.1038/s41467-021-23866-7

Marconi, V. C., Ramanan, A. V., de Bono, S., Kartman, C. E., Krishnan, V., Liao, R., Piruzeli, M. L. B., Goldman, J. D., Alatorre-Alexander, J., de Cassia Pellegrini, R., Estrada, V., Som, M., Cardoso, A., Chakladar, S., Crowe, B., Reis, P., Zhang, X., Adams, D. H.,

& Esteban, A. (2021). Efficacy and safety of baricitinib for the treatment of hospitalised adults with COVID-19 (COV-BARRIER): A randomised, double-blind, parallel-group, placebo-controlled phase 3 trial. *The Lancet Respiratory Medicine*, *9*(12), 1407–1418. https://doi.org/10.1016/S2213-2600(21)00331-3

Maslo, C., Friedland, R., Toubkin, M., Laubscher, A., Akaloo, T., & Kama, B. (2022). Characteristics and outcomes of hospitalized patients in South Africa during the COVID-19 Omicron wave compared with previous waves. *JAMA*, *327*(6), 583–584. https://doi.org/10.1001/jama.2021.24868

Mathieu, E., Ritchie, H., Rodés-Guirao, L., Appel, C., Gavrilov, D., Giattino, C., Hasell, J., Macdonald, B., Dattani, S., Beltekian, D., Ortiz-Ospina, E., & Roser, M. (2020a). *COVID-19 pandemic*. Our World in Data. https://ourworldindata.org/coronavirus

Mathieu, E., Ritchie, H., Rodés-Guirao, L., Appel, C., Gavrilov, D., Giattino, C., Hasell, J., Macdonald, B., Dattani, S., Beltekian, D., Ortiz-Ospina, E., & Roser, M. (2020b). *Excess mortality during the coronavirus pandemic (COVID-19)*. Our World in Data. https://ourworldindata.org/excess-mortality-covid

Mathieu, E., Ritchie, H., Ortiz-Ospina, E., Roser, M., Hasell, J., Appel, C., Giattino, C., & Rodés-Ospina, L. (2023). A global database of COVID-19 vaccinations. *Nature Human Behaviour*, *5*, 947–953. https://doi.org/10.1038/s41562-021-01122-8

Medema, G., Heijnen, L., Elsinga, G., Italiaander, R., & Brouwer, A. (2020). Presence of SARS-coronavirus-2 in sewage and correlation with reported COVID-19 prevalence in the early stage of the epidemic in the Netherlands. *Environmental Science & Technology Letters*, *7*(7), 511–516. https://doi.org/10.1021/acs.estlett.0c00357

Mehandru, S., & Merad, M. (2022). Pathological sequelae of long-haul COVID. *Nature Immunology*, *23*(2), 194–202. https://doi.org/10.1038/s41590-021-01104-y

Mena, G. E., Martínez, P. P., Mahmud, A. S., Marquet, P. A., Buckee, C. O., & Santillana, M. (2021). Socioeconomic status determines COVID-19 incidence and related mortality in Santiago, Chile. *Science*, *372*(6545), eabg5298. https://doi.org/10.1126/science.abg5298

Merow, C., & Urban, M. C. (2020). Seasonality and uncertainty in global COVID-19 growth rates. *Proceedings of the National Academy of Sciences*, *117*(44), 27456–27464. https://doi.org/10.1073/pnas.2008590117

Moriyama, M., Hugentobler, W. J., & Iwasaki, A. (2020). Seasonality of respiratory viral infections. *Annual Review of Virology*, *7*, 83–101. https://doi.org/10.1146/annurev-virology-012420-022445

Moustsen-Helms, I. R., Bager, P., Larsen, T. G., Møller, F. T., Vestergaard, L. S., Christiansen, L. E., Valentiner-Branth, P., & Hansen, C. H. (2024). Relative vaccine protection, disease severity and symptoms associated with infection with SARS-CoV-2 Omicron subvariant Ba.2.86 and descendent Jn.1: A Danish nationwide register-based study. *SSRN*. https://doi.org/10.2139/ssrn.4716761

National Institutes of Health (NIH). (2024). COVID-19 treatment guidelines. https://www.ncbi.nlm.nih.gov/books/NBK570371/pdf/Bookshelf_NBK570371.pdf

Naughton, C. C., Roman, F. A., Alvarado, A. G. F., Tariqi, A. Q., Deeming, M. A., Kadonsky, K. F., Bibby, K., Bivins, A., Medema, G., Ahmed, W., Katsivelis, P., Allan, V., Sinclair, R., & Rose, J. B. (2023). Show us the data: Global COVID-19 wastewater monitoring efforts, equity, and gaps. *FEMS Microbes*, *4*, xtad003. https://doi.org/10.1093/femsmc/xtad003

Navarro, A., Gómez, L., Sanseverino, I., Niegowska, M., Roka, E., Pedraccini, R., Vargha, M., & Lettieri, T. (2021). SARS-CoV-2 detection in wastewater using multiplex quantitative PCR. *Science of the Total Environment*, 797, 148890. https://doi.org/10.1016/j.scitotenv.2021.148890

Nemudryi, A., Nemudraia, A., Wiegand, T., Surya, K., Buyukyoruk, M., Cicha, C., Vanderwood, K. K., Wilkinson, R., & Wiedenheft, B. (2020). Temporal detection and phylogenetic assessment of SARS-CoV-2 in municipal wastewater. *Cell Reports Medicine*, *1*(6), 100098. https://doi.org/10.1016/j.xcrm.2020.100098

NIH RECOVER Initiative. (2024, December 17). *Reviewing RECOVER's impact in 2024: Understanding, treating, and preventing Long COVID*. RECOVER Initiative, National Institutes of Health. Retrieved from https://recovercovid.org/news/reviewing-recovers-impact-2024

Nyberg, T., Ferguson, N. M., Nash, S. G., Webster, H. H., Flaxman, S., Andrews, N., Hinsley, W., Bernal, J. L., Kall, M., Bhatt, S., Needham, K., Obi, C., Zambon, M., Funk, S., Chand, M., Brown, C. S., United Kingdom Health Security Agency, COVID-19 National Infection Service Surveillance Team, Ramsay, M., … Thelwall, S. (2022). Comparative analysis of the risks of hospitalisation and death associated with SARS-CoV-2 omicron (B.1.1.529) and delta (B.1.617.2) variants in England: A cohort study. *The Lancet*, *399*(10332), 1303–1312. https://doi.org/10.1016/S0140-6736(22)00462-7

O'Toole, Á, Scher, E., Underwood, A., Jackson, B., Hill, V., McCrone, J. T., Colquhoun, R., Ruis, C., Abu-Dahab, K., Taylor, B., Yeats, C., du Plessis, L., Maloney, D., Medd, N., Attwood, S. W., Aanensen, D. M., Holmes, E. C., Pybus, O. G., & Rambaut, A. (2021). Assignment of epidemiological lineages in an emerging pandemic using the pangolin tool. *Virus Evolution*, *7*(2), veab064. https://doi.org/10.1093/ve/veab064

Peccia, J., Zulli, A., Brackney, D. E., Grubaugh, N. D., Kaplan, E. H., Casanovas-Massana, A., Ko, A. I., Malik, A. A., Wang, D., Wang, M., Warren, J. L., Weinberger, D. M., Arnold, W., & Omer, S. B. (2020). Measurement of SARS-CoV-2 RNA in wastewater tracks community infection dynamics. *Nature Biotechnology*, *38*(10), 1164–1167. https://doi.org/10.1038/s41587-020-0684-z

Petherick, A., Goldszmidt, R., Andrade, E. B., Furst, R., Hale, T., Pott, A., & Wood, A. (2021). A worldwide assessment of changes in adherence to COVID-19 protective behaviours and hypothesized pandemic fatigue. *Nature Human Behaviour*, *5*(9), 1145–1160. https://doi.org/10.1038/s41562-021-01181-x

Phua, J., Weng, L., Ling, L., Egi, M., Lim, C. M., Divatia, J. V., Shrestha, B. R., Arabi, Y. M., Ng, J., Gomersall, C. D., Nishimura, M., Koh, Y., & Du, B. (2020). Intensive care management of coronavirus disease 2019 (COVID-19): Challenges and recommendations. *The Lancet Respiratory Medicine*, *8*(5), 506–517. https://doi.org/10.1016/S2213-2600(20)30161-2

Plante, J. A., Liu, Y., Liu, J., Xia, H., Johnson, B. A., Lokugamage, K. G., Zhang, X., Muruato, A. E., Zou, J., Fontes-Garfias, C. R., Mirchandani, D., Scharton, D., Bilello, J. P., Ku, Z., An, Z., Kalveram, B., Freiberg, A. N., Menachery, V. D., Xie, X., … Shi, P. Y. (2021). Spike mutation D614G alters SARS-CoV-2 fitness. *Nature*, *592*(7852), 116–121. https://doi.org/10.1038/s41586-020-2895-3

Pochtovyi, A. A., Kustova, D. D., Siniavin, A. E., Dolzhikova, I. V., Shidlovskaya, E. V., Shpakova, O. G., Vasilchenko, L. A., Glavatskaya, A. A., Kuznetsova, N. A., Iliukhina, A. A., Shelkov, A. Y., Grinkevich, O. M., Komarov, A. G., Logunov, D. Y., Gushchin, V. A., & Gintsburg, A. L. (2023). In vitro efficacy of antivirals and monoclonal antibodies against SARS-CoV-2 Omicron lineages XBB.1.9.1, XBB.1.9.3, XBB.1.5, XBB.1.16, XBB.2.4, BQ.1.1.45, CH.1.1, and CL.1. *Vaccines*, *11*(10), 1533. https://doi.org/10.3390/vaccines11101533

Polack, F. P., Thomas, S. J., Kitchin, N., Absalon, J., Gurtman, A., Lockhart, S., Perez, J. L., Pérez Marc, G., Moreira, E. D., Zerbini, C., Bailey, R., Swanson, K. A., Roychoudhury, S., Koury, K., Li, P., Kalina, W. V., Cooper, D., Frenck, R. W., Hammitt, L. L., … C4591001 Clinical Trial Group. (2020). Safety and efficacy of the BNT162b2 mRNA COVID-19 vaccine. *New England Journal of Medicine*, *383*(27), 2603–2615. https://doi.org/10.1056/NEJMoa2034577

Pouwels, K. B., Pritchard, E., Matthews, P. C., Stoesser, N., Eyre, D. W., Vihta, K.-D., House, T., Hay, J., Bell, J. I., Newton, J. N., Farrar, J., Crook, D., Cook, D., Rourke, E., Studley, R., Peto, T. E. A., Diamond, I., & Walker, A. S. (2021). Effect of delta variant on viral burden and vaccine effectiveness against new SARS-CoV-2 infections in the UK. *Nature Medicine*, *27*(12), 2127–2135. https://doi.org/10.1038/s41591-021-01548-7

Rader, B., Scarpino, S. V., Nande, A., Hill, A. L., Adlam, B., Reiner, R. C., Pigott, D. M., Gutierrez, B., Zarebski, A. E., Shrestha, M., Brownstein, J. S., Castro, M. C., Dye, C., Tian, H., Pybus, O. G., & Kraemer, M. U. G. (2020). Crowding and the shape of COVID-19 epidemics. *Nature Medicine*, *26*(12), 1829–1834. https://doi.org/10.1038/s41591-020-1104-0

Rambaut, A., Holmes, E. C., O'Toole, Á., Hill, V., McCrone, J. T., Ruis, C., du Plessis, L., & Pybus, O. G. (2020). A dynamic nomenclature proposal for SARS-CoV-2 lineages to assist genomic epidemiology. *Nature Microbiology*, *5*(11), 1403–1407. https://doi.org/10.1038/s41564-020-0770-5

RECOVERY Collaborative Group. (2020). Effect of hydroxychloroquine in hospitalized patients with COVID-19. *New England Journal of Medicine*, *383*(21), 2030–2040. https://doi.org/10.1056/NEJMoa2022926

RECOVERY Collaborative Group. (2021a). Dexamethasone in hospitalized patients with COVID-19. *New England Journal of Medicine*, *384*(8), 693–704. https://doi.org/10.1056/NEJMoa2021436

RECOVERY Collaborative Group. (2021b). Tocilizumab in patients admitted to hospital with COVID-19 (RECOVERY): A randomised, controlled, open-label, platform trial. *The Lancet*, *397*(10285), 1637–1645. https://doi.org/10.1016/S0140-6736(21)00676-0

RECOVERY Collaborative Group. (2022). Baricitinib in patients admitted to hospital with COVID-19 (RECOVERY): A randomised, controlled, open-label, platform trial and updated meta-analysis. *The Lancet*, *400*(10349), 359–368. https://doi.org/10.1016/S0140-6736(22)01109-6

Rey, D., Fafi-Kremer, S., Hantz, S., Karrer, U., Lina, B., Martin-Blondel, G., Pawlotsky, J. M., Schwartz, O., Seguin-Devaux, C., Thibault, V., & Molina, J. M. (2024, April 30). COVID-19: Which monoclonal antibodies should be used for vulnerable individuals? *Institut Pasteur Research Journal*. https://www.pasteur.fr/en/research-journal/reports/covid-19-which-monoclonal-antibodies-should-be-used-vulnerable-individuals

Richardson, D. B., Bai, J., Zhang, Q., Zeng, C., Xue, T., Wang, Q., Cui, X., Pierce, J., Wang, Q., Liu, Y., & Song, G. (2023). Global to USA county scale analysis of weather, urban density, mobility, homestay, and mask use on COVID-19. *International Journal of Health Geographics*, *22*(1), 15. https://doi.org/10.1186/s12942-023-00328-5

Roberts, J. A., Baker, M. A., & Klompas, M. (2022). COVID-19 treatment: A review of early and emerging options. *Cleveland Clinic Journal of Medicine*, *89*(5), 247–256. https://doi.org/10.3949/ccjm.89a.21046

Sajadi, M. M., Habibzadeh, P., Vintzileos, A., Shokouhi, S., Miralles-Wilhelm, F., & Amoroso, A. (2020). Temperature, humidity, and latitude analysis to estimate potential spread and seasonality of coronavirus disease 2019 (COVID-19). *JAMA Network Open*, *3*(6), e2011834. https://doi.org/10.1001/jamanetworkopen.2020.11834

Sandoval, C., Heitman, J., Ramirez, R., Griffin, K., Sattui, S. E., Sparks, J. A., & Harrison, L. B. (2023). Effectiveness of mRNA, protein subunit vaccine and viral vectors vaccines against SARS-CoV-2 in people over 18 years old: A systematic review. *Expert Review of Vaccines*, *22*(3), 303–315. https://doi.org/10.1080/14760584.2023.2156861

Schmidt, M., Hajage, D., Lebreton, G., Monsel, A., Voiriot, G., Levy, D., Baron, E., Beurton, A., Chommeloux, J., Meng, P., Nemlaghi, S., Bay, P., Leprince, P., Demoule, A., Guidet, B., Constantin, J. M., Fartoukh, M., Dres, M., & Combes, A. (2020). Extracorporeal membrane oxygenation for severe acute respiratory distress syndrome associated with COVID-19: A retrospective cohort study. *The Lancet Respiratory Medicine*, *8*(11), 1121–1131. https://doi.org/10.1016/S2213-2600(20)30328-3

Self, W. H., Tenforde, M. W., Gaglani, M., Ginde, A. A., Douin, D. J., Talbot, H. K., Casey, J. D., Mohr, N. M., Zepeski, A., McNeal, T., Ghamande, S., Gibbs, K. W., Files, D. C., Hager, D. N., Shehu, A., Prekker, M. E., Erickson, H. L., Exline, M. C., Gong, M. N., … Patel, M. M. (2024). Effectiveness of updated 2023-2024 (monovalent XBB.1.5)

COVID-19 vaccination against SARS-CoV-2 Omicron XBB and BA.2.86/JN.1 lineage hospitalization and a comparison of clinical severity-IVY network, 26 hospitals, October 18, 2023-March 9, 2024. *Clinical Infectious Diseases*, *78*(8), 1146–1155. https://doi.org/10.1093/cid/ciad642

Sharma, M., Mindermann, S., Rogers-Smith, C., Leech, G., Snodin, B., Ahuja, J., Sandbrink, J. B., Monrad, J. T., Altman, G., Dhaliwal, G., Finnveden, L., Norman, A. J., Oehm, S. B., Sandkühler, J. F., Verdecchia, M., Gal, Y., Kulveit, J., & Brauner, J. M. (2021). Understanding the effectiveness of government interventions in Europe's second wave of COVID-19. *Nature Communications*, *12*(1), 5820. https://doi.org/10.1038/s41467-021-26013-4

Sheikh, A., McMenamin, J., Taylor, B., & Robertson, C. (2021). SARS-CoV-2 Delta VOC in Scotland: Demographics, risk of hospital admission, and vaccine effectiveness. *The Lancet*, *397*(10293), 2461–2462. https://doi.org/10.1016/S0140-6736(21)01358-1

Sheikh, A., Robertson, C., & Taylor, B. (2023). BNT162b2 and ChAdOx1 nCoV-19 vaccine effectiveness against death from the delta variant. *New England Journal of Medicine*, *385*(23), 2195–2197. https://doi.org/10.1056/NEJMc2113864

Sil, D., Gautam, S., Saxena, S., Joshi, S., Kumar, D., Mehta, A., Jindal, P., Sharma, S., Pandey, P., Diksha, & Singh, A. (2024). Comprehensive analysis of Omicron subvariants: EG.5 rise, vaccination strategies, and global impact. *Current Drug Targets*, *25*(8), 517–525. https://doi.org/10.2174/0113894501296586240430061915

Sluvkin, I. I., Khavrutskii, I., Kurauchi, K., Glembo, T., Sarkar, D., Khavinson, K., Natzle, N., Horton, L., Lopez, O., Alvarado, A., Gundlapalli, S., Patel, M., Madeira, F., Mir, P., Pueyo, J. D., Thomas, P., Nambiar, K., & Gupta, S. (2024). Distinct evolution of SARS-CoV-2 Omicron XBB and BA.2.86/JN.1 lineages combining increased fitness and antibody evasion. *Nature Communications*, *15*(1), 3242. https://doi.org/10.1038/s41467-024-46490-7

Sweeney, D. A., Lobo, S. M., Póvoa, P., & Kalil, A. C. (2024). Choosing immunomodulating therapies for the treatment of COVID-19: Recommendations based on placebo-controlled trial evidence. *Current Opinion in Critical Care*, *30*(1), 36–42. https://doi.org/10.1097/MCC.0000000000001080

Takashita, E., Yamayoshi, S., Fukushi, S., Suzuki, T., Ito, M., Furusawa, Y., Hashimoto, R., Lopes, T. J. S., Lim, C. K., Uno, M., Ujike, M., Deguchi, S., Yamamoto, S., Ichihara, K., Sakai-Tagawa, Y., Saito, M., Noda, M., & Kawaoka, Y. (2022). Efficacy of antiviral agents against the Omicron subvariant BA.2.75. *New England Journal of Medicine*, *387*(13), 1236–1238. https://doi.org/10.1056/NEJMc2207519

Tartof, S. Y., Slezak, J. M., Frankland, T. B., Puzniak, L., Hong, V., Ackerson, B. K., Stern, J. A., Zamparo, J., Simmons, S., Jodar, L., & McLaughlin, J. M. (2024). Estimated effectiveness of the BNT162b2 XBB vaccine against COVID-19. *JAMA Internal Medicine*, *184*(8), 932–940. https://doi.org/10.1001/jamainternmed.2024.1640

Tenforde, M. W., Self, W. H., Adams, K., Gaglani, M., Ginde, A. A., McNeal, T., Ghamande, S., Douin, D. J., Talbot, H. K., Casey, J. D., Mohr, N. M., Zepeski, A., Hager, D. N., Qadir, N., Shehu, A., Prekker, M. E., Erickson, H. L., Brown, S. M., Peltan, I. D., ... IVY Network. (2021). Association between mRNA vaccination and COVID-19 hospitalization and disease severity. *JAMA*, *326*(20), 2043–2054. https://doi.org/10.1001/jama.2021.19499

Thomas, S. J., Moreira, E. D., Jr., Kitchin, N., Absalon, J., Gurtman, A., Lockhart, S., Perez, J. L., Pérez Marc, G., Polack, F. P., Zerbini, C., Bailey, R., Swanson, K. A., Xu, X., Roychoudhury, S., Koury, K., Bouguermouh, S., Kalina, W. V., Cooper, D., Frenck, R. W., Jr., … C4591001 Clinical Trial Group. (2021). Safety and efficacy of the BNT162b2 mRNA COVID-19 vaccine through 6 months. *New England Journal of Medicine*, *385*(19), 1761–1773. https://doi.org/10.1056/NEJMoa2110345

Tian, H., Liu, Y., Li, Y., Wu, C. H., Chen, B., Kraemer, M. U. G., Li, B., Cai, J., Xu, B., Yang, Q., Wang, B., Yang, P., Cui, Y., Song, Y., Zheng, P., Wang, Q., Bjornstad, O. N., Yang, R., Grenfell, B. T., … Dye, C. (2020). An investigation of transmission control measures during the first 50 days of the COVID-19 epidemic in China. *Science*, *368*(6491), 638–642. https://doi.org/10.1126/science.abb6105

Tobin, M. J., Laghi, F., & Jubran, A. (2020). Why COVID-19 silent hypoxemia is baffling to physicians. *American Journal of Respiratory and Critical Care Medicine*, *202*(3), 356–360. https://doi.org/10.1164/rccm.202006-2157CP

Twohig, K. A., Nyberg, T., Zaidi, A., Thelwall, S., Sinnathamby, M. A., Aliabadi, S., Seaman, S. R., Harris, R. J., Hope, R., Lopez-Bernal, J., Gallagher, E., Charlett, A., de Angelis, D., The COVID-19 Genomics UK (COG-UK) consortium, Presanis, A. M., & Dabrera, G. (2022). Hospital admission and emergency care attendance risk for SARS-CoV-2 delta (B.1.617.2) compared with alpha (B.1.1.7) variants of concern: A cohort study. *The Lancet Infectious Diseases*, *22*(1), 35–42. https://doi.org/10.1016/S1473-3099(21)00475-8

UK Health Security Agency. (2023-2024). *COVID-19 vaccine surveillance reports*. https://www.gov.uk/government/publications/covid-19-vaccine-weekly-surveillance-reports

Umunnakwe, C. N., Makatini, Z. N., Maphanga, M., Mdunyelwa, A., Mlambo, K. M., Manyaka, P., Nijhuis, M., Wensing, A., & Tempelman, H. A. (2022). Evaluation of a commercial SARS-CoV-2 multiplex PCR genotyping assay for variant identification in resource-scarce settings. *PLOS ONE*, 17(6), e0269071. https://doi.org/10.1371/journal.pone.0269071

University of California San Francisco. (2024). *Extended Paxlovid may help some people with Long COVID*. UCSF News. https://www.ucsf.edu/news/2024/12/429266/extended-paxlovid-may-help-some-people-long-covid

Vanderbilt University Medical Center. (2024). *NIH-funded trial to determine if immunomodulation can improve brain and cardiovascular dysfunction in Long COVID*. VUMC News. https://news.vumc.org/2024/02/22/nih-funded-trial-to-determine-if-immunomodulation-can-improve-brain-and-cardiovascular-dysfunction-in-long-covid/

Vogels, C. B. F., Breban, M. I., Ott, I. M., Alpert, T., Petrone, M. E., Watkins, A. E., Kalinich, C. C., Earnest, R., Rothman, J. E., Goes de Jesus, J., Aguero-Rosenfeld, M. E., Rice, P., Hoxie, I., Santangelo, R., Fauver, J. R., Grubaugh, N. D., & the Yale SARS-CoV-2 Genomic Surveillance Initiative. (2021). Multiplex qPCR discriminates variants of concern to enhance global surveillance of SARS-CoV-2. *PLOS Biology*, *19*(5), e3001236. https://doi.org/10.1371/journal.pbio.3001236

Volz, E., Hill, V., McCrone, J. T., Price, A., Jorgensen, D., O'Toole, Á, Southgate, J., Johnson, R., Jackson, B., Nascimento, F. F., Rey, S. M., Nicholls, S. M., Colquhoun, R. M., da Silva Filipe, A., Shepherd, J., Pascall, D. J., Shah, R., Jesudason, N., Li, K., … COVID-19 Genomics UK (COG-UK) Consortium. (2021). Evaluating the effects of SARS-CoV-2 spike mutation D614G on transmissibility and pathogenicity. *Cell*, *184*(1), 64–75.e11. https://doi.org/10.1016/j.cell.2020.11.020

Volz, E., Mishra, S., Chand, M., Barrett, J. C., Johnson, R., Geidelberg, L., Hinsley, W. R., Laydon, D. J., Dabrera, G., O'Toole, Á., Amato, R., Ragonnet-Cronin, M., Harrison, I., Jackson, B., Ariani, C. V., Boyd, O., Loman, N. J., McCrone, J. T. Gonçalves, S., … COVID-19 Genomics UK (COG-UK) consortium (2021). Assessing transmissibility of SARS-CoV-2 lineage B.1.1.7 in England. *Nature*, *593*(7858), 266–269. https://doi.org/10.1038/s41586-021-03470-x

Voysey, M., Clemens, S. A. C., Madhi, S. A., Weckx, L. Y., Folegatti, P. M., Aley, P. K., Angus, B., Baillie, V. L., Barnabas, S. L., Bhorat, Q. E., Bibi, S., Briner, C., Cicconi, P., Collins, A. M., Colin-Jones, R., Cutland, C. L., Darton, T. C., Dheda, K., Duncan, C. J. A., … Oxford COVID Vaccine Trial Group. (2021). Safety and efficacy of the ChAdOx1 nCoV-19 vaccine (AZD1222) against SARS-CoV-2: An interim analysis of four randomised controlled trials in Brazil, South Africa, and the UK. *The Lancet*, *397*(10269), 99–111. https://doi.org/10.1016/S0140-6736(20)32661-1

Wang, C., Liu, B., Zhang, S., Huang, N., Zhao, T., Lu, Q. B., & Cui, F. (2022). Differences in incidence and fatality of COVID-19 by SARS-CoV-2 Omicron variant versus Delta variant in relation to vaccine coverage: A world-wide review. *Journal of Medical Virology*, *95*(1), e28118. https://doi.org/10.1002/jmv.28118

Wang, P., Nair, M. S., Liu, L., Iketani, S., Luo, Y., Guo, Y., Wang, M., Yu, J., Zhang, B., Kwong, P. D., Graham, B. S., Mascola, J. R., Chang, J. Y., Yin, M. T., Sobieszczyk, M., Kyratsous, C. A., Shapiro, L., Sheng, Z., Huang, Y., & Ho, D. D. (2021). Antibody resistance of SARS-CoV-2 variants B.1.351 and B.1.1.7. *Nature*, *593*(7857), 130–135. https://doi.org/10.1038/s41586-021-03398-2

Wang, Q., Berger, N. A., & Xu, R. (2021). Increased risk for COVID-19 breakthrough infection in fully vaccinated patients with substance use disorders in the United States between December 2020 and August 2021. *World Psychiatry*, *20*(3), 427–430. https://doi.org/10.1002/wps.20921

Wang, Q., Iketani, S., Li, Z., Liu, L., Guo, Y., Huang, Y., Bowen, A. D., Liu, M., Wang, M., Yu, J., Valdez, R., Lauring, A. S., Sheng, Z., Wang, H. H., Gordon, A., Liu, L., & Ho, D. D. (2023). Alarming antibody evasion properties of rising SARS-CoV-2 BQ and XBB subvariants. *Cell*, *186*(2), 279–286.e8. https://doi.org/10.1016/j.cell.2022.12.018

Wang, Q., Guo, Y., Bowen, A., Mellis, I. A., Valdez, R., Gherasim, C., Gordon, A., Liu, L., & Ho, D. D. (2024). XBB.1.5 monovalent mRNA vaccine booster elicits robust neutralizing antibodies against XBB subvariants and JN.1. *Cell Host & Microbe*, *32*(3), 315–321.e3. https://doi.org/10.1016/j.chom.2024.01.014

Wang, Q., Guo, Y., Liu, L., Schwarz, L. T., Li, Z., Nair, M. S., Liu, H., Ellis, D., Ho, D. D., & Bieniasz, P. D. (2023). XBB.1.5 monovalent mRNA vaccine booster elicits robust neutralizing antibodies against XBB subvariants and JN.1. *Cell Host & Microbe*, *10*, S1931–S3128. https://doi.org/10.1016/j.chom.2023.12.003

Wang, Y., Zhang, D., Du, G., Du, R., Zhao, J., Jin, Y., Fu, S., Gao, L., Cheng, Z., Lu, Q., Hu, Y., Luo, G., Wang, K., Lu, Y., Li, H., Wang, S., Ruan, S., Yang, C., Mei, C., … Wang, C. (2020). Remdesivir in adults with severe COVID-19: A randomised, double-blind, placebo-controlled, multicentre trial. *The Lancet*, *395*(10236), 1569–1578. https://doi.org/10.1016/S0140-6736(20)31022-9

Weinreich, D. M., Sivapalasingam, S., Norton, T., Ali, S., Gao, H., Bhore, R., Xiao, J., Hooper, A. T., Hamilton, J. D., Musser, B. J., Rofail, D., Hussein, M., Im, J., Atmodjo, D. Y., Perry, C., Pan, C., Mahmood, A., Hosain, R., Davis, J. D., … Yancopoulos, G. D. (2021). REGEN-COV antibody combination and outcomes in outpatients with COVID-19. *New England Journal of Medicine*, *385*(23), e81. https://doi.org/10.1056/NEJMoa2108163

Wiersinga, W. J., Rhodes, A., Cheng, A. C., Peacock, S. J., & Prescott, H. C. (2020). Pathophysiology, transmission, diagnosis, and treatment of coronavirus disease 2019 (COVID-19): A review. *JAMA*, *324*(8), 782–793. https://doi.org/10.1001/jama.2020.12839

Wikramaratna, P., Paton, R. S., Ghafari, M., & Lourenço, J. (2020). Estimating false-negative detection rate of SARS-CoV-2 by RT-PCR. *medRxiv*. https://doi.org/10.1101/2020.04.05.20053355

Woloshin, S., Patel, N., & Kesselheim, A. S. (2020). False negative tests for SARS-CoV-2 infection—Challenges and implications. *New England Journal of Medicine*, *383*(6), e38. https://doi.org/10.1056/NEJMp2015897

Wolter, N., Jassat, W., Walaza, S., Welch, R., Moultrie, H., Groome, M., Amoako, D. G., Everatt, J., Bhiman, J. N., Scheepers, C., Tebeila, N., Chiwandire, N., du Plessis, M., Govender, N., Ismail, A., Glass, A., Mlisana, K., Stevens, W., Treurnicht, F. K., … von Gottberg, A. (2022). Early assessment of the clinical severity of the SARS-CoV-2 omicron variant in South Africa: A data linkage study. *The Lancet*, *399*(10322), 437–446. https://doi.org/10.1016/S0140-6736(22)00017-4

Woodrow, M., Carey, C., Ziauddeen, N., Ibarra-Moreno, A., Richter, A., Welch, A. A., & Khaw, K. T. (2023). Systematic review of the prevalence of long COVID. *Open Forum Infectious Diseases*, *10*(7), ofad233. https://doi.org/10.1093/ofid/ofad233

World Bank. (2024). *World Bank financing for COVID-19 vaccine rollout and pandemic preparedness*. https://www.worldbank.org/en/topic/health/brief/world-bank-support-to-covid-19-vaccine-development

World Health Organization (WHO). (2021a). *Classification of Omicron (B.1.1.529): SARS-CoV-2 variant of concern*. https://www.who.int/news/item/26-11-2021-classification-of-omicron-(b.1.1.529)-sars-cov-2-variant-of-concern

World Health Organization (WHO). (2021b). *Strategy to achieve global COVID-19 vaccination by mid-2022*. https://www.who.int/publications/m/item/strategy-to-achieve-global-covid-19-vaccination-by-mid-2022

World Health Organization (WHO). (2022a). *COVID-19 weekly epidemiological update*, January 2022. Retrieved from https://www.who.int/emergencies/diseases/novel-coronavirus-2019/situation-reports

World Health Organization (WHO). (2022b). *Interim statement on COVID-19 vaccination for children*. https://www.who.int/news/item/11-08-2022-interim-statement-on-covid-19-vaccination-for-children

World Health Organization (WHO). (2023a). *COVID-19 wastewater environmental surveillance*. https://data.who.int/dashboards/covid19/wastewater

World Health Organization (WHO). (2023b). *Therapeutics and COVID-19: Living Guideline*. WHO/2019-nCoV/therapeutics/2022.5. https://www.who.int/publications/i/item/WHO-2019-nCoV-therapeutics-2023.2

World Health Organization (WHO). (2024). *COVID-19 vaccination dashboard*. https://data.who.int/dashboards/covid19/vaccines

World Health Organization (WHO). (2025a). *COVID-19 epidemiological updates* (Editions 170–177). https://www.who.int/emergencies/diseases/novel-coronavirus-2019/situation-reports

World Health Organization (WHO). (2025b). *Tracking SARS-CoV-2 variants*. https://www.who.int/activities/tracking-SARS-CoV-2-variants

Worldometer. (2020). *Coronavirus testing criteria and numbers by country*. https://www.worldometers.info/coronavirus/covid-19-testing/

Worldometer. (2024, April 13). *COVID-19 coronavirus pandemic*. https://www.worldometers.info/coronavirus/#countries

Wu, X., Xu, K., Zhan, P., Chen, K., Chen, R., Zhao, L., Chen, M., Zhang, M., Li, X., & Zhang, Z. (2024). Comparative efficacy and safety of COVID-19 vaccines in phase III trials: A network meta-analysis. *BMC Infectious Diseases*, *24*, 234. https://doi.org/10.1186/s12879-023-08754-3

Yale Medicine. (2024a). 13 Things to know about Paxlovid, the latest COVID-19 pill. *Yale Medicine News*. https://www.yalemedicine.org/news/13-things-to-know-paxlovid-covid-19

Yale Medicine. (2024b). *What to know about the updated 2024-2025 COVID vaccines*. https://www.yalemedicine.org/news/updated-2024-2025-covid-vaccines

Yang, T.-C., Kim, S., Zhao, Y., & Choi, S.-W. (2021). Examining ZIP code–level disparities in COVID-19 testing and positivity in New York City: A spatial modeling approach. *Health & Place*, *69*, 102574. https://doi.org/10.1016/j.healthplace.2021.102574

Yisimayi, A., Song, W., Wang, J., Jian, F., Yu, Y., Chen, X., Fu, L., Wu, N., Li, Z., Qian, K., Wang, Q., Ju, B., Wang, Y., & Gao, G. F. (2024). Repeated Omicron exposures override ancestral SARS-CoV-2 immune imprinting. *Nature*, *625*, 148–156. https://doi.org/10.1038/s41586-023-06753-7

Yoshikawa, R., Abe, H., Igasaki, Y., Asano, K., & Shibasaki, S. (2020). Development and evaluation of a rapid and simple diagnostic assay for COVID-19 based on loop-mediated isothermal amplification. *PLOS Neglected Tropical Diseases*, *14*(11), e0008855. https://doi.org/10.1371/journal.pntd.0008855

You, J. (2020). Lessons from South Korea's COVID-19 policy response. *American Review of Public Administration*, *50*(6–7), 801–808. https://doi.org/10.1177/0275074020943708

You, S. H., Baek, M. S., Kim, T. W., Jung, S. Y., & Kim, W. Y. (2025). Influence of SARS-CoV-2 variants and corticosteroid use on the effectiveness of baricitinib therapy in critical COVID-19. *Critical Care*, *29*(1), 131. https://doi.org/10.1186/s13054-025-05367-x

Zhang, L., Jackson, C. B., Mou, H., Ojha, A., Peng, H., Quinlan, B. D., Rangarajan, E. S., Pan, A., Vanderheiden, A., Suthar, M. S., Li, W., Izard, T., Rader, C., Farzan, M., & Choe, H. (2020). SARS-CoV-2 spike-protein D614G mutation increases virion spike density and infectivity. *Nature Communications*, *11*(1), 6013. https://doi.org/10.1038/s41467-020-19808-4

Zhou, Y., Wu, J., Zeng, X., Xiong, X., Guo, X., Zhang, S., Huang, S., Zhao, J., & Luo, L. (2020). Effects of human mobility restrictions on the spread of COVID-19 in Shenzhen, China: A modelling study using mobile phone data. *The Lancet Digital Health*, *2*(8), e417–e424. https://doi.org/10.1016/S2589-7500(20)30165-5

10 Structural Foundations

How Systems and Institutions Shaped the Pandemic Response

As we descend into the pandemic's deeper layers, we encounter the structural foundations that shaped both visible events and underlying patterns (Figure 10.1). Like the submerged mass of an iceberg, these systems—from healthcare infrastructure to supply chains to information management—formed the hidden base through which responses were mobilized.

The pandemic exposed critical vulnerabilities in these frameworks while revealing which elements proved most resilient. Healthcare systems, supply networks, and public institutions faced unprecedented strain, forcing rapid adaptation and spotlighting long-neglected weaknesses. Just as the Titanic's fate was sealed by flaws in its hull, COVID-19's impact was amplified by systemic fragilities long left unaddressed.

This section examines the key structural forces that shaped the global response:

- ***Health Systems Resilience and Preparedness***
- ***Vaccine Manufacturing and Supply Chain Challenges***
- ***Global Vaccine Equity and Distribution Disparities***
- ***Socioeconomic and Policy Interventions During the Pandemic***
- ***Communication Breakdowns and the Rise of Misinformation***

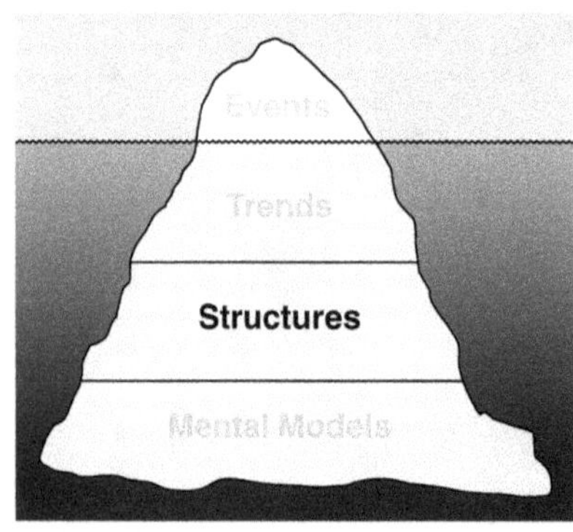

Figure 10.1 Iceberg Model—Structures.

DOI: 10.4324/9781003595564-13

Health Systems Resilience and Preparedness

The COVID-19 pandemic served as a stress test for global healthcare systems, revealing dramatic disparities in preparedness and exposing both infrastructural and human resource limitations. Some nations, particularly those that had faced recent epidemics like SARS or MERS, demonstrated remarkable resilience through strong healthcare infrastructure, well-defined public health policies, and a stable clinical workforce. Others, despite their apparent advantages in resources and technology, struggled with fragmented responses, workforce shortages, and widespread burnout.

Regional Approaches to Pandemic Preparedness

Asia: The region's pandemic response was significantly shaped by prior experiences with SARS and MERS, which informed early preparedness and public receptivity to health measures (Jamison & Wu, 2021). China implemented a sweeping "zero-COVID" strategy, marked by strict lockdowns, mass testing, and centralized contact tracing. The lockdown of Wuhan in January 2020 became a global

Table 10.1 Regional Pandemic Strategies, Strengths, and Challenges During COVID-19

Region	*Primary Strategies*	*Key Strengths*	*Key Challenges*
Asia *(e.g., China, South Korea, Japan, Taiwan)*	Containment through testing, tracing, isolation	Rapid response; effective containment; fewer deaths	Varying restrictions on individual freedom
Europe *(e.g., U.K., Germany, Sweden, France)*	Mixed approaches; strict lockdowns to voluntary	Strong vaccination campaigns; adaptable responses	Coordination challenges; healthcare system strain
North America *(e.g., U.S., Canada, Mexico)*	Decentralized responses; vaccine development	Vaccine development speed; high resources	Initial testing delays; coordination issues
South America *(e.g., Brazil, Argentina, Peru)*	Varied policies; economic constraints	Innovative regional solutions	Federal-state tensions; socioeconomic challenges
Africa *(e.g., Rwanda, South Africa)*	Innovation with limited resources	Leveraged existing disease infrastructure	Resource constraints; limited healthcare capacity
Oceania *(e.g., New Zealand, Australia)*	Elimination strategies	Extended periods of zero transmission	Economic impacts of prolonged isolation

Sources: El Bcheraoui et al. (2020); Assefa et al. (2022); Jamison and Wu (2021); da Silva and Pena (2021); Wang et al. (2020); World Health Organization (WHO) (2024); Ramírez Varela et al. (2023); Brusselaers et al. (2022); Baker et al. (2020); Chen and Fang (2024); Chung and Soh (2020); McKee et al. (2021); Madhi et al. (2022); Oshitani et al. (2020); Roux et al. (2023); Bautista-Reyes et al. (2023); Edwards et al. (2022).

reference point for containment efforts (Ba et al., 2023; Hu & Zhang, 2024). Taiwan, just 130 kilometers from China, took a markedly different approach. Drawing on lessons from SARS, it quickly mobilized testing, contact tracing, and digital surveillance tools—achieving "COVID-19 zero" without full-scale lockdowns and while maintaining relative economic stability (Chen & Fang, 2024; Wang et al., 2020). South Korea also responded swiftly, implementing drive-through testing centers and digital contact tracing systems that became global models (Chung & Soh, 2020). Japan pursued a more restrained strategy, relying heavily on public cooperation, targeted restrictions, and cluster-based contact tracing rather than blanket mandates. Though less aggressive than some of its neighbors, Japan's approach emphasized cultural norms of compliance and risk aversion, which helped mitigate transmission despite limited testing in the early phase (Oshitani et al., 2020).

Europe: European countries took divergent paths in responding to the pandemic, shaped by their political systems, public health infrastructure, and societal values. The United Kingdom's National Health Service (NHS) was overwhelmed during the early waves, with high mortality in care homes and significant strain on hospitals. However, the country later mounted one of the world's fastest and most efficient vaccination rollouts, aided by early procurement and centralized coordination (El Bcheraoui et al., 2020; McKee et al., 2021). Germany initially managed the crisis well, leveraging a strong healthcare infrastructure and extensive testing. Yet over time, coordination challenges between the federal government and the Länder (states) complicated response consistency. Sweden took a markedly different path, opting for voluntary guidelines rather than mandatory lockdowns. This approach, aimed at long-term sustainability and preserving civil liberties, sparked international debate and led to higher early death rates compared to its Nordic neighbors (Brusselaers et al., 2022; Irwin, 2020; Ludvigsson, 2020). France pursued a more centralized model, implementing strict nationwide lockdowns and widespread testing. Government-led coordination and communication helped enforce containment measures, though compliance varied and public fatigue grew over time (Roux et al., 2023).

North America: Different healthcare systems produced varying outcomes across the region. The United States struggled with early testing failures, inconsistent messaging, and a fragmented federal response. However, it later became a leader in vaccine development and distribution, particularly through Operation Warp Speed (El Bcheraoui et al., 2020). Canada's response benefited from more effective federal-provincial coordination and a universal public healthcare system, which helped facilitate access to care and public compliance with mitigation measures (Allin et al., 2021). Mexico, by contrast, faced considerable challenges in implementing consistent nationwide policies. Limited healthcare infrastructure, especially in rural areas, constrains testing and treatment capacity. In addition, economic pressures and a high proportion of informal labor made lockdowns and distancing measures harder to sustain. The country's decentralized governance structure also contributed to uneven enforcement and public health messaging across states (Bautista-Reyes et al., 2023).

South America: The region faced a series of daunting challenges during the pandemic. In Brazil, the federal government downplayed the severity of COVID-19, with President Bolsonaro opposing lockdowns, promoting unproven treatments, and undermining public health messaging. In response, state governments were forced to act independently, resulting in a fragmented national strategy (da Silva & Pena, 2021). Ongoing power struggles between the federal executive and state governors further obstructed coordination (Bigoni et al., 2022). Argentina imposed one of the earliest and strictest lockdowns, which remained in effect through November 2020, but the country was unable to sustain it economically. A large share of the workforce operated in the informal sector, making prolonged lockdowns especially damaging to livelihoods (International Monetary Fund, 2021b). Peru implemented some of the world's most stringent restrictions, yet still recorded the highest per capita death rate. High levels of poverty, a heavily informal economy, an underfunded healthcare system, and overcrowded living conditions combined to severely limit the effectiveness of public health interventions (National Public Radio (NPR), 2021). Across the region, the prevalence of informal labor made strict public health measures difficult to enforce and sustain (Ramírez Varela et al., 2023).

Africa: Despite limited resources, many African countries responded with agility, drawing on past experiences with epidemics and leveraging innovative strategies. Rwanda exemplified this approach by deploying drones to deliver medical supplies and using robots in hospitals to reduce health worker exposure, as well as for public health messaging (Assefa et al., 2022; Musanabaganwa et al., 2020). The country's prior experience with Ebola and investment in digital health infrastructure enabled rapid adaptation to the demands of the COVID-19 crisis (WHO Africa, 2020). South Africa, facing high burdens of HIV and tuberculosis, repurposed its existing disease surveillance and laboratory infrastructure to expand COVID-19 testing and care. Its genomic research capacity, built over decades of HIV/TB work, made the country a global leader in identifying and tracking new variants, including the Beta and Omicron variants (Madhi et al., 2022; Wilkinson et al., 2021). While resource limitations posed serious challenges across the continent, these examples show how historical public health investments and innovation under constraint shaped Africa's pandemic response in uniquely adaptive ways.

Oceania: Countries in Oceania pursued elimination rather than mitigation strategies during the early stages of the pandemic. New Zealand responded swiftly with early border closures, nationwide lockdowns, and transparent communication from executive leadership. These measures, supported by strong public trust and clear health messaging, allowed the country to achieve months of zero community transmission (Baker et al., 2020; Jamison & Wu, 2021). The combination of decisive policy action and cohesive public cooperation enabled New Zealand to keep the virus at bay until vaccines became widely available (Summers et al., 2020). Australia adopted a similarly aggressive approach, but its federal system meant that states exercised significant autonomy in managing outbreaks. States like Victoria and New South Wales implemented region-specific lockdowns and contact tracing strategies, while national coordination supported vaccine procurement and broad health messaging. This flexible model allowed for tailored responses but occasionally led to intergovernmental tension and policy inconsistencies (Edwards et al., 2022). Nonetheless, both countries initially succeeded in minimizing deaths and transmission compared to much of the world.

Overall, these regional case studies highlight the wide range of strategies employed in managing the COVID-19 pandemic, each shaped by distinct political structures, public health capacities, and socioeconomic conditions. Some nations successfully leveraged existing health infrastructure and technological innovation, while others devised context-specific solutions to navigate severe resource limitations. These varied experiences exposed significant disparities in pandemic preparedness and response—not always aligned with conventional expectations about system strength. While certain countries demonstrated agility, coordination, and adaptability under pressure, others struggled to translate infrastructure or past experience into effective action. In the end, the pandemic challenged longstanding assumptions about which health systems were truly equipped to confront a global crisis (Abbey et al., 2020).

The "Preparedness Paradox": How Nations Faced the Reality of Pandemic Response

As the pandemic unfolded, it became increasingly clear that formal pandemic preparedness plans, while essential, were only as effective as a nation's ability to implement them swiftly and decisively (Mahajan, 2021). Countries that had weathered previous outbreaks often proved more adaptable and responsive, while those with fragmented healthcare systems or political hesitancy faced widespread challenges, regardless of their theoretical preparedness levels (Jamison & Wu, 2021).

The global health security (GHS) Index, first published in 2019, offered a pre-pandemic assessment of countries' preparedness based on various indicators, including healthcare infrastructure, early detection capabilities, and emergency response plans (Johns Hopkins Center for Health Security et al., 2021). However, when the COVID-19 pandemic struck, these theoretical frameworks were tested, and the results challenged many assumptions about pandemic readiness (Abbey et al., 2020).

The before and after data revealed a striking pattern: many of the highest-ranked nations on paper struggled most visibly with COVID-19 response (Abbey et al., 2020). The United Kingdom's performance particularly highlighted this disconnect, dropping from second to seventh place with the steepest decline (−10.7 points). The United States, while maintaining its top ranking, also saw a significant drop (−7.6 points). Other highly ranked nations like the Netherlands (−10.9) and Sweden (−7.2) experienced substantial drops as well. While GHS has since updated its scoring criteria to account for these broader gaps between theoretical preparedness and execution, these declines reflected the significant challenges these nations faced in implementing their pandemic response plans effectively (Johns Hopkins Center for Health Security et al., 2021).

Table 10.2 Global Health Security Index Rankings of Theoretical Health System Preparedness, Pre-Pandemic (2019) vs. Pandemic (2021)

Country	*2019 Rank*	*2019 Score*	*2021 Rank*	*2021 Score*	*Score Change*
The United States	**1**	**83.5**	**1 (--)**	**75.9**	**−7.6**
The United Kingdom	**2**	**77.9**	**7 (↓)**	**67.2**	**−10.7**
The Netherlands	**3**	**75.6**	**11 (↓)**	**64.7**	**−10.9**
Australia	**4**	**75.5**	**2 (↑)**	**71.1**	**−4.4**
Canada	**5**	**75.3**	**4 (↑)**	**69.8**	**−5.5**
Thailand	**6**	**73.2**	**5 (↑)**	**68.2**	**−5.0**
Sweden	**7**	**72.1**	**10 (↓)**	**64.9**	**−7.2**
Denmark	**8**	**70.4**	**12 (↓)**	**64.4**	**−6.0**
South Korea	**9**	**70.2**	**9 (--)**	**65.4**	**−4.8**
Finland	**10**	**68.7**	**3 (↑)**	**70.9**	**+2.2**
France	**11**	**68.2**	**14 (↓)**	**61.9**	**−6.3**
Slovenia	**12**	**67.2**	**6 (↑)**	**67.8**	**+0.6**
Switzerland	**13**	**67.0**	**23 (↓)**	**58.8**	**−8.2**
Germany	**14**	**66.0**	**8 (↑)**	**65.5**	**−0.5**
Spain	**15**	**65.9**	**17 (↓)**	**60.9**	**−5.0**

Sources: Johns Hopkins Center for Health Security et al. (2021); Johns Hopkins Center for Health Security et al. (2019–2021); Nuclear Threat Initiative (NTI) (2020); Abbey et al. (2020); Mahajan (2021).

The "preparedness paradox" manifested most clearly in the experiences of the U.S. and U.K. (Mahajan, 2021). The U.S. case proved particularly telling—despite its comprehensive pandemic framework and leading position in health security, many critical weaknesses emerged early. The Strategic National Stockpile (SNS) proved inadequately maintained, leading to devastating PPE and ventilator shortages during the first wave (NTI, 2020). More fundamentally, inconsistent communication between federal and state governments, coupled with delayed testing and containment efforts, undermined the country's ability to execute its preparedness plans uniformly.

The U.K. faced similar challenges, entering the pandemic with a well-regarded healthcare system, but that had been undermined by years of austerity measures (El Bcheraoui et al., 2020). Early political indecision and inconsistent public health messaging delayed crucial interventions, while the NHS struggled with longstanding staffing and resource constraints. These two examples of well-resourced nations demonstrated that merely having sophisticated plans on paper means little without the political commitment and public health infrastructure investment measures needed to implement them effectively (Mahajan, 2021).

In contrast, several nations with lower GHS rankings, but with recent epidemic experience, demonstrated how well-maintained preparedness frameworks backed by decisive leadership and public trust could effectively manage the crisis (Jamison & Wu, 2021). Countries like Taiwan (not formally ranked), Japan (+0.7), South Korea (−4.8), and New Zealand (+10.4) largely succeeded and minimized the pandemic's impact through three key factors: clear, consistent communication with the public; effective use of technology for tracking and response; and swift, decisive intervention when threats emerged (Wang et al., 2020). These nations not only had strong plans in place but also possessed the political will and infrastructure needed for rapid implementation.

Healthcare Workforce Capacity and Burnout: The Human Core of System Resilience

The pandemic revealed that healthcare workers form the essential foundation of system resilience, with their capacity and wellbeing directly determining response effectiveness (Assefa et al., 2022). Even before COVID-19, healthcare professionals faced significant rates of burnout, but the pandemic amplified these pressures to unprecedented crisis levels. A comprehensive global meta-analysis examining burnout among healthcare workers found a pooled overall prevalence of 52% during the COVID-19 pandemic (95% CI 40–63%), based on 30 observational studies covering 32,724 healthcare workers (Ghahramani et al., 2021). Another meta-analysis examining burnout among the public health workforce found rates rising to 42% during the pandemic compared to 35% in pre-pandemic periods—demonstrating a marked increase in workforce strain during the crisis (Nagarajan et al., 2024). This trend is further illustrated in the following comparison of global burnout rates across several major studies.

Table 10.3 Global Burnout Rates Among Healthcare Workers During the COVID-19 Pandemic

Measurement Period	*Global Burnout Rate*	*Sample Size*	*Notes/Source*
Pre-pandemic period	35% (95% CI: 10–60%)	Part of 215,787 total sample	*Meta-analysis of 8 studies; baseline rates before pandemic (Nagarajan et al., 2024)*
During COVID-19 pandemic	42% (95% CI: 17–66%)	Part of 215,787 total sample	*Observed 7% increase during pandemic (Nagarajan et al., 2024)*
Overall pooled data	39% (95% CI: 25–53%)	215,787 healthcare workers	*Global meta-analysis (Nagarajan et al., 2024)*
Overall burnout during COVID-19	52% (95% CI: 40–63%)	32,724 healthcare workers	*Meta-analysis of 30 studies during pandemic (Ghahramani et al., 2021)*
60-country international survey	51% reported burnout	2,707 healthcare professionals	*International survey of 60 countries (Morgantini et al., 2020)*

Sources: Nagarajan et al. (2024); Ghahramani et al. (2021); Morgantini et al. (2020).

The impact of burnout fell particularly hard on frontline workers in intensive care units and emergency departments, who faced relentless waves of critically ill patients while working under extreme conditions. A large-scale international study spanning 60 countries found that 51% of healthcare professionals reported experiencing burnout during the pandemic, with the United States showing the highest rates at nearly 63%—demonstrating significant regional variation in workforce strain (Morgantini et al., 2020). The crisis was so severe that by late 2022, the U.S. Surgeon General issued an advisory acknowledging that health workers were facing a mental health crisis, with burnout rates reaching historically high levels (U.S. Department of Health and Human Services, 2022). Surveys by the end of 2022 revealed that over 60% of nurses in high-intensity care units reported moderate to severe burnout, with approximately 30% considering leaving their positions entirely (Rotenstein et al., 2023).

The working conditions that contributed to this crisis were unheard of in modern healthcare. Nurses and doctors often worked extended shifts while wearing full personal protective equipment (PPE) which limited their ability to take breaks or even maintain basic human comforts like drinking water or using the bathroom. The isolation from patients and colleagues, combined with the emotional burden of high mortality rates, created an environment of profound psychological stress. In the United States, CDC data revealed a dramatic increase in healthcare worker burnout, with 46% reporting feeling burned out often or very often in 2022, compared to 32% in 2018—a significant increase not seen in other worker groups during this period (Centers for Disease Control and Prevention (CDC), 2023).

The implications of this widespread burnout threaten to reshape the healthcare workforce for years to come. According to the 2022 National Sample Survey of Registered Nurses, nearly a quarter (23%) of RNs working in outpatient, ambulatory, and clinical settings plan to retire by 2025, with job dissatisfaction and burnout cited as major factors (American Association of Colleges of Nursing (AACN), 2024). This exodus is already creating critical staffing shortages, particularly in rural and underserved areas. A global systematic review examining healthcare worker turnover intention during the pandemic found that intention to leave varied widely by region—from 15.0% in the Eastern Mediterranean to 28.7% in the Western Pacific—with workplace stress, burnout, and job dissatisfaction identified as key drivers (Lim et al., 2022). Expert panels have warned that this workforce crisis represents one of the most significant threats to GHS, requiring urgent intervention at both national and international levels (Davino-Ramaya et al., 2023).

The relationship between workforce capacity and overall system resilience became evident across regions (Assefa et al., 2022). Countries that prioritized healthcare worker protection and support—both physically through adequate PPE and psychologically through mental health resources—demonstrated greater overall resilience. South Korea's comprehensive approach to healthcare worker safety, including dedicated rest facilities and routine mental health check-ins, contrasted sharply with countries where frontline workers faced shortages of basic PPE (Jamison & Wu, 2021). Similarly, Taiwan's effective management of healthcare

Table 10.4 Factors Associated with Increased Burnout Risk Among Healthcare Workers

Risk Factor	*Key Finding*	*Source*
Professional role	Highest burnout among nurses and/or physicians (66%) during pandemic	Ghahramani et al. (2021)
Workplace harassment	A total of 60% of harassed workers reported depression vs. 31% of non-harassed workers	Centers for Disease Control and Prevention (CDC) (2023)
Feeling undervalued	Only 46% of healthcare workers felt highly valued by their organization during the pandemic	Centers for Disease Control and Prevention (CDC) (2023)
Work overload	Work overload doubled odds of burnout and intent to leave by 68% (OR=2.14, 95% CI 1.99–2.30); (OR=1.68, 95% CI 1.56–1.82)	Rotenstein et al. (2023)
Work-life impact	Work interfering with household activities associated with 57% higher burnout risk	Morgantini et al. (2020)
Feeling pushed beyond training	Associated with 32% higher burnout risk	Morgantini et al. (2020)
COVID-19 exposure	Direct patient exposure associated with 18% higher burnout risk	Morgantini et al. (2020)

Sources: CDC (2023); Ghahramani et al. (2021); Rotenstein et al. (2023); Morgantini et al. (2020); MacGillivray et al. (2023); Harvard Gazette (2023).

worker capacity through strategic resource allocation and rotation policies prevented the widespread burnout seen in other regions (Wang et al., 2020).

Research has shown that workplace conditions significantly influence burnout rates, with harassment being a particularly damaging factor (Kekatos, 2023). Healthcare workers who experienced workplace harassment were nearly twice as likely to report depression (60% vs. 31% for those who did not experience harassment)—highlighting how workplace safety directly impacts workforce resilience (CDC, 2023). A comprehensive study during COVID-19 found that work overload was strongly associated with both burnout and intent to leave, with perceived work overload doubling the odds of burnout (OR=2.14, 95% CI 1.99–2.30) and increasing intent to leave by 68% (OR=1.68, 95% CI 1.56–1.82) (Rotenstein et al., 2023). Studies across 48 countries further revealed that excessive workload was a dominant factor in healthcare worker burnout globally, with the three countries producing the most research on this crisis being the United States, Spain, and China—reflecting both the universal nature of the challenge and regional variations in its severity (Sanghera et al., 2020).

Building Preparedness Resilience: Lessons for the Future of Public Health

The pandemic has fundamentally reshaped our understanding of what healthcare system resilience looks like. Drawing from both successful responses, like South

Korea's technological innovation and catastrophic failures seen in various regions, it became clear that true resilience extends far beyond having advanced medical technologies or adequate hospital capacity. It requires a robust, integrated public health infrastructure—the complex network of healthcare facilities, trained personnel, surveillance systems, and emergency response capabilities that enable effective crisis management.

This infrastructure must be supported by strong leadership willing to act decisively based on scientific evidence rather than political motivation, as demonstrated by New Zealand's communication strategy. It requires flexible systems that can adapt quickly to evolving threats, exemplified by Taiwan's rapid mobilization of resources and South Korea's extensive contact tracing efforts. Most crucially, it demands maintaining public trust through transparent and consistent messaging.

Critical to this resilience is sustained investment in healthcare worker wellbeing and capacity. The pandemic demonstrated that without adequate support for the clinical workforce, even well-designed response plans falter. Countries must develop comprehensive strategies for maintaining workforce capacity during crises, including mental health support, adequate protective equipment, and sustainable staffing models that prevent system-wide burnout.

Moving forward, COVID-19 has established that effective pandemic preparedness requires nations to strengthen foundational public health infrastructure—enhancing ICU capacity, securing essential supplies, implementing advanced surveillance systems, and optimizing coordination—while integrating strategic planning, infrastructure development, political will, and public engagement. The U.S. and U.K. experiences demonstrate the necessity of maintaining these systems even during periods of relative stability. Only through sustained investment during non-crisis periods can healthcare systems develop the comprehensive resilience necessary to address inevitable future global health challenges.

Vaccine Manufacturing and Supply Chain Challenges

The global response to COVID-19 exposed significant weaknesses in medical supply chains. As pharmaceutical companies raced to meet worldwide vaccine demand, limitations in manufacturing production capacity, intellectual property frameworks, and distribution infrastructure quickly became apparent. The emergence of vaccine supply chains during the pandemic revealed how geopolitical factors, export controls, and manufacturing concentration created bottlenecks that hindered global distribution.

Bottlenecks and Breakdowns: The Global Struggles of Vaccine Manufacturing

The unprecedented scale of COVID-19 vaccine production revealed critical weaknesses in global pharmaceutical manufacturing capacity. While multiple companies successfully developed effective vaccines in record time, producing billions of doses proved to be an entirely different challenge, underscoring the gap between vaccine development and large-scale manufacturing capabilities. A comprehensive analysis of vaccine manufacturing scale-up identified multiple critical bottlenecks, including raw material shortages, limited production facilities, and insufficient technology transfer mechanisms that constrained global production capacity (Feddema et al., 2023).

mRNA Vaccine Constraints

Manufacturers of mRNA vaccines faced unique technical hurdles in scaling up this novel technology. The production process required specialized ingredients and equipment, with lipid nanoparticles proving particularly challenging to source. These microscopic fatty molecules – essential for protecting and delivering mRNA into human cells – were manufactured by only a handful of companies worldwide before the pandemic (Schmidt, 2021).

In early 2021, experts noted that no one had ever envisioned a scenario requiring lipid nanoparticle formulation for billions of doses, emphasizing that the industry had not invented a process for producing these components at scale (Pradhan & Allen, 2021). The challenges of scaling up novel vaccine platforms like mRNA were compounded by the lack of established manufacturing infrastructure and expertise, particularly in regions that traditionally focused on conventional vaccine production (Feddema et al., 2023). Similarly, the enzymes needed to synthesize mRNA became critically scarce as manufacturers scaled up production. Biotechnology executives identified certain enzymes—particularly the vaccinia capping enzyme—as critical raw materials in short supply, with extremely limited global manufacturing capacity. Companies like Moderna warned that shortages of raw materials and reagents could significantly delay their production timelines (Nelson, 2021). The combined scarcity of lipid nanoparticles and enzymes created major bottlenecks that hampered mRNA vaccine output worldwide.

Traditional Vaccine Challenges

Manufacturers of more traditional vaccines encountered different but equally significant obstacles. AstraZeneca's production issues in Europe illustrated how slight variations in biological manufacturing conditions could drastically impact vaccine yield. In early 2021, one AstraZeneca facility in Belgium reported significantly lower output due to reduced cell culture yields, contributing to a 60% shortfall of expected doses for the European Union (Politico, 2021). Company officials revealed that some production plants were yielding up to three times as much vaccine as others, reflecting the inherent variability in complex biologic processes (The Guardian, 2021).

Johnson & Johnson's rollout was similarly disrupted by quality control failures at its subcontractor, Emergent BioSolutions. In March 2021, a contamination error at Emergent's Baltimore plant ruined up to 15 million doses of J&J's vaccine (Chappell & Wamsley, 2021). This mishap forced regulators to halt production there, ultimately leading to the discard of tens of millions of doses and significant delays in J&J's delivery schedule (Fierce Pharma, 2021). This exposed a key vulnerability: relying on a single facility for large-scale production meant that a single point of failure had global repercussions for vaccine supply.

The Serum Institute Story

A particularly illuminating example is the Serum Institute of India (SII). As the world's largest vaccine manufacturer by volume, SII was positioned as a key supplier for global vaccine distribution. Yet in 2021, its production was severely constrained by shortages of critical raw materials after the U.S. government invoked the Defense Production Act (DPA) (Das & Monnappa, 2021). The DPA gave U.S. vaccine makers priority access to supplies like specialized filters, bioreactor bags, and reagents, effectively limiting exports of those items (Pradhan & Allen, 2021). This policy decision reflected broader supply chain nationalism that emerged during the pandemic, as countries prioritized domestic vaccine production (Bown & Bollyky, 2022).

SII's CEO publicly appealed to the U.S. to lift its export embargo on vaccine inputs, warning that such restrictions were directly hurting production of COVID-19 shots (Reuters, 2021a). Ultimately, the raw material crunch forced SII to scale back output of the Oxford/AstraZeneca vaccine (branded "Covishield"), further emphasizing how export controls from a single source could create cascading disruptions throughout global vaccine manufacturing networks (Kansteiner, 2021).

Intellectual Property vs. Public Health Responsibility: The Vaccine Patent Debate

Tension between intellectual property rights and global vaccine access emerged as a central controversy during the pandemic. In October 2020, India and South Africa submitted a proposal to the World Trade Organization seeking a waiver of certain provisions of the TRIPS Agreement for COVID-19 products (WTO, 2020). This TRIPS waiver initiative aimed to temporarily suspend patent protections on COVID-19 vaccines, treatments, and related technologies to enable broader manufacturing capabilities.

India's advocacy was especially notable given the capacity of institutes like SII, but also their limited ability to produce newer vaccines like mRNA shots without technology transfer. The international response to the proposed waiver exposed deep divisions. Pharmaceutical companies and many high-income countries initially opposed the patent waiver, arguing that protecting intellectual property was essential for innovation and that quality and safety could be compromised if vaccines were produced by inexperienced manufacturers (PhRMA, 2022).

Germany's response echoed this in May 2021 when they warned that giving away patents wasn't the solution, expressing concern that uncontrolled production could diminish quality and create more risk than opportunity (Nasr, 2021). Industry groups like PhRMA likewise contended that a waiver would undermine the incentives that spurred vaccine development and potentially introduce quality issues. Prior to 2021, the U.S., the EU, the U.K., and others had blocked discussions of the waiver at the WTO, reflecting these concerns.

The landscape shifted dramatically in May 2021 when the Biden administration announced U.S. support for a temporary TRIPS waiver for vaccines. This marked a dramatic reversal of the previous U.S. stance and injected new momentum into the debate (Shalal et al., 2021). WTO deliberations on the waiver gained urgency with backing from over 100 countries and vocal support from global health advocates.

However, the EU remained a staunch holdout. The EU resisted comprehensive patent waivers, instead proposing alternative solutions such as voluntary licensing arrangements, limited compulsory licensing, and technology transfer partnerships (Chalmers & Strupczewski, 2021). EU leaders argued that manufacturing capacity and supply chain issues, rather than patents, were the real bottlenecks. France stated that the main issue was the distribution of doses, suggesting that knowledge and resources to produce vaccines couldn't be conjured overnight by waiving intellectual property alone (Reuters, 2021).

Critics of the EU's position accused it of protecting its own pharmaceutical industry's interests under the guise of these arguments (Human Rights Watch, 2021). Commentators noted that the countries opposing the waiver were those hosting major vaccine companies and enjoying ample vaccine supplies at home. Despite intense public pressure and negotiations, a broad consensus on the TRIPS waiver proved elusive in 2021. A narrow waiver for vaccines was eventually agreed in 2022, though observers questioned its efficacy in addressing the fundamental issues (Devex, 2022).

The patent debate during COVID-19 revealed deeper structural issues: even if IP barriers were removed, many low-income countries lacked the technical infrastructure and know-how to produce complex vaccines like mRNA shots at scale. This recognition has since driven new initiatives—such as the WHO's mRNA Technology Transfer Hub in South Africa – to build manufacturing capacity in the Global South, though these efforts face significant challenges without the cooperation of major vaccine developers (Roelf, 2023).

The Cold Chain Crisis: Distribution Barriers Hinder Vaccine Access

Temperature-controlled supply chains emerged as another critical bottleneck in global vaccination efforts. The requirements were especially demanding for mRNA vaccines, with Pfizer-BioNTech's formulation initially requiring storage at −70°C, far colder than traditional vaccine storage conditions (FDA, 2021). This necessitated specialized ultra-cold freezers, continuous temperature monitoring systems, and carefully coordinated transportation networks to keep doses viable during transit.

In late 2020, many countries rapidly invested in ultra-cold chain infrastructure. Hospitals and states in the U.S. scrambled to procure freezers capable of −70°C storage, with costs ranging from $10,000 to $20,000 each, in preparation for Pfizer's vaccine (CNBC, 2020; Reuters, 2020). The technical requirements for maintaining ultra-cold temperatures presented significant logistical challenges, particularly in regions with limited infrastructure (Wright et al., 2021).

Infrastructure challenges varied significantly by region. Health facilities in rural areas often faced unreliable electricity supplies, making consistent vaccine refrigeration technically challenging. In sub-Saharan Africa, only about 28% of health facilities have access to reliable electricity, creating significant operational constraints for maintaining cold chain requirements (Adair-Rohani et al., 2013; World Bank, 2022). This infrastructure gap meant that many clinics couldn't maintain the stable temperatures required for vaccine storage.

International organizations scrambled to address these cold chain disparities. COVAX, the global vaccine-sharing initiative, launched a large-scale effort to supply ultra-cold storage equipment to participating countries. UNICEF, on behalf of COVAX, set up an Ultra-Cold Chain Equipment Support Package, deploying hundreds of ultra-low temperature freezers to nations in Africa, Asia, and Latin America in 2021 (UNICEF, 2021). This represented the largest ever expansion of ultra-cold chain capacity worldwide. In parallel, COVAX and Gavi worked with manufacturers on specialized thermal shipping containers – essentially high-tech cold boxes packed with dry ice – to transport mRNA vaccines to remote regions while maintaining required temperatures (Gavi, 2021b).

Vaccine producers also began introducing more thermally stable formulations. By mid-2021, regulatory approvals allowed the Pfizer-BioNTech vaccine to be stored at standard freezer temperatures (around –20°C) for up to two weeks, and later under regular refrigerated conditions (2–8°C) for up to one month (FDA, 2021; Pfizer, 2021). Moderna's vaccine required –20°C storage by design (an easier requirement), and Novavax's protein-based vaccine was stable at ordinary refrigerator temperatures. These developments gradually eased the cold chain burden, especially as newer data showed some mRNA vaccines could tolerate less extreme conditions for short periods.

Despite these improvements, cold chain requirements continued to influence global vaccination patterns and contributed to inequity between nations. The high cost and technical complexity of ultra-cold logistics delayed mRNA vaccine roll-outs in many low-income countries in 2021, forcing those countries to rely more on vaccines like AstraZeneca or Johnson & Johnson that could be handled in normal cold chains (2–8°C). Programs to distribute ultra-cold freezers encountered implementation hurdles – not only the expense of the equipment, but also the need for training staff, ensuring maintenance, and securing a continuous power supply (WHO, 2021a; WHO, 2021b). Even when equipment was provided through donations, some countries faced delays in delivery and installation. For instance, a country might receive freezers but lack sufficient dry ice production or expertise to effectively deploy them in rural clinics.

By late 2021, manufacturers and global agencies were actively mitigating cold chain constraints. Pfizer developed insulated shipping containers that could keep vaccines at ultra-low temperatures for up to 30 days with dry ice refills (Pharmaceutical Commerce, 2020). Additionally, expanded global production of mRNA vaccines in 2022 and newer vaccine versions that tolerate higher temperatures

Table 10.5 Cold Chain Requirements by COVID-19 Vaccine Technology

Vaccine Technology	*Storage Temperature*	*Maximum Storage Duration*	*Special Equipment Needed*
mRNA *(Pfizer-BNT, Moderna)*	−70°C to −20°C (−94°F to −4°F) • *Pfizer: −70°C (−94°F)* • *Moderna: −20°C (−4°F)*	• Up to 6 months *(ultra-cold/frozen temperature)* • 5–30 days at 2–8°C	• Ultra-cold freezers or dry ice • Temperature monitoring • Complex cold chain logistics
Viral Vector *(AstraZeneca, J&J)*	2–8°C (36–46°F) • *Some require −20°C for shipping*	3–6 months at 2–8°C *(standard refrigeration)*	• Standard medical refrigeration
Protein Subunit *(Novavax)*	2–8°C (36–46°F)	• 6+ months at 2–8°C *(standard refrigeration)* • Up to 24 hours *(room temperature)*	• Standard medical refrigeration
Inactivated Virus *(Sinovac, Sinopharm)*	2–8°C (36–46°F)	• Up to 3 years at 2–8°C *(standard refrigeration)*	• Standard medical refrigeration • Some require heat monitors

Sources: WHO (2021); FDA (2021); Gavi (2021).

began to reduce dependence on ultra-cold storage at the last mile. Nonetheless, the "cold chain crisis" of 2021 provides a cautionary lesson: logistical capacity can be as important as scientific capacity in a pandemic response. Going forward, strengthening cold chain infrastructure—from reliable electricity in clinics to regional freezer farms—is seen as a priority for improving preparedness and ensuring that life-saving vaccines reach everyone who needs them, not just those in wealthy nations (Golumbeanu & Knuckles, 2022).

Building Resilient Supply Systems for the Future

The pandemic exposed critical vulnerabilities in global medical supply chains that require comprehensive reforms. The convergence of manufacturing constraints, intellectual property disputes, and cold chain limitations created multiple bottlenecks that hampered vaccine distribution worldwide. These challenges revealed that the global health infrastructure was designed primarily for routine medical needs rather than the intense demands of a worldwide health emergency. The rapid emergence of vaccine supply chains during COVID-19 demonstrated both the potential for expedient innovation and the need for more resilient manufacturing and distribution systems going forward (Bown & Bollyky, 2022).

Key priorities include diversifying manufacturing capacity geographically, developing more flexible IP frameworks for health emergencies, and investing in cold chain infrastructure. Building resilient supply chains requires addressing multiple systemic weaknesses simultaneously, including establishing emergency manufacturing protocols, developing frameworks for swift intellectual property sharing during crises, and strengthening international cooperation mechanisms. These reforms are crucial not only for managing ongoing pandemic responses but also for preparing for future global health crises.

Global Vaccine Equity and Distribution Disparities

The global race to develop COVID-19 vaccines quickly evolved into an equally challenging race to distribute them, revealing deep inequities in global health access. As vaccines emerged as the key to ending the pandemic, wealthy nations leveraged their financial resources and political influence to secure the majority of early supplies – engaging in what became known as "vaccine nationalism," prioritizing their own populations over global distribution through direct negotiations with manufacturers. This approach created immediate disparities, with wealthier countries rapidly accumulating vaccines while low- and middle-income countries struggled to gain access. In response to these emerging inequities, the international community launched initiatives like COVAX to address the imbalance, though these efforts faced significant logistical, political, and financial hurdles. Meanwhile, the distribution challenge gave rise to new geopolitical dynamics, with countries like China and Russia using vaccine access as a diplomatic tool to extend their global influence.

COVAX and Vaccine Equity: A Struggle Against Supply and Sovereignty

The launch of the COVID-19 Vaccines Global Access program (COVAX) in 2020 represented an ambitious attempt to ensure equitable access to COVID-19 vaccines worldwide. Co-led by the WHO, Gavi, and the Coalition for Epidemic Preparedness Innovations (CEPI), the initiative aimed to pool resources and secure vaccines for the world's most vulnerable populations, particularly in low- and middle-income countries that lacked the means to negotiate large vaccine contracts directly with pharmaceutical companies.

COVAX set an initial goal of delivering 2 billion vaccine doses by the end of 2021 and aimed to cover at least 20% of each participating country's population, prioritizing healthcare workers and high-risk groups (Berkley, 2020). However, the initiative fell significantly short of these objectives. By January 2022, COVAX had delivered only about 1 billion doses—barely half of its original target (Guarascio, 2022). This amounted to less than 10% of the total ~8 billion vaccine doses administered globally by that time (WHO, 2021d, 2022b). Coverage in most low-income countries remained in the single digits (often under 5% of the population vaccinated), falling roughly 50% short of the 20% coverage goal in many of the hardest-hit regions. In terms of geographic reach, COVAX also underperformed: while it aspired to serve over 190 participating nations, only 144 countries had received vaccines via COVAX by early 2022 (WHO, 2022b).

Even as COVAX began its work, wealthy nations had already secured much of the early vaccine supply through bilateral agreements with manufacturers. The inequitable distribution was not merely a matter of purchasing power, but also reflected deeper structural disparities in how vaccine supply chains emerged during the pandemic. Wealthy nations leveraged their existing pharmaceutical infrastructure and relationships to secure priority access to limited production capacity (Bown & Bollyky, 2022). The United States, United Kingdom, and European Union members claimed millions of doses before COVAX could establish its distribution network, weakening the initiative's purchasing power and ability to negotiate effectively with pharmaceutical companies.

These challenges multiplied when India halted vaccine exports during its devastating second wave in early 2021. This decision significantly impacted COVAX's distribution plans, as the program heavily relied on the SII for a large share of its supply. COVAX had to revise its forecasted 2021 deliveries downward by approximately 25% mid-year due to the sudden shortfall (Gavi, 2021a). In addition to these supply disruptions, many recipient countries faced formidable operational challenges. The ultra-cold storage requirements for mRNA vaccines like Pfizer-BioNTech's demanded large investments in infrastructure, which were often beyond reach in lower-income settings (Khairi et al., 2022).

COVAX's financial model—dependent on advance purchase agreements and voluntary donations – also proved fragile in the face of shifting political priorities and rising vaccine nationalism. Rich countries largely sidestepped COVAX's pooled procurement in 2021 by pursuing their own deals or even donating doses outside of COVAX, which reduced the volumes COVAX could deliver in its early phase (Wouters et al., 2021). Critics argued that the international community needed to look beyond COVAX for comprehensive solutions to vaccine inequity, as the initiative alone was insufficient to address the scale of global disparities (The Lancet, 2021). When vaccines became more widely available in late 2021, logistical issues such as limited healthcare workforce capacity, vaccine hesitancy, and last-mile delivery bottlenecks further constrained uptake. Despite its shortcomings, COVAX marked a crucial step toward global solidarity – but its struggles highlighted the persistent inequalities in global health systems and the tensions between sovereignty, supply, and shared responsibility. The initiative remained central to WHO's broader vaccine equity campaign, which emphasized that equitable access was both a moral imperative and a practical necessity for ending the pandemic (WHO, 2022a).

Vaccine Diplomacy: Geopolitical Power Plays in a Global Health Crisis

As COVAX struggled to meet its distribution goals, a new form of international relations emerged through vaccine diplomacy, where nations wielded vaccine access as a tool for extending their global influence and strengthening diplomatic ties. This practice became particularly evident in the strategies employed by China and Russia, who saw an opportunity to fill the vacuum created by Western nations' focus on domestic vaccination campaigns.

China, already pursuing global influence through its Belt and Road Initiative, strategically positioned its vaccine exports as part of a broader diplomatic outreach program. The country's two major vaccines, Sinopharm and Sinovac, became powerful instruments of soft power, particularly in regions struggling to secure doses through traditional channels. China distributed millions of doses across Africa, Latin America, and Southeast Asia, creating closer ties with these regions and positioning itself as a reliable partner in global health crises. Early in 2021, China's government provided free vaccine doses to 69 countries and sold doses to 28 others as part of this "vaccine diplomacy" effort (Huang, 2021). However, this diplomatic success was tempered by growing concerns over the efficacy of Chinese vaccines, as studies emerged suggesting lower effectiveness compared to mRNA alternatives.

Russia pursued a similar strategy with its Sputnik V vaccine, targeting countries that found themselves at the back of the queue for Western vaccines. The Russian vaccine gained particular traction in nations like Argentina, India, and parts of Eastern Europe, where Russia framed its exports as a viable alternative to Western vaccines. However, Russia's vaccine diplomacy efforts faced their own challenges, including production delays and questions about data transparency, which ultimately limited Sputnik V's global impact.

The pandemic initiated the emergence of vaccine diplomacy and created new avenues for geopolitical competition and influence. While these diplomatic efforts helped fill critical gaps in global vaccine distribution, they also raised concerns about the increasing politicization of public health initiatives. The transformation of vaccines from medical necessities to diplomatic tools reflected the broader failure of global cooperation in ensuring equitable access (Khairi et al., 2022). Vaccines became not just necessary medical interventions but powerful tools of international relations, capable of reshaping diplomatic alignments and regional partnerships.

Vaccine Hoarding: How Wealthy Nations Prolonged Global Inequity

Perhaps the most striking manifestation of global inequity during the vaccine rollout emerged through the practice of vaccine hoarding by wealthy nations. This systematic stockpiling of vaccines by high-income countries, who secured and stored more doses than their populations required, created a profound imbalance in global access. The practice began even before vaccines gained regulatory approval, as wealthy nations used their financial and political leverage to establish advance purchase agreements with pharmaceutical companies. The ability to secure these early agreements was facilitated by existing supply chain relationships and infrastructure advantages that high-income countries possessed (Bown & Bollyky, 2022).

The scale of this hoarding became apparent by early 2021. Wealthy Western countries like the United States, Canada, Australia, and the United Kingdom had secured enough doses to vaccinate their entire populations multiple times over (Kirk et al., 2021). For example, by early 2021, Canada had secured vaccine doses equivalent to roughly 5 times its population, and the United Kingdom enough for

Table 10.6 Initial COVID-19 Vaccine Procurement by Selected High-Income Countries

Country/Region	*Doses Secured*	*Population (2021)*	*Full Vaccination Courses Possible*	*Times Population Could Be Fully Vaccinated*
Australia	~280 million	~25 million	~140 million	**5.6×**
Canada	~362 million	~38 million	~181 million	**4.8×**
The United Kingdom	~457 million	~67 million	~228.5 million	**3.4×**
European Union	~2.6 billion	~447 million	~1.3 billion	**2.9×**
Japan	~564 million	~126 million	~282 million	**2.2×**
The United States	~1.2 billion	~331 million	~600 million	**1.8×**
South Korea	~190 million	~52 million	~95 million	**1.8×**

Sources: Procurement data compiled from Duke Global Health Innovation Center (Kirk et al., 2021).

about three to five times its population (Kirk et al., 2021). Such early hoarding by a handful of wealthy nations (making up only ~16% of the world's people) accounted for at least 4.2 billion reserved doses – over half the global vaccine supply at that time. These aggressive procurement strategies effectively locked up large portions of the global vaccine supply, leaving fewer doses available for both COVAX and low-income nations attempting to secure their own supplies through direct purchases.

The consequences of this inequitable distribution manifested clearly in vaccination statistics. By September 2021, while roughly 65–70% of populations in high-income countries had received full vaccination courses, vaccination rates in low-income countries were still below 5% (Rouw et al., 2021). The disparity was even more severe in regions like Africa, which had fully vaccinated no more than 3% of its population by September 2021 (AFRO WHO, 2021). Research revealed that these disparities were mediated not just by supply availability but also by vaccination policy differences between countries of different income levels (Duan et al., 2021).

The UNDP's Global Dashboard for Vaccine Equity tracked these disparities in real-time, revealing the deep contrasts in vaccination progress across income groups (UNDP, 2021). Systematic reviews of vaccine distribution patterns confirmed persistent inequalities, with high-income countries maintaining significantly higher vaccination rates throughout the pandemic (Bayati et al., 2022). Researchers have measured this global inequality using the Gini coefficient (where 0 represents perfect equality and 1 represents maximum inequality), finding values of 0.91 in June 2021 and 0.88 in December 2021—indicating extreme vaccine inequality throughout the year (Tatar et al., 2022).

The practice of vaccine hoarding extended beyond inequity in distribution and created significant public health risks on a global scale. As the virus continued to circulate freely in under-vaccinated regions, it gained more opportunities to mutate and evolve. Modeling studies demonstrated that vaccine nationalism not only

Table 10.7 Cumulative COVID-19 Vaccination Coverage by Country Income Level (2021 vs. 2025)

Country Income Level	*Population Fully Vaccinated (%)—2021*	*Population Fully Vaccinated (%)—2025*	*Current Status*
High-income	Approx. 65–70	Approx. 75–77	Plateau reached
Upper-middle-income	Approx. 50–55	Approx. 78–80	Surpassed HICs; strong growth
Lower-middle-income	Approx. 22–30	Approx. 60	Significant improvement
Low-income	Approx. 2–3	Approx. 33	Still lagging significantly

Sources: Vaccination coverage data for 2021 from WHO and Our World in Data; 2025 figures from WHO COVID-19 Dashboard.

prolonged the pandemic but also increased the likelihood of variant emergence that could evade immunity (Wagner et al., 2021). The emergence of new variants in regions with limited vaccine access demonstrated the interconnected nature of GHS (Khairi et al., 2022). A report from October 2021 estimated that high-income countries were holding approximately 870 million excess vaccine doses, with G7 and EU countries alone at risk of wasting 241 million doses by the end of 2021 (MSF, 2021). This dynamic became painfully evident with the emergence of new variants like Delta and Omicron, which developed in regions with lower vaccination rates before spreading globally. As health experts warned, the failure to achieve global vaccine equity would have dire consequences for all nations (Goldstein, 2021). These variants not only prolonged the pandemic but also demonstrated how vaccine hoarding by wealthy nations ultimately undermined their own efforts to control the virus within their own borders.

UN Secretary-General António Guterres succinctly put it: “if the virus is allowed to spread like wildfire in the global South, it will mutate again and again… enabling the virus to come back to plague the global North” (United Nations, 2021). This prescient warning underscored the principle that “no one is safe until everyone is safe”—a mantra that should guide global health policy. The WHO’s vaccine equity campaign repeatedly emphasized this interconnected nature of GHS, arguing that vaccine hoarding ultimately undermined the pandemic response for all nations (WHO, 2022b).

Beyond the Pandemic: Lessons and Reforms for Global Health Equity

These disparities in vaccine access during the COVID-19 pandemic have left lasting imprints on global health systems and international relations. The practice of vaccine hoarding by wealthy nations, combined with the limitations of initiatives like COVAX and the emergence of vaccine diplomacy, exposed fundamental weaknesses in the global health infrastructure that require systematic reform.

Trust between high-income and low- and middle-income countries suffered significant damage during the pandemic response. Many nations in the Global South viewed the Western approach to vaccine distribution as selfish and a betrayal of principles of global solidarity. Leaders from Africa, Asia, and Latin America openly criticized how a few rich countries monopolized early vaccine supplies and refused to waive intellectual property rights, despite pleas from the developing world (Al Jazeera, 2021). This erosion of trust may have lasting consequences for global health governance, particularly in responding to future pandemics where rapid information sharing and collaborative action are essential.

The economic and social instability caused by uneven vaccine access continues to reverberate through the global economy. Countries with lower vaccination rates have experienced prolonged periods of disease burden, leading to greater economic disruption and slower recovery. Modeling studies estimated the significant impact of vaccine inequities on global health outcomes, demonstrating how unequal distribution prolonged the pandemic for all nations (Gozzi et al., 2023). This disparity has further widened the gap between wealthy and poor nations, potentially setting back global development goals by years or even decades. Estimates from the IMF and other analyses showed that ensuring vaccines for lower-income countries would have had high returns by speeding the end of the pandemic for everyone.

Moving forward, the international community must address these systemic inequities by strengthening institutions like COVAX, developing more robust global supply chains, and establishing clear protocols for equitable distribution during health emergencies. The pandemic revealed how existing supply chain structures inherently favored wealthy nations with established pharmaceutical infrastructure (Bown & Bollyky, 2022). The WHO's vaccine equity framework highlighted the need for binding international commitments and sustainable financing mechanisms to prevent future inequities (WHO, 2022a). Initiatives are underway to bolster manufacturing capacity in the Global South—for instance, mRNA vaccine production hubs in Africa – so that poorer regions are not entirely dependent on charity or external supply in the next crisis. Likewise, proposals for a pandemic treaty at the WHO include provisions on the sharing of vaccines, technology transfer, and financing mechanisms to avoid a repeat of the 2021 vaccine apartheid.

These reforms represent essential investments in GHS, recognizing that in an interconnected world, the vulnerability of any population ultimately threatens the health and safety of all. The pandemic demonstrated the need to transition from vaccine nationalism to vaccine equity, requiring both immediate actions and long-term structural changes (Katz et al., 2021). The hope is that these lessons will spur genuine changes—in financing global public goods, strengthening institutions like the WHO, and fostering a mindset that global problems require global solutions based on solidarity rather than scarcity and competition.

Socioeconomic and Policy Interventions During the Pandemic

The COVID-19 pandemic triggered a profound socioeconomic crisis that forced governments worldwide to rapidly implement economic stimulus and support programs. As businesses shuttered and unemployment soared, countries scrambled to protect their economies and citizens from financial devastation. However, the effectiveness of these responses varied considerably, shaped by each nation's

Table 10.8 Initial Pandemic Economic Response by Country (2020–2021)

Region	*Stimulus as % of GDP*	*Policy Focus*	*Social Safety Net Strength*
The United States	25.5–27.0	Broad economic stimulus	Limited
The United Kingdom	18.5–20.0	Employment preservation	Moderate
Germany	14.8–16.0	Employment preservation	Strong
France	8.8–9.6	Employment support and economic recovery	Strong
South Korea	6.4–7.0	Coordinated health and economic strategy	Moderate
Japan	16.7–18.0	Universal support	Strong
China	4.4–6.0	Industrial recovery; infrastructure investment	Limited/Fragmented
Taiwan	3.5–4.0	Consumer spending; enterprise protection	Moderate
Brazil	8.0–9.2	Expanded social protection	Moderate/Targeted
India	3.9–4.5	Multi-faceted; federalized	Limited/Fragmented
South Africa	4.8–5.3	Social protection expansion	Limited
Mexico	0.7–1.3	Fiscal conservatism	Limited

Sources: International Monetary Fund (IMF) (2021a, 2021b); Hale et al. (2021); OECD (2020); World Bank (2021).

existing economic structure, social safety nets, and political priorities. Meanwhile, the pandemic further exposed and deepened long-standing socioeconomic inequalities, with marginalized communities bearing a disproportionate burden of both health risks and economic hardship.

The American Response: Stimulus Programs and Structural Inequities

In the United States, the federal government's response centered on massive stimulus packages, beginning with the $2.3 trillion CARES Act in March 2020. The scale of U.S. fiscal intervention was among the largest globally, representing approximately 25.5% of GDP across various relief measures (IMF, 2021a, 2021b). While unmatched in scale, these programs revealed deep structural inequities in the American economy. Real-time economic data demonstrated how different segments of the population experienced vastly different economic impacts, with low-wage workers suffering disproportionate job losses while high-income workers largely maintained employment (Chetty et al., 2024). The Paycheck Protection Program (PPP) demonstrated how existing banking relationships determined access to support, with large corporations, well-connected firms, and even billionaires' companies securing funds quickly while many small businesses—particularly those in minority and low-income communities—faced delays or denials. Financial institutions prioritized their wealthiest clients, leading to significant disparities in aid distribution (National Community Reinvestment Coalition (NCRC), 2020).

Furthermore, inadequate verification requirements and oversight enabled widespread fraud, with scammers, large corporations, and politically connected individuals diverting billions in taxpayer funds. Some businesses inflated payroll figures, while others created fictitious companies to obtain relief money. Concurrently, the federal government weakened key accountability measures, exemplified by the Trump administration's removal of the inspector general responsible for monitoring relief funds. Publicly traded companies and large restaurant chains exploited regulatory gaps to qualify for funds intended for small businesses, often returning the money only after public outcry and scrutiny. According to investigations, at least 75 public companies obtained PPP loans through affiliate rules (Observer, 2020), and an estimated $80 billion (roughly 10% of all PPP funds) may have been obtained fraudulently (Fitzpatrick & Strickler, 2023).

Direct payments and unemployment benefits, though vital, further exposed significant gaps in the U.S. social safety net. Many low-income workers, particularly undocumented immigrants, gig workers, and those in informal employment, struggled to access relief or were excluded entirely (Narea, 2020). The enhanced Child Tax Credit under the American Rescue Plan in 2021 temporarily lifted millions out of poverty, demonstrating both the effectiveness of direct economic support and the inadequacy of previous policies in addressing modern workforce realities. During the six months of expanded monthly CTC payments, the U.S. child poverty rate dropped by an estimated 30–46%, hitting historically low levels. However, when pandemic-era measures expired, economic vulnerabilities reemerged—the child poverty rate spiked in 2022, more than doubling back to pre-pandemic levels, reinforcing systemic inequities in financial aid distribution (Sy & Cuevas, 2023).

While the U.S. response was substantial in magnitude, its implementation reflected institutional biases favoring more affluent individuals, corporations, and those with established connections, rather than ensuring equitable relief across all affected populations.

European Response: Labor Market Protection Strategies

European nations prioritized employment preservation through wage subsidies and furlough programs, revealing a distinct policy approach from the U.S. model (Birnbaum, 2020). The European strategy focused on maintaining employer-employee relationships through short-time work schemes rather than allowing mass layoffs followed by rehiring, a policy choice that reflected different institutional frameworks and labor market philosophies (OECD, 2020). Analysis of wage inequality impacts across European countries showed that social distancing measures had differential effects on income distribution, with lower-wage workers experiencing greater economic hardship despite protective policies (Rodríguez et al., 2020). While generally effective at workforce stabilization, these programs exposed persistent challenges in addressing labor market inequalities, particularly for non-standard employment arrangements and the informal sector. Recent comprehensive research on EU small and medium-sized enterprises revealed how fiscal

Table 10.9 Initial Pandemic Household and Business Support Measures (2020–2021)

Region	*Household Support*	*Business Support*
The United States	Direct cash support *(stimulus checks, enhanced unemployment)*	Business loans and bailouts (PPP)
The United Kingdom	Unemployment wage protection *(Furlough Schemes)*	Business loans and tax deferrals
Germany	Unemployment wage protection *(Kurzarbeit)*	Liquidity assistance
France	Unemployment wage protection *(Chômage Partiel)*	State-backed loans; small business grants
South Korea	Targeted cash support *(Emergency Disaster Relief Payments)*	Small/medium enterprise support programs
Japan	Universal cash support *(Special Cash Payments)*	Employment subsidies
China	Consumer stimulus support *(Digital vouchers for household spending)*	Tax relief and low-interest loans
Taiwan	Consumer stimulus support *(Triple Stimulus Voucher Program)*	Business subsidies and sectoral support
Brazil	Direct cash support *(Auxílio Emergencial)*	Credit programs for small businesses
India	Targeted cash and food support *(PM-GKY, PDS)*	Credit guarantees
South Africa	Direct cash support *(Social Relief of Distress)*	Loan guarantees
Mexico	Limited direct support	Limited

Sources: IMF (2021a); Gentilini et al. (2022); Lacey et al. (2021); national government reports.

policy responses varied in effectiveness across different business sectors and regions (LSE-EIF Capstone Project, 2024).

The United Kingdom's response exemplified this approach through its *Coronavirus Job Retention Scheme*, providing up to 80% wage coverage for furloughed workers. By October 2020, over 8 million U.K. workers were on furlough, and ultimately, 11.7 million jobs (one-third of the workforce) had been supported by the scheme's end in 2021 (ONS, 2021). The scheme's structure and implementation details demonstrated the U.K. government's commitment to employment preservation, though its design evolved over time to address emerging challenges (Institute for Government, 2022). While the program prevented widespread unemployment, its structure revealed significant limitations. *The Self-Employment Income Support Scheme* attempted to address gaps in coverage, but eligibility requirements excluded recent entrepreneurs and various freelance categories. An estimated 1.8 million self-employed people (around one-quarter of the U.K.'s self-employed) were not eligible due to criteria such as recent business establishment or income thresholds (Cribb et al., 2021). The government's subsequent stimulus measures, including targeted VAT reductions and consumption incentives, demonstrated the challenge of balancing immediate relief with longer-term economic stability.

Germany expanded its established *Kurzarbeit* program, enabling firms to reduce employee hours while maintaining employment relationships. This system proved particularly effective for industrial employment stability but struggled to support workers in marginal employment arrangements. Many part-time and informal workers in "mini-jobs" were left without wage support despite the broad success of the program for standard employees. The government's supplementary stimulus packages, including significant allocations for energy cost relief and economic stabilization through the €130 billion Konjunkturpaket, illustrated the challenge of providing comprehensive support while addressing emerging crisis impacts (Bundesregierung, 2022).

France's partial unemployment scheme (*Chômage Partiel*) followed the broader European pattern while introducing unique elements through broader investment strategies like their *France Relance* industrial recovery plan (Kirchner, 2022). This multifaceted approach achieved significant economic stabilization—the recession in 2020, though sharp (−8% GDP), could have been worse without these measures, and by late 2021 France's GDP had nearly regained its pre-crisis level (IMF, 2021b). The distribution of benefits reflected institutional structures: larger firms and those in the formal sector were reached quickly, whereas some smaller enterprises and informal workers experienced delays or difficulties accessing aid.

Table 10.10 Pandemic Economic Response Implementation Gaps and Access Barriers by Region

Region	*Most Excluded Groups*	*Access Barriers*	*Digital Challenges*	*Distribution Efficiency*
North America	Undocumented, gig workers	Banking ties, ID requirements	Urban–rural divide	High *(formal sectors)*
Europe	Self-employed, new entrepreneurs	Eligibility rules, bureaucracy	Limited access for elderly	High overall
East Asia	Rural, non-standard workers	Administrative hurdles	Urban–rural divide	Very High *(urban areas)*
Latin America	Informal, unbanked workers	Digital sign-up, formal banking	Coverage gaps	Moderate
South Asia	Informal workers, migrants	Digital literacy, ID issues	Urban–rural divide	Limited
Africa	Rural, informal workers	Banking access, digital skills	Infrastructure constraints	Limited

Sources: IMF (2021a, 2021b); World Bank (2021); Gentilini et al. (2022); Abidoye et al. (2021); LSE-EIF Capstone Project (2024).

East Asian Responses: Integrated Economic and Public Health Approaches

East Asian economies demonstrated distinct policy frameworks that integrated public health measures with economic stabilization strategies, often leveraging digital technologies for rapid benefit distribution (Blavatnik School of Government, 2021). A common challenge across the region was the digital divide between urban and rural areas, affecting benefit distribution efficiency. Additionally, while these nations generally showed sophisticated technological implementation, traditional administrative requirements often created barriers for non-standard workers and small enterprises.

South Korea implemented a technology-driven response centered on targeted household support and business stabilization. According to the Oxford COVID-19 Government Response Tracker, South Korea's integrated approach combined stringent health measures with selective economic support (Hale et al., 2021). Its *Emergency Disaster Relief Payment* program strategically excluded the top 30% income bracket, while the Bank of Korea complemented these measures through monetary policy adjustments and enhanced small and medium enterprise lending support. The government's comprehensive relief package, totaling 53.7 trillion won, demonstrated high operational efficiency in urban areas while revealing persistent institutional barriers for specific demographic segments (Korea Herald, 2020).

Japan adopted a more conservative fiscal approach, implementing universal rather than targeted support through its *Special Cash Payments* program. While this approach ensured broad coverage, including foreign residents with valid status, reliance on traditional administrative mechanisms created operational inefficiencies. The employment adjustment subsidies effectively supported major industrial employers but revealed structural limitations in addressing labor market segmentation, particularly affecting female workers in non-standard employment arrangements.

China's centralized response emphasized direct market interventions and structural adjustments, combining tax relief, interest-free loans, and digital payment platforms for consumer vouchers. The government's stimulus measures included significant infrastructure investment and industrial recovery programs, with policies focused on maintaining employment and stabilizing supply chains (China Briefing, 2022). While this approach effectively stabilized formal economic sectors, it highlighted rural-urban disparities and demonstrated limited efficacy in addressing informal economy needs. The government's emphasis on infrastructure investment paralleled its 2008 crisis response, successfully maintaining formal economic stability while revealing persistent institutional challenges in providing comprehensive social protection.

Taiwan's response centered on innovative consumer-driven recovery through its *Triple Stimulus Voucher* program, achieving high participation rates while balancing technological efficiency with traditional access methods. The program's design effectively stimulated domestic consumption through sector-specific targeting, though smaller cash-dependent vendors faced operational challenges. This approach demonstrated how policy design could maximize economic impact while working within existing institutional frameworks.

Developing Nations: Resource Constraints and Structural Limitations

Developing economies faced distinct challenges in implementing emergency economic measures under resource constraints. Common obstacles included limited institutional capacity, large informal sectors, and inadequate digital infrastructure. These structural limitations often resulted in significant gaps between policy design and implementation effectiveness, particularly affecting the most vulnerable populations. The World Bank's comprehensive review of social protection responses documented how these constraints shaped policy outcomes across the developing world (Gentilini et al., 2022).

Brazil's *Auxílio Emergencial* program marked a substantial expansion of social protection, reaching over 67 million recipients and representing one of the largest emergency cash transfer programs globally (Lacey et al., 2021). While integration with existing programs like *Bolsa Família* facilitated distribution, digital registration requirements created systematic exclusion patterns. A comprehensive analysis of Brazil's pandemic response revealed how pre-existing socioeconomic inequalities and health system vulnerabilities shaped policy outcomes, with marginalized communities experiencing disproportionate impacts despite the scale of government intervention (Rocha et al., 2021). The government's complementary measures for small enterprises revealed the challenges of extending support through formal banking systems in economies with significant informal sectors.

India's multi-faceted response operated within complex federal structures, combining direct transfers, food security measures, and economic support through programs like the *Atmanirbhar Bharat Abhiyan.* The government announced a comprehensive ₹20 lakh crore stimulus package, representing approximately 10% of GDP, though critics noted that much of this included previously announced measures and credit guarantees rather than direct fiscal spending (Chawa, 2020). The *Emergency Credit Line Guarantee Scheme* highlighted the persistent challenge of supporting informal enterprises, while the crisis particularly exposed the limitations of state-based welfare systems in accommodating inter-state mobility. Rural infrastructure projects attempted to address return migration, though implementation faced significant coordination challenges.

South Africa's stimulus package demonstrated the complexities of implementing large-scale economic support in a developing economy context. The *COVID-19 Social Relief of Distress* grant revealed how digital application requirements and formal banking prerequisites created significant access barriers, particularly in informal settlements and rural areas (IMF, 2021a).

Mexico's conservative fiscal response prioritized stability over expansive relief measures, with crisis spending limited to approximately less than 1% of total GDP (Dallas Federal Reserve, 2021). This approach particularly affected informal sector workers, who comprise a substantial portion of the labor force yet received minimal direct support.

Global Economic Responses and Long-Term Socioeconomic Implications

The COVID-19 pandemic triggered unprecedented economic interventions worldwide while simultaneously exposing and deepening structural inequalities across societies (Ferreira, 2021). The Lancet Commission's comprehensive analysis highlighted how pandemic responses reflected and often amplified existing societal fault lines (Sachs et al., 2022). The tension between health protection and economic preservation created difficult policy tradeoffs, with distributional consequences that varied significantly across income levels and demographic groups (Ríos-Rull et al., 2020). Despite varied approaches between regions, common patterns emerged in how existing socioeconomic structures determined both immediate crisis responses and long-term recovery trajectories.

Across all regions, certain vulnerable populations consistently faced exclusion from support systems. Undocumented immigrants, informal sector workers, and gig economy participants frequently fell through coverage gaps, despite often working in essential industries during the height of the pandemic. Digital infrastructure limitations and complex application processes created additional barriers, while established businesses and individuals with strong institutional relationships gained easier access to support. The Oxfam report "The Inequality Virus" documented how these disparities widened wealth gaps globally, with billionaires increasing their wealth while the poorest faced deepening poverty (Berkhout et al., 2021). The recovery has followed these same fault lines—in wealthy nations, technology and financial sectors have flourished while service industry workers continue to struggle with financial instability (Federal Reserve Board, 2024). Developing nations face even steeper challenges, with mounting debt and economic contraction threatening years of development. The World Bank estimated that the pandemic pushed 120 million additional people into extreme poverty in 2020–2021, eroding hard-won gains in poverty reduction (World Bank, 2021). The pandemic's impact on achieving the Sustainable Development Goals has been particularly severe, with setbacks across multiple dimensions including health, education, and economic development (Abidoye et al., 2021).

The pandemic's impact on public health revealed an equally troubling divide. Communities that faced delayed access to vaccines and higher infection rates now confront increased risks of long-term health complications. These same communities often lack the resources for ongoing medical care, creating a cycle of worsening health outcomes. Empirical assessments have confirmed the disproportionate socioeconomic burden on marginalized communities (Gupta et al., 2022). The global distribution of healthcare resources—from protective equipment to vaccines – has followed patterns of existing economic inequality. By mid-2021, for example, only about 0.3% of COVID-19 vaccine doses administered worldwide had gone to people in low-income countries (WHO, 2021c), with devastating consequences for populations in resource-limited settings.

These challenges are substantial but not insurmountable. The diverse policy responses implemented during the crisis offer valuable insights for building more resilient and equitable systems. Research on vulnerable communities has identified specific lessons for improving crisis response systems to better serve those with the greatest socioeconomic vulnerabilities (Sheikhattari et al., 2023). Success requires sustained commitment to reform and willingness to learn from both achievements and failures. Future crisis response systems must be designed with structural vulnerabilities in mind, ensuring that emergency aid reaches those most in need rather than those best positioned to access it. Most importantly, preparation for future crises cannot wait for the next emergency to catch us off guard—it must begin with addressing the fundamental inequities that shape our current systems.

Communication Breakdowns and the Rise of Misinformation

The COVID-19 pandemic marked a unique challenge in public health communication, as authorities struggled to provide accurate, timely guidance while combating a rising tide of misinformation. Public health agencies like the CDC, WHO, and national bodies worldwide faced the complex task of communicating evolving scientific understanding while maintaining public trust. This challenge was further complicated by the rapid spread of conspiracy theories and false information across social media platforms, creating what the WHO termed an "infodemic"—an overwhelming volume of information that made it difficult for people to find reliable guidance when they needed it.

From Clarity to Confusion: The Challenges of Pandemic Communication

In the pandemic's early stages, public health agencies achieved notable successes in raising global awareness and mobilizing international containment efforts upon the WHO January 2020 Public Health Emergency of International Concern (PHEIC) declaration. Initial public health campaigns promoting basic prevention measures like hand hygiene, respiratory etiquette, and social distancing gained significant traction. This was particularly evident in parts of East Asia, where clear and consistent messaging by officials led to high compliance rates (Hotez, 2023; Razai et al., 2021).

However, as the pandemic evolved and scientific knowledge grew, maintaining consistent and accurate communication became increasingly difficult. The most notable example of this challenge emerged around mask guidance. In the initial phase of the outbreak, organizations like the WHO and CDC advised against widespread mask usage by the general public. This early guidance was given for several reasons: authorities were concerned about limited supplies of certified masks (which needed to be reserved for healthcare workers), and at the time there was incomplete evidence about transmission routes—with an early emphasis on fomite (surface) transmission over respiratory or aerosol spread (Missoni et al., 2020; Peeples, 2020).

As evidence mounted that COVID-19 was primarily transmitted through respiratory droplets, health agencies reversed their stance, advocating for universal mask usage by April 2020 for the CDC and June 2020 for the WHO. This abrupt shift, though scientifically justified, created widespread public confusion and skepticism (Schünemann et al., 2020). CDC Director Robert Redfield's testimony that 95% mask adoption occurred early in the pandemic, deaths could have been reduced by over 100,000, further highlighting the stakes of this communication failure (Peeples, 2020; Razai et al., 2021).

The situation was further complicated by inconsistent messaging from political leaders, some of whom actively questioned mask effectiveness. In the United States, high-profile figures refused to wear masks and downplayed their utility, sending mixed signals that contradicted public health experts (Gonsalves & Yamey, 2020). Analysis of local news coverage throughout the pandemic revealed how face coverings became increasingly politicized, with media framing shifting from public health necessity to partisan talking points (Neumann et al., 2023). What should have been a straightforward public health measure instead became a symbol of deeper ideological divisions, with mask-wearing increasingly viewed through a political rather than medical lens. Research confirmed that mask usage and attitudes were split rather unambiguously along these partisan lines, mostly fueled by cues from media figureheads and government leadership (Gonsalves & Yamey, 2020; Razai et al., 2021). The politicization of science in COVID-19 communication was particularly evident when comparing messages from politicians, medical experts, and government agencies, with significant divergence in how each group framed vaccine and prevention measures (Zhou et al., 2023).

Navigating Vaccine Hesitancy and Public Trust

The rollout of COVID-19 vaccines presented another critical test for public health communication. While the rapid development of effective vaccines marked a scientific milestone, public health bodies struggled to address mounting concerns about vaccine safety. This challenge became particularly evident in the case of the AstraZeneca vaccine, where reports of rare blood clots led to temporary suspensions in several European countries. The varying responses to these safety concerns—with some nations pausing distribution altogether while others continued—created a ripple effect of confusion and hesitancy that extended far beyond Europe's borders (Jain & Lorgelly, 2022; Subramanian, 2020).

The impact was especially pronounced in low-income countries, many of which relied heavily on the AstraZeneca vaccine through the COVAX initiative. Public confidence plummeted in these regions, significantly slowing vaccination campaigns at a critical time. The Africa CDC warned in March 2021 that Africa's reliance on AstraZeneca meant that misinformation and panic over these reports could have "particularly damaging consequences" on the continent (Swindells, 2021).

When wealthier nations publicized safety concerns and halted AstraZeneca's rollout, it indirectly sent a message to populations elsewhere that the vaccine might be unsafe, despite its overwhelmingly positive risk-benefit ratio (Swindells, 2021). Pre-existing vaccine skepticism and anti-vaccine movements seized on the AstraZeneca clot controversy to spread new waves of fear about all COVID-19 vaccines, particularly via social media channels that easily transmitted alarmist narratives across borders (Hotez, 2023).

To rebuild trust, many countries had to engage in proactive outreach, enlist community leaders, and increase transparency about vaccine safety monitoring. However, inconsistent policies (one country pausing a vaccine while another declared it safe) gave an appearance of disarray, which was exploited by anti-vaccine campaigners to cast doubt on vaccine uptake in general (Razai et al., 2021).

The Rise of Misinformation and the Battle for Public Trust

As public health agencies worked to communicate scientific guidance, a parallel narrative ecosystem emerged across social media platforms, characterized by widespread misinformation and conspiracy theories. Social media's role proved double-edged: while platforms like Facebook, Twitter, TikTok, and YouTube were crucial for disseminating public health information, they also became powerful vectors for false narratives and dangerous medical claims. Studies have shown that false news spreads faster and farther online than true news, because it tends to be more novel or emotionally evocative (Vosoughi et al., 2018). The COVID-19 infodemic on social media was characterized by a massive and rapid spread of misinformation that often outpaced official communications (Cinelli et al., 2020).

The promotion of unproven treatments became a particularly dangerous manifestation of this trend. Early in the pandemic, hydroxychloroquine, a drug traditionally used for malaria and autoimmune conditions, was widely touted as a potential COVID-19 miracle cure. High-profile political figures, including the presidents of the U.S. and Brazil, amplified claims about the drug's effectiveness, citing small, non-randomized studies that suggested possible benefits (Casarões & Magalhães, 2021; Rome et al., 2021). News outlets played a significant role in amplifying these unsubstantiated claims, with media coverage contributing substantially to the rise of hydroxychloroquine as a conspiracy theory in the early days of the pandemic (Dickinson et al., 2024).

Though the FDA initially issued an EUA in March 2020 based on limited evidence, larger clinical trials soon revealed no benefit in treating COVID-19, leading to the EUA's revocation by June 2020 (RECOVERY Collaborative Group, 2020). However, the damage was already done—public demand for hydroxychloroquine had surged, leading to shortages for patients who needed it for legitimate medical conditions. Surveys in April 2020 found that over half of lupus patients had difficulty refilling their prescriptions due to sudden spikes in demand and supply disruptions (CDC, 2021).

A similar pattern emerged with ivermectin, an antiparasitic medication. Despite early in vitro studies showing potential effects against SARS-CoV-2 only at concentrations far exceeding safe human dosage levels, the drug gained a devoted following through social media promotion and endorsements from public figures. The consequences were severe, with numerous reports of poisoning from people consuming veterinary formulations of the drug. By mid-2021, U.S. poison control centers were seeing a sharp spike in calls related to ivermectin overdose—one CDC advisory noted a several-fold increase compared to pre-pandemic baselines (CDC, 2021).

Public health agencies found themselves in the unusual position of having to issue warnings like the FDA's now-famous advisory, "*You are not a horse. You are not a cow*" (CDC, 2021). This striking message encapsulated the exasperation of the medical community and highlighted how widespread the misuse had become.

The Infodemic: How Information Overload Undermined Pandemic Response

The sheer volume of information circulating during the pandemic – both accurate and false—created what the WHO termed an "infodemic." This oceanic flood of content overwhelmed traditional fact-checking systems and made it increasingly difficult for individuals to discern reliable guidance from misleading or harmful information (WHO, 2020; Zarocostas, 2020). The psychological impact of this information overload was significant, with people experiencing increased anxiety and decision paralysis when faced with contradictory information. Social media algorithms, designed to amplify engaging content regardless of accuracy, often elevate sensational or misleading posts over more measured scientific communication. The overall impact of COVID-19 misinformation was profound, directly contributing to preventable deaths, vaccine hesitancy, and undermining public health measures (Ferreira Caceres et al., 2022).

One notorious conspiracy theory linked 5G wireless technology to COVID-19, despite having no scientific basis. These theories gained significant traction across multiple countries, eventually culminating in attacks on telecommunications infrastructure. In the United Kingdom, at least 61 suspected arson attacks targeted telephone masts in early 2020. The Netherlands experienced over 20 such incidents, with several cell towers set ablaze amid fears that 5G technology was linked to the virus (Cerulus, 2020; Subramanian, 2020).

Another example is the *Plandemic* documentary phenomenon in May 2020 that further illustrated the challenge. The video propagated a range of false claims, including allegations that COVID-19 was a planned conspiracy. Within the first two days of its release, the video garnered 4.7 million views on YouTube, and some estimates suggest it ultimately achieved over 9 million views, with related content generating more than 16 million engagements on Facebook (Kaplan, 2020).

Marginalized communities proved especially vulnerable to the effects of the infodemic (WHO, 2021e). Historical mistrust of healthcare systems, language barriers, and targeted disinformation campaigns all contributed to higher rates of vaccine hesitancy among minority populations in many countries. Online misinformation specifically targeted these communities, exploiting existing medical mistrust to amplify vaccine hesitancy (Garrett & Young, 2021). For instance, by late 2020, polls indicated that Black Americans were less likely than white Americans to say they'd get vaccinated, often citing distrust as a key reason (Malik et al., 2020). This pattern was particularly pronounced among communities with histories of medical discrimination, where COVID-19 vaccine hesitancy was strongly predicted by medical mistrust and perceived discrimination (Morgan et al., 2023). Similarly in the U.K., initial vaccine uptake among elderly Black and South Asian Britons lagged significantly behind that of white Britons (Razai et al., 2021).

Table 10.11 Common Misinformation and Conspiracies Spread Throughout the COVID-19 Pandemic, with Corresponding Explanations

Misinformation Claim	*Explanation*
"COVID-19 was intentionally created in a lab as a bioweapon."	While the lab leak theory remains a possible origin scenario, there is no evidence that COVID-19 was intentionally engineered as a bioweapon.
"Gain-of-function research was used to make COVID-19 more dangerous."	Genetic analyses show no clear signs of artificial manipulation of SARS-CoV-2 via gain-of-function research.
"5G networks spread COVID-19."	COVID-19 spread correlates with human movement and transmission, not wireless networks via electromagnetic waves.
"Wearing masks causes carbon dioxide poisoning."	Masks are designed to allow airflow while filtering out respiratory droplets. CO_2 molecules are too small to be trapped by masks.
"Natural immunity is superior to vaccine-induced immunity."	Natural immunity helps, but vaccine-induced immunity is more predictable and protective, especially against severity and/or reinfection.
"Ivermectin and hydroxychloroquine are effective treatments for COVID-19."	Extensive trials found that neither ivermectin nor hydroxychloroquine provided significant benefits in treating COVID-19.
"COVID-19 vaccines alter DNA."	mRNA vaccines do not alter DNA. They instruct cells to produce a harmless spike protein to trigger an immune response.
"COVID-19 vaccines cause infertility."	No scientific evidence supports claims that COVID-19 vaccines cause infertility.
"COVID-19 vaccines contain microchips."	There are no microchips in COVID-19 vaccines. The claim spread as an unfounded conspiracy theory with no basis in evidence.
"The vaccines were rushed and unsafe."	While developed quickly, COVID-19 vaccines underwent rigorous trials and regulatory reviews to ensure high safety and efficacy.
"PCR tests give false positives due to detecting common cold viruses."	PCR tests specifically detect SARS-CoV-2, not common cold viruses. The claim is based on the misunderstanding of test sensitivity.
"COVID-19 was planned as part of a global population control scheme."	There is no credible evidence supporting claims that COVID-19 was planned as a global population control scheme.

Sources: CDC (2021); Ferreira Caceres et al. (2022); RECOVERY Collaborative Group (2020); Razai et al. (2021); WHO (2020).

Strengthening Public Health Communication in the Digital Age

The COVID-19 pandemic fundamentally reshaped our understanding of public health communication in the digital era, exposing critical shortcomings in current approaches while pointing toward necessary reforms. Public health agencies must develop more sophisticated strategies for maintaining clear, consistent messaging across borders while actively countering misinformation.

The challenge of combating misinformation demands multifaceted solutions that combine technological tools with community engagement. Some social media platforms have begun investing in AI-driven tools to detect and flag false information more quickly, while also expanding partnerships with fact-checkers across different languages and regions. However, technology alone cannot solve the problem—particularly when the flow of information is shaped by corporate or political interests, such as social media algorithms prioritizing engagement over accuracy, or when commercial and institutional actors shape the visibility of health guidance in ways that reflect ideological or strategic agendas rather than public health priorities.

Research on interventional fact-checking effectiveness has revealed a paradox: while COVID-19 vaccine fact-checking posts from hospitals yielded more positive attitudes toward vaccination than other sources, these trusted institutions received significantly less engagement (Xue et al., 2022). This paradox highlights a fundamental problem in public health communication—the most credible sources often struggle to compete with sensational content for public attention. As the pandemic progressed, third-party fact-checkers played an increasingly larger role in posting vaccine-related fact-checks, though the overall percentage of fact-checking posts steadily decreased after May 2020 (Xue et al., 2022).

The recent example of X (formerly Twitter) rolling back content moderation policies demonstrates how platforms can become "echo chambers" for misinformation under the guise of protecting "free speech" or open discourse. Similarly, Facebook's decision to scale back fact-checking initiatives and deprioritize combating misinformation reflects a troubling pivot toward prioritizing engagement metrics over public trust and safety. These actions illustrate how corporate interests may converge with political opportunism, often undermining public trust in the process.

As we've witnessed, the rapid abandonment of trust initiatives by these platforms highlights the vulnerability of our information ecosystem to political pressures. Such actions emphasize the foundational role that government institutions and independent media play in maintaining public trust during crises. When these institutions are undermined, hollowed out, or weaponized for political clout, the resulting erosion of trust can cause severe harm to populations worldwide. Addressing these conflicts will require greater transparency and accountability from platforms, along with independent oversight to ensure that public health priorities always remain at the forefront.

As it stands, public health agencies face a delicate balance in crisis communication: maintaining credibility while adapting to evolving scientific understanding. When guidance changes—as it inevitably does during an emerging crisis—clear, contextual explanations must accompany these shifts. Effective communication requires acknowledging uncertainty while still providing actionable guidance that inspires public trust and adherence. Ultimately, successful public health messaging should prioritize trust-building over coercion.

These communication breakdowns and the resulting infodemic fundamentally altered how individuals and societies conceptualized the pandemic. Institutional erosion, the politicization of health measures, and persistent misinformation didn't just affect information flow—they created entirely new frameworks through which people understood COVID-19 and public health authority itself. But to fully comprehend why communication collapsed so catastrophically, we must look deeper than institutional failings or technological shortcomings. The pandemic revealed something more profound: how our underlying mental models—individual, collective, and institutional—determined not just what information we trusted, but how we processed reality itself during this generation-defining global crisis.

References

Abbey, E. J., Khalifa, B. A. A., Oduwole, M. O., Ayeh, S. K., Nudotor, R. D., & Salia, E. L. (2020). The Global Health Security Index is not predictive of coronavirus pandemic responses among Organization for Economic Cooperation and Development countries. *PLoS ONE, 15*(10), e0239398. https://doi.org/10.1371/journal.pone.0239398

Abidoye, B., Felix, J., Kapto, S., & Patterson, L. (2021). *Leaving no one behind: Impact of COVID-19 on the sustainable development goals (SDGs)*. United Nations Development Programme and Frederick S. Pardee Center for International Futures.

Adair-Rohani, H., Zukor, K., Bonjour, S., Wilburn, S., Kuesel, A. C., Hebert, R., & Fletcher, E. (2013). Limited electricity access in health facilities of sub-Saharan Africa: A systematic review of data on electricity access, sources, and reliability. *Global Health: Science and Practice*, *1*(2), 249–261. https://doi.org/10.9745/GHSP-D-13-00037

AFRO WHO. (2021, September 2). *Opening statement, COVID-19 press conference*. World Health Organization Regional Office for Africa. https://www.afro.who.int/regional-director/speeches-messages/opening-statement-covid-19-press-conference-2-september-2021

Al Jazeera. (2021, September 30). *Vaccine apartheid: The global South fights back*. Al Jazeera. https://www.aljazeera.com/opinions/2021/9/30/vaccine-apartheid-the-global-south-fights-back

Allin, S., Fitzpatrick, T., Marchildon, G., & Quesnel-Vallée, A. (2021). The federal government and Canada's COVID-19 response: From 'we're ready, we're prepared' to 'fires are burning'. *Health Economics, Policy and Law*, 1–16. https://doi.org/10.1017/S1744133121000220

American Association of Colleges of Nursing (AACN). (2024, May). *Nursing shortage fact sheet*. https://www.aacnnursing.org/news-data/research-data-center/nursing-shortage-fact-sheet

Assefa, Y., Gilks, C. F., Reid, S., van de Pas, R., Williams, O. D., & Hill, P. S. (2022). Analysis of the COVID-19 pandemic: Lessons towards a more effective response to public health emergencies. *Global Health, 18*, 10. https://doi.org/10.1186/s12992-022-00805-9

Ba, Z., Li, Y., Ma, J., Qin, Y., Tian, J., Meng, Y., Yi, J., Zhang, Y., & Chen, F. (2023). Reflections on the dynamic zero-COVID policy in China. *Preventive Medicine Reports*, *36*, 102466. https://doi.org/10.1016/j.pmedr.2023.102466

Baker, M. G., Wilson, N., & Anglemyer, A. (2020). Successful elimination of COVID-19 transmission in New Zealand. *New England Journal of Medicine*, *383*(8), e56. https://doi.org/10.1056/NEJMc2025203

Bautista-Reyes, D., Werner-Sunderland, J., Aragón-Gama, A. C., Duran, J. R. C., Medina, K. D. C., Urbina-Fuentes, M., & Bautista-González, E. (2023). Health-care policies during the COVID-19 pandemic in Mexico: A continuous case of heterogeneous, reactive, and unequal response. *Health Policy Open*, *5*, 100100. https://doi.org/10.1016/j.hpopen.2023.100100

Bayati, M., Noroozi, R., Ghanbari-Jahromi, M., Jalali, F. S., Saboori, H., Salehi, M., Lohivash, S., Yaghoubi, S., Lohivash, S., & Aarabi, M. (2022). Inequality in the distribution of Covid-19 vaccine: A systematic review. *International Journal for Equity in Health, 21*, 122. https://doi.org/10.1186/s12939-022-01729-x

Berkhout, E., Galasso, N., Lawson, M., Rivero Morales, P. A., Taneja, A., & Vázquez Pimentel, D. A. (2021). *The inequality virus: Bringing together a world torn apart by coronavirus through a fair, just and sustainable economy*. Oxfam International. https://policy-practice.oxfam.org/resources/the-inequality-virus-bringing-together-a-world-torn-apart-by-coronavirus-throug-621149/

Berkley, S. (2020, September 3). COVAX explained. *Gavi, the Vaccine Alliance*. https://www.gavi.org/vaccineswork/covax-explained

Bigoni, A., Malik, A. M., Tasca, R., Carrera, M. B. M., Schiesari, L. M. C., Gambardella, D. D., & Massuda, A. (2022). Brazil's health system functionality amidst of the COVID-19 pandemic: An analysis of resilience. *The Lancet Regional Health – Americas, 10*, 100222. https://doi.org/10.1016/j.lana.2022.100222

Birnbaum, M. (2020, April 30). *Coronavirus hits European economies but governments help shield workers*. The Washington Post. https://www.washingtonpost.com/world/europe/joblessness-is-rising-far-more-slowly-in-europe-than-in-the-us-during-the-pandemic-new-figures-show/2020/04/30/7a5a050a-8a5a-11ea-80df-d24b35a568ae_story.html

Blavatnik School of Government. (2021). *COVID-19 policy briefs*. University of Oxford. Retrieved from https://www.bsg.ox.ac.uk/research/covid-19-government-response-tracker

Bown, C. P., & Bollyky, T. J. (2022). How COVID-19 vaccine supply chains emerged in the midst of a pandemic. *The World Economy, 45*(2), 468–522. https://doi.org/10.1111/twec.13183

Brusselaers, N., Steadson, D., Bjorklund, K., Breland, S., Stilhoff Sörensen, J., Ewing, A., Bergmann, S., & Steineck, G. (2022). Evaluation of science advice during the COVID-19 pandemic in Sweden. *Humanities and Social Sciences Communications, 9*, 91. https://doi.org/10.1057/s41599-022-01097-5

Bundesregierung. (2022). *Third relief package to address energy prices*. https://www.bundesregierung.de/breg-en/news/third-relief-package-2123130

Casarões, G., & Magalhães, D. (2021). The hydroxychloroquine alliance: How far-right leaders and alt-science preachers came together to promote a miracle drug. *Revista De Administração Pública, 55*(1), 197–214. https://doi.org/10.1590/0034-761220200556

Centers for Disease Control and Prevention (CDC). (2021, August 26). *Rapid increase in ivermectin prescriptions and reports of severe illness associated with use of products containing ivermectin to prevent or treat COVID-19 (CDC Health Advisory No. 449)*. CDC Health Alert Network. https://stacks.cdc.gov/view/cdc/109271

Centers for Disease Control and Prevention (CDC). (2023, October 24). *Health workers face a mental health crisis: Vital signs*. https://www.cdc.gov/vitalsigns/health-worker-mental-health/index.html

Cerulus, L. (2020, April 23). *5G mast torchers turn up in Continental Europe*. Politico. https://www.politico.eu/article/5g-mast-torchers-turn-up-in-continental-europe/

Chalmers, J., & Strupczewski, J. (2021, May 7). *Key EU countries rebuff Biden on sharing COVID vaccine patents*. Reuters. https://www.reuters.com/world/europe/eu-split-vaccine-waiver-idea-unlikely-take-clear-stance-2021-05-07/

Chappell, B., & Wamsley, L. (2021, April 1). *Johnson & Johnson says contractor botched part of vaccine production*. NPR. https://www.npr.org/2021/04/01/983380847/johnson-johnson-says-contractor-botched-part-of-vaccine-production

Chawla, D. (2020, May 13). *Invest India*. Investindia.gov.in. https://www.investindia.gov.in/team-india-blogs/finance-minister-announces-details-indias-20-lakh-crore-economic-package

Chen, Y.-H., & Fang, C.-T. (2024). Achieving COVID-19 zero without lockdown, January 2020 to March 2022: The Taiwan model explained. *Journal of the Formosan Medical Association, 123*(Suppl 1), S8–S16. https://doi.org/10.1016/j.jfma.2023.09.001

Chetty, R., Friedman, J. N., Stepner, M., & Opportunity Insights Team. (2024). The economic impacts of COVID-19: Evidence from a new public database built using private sector data. *The Quarterly Journal of Economics*, *139*(2), 829–889. https://doi.org/10.1093/qje/qjad048

China Briefing. (2022, June 10). *China's economic stimulus explained – understanding China's monetary and fiscal policy*. https://www.china-briefing.com/news/chinas-economic-stimulus-explained-monetary-fiscal-policy/

Chung, D., & Soh, H. S. (2020, March 23). *Korea's response to COVID-19: Early lessons in tackling the pandemic*. World Bank Blogs. https://blogs.worldbank.org/en/eastasiapacific/koreas-response-covid-19-early-lessons-tackling-pandemic

Cinelli, M., Quattrociocchi, W., Galeazzi, A., Valensise, C. M., Brugnoli, E., Schmidt, A. L., Zola, P., Zollo, F., & Scala, A. (2020). The COVID-19 social media infodemic. *Scientific Reports*, *10*, 16598. https://doi.org/10.1038/s41598-020-73510-5

CNBC. (2020, November 24). *Ford orders 12 ultra-cold freezers to distribute COVID-19 vaccines*. https://www.cnbc.com/2020/11/24/ford-orders-12-ultra-cold-freezers-to-distribute-covid-19-vaccines-.html

Cribb, J., Delestre, I., & Johnson, P. (2021). *Who is excluded from the government's Self Employment Income Support Scheme and what could the government do about it?*. London: IFS. Available at: https://ifs.org.uk/publications/who-excluded-governments-self-employment-income-support-scheme-and-what-could

da Silva, S. J. R., & Pena, L. (2021). Collapse of the public health system and the emergence of new variants during the second wave of the COVID-19 pandemic in Brazil. *One Health*, *13*, 100287. https://doi.org/10.1016/j.onehlt.2021.100287

Dallas Federal Reserve. (2021). COVID-19 poses stubborn challenge to economic growth in Mexico. *Southwest Economy* (1). Federal Reserve Bank of Dallas. https://www.dallasfed.org/research/swe/2021/swe2101/swe2101c

Das, K. N., & Monnappa, C. (2021, April 16). *Indian vaccine maker Serum Institute appeals to Biden to lift embargo on raw material exports*. Reuters. https://www.reuters.com/article/health-coronavirus-india-vaccines-idUSKBN2C30ZR

Davino-Ramaya, C. M., Hostetler Lippy, S., Naturale, A., Feist, J. C., Cipriano, P., & Clark, D. (2023). Burnout and the effect on the global health care workforce crisis: An expert panel discussion. *The Permanente Journal*, 27(2), Article 23.053. https://doi.org/10.7812/TPP/23.053

Devex. (2022, June 17). *WTO finally agrees on a TRIPS deal. But not everyone is happy*. https://www.devex.com/news/wto-finally-agrees-on-a-trips-deal-but-not-everyone-is-happy-103476

Dickinson, R., Makowski, D., van Marwijk, H., & Ford, E. (2024). *Exploring the role of news outlets in the rise of a conspiracy theory: Hydroxychloroquine in the early days of COVID-19*. *COVID*, *4*(12), 1873–1896. https://doi.org/10.3390/covid4120132

Doctors Without Borders (MSF). (2021, October 18). *High-income countries must stop hoarding 870 million excess COVID-19 vaccine doses and redistribute them to save lives* [Press release]. Médecins Sans Frontières Access Campaign. https://www.doctorswithoutborders.ca

Duan, Y., Shi, J., Wang, Z., Zhou, S., Jin, Y., & Zheng, Z.-J. (2021). Disparities in COVID-19 vaccination among low-, middle-, and high-income countries: The mediating role of vaccination policy. *Vaccines*, *9*(8), 905. https://doi.org/10.3390/vaccines9080905

Economic Times. (2020, May 13). *Top highlights of Finance Minister Nirmala Sitharaman's speech on Modi's ₹20 lakh crore COVID-19 stimulus*. https://economictimes.indiatimes.com/news/economy/policy/top-highlights-of-finance-minister-nirmala-sitharaman-speech-on-modi-20-lakh-crore-covid-19-stimulus/articleshow/75714287.cms

Edwards, B., Barnes, R., Rehill, P., Ellen, L., Zhong, F., Killigrew, A., Riquelme Gonzalez, P., Sheard, E., Zhu, R., & Philips, T. (2022). *Variation in policy response to*

COVID-19 across Australian states and territories [BSG Working Paper Series No. BSG-WP-2022/046]. Blavatnik School of Government, University of Oxford. https://www.bsg.ox.ac.uk/covidtracker

El Bcheraoui, C., Weishaar, H., Pozo-Martin, F., & Hanefeld, J. (2020). Assessing COVID-19 through the lens of health systems' preparedness: Time for a change. *Global Health, 16*, 112. https://doi.org/10.1186/s12992-020-00645-5

FDA. (2021, May 19). *FDA brief: FDA authorizes longer time for refrigerator storage of thawed Pfizer-BioNTech COVID-19 vaccine*. U.S. Food and Drug Administration. https://www.fda.gov/news-events/press-announcements/fda-brief-fda-authorizes-longer-time-refrigerator-storage-thawed-pfizer-biontech-covid-19-vaccine

Feddema, J. J., Fernald, K. D. S., Schikan, H. G. C. P., & van de Burgwal, L. H. M. (2023). Upscaling vaccine manufacturing capacity – Key bottlenecks and lessons learned. *Vaccine, 41*(30), 4359–4368. https://doi.org/10.1016/j.vaccine.2023.05.027

Federal Reserve Board. (2024, May 17). *Why is the U.S. GDP recovering faster than other advanced economies?* [FEDS Notes]. Board of Governors of the Federal Reserve System. https://www.federalreserve.gov/econres/notes/feds-notes/why-is-the-u-s-gdp-recovering-faster-than-other-advanced-economies-20240517.html

Ferreira, F. H. G. (2021). Inequality in the time of COVID-19. *Finance & Development, 58*(2). International Monetary Fund. https://www.imf.org/en/Publications/fandd/issues/2021/06/inequality-and-covid-19-ferreira

Ferreira Caceres, M. M., Sosa, J. P., Lawrence, J. A., Sestacovschi, C., Tidd-Johnson, A., Rasool, M. H. U., Gadamidi, V. K., Ozair, S., Pandav, K., Cuevas-Lou, C., Parrish, M., Rodriguez, I., & Fernandez, J. P. (2022). The impact of misinformation on the COVID-19 pandemic. *AIMS Public Health, 9*(2), 262–277. https://doi.org/10.3934/publichealth.2022018

Fierce Pharma. (2021, August 30). *How did 75M J&J vaccines get ruined? FDA details the manufacturing woes at Emergent's beleaguered site*. https://www.fiercepharma.com/manufacturing/some-j-j-covid-19-doses-now-cleared-from-emergent-but-several-countries-are-already

Fitzpatrick, S., & Strickler, L. (2023, January 17). In new oversight role, House Republicans target billions lost to Covid relief fraud. *NBC News*. https://www.nbcnews.com/politics/congress/billions-covid-loans-questionable-social-security-numbers-rcna68296

Garrett, R., & Young, S. D. (2021). Online misinformation and vaccine hesitancy. *Translational Behavioral Medicine, 11*(12), 2194–2199. https://doi.org/10.1093/tbm/ibab128

Gavi. (2021a). *COVAX: The forecast for vaccine supply*. Gavi, the Vaccine Alliance. https://www.gavi.org/vaccineswork/covax-forecast-vaccine-supply

Gavi. (2021b, July). *Q&A: Cold chain experts on keeping vaccines cool*. Gavi, the Vaccine Alliance. https://www.gavi.org/vaccineswork/qa-cold-chain-experts-keeping-vaccines-cool

Gentilini, U., Almenfi, M. B. A., Iyengar, T. M. M., Okamura, Y., Downes, J. A., Dale, P., Weber, M., Newhouse, D. L., Rodriguez Alas, C. P., Kamran, M., Mujica Canas, I. V., Fontenez, M. B., Asieduah, S., Mahboobani Martinez, V. R., Reyes Hartley, G. J., Demarco, G. C., Abels, M., Zafar, U., Urteaga, E. R., Valleriani, G., Muhindo, J. V., & Aziz, S. (2022). *Social protection and jobs responses to COVID-19: A real-time review of country measures*. World Bank. https://hdl.handle.net/10986/37186

Ghahramani, S., Lankarani, K. B., Yousefi, M., Heydari, K., Shahabi, S., & Azmand, S. (2021). A systematic review and meta-analysis of burnout among healthcare workers during COVID-19. *Frontiers in Psychiatry, 12*, Article 758849. https://doi.org/10.3389/fpsyt.2021.758849

Goldstein, A. (2021). Failure to achieve global vaccine equity will have dire consequences. *BMJ, 372*, n712. https://doi.org/10.1136/bmj.n712

Golumbeanu, R., & Knuckles, J. (2022, October 5). *Powering health facilities in the aftermath of the pandemic*. World Bank Blogs. https://blogs.worldbank.org/energy/powering-health-facilities-aftermath-pandemic

Gonsalves, G., & Yamey, G. (2020). Political interference in public health science during COVID-19. *BMJ*, *371*, m3878. https://doi.org/10.1136/bmj.m3878

Gozzi, N., Chinazzi, M., Dean, N. E., Longini, I. M. Jr., Halloran, M. E., Perra, N., & Vespignani, A. (2023). Estimating the impact of COVID-19 vaccine inequities: A modeling study. *Nature Communications*, *14*(1), 3272. https://doi.org/10.1038/s41467-023-39098-w

Guarascio, F. (2022, January 15). *Global vaccine-sharing programme reaches milestone of 1 billion doses*. Reuters. https://www.reuters.com/world/global-vaccine-sharing-programme-reaches-milestone-1-billion-doses-2022-01-15/

Gupta, V., Santosh, K. C., Arora, R., Ciano, T., Kalid, K. S., & Mohan, S. (2022). Socioeconomic impact due to COVID-19: An empirical assessment. *Information Processing & Management*, *59*(2), 102810. https://doi.org/10.1016/j.ipm.2021.102810

Hale, T., Angrist, N., Goldszmidt, R., Kira, B., Petherick, A., Phillips, T., Webster, S., Cameron-Blake, E., Hallas, L., Majumdar, S., & Tatlow, H. (2021). A global panel database of pandemic policies (Oxford COVID-19 Government Response Tracker). *Nature Human Behaviour*, *5*(4), 529–538. https://doi.org/10.1038/s41562-021-01079-8

Harvard Gazette. (2023, November 9). *COVID burnout hitting all levels of healthcare workforce*. https://news.harvard.edu/gazette/story/2023/03/covid-burnout-hitting-all-levels-of-health-care-workforce/

Hotez, P. J. (2023). Confronting the evolution and expansion of anti-vaccine activism in the USA in the COVID-19 era. *The Lancet*, *401*(10379), 1139–1140. https://doi.org/10.1016/S0140-6736(23)00136-8

Hu, K., & Zhang, L. (2024). Challenges and opportunities associated with lifting the zero COVID-19 policy in China. *Exploration of Research and Hypothesis in Medicine*, *9*(1), 71–75. https://doi.org/10.14218/erhm.2023.00002

Huang, Y. (2021, March 5). *Vaccine diplomacy is paying off for China*. Foreign Affairs. https://www.foreignaffairs.com

Human Rights Watch. (2021, June 3). *Seven reasons the EU is wrong to oppose the TRIPS waiver*. https://www.hrw.org/news/2021/06/03/seven-reasons-eu-wrong-oppose-trips-waiver

Institute for Government. (2022, March 31). *Coronavirus job retention scheme (CJRS) explained*. https://www.instituteforgovernment.org.uk/explainer/coronavirus-economic-support-individuals

International Monetary Fund (IMF). (2021a). *Fiscal monitor database of country fiscal measures in response to the COVID-19 pandemic*. Retrieved from https://www.imf.org/en/Topics/imf-and-covid19/Fiscal-Policies-Database-in-Response-to-COVID-19

International Monetary Fund (IMF). (2021b). *Policy responses to COVID-19*. https://www.imf.org/en/Topics/imf-and-covid19/Policy-Responses-to-COVID-19

Irwin, R. E. (2020). Misinformation and de-contextualization: International media reporting on Sweden and COVID-19. *Globalization and Health*, *16*, 62. https://doi.org/10.1186/s12992-020-00588-x

Jain, V., & Lorgelly, P. (2022). The impact of pausing the Oxford-AstraZeneca COVID-19 vaccine on uptake in Europe: A difference-in-differences analysis. *European Journal of Public Health*, *32*(4), 648–654. https://doi.org/10.1093/eurpub/ckac039

Jamison, D. T., & Wu, K. B. (2021). The East–West divide in response to COVID-19. *Engineering*, *7*(7), 936–947. https://doi.org/10.1016/j.eng.2021.05.008

Johns Hopkins Center for Health Security, Nuclear Threat Initiative, & Economist Impact. (2019-2021). *Global Health Security Index*. Retrieved February 12, 2025, from https://ghsindex.org/

Johns Hopkins Center for Health Security, Nuclear Threat Initiative, & Economist Impact. (2021, December 8). 2021 Global Health Security Index finds all countries remain dangerously unprepared for future epidemic and pandemic threats. *Global Health Security Index*. https://ghsindex.org/news/2021-global-health-security-index-finds-all-countries-remain-dangerously-unprepared-for-future-epidemic-and-pandemic-threats/

Kansteiner, F. (2021, April 19). *Serum Institute nears $400M grant to boost AstraZeneca COVID shot production—Just as material shortages mount*. Fierce Pharma. https://www.fiercepharma.com/manufacturing/serum-institute-homes-400m-grant-to-make-az-shot-as-supply-shortages-mount

Kaplan, A. (2020, May 7). A coronavirus conspiracy theory film attacking vaccines has racked up millions of views and engagements on YouTube and Facebook. *Media Matters for America*. https://www.mediamatters.org/coronavirus-covid-19/coronavirus-conspiracy-theory-film-attacking-vaccines-has-racked-millions

Katz, I. T., Weintraub, R., Bekker, L.-G., & Brandt, A. M. (2021). From vaccine nationalism to vaccine equity—Finding a path forward. *New England Journal of Medicine*, *384*(14), 1281–1283. https://doi.org/10.1056/NEJMp2103614

Kekatos, M. (2023, October 24). Health care workers report increase in burnout, harassment since the COVID pandemic: CDC. *ABC News*. https://abcnews.go.com/Health/health-care-workers-report-increase-burnout-harassment-covid/story?id=104250554

Khairi, L. N. H. M., Fahrni, M. L., & Lazzarino, A. I. (2022). The race for global equitable access to COVID-19 vaccines. *Vaccines (Basel)*, *10*(8), 1306. https://doi.org/10.3390/vaccines10081306

Kirchner, A. (2022, March 10). *Zooming in on French Industrial Policy*. Institut Montaigne. https://www.institutmontaigne.org/en/expressions/zooming-french-industrial-policy

Kirk, A., Sheehy, F., & Levett, C. (2021, January 29). Canada and UK among countries with most COVID vaccine doses ordered per person. *The Guardian*. https://www.theguardian.com/world/2021/jan/29/canada-and-uk-among-countries-with-most-vaccine-doses-ordered-per-person

Korea Herald. (2020, April 8). *53.7 trillion won relief package*. https://www.koreaherald.com/view.php?ud=20200408000825

Lacey, E., Massad, J., & Utz, R. (2021). *A review of fiscal policy responses to COVID-19 (equitable growth, finance and Institutions insight)*. World Bank. http://hdl.handle.net/10986/35904

Lim, W. Y., Ong, J., Ong, S., Tan, Y. X., Le Cam, S., Chin, H. X., & Car, J. (2022). A global overview of healthcare workers' turnover intention amid COVID-19 pandemic: A systematic review with future directions. *Human Resources for Health*, 20(1), Article 70. https://doi.org/10.1186/s12960-022-00764-7

LSE-EIF Capstone Project. (2024, March). *The COVID-19 impact and fiscal policy response on EU small and medium-sized enterprises: A public policy perspective*. London School of Economics and Political Science; European Investment Fund.

Ludvigsson, J. F. (2020). The first eight months of Sweden's COVID-19 strategy and the key actions and actors that were involved. *Acta Paediatrica*, *109*(12), 2459–2471. https://doi.org/10.1111/apa.15582

MacGillivray, E. M., Smith, M., Zalis, M., Seymour, P., Berenson, C., Truong, K. K., Sarkisian, R., Levine, Z. G., Chen, S. R., Simoes, M., Dunbar, M., Joseph, T. B., Miller, L. G., Hinson, J. S., Dooley, K. E., & Regenold, W. T. (2023). *COVID-19 pandemic impacts on mental health, burnout, and longevity in the workplace among healthcare workers: A mixed methods study*. PMC. https://pmc.ncbi.nlm.nih.gov/articles/PMC10248469/

Madhi, S. A., Kwatra, G., Myers, J. E., Jassat, W., Dhar, N., Mukendi, C. K., Nana, A. J., Blumberg, L., Welch, R., Ngorima-Mabhena, N., & Mutevedzi, P. C. (2022). Population immunity and COVID-19 severity with Omicron variant in South Africa. *New England Journal of Medicine*, *386*(14), 1314–1326. https://doi.org/10.1056/NEJMoa2119658

Mahajan, M. (2021). Casualties of preparedness: The Global Health Security Index and COVID-19. *International Journal of Law in Context*, *17*(2), 204–214. https://doi.org/10.1017/S1744552321000288

Malik, A. A., McFadden, S. M., Elharake, J., & Omer, S. B. (2020). Determinants of COVID19 vaccine acceptance in the US. *EClinicalMedicine*, *26*. https://doi.org/10.1016/j.eclinm.2020.100495

McKee, M., Dunnell, K., Anderson, M., Brayne, C., Charlesworth, A., Johnston-Webber, C., Knapp, M., McGuire, A., Newton, J. N., Taylor, D., & Watt, R. G. (2021). The changing health needs of the UK population. *The Lancet, 397*(10288), 1991–2001. https://doi.org/10.1016/S0140-6736(21)00229-4

Missoni, E., Armocida, B., & Formenti, B. (2020). Face masks for all and all for face masks in the COVID-19 pandemic: Community level production to face the global shortage and shorten the epidemic. *Disaster Medicine and Public Health Preparedness, 15*(e29–e33), e29–e33. https://doi.org/10.1017/dmp.2020.207

Morgan, K. M., Maglalang, D. D., Monnig, M. A., Stein, M. D., Borsari, B., Alexander-Scott, N., Rich, J. D., & Ahluwalia, J. S. (2023). Medical mistrust, perceived discrimination, and race: A longitudinal analysis of predictors of COVID-19 vaccine hesitancy in US adults. *Journal of Racial and Ethnic Health Disparities, 10*, 1846–1855. https://doi.org/10.1007/s40615-022-01368-6

Morgantini, L. A., Naha, U., Wang, H., Francavilla, S., Acar, Ö., Flores, J. M., Crivellaro, S., Moreira, D., Abern, M., Eklund, M., Vigneswaran, H. T., & Weine, S. M. (2020). Factors contributing to healthcare professional burnout during the COVID-19 pandemic: A rapid turnaround global survey. *PLoS ONE, 15*(9). https://journals.plos.org/plosone/article?id=10.1371/journal.pone.0238217

Musanabaganwa, C., Semakula, M., Mazarati, J. B., Nyamusore, J., Uwimana, A., Kayumba, M., Umutesi, F., Uwizihiwe, J. P., Muhire, A., Nyatanyi, T., Thom, H., Hitimana, N., Byiringiro, F., Mutesa, L., & Nsanzimana, S. (2020). Use of technologies in COVID-19 containment in Rwanda. *Rwanda Public Health Bulletin, 2*(2), 4–9.

Nagarajan, R., Ramachandran, P., Dilipkumar, R., & Kaur, P. (2024). Global estimate of burnout among the public health workforce: A systematic review and meta-analysis. *Human Resources for Health, 22*(1), 30. https://doi.org/10.1186/s12960-024-00917-w

Narea, N. (2020, May 5). *For immigrants without legal status, federal coronavirus relief is out of reach.* Vox. https://www.vox.com/2020/5/5/21244630/undocumented-immigrants-coronavirus-relief-cares-act

Nasr, J. (2021, May 8). *Vaccine patent waiver could impact quality of shots – Merkel.* Reuters. https://www.reuters.com/article/health-coronavirus-eu-merkel-idUSS8N2D400S

National Community Reinvestment Coalition (NCRC). (2020). *Lending discrimination during COVID-19: Black and Hispanic women-owned businesses.* Retrieved from https://ncrc.org/lending-discrimination-during-covid-19-black-and-hispanic-women-owned-businesses/

National Public Radio (NPR). (2021, November 27). *The highest COVID death rate in the world is in Peru. How did that happen?* NPR. https://www.npr.org/sections/goatsandsoda/2021/11/27/1057387896/peru-has-the-worlds-highest-covid-death-rate-heres-why

Nelson, M. (2021, January 14). *Moderna has the capacity but cannot guarantee the supply of COVID-19 vaccine.* BioProcess Insider. https://www.bioprocessintl.com/bioprocess-insider/moderna-has-the-capacity-but-cannot-guarantee-the-supply-of-covid-19-vaccine

Neumann, M., Moore, S. T., Baum, L. M., Oleinikov, P., Xu, Y., Niederdeppe, J., & Fowler, E. F. (2023). Politicizing masks? Examining the volume and content of local news coverage of face coverings in the U.S. through the COVID-19 pandemic. *Political Communication, 41*(1), 66–106. https://doi.org/10.1080/10584609.2023.2239181

Nuclear Threat Initiative (NTI). (2020, April 21). *The U.S. and COVID-19: Leading the world by GHS Index score, not by response.* https://www.nti.org/risky-business/us-and-covid-19-leading-world-ghs-index-score-not-response/

Observer. (2020, April 21). 75 public companies took COVID-19 loans meant for small businesses: Investigation (S. Cao). *The New York Observer.* https://observer.com/2020/04/public-large-companies-take-small-business-loan-coronavirus-relief-package/

OECD. (2020). Tax and fiscal policy in response to the Coronavirus crisis: Strengthening confidence and resilience. In *OECD policy responses to Coronavirus (COVID-19).* OECD Publishing. https://doi.org/10.1787/60f640a8-en

Oshitani, H., & Expert Members of The National COVID-19 Cluster Taskforce at The Ministry of Health, Labour and Welfare, Japan. (2020). Cluster-based approach to coronavirus disease 2019 (COVID-19) response in Japan, from February to April 2020. *Japanese Journal of Infectious Diseases*, *73*(6), 491–493. https://doi.org/10.7883/yoken.JJID.2020.363

Peeples, L. (2020). Face masks: What the data say. *Nature*, *586*(7828), 186–189. https://doi.org/10.1038/d41586-020-02801-8

Pfizer. (2021, May 31). *EMA approves new storage option for Pfizer-BioNTech vaccine*. https://www.pfizer.com/news/press-release/press-release-detail/ema-approves-new-storage-option-pfizer-biontech-vaccine

Pharmaceutical Commerce. (2020, December 14). *Meeting the challenges of rapid COVID-19 vaccine cold chain deployment*. https://www.pharmaceuticalcommerce.com/view/meeting-the-challenges-of-rapid-covid-19-vaccine-cold-chain-deployment

PhRMA. (2022, March 15). *PhRMA statement on WTO TRIPS intellectual property waiver*. Pharmaceutical Research and Manufacturers of America. https://www.phrma.org/resources/phrma-statement-on-wto-trips-waiver-negotiations

Politico. (2021, January 26). *AstraZeneca: Coronavirus vaccine deliveries to EU reduced*. https://www.politico.eu/article/astrazeneca-coronavirus-vaccine-deliveries-to-eu-reduced/

Pradhan, R., & Allen, A. (2021, April 9). After billions of dollars and dozens of wartime declarations, why are vaccines still in short supply? *KFF Health News*. https://kffhealthnews.org/news/article/after-billions-of-dollars-and-dozens-of-wartime-declarations-why-are-vaccines-still-in-short-supply/

Ramírez Varela, A., Touchton, M., Miranda, J. J., Mejía Grueso, J., Laajaj, R., Carrasquilla, G., Vives Florez, M., Vesga Gaviria, A. M., Ortiz Hoyos, A. M., Vanegas Duarte, E. O., Velásquez Morales, A., Velasco, N., & Restrepo Restrepo, S. (2023). Assessing pandemic preparedness, response, and lessons learned from the COVID-19 pandemic in four South American countries: Agenda for the future. *Frontiers in Public Health*, *11*, 1274737. https://doi.org/10.3389/fpubh.2023.1274737

Razai, M. S., Osama, T., McKechnie, D. G. J., & Majeed, A. (2021). Covid-19 vaccine hesitancy among ethnic minority groups. *BMJ*, *372*, n513. https://doi.org/10.1136/bmj.n513

RECOVERY Collaborative Group. (2020). Effect of hydroxychloroquine in hospitalized patients with COVID-19 (RECOVERY trial). *New England Journal of Medicine*, *383*(21), 2030–2040. https://doi.org/10.1056/NEJMoa2022926

Reuters. (2020, November 10). *U.S. states race to buy ultra cold vaccine freezers, fueling supply worries*. https://www.reuters.com/article/business/healthcare-pharmaceuticals/us-states-race-to-buy-ultra-cold-vaccine-freezers-fueling-supply-worries-idUSKBN27T2S5

Reuters. (2021a, April 16). *Serum Institute CEO appeals to Biden on raw material exports*. https://www.reuters.com/article/business/healthcare-pharmaceuticals/indian-vaccine-maker-serum-institute-appeals-to-biden-to-lift-embargo-on-raw-mat-idUSKBN2C30ZR/

Reuters. (2021b, May 8). *France's Macron on vaccine patent waivers*. https://www.reuters.com/article/health-coronavirus-eu-macron-idUSS8N2D400T

Ríos-Rull, J., Heathcote, J., Krueger, D., & Glover, A. (2020). *Health versus wealth: On the distributional effects of controlling a pandemic*. COVID economics, 6. CEPR Press. https://cepr.org/publications/covid-economics-issue-6#392514_392882_391017

Rocha, R., Atun, R., Massuda, A., Rache, B., Spinola, P., Nunes, L., Lago, M., & Castro, M. C. (2021). Effect of socioeconomic inequalities and vulnerabilities on health-system preparedness and response to COVID-19 in Brazil: A comprehensive analysis. *The Lancet Global Health*, *9*(6), e782–e792. https://doi.org/10.1016/S2214-109X(21)00081-4

Rodríguez, J., Sebastián, R., & Palomino, J. C. (2020). *Wage inequality and poverty effects of social distancing in Europe*. Covid economics: Vetted and real-time papers, 25, 90–108. CEPR Press. https://cepr.org/publications/covid-economics-issue-25#392514_392901_390498

Roelf, W. (2023, April 21). WHO launches mRNA vaccine hub in Cape Town. *Reuters*. https://www.reuters.com/business/healthcare-pharmaceuticals/who-officially-launches-mrna-vaccine-hub-cape-town-2023-04-20/

Rome, B. N., Avorn, J., & Kesselheim, A. S. (2021). Characteristics of US patients and prescribers using hydroxychloroquine during the COVID-19 pandemic. *Journal of General Internal Medicine*, *36*(12), 3918–3921. https://doi.org/10.1007/s11606-021-07144-2

Rotenstein, L. S., Brown, R., Sinsky, C., Linzer, M., Poplau, S., & Seixas, N. (2023). The association of work overload with burnout and intent to leave the job across the healthcare workforce during COVID-19. *Journal of General Internal Medicine*, *38*, 1920–1927. https://doi.org/10.1007/s11606-023-08153-z

Rouw, A., Kates, J., Wexler, A., & Michaud, J. (2021, September 22). *Tracking Global COVID-19 Vaccine Equity: An Update*. KFF. https://www.kff.org/coronavirus-covid-19/issue-brief/tracking-global-covid-19-vaccine-equity-an-update/

Roux, J., Massonnaud, C. R., Colizza, V., & colleagues (2023). Modeling the impact of national and regional lockdowns on the 2020 spring wave of COVID-19 in France. *Scientific Reports*, *13*, 1834. https://doi.org/10.1038/s41598-023-28687-w

Sachs, J. D., Karim, S. S. A., Aknin, L., Allen, J., Brosbøl, K., Colombo, F., Barron, G. C., Espinosa, M. F., Gaspar, V., Gaviria, A., Haines, A., Hotez, P. J., Koundouri, P., Bascuñán, F. L., Lee, J.-K., Pate, M. A., Ramos, G., Srinath, R. K., Serageldin, I., … & Michie, S. (2022). The Lancet Commission on lessons for the future from the COVID-19 pandemic. *The Lancet*, *400*(10359), 1224–1280. https://doi.org/10.1016/S0140-6736(22)01585-9

Sanghera, J., Pattani, N., Hashmi, Y., Varley, K. F., Cheruvu, M. S., Bradley, A., & Burke, J. R. (2020). The impact of SARS-CoV-2 on the mental health of healthcare workers in a hospital setting—A systematic review. *Journal of Occupational Health*, *62*(1), e12175. https://doi.org/10.1002/1348-9585.12175

Schmidt, C. (2021, February 5). *New COVID vaccines need absurd amounts of material and labor*. Scientific American. https://www.scientificamerican.com/article/new-covid-vaccines-need-absurd-amounts-of-material-and-labor/

Shalal, A., Mason, J., & Lawder, D. (2021, May 5). *U.S. reverses stance, backs giving poorer countries access to COVID vaccine patents*. Reuters. https://www.reuters.com/business/healthcare-pharmaceuticals/biden-says-plans-back-wto-waiver-vaccines-2021-05-05/

Sheikhattari, P., Barsha, R. A. A., Shaffer, E., Goodman, R. M., Beane, M., & Gielen, A. C. (2023). Lessons learned to improve COVID-19 response in communities with greatest socio-economic vulnerabilities. *BMC Public Health*, *23*, 659. https://doi.org/10.1186/s12889-023-15479-0

Subramanian, S. (2020, May 18). *In Europe, they're burning witches again*. Politico. https://www.politico.eu/article/coronavirus-5g-conspiracy-mast-burning/

Summers, J., Cheng, H. Y., Lin, H. H., Barnard, L. T., Kvalsvig, A., Wilson, N., & Baker, M. G. (2020). Potential lessons from the Taiwan and New Zealand health responses to the COVID-19 pandemic. *The Lancet Regional Health - Western Pacific*, *4*, 100044. https://doi.org/10.1016/j.lanwpc.2020.100044

Swindells, K. (2021, March 19). Why Europe's vaccine debacle could hurt Africa most. *New Statesman*. https://www.newstatesman.com/world/2021/03/why-europe-s-vaccine-debacle-could-hurt-africa-most

Sy, S., & Cuevas, K. (2023, September 12). Child poverty increases sharply following expiration of expanded tax credit [Television broadcast transcript]. *PBS NewsHour*.https://www.pbs.org/newshour/show/child-poverty-increases-sharply-following-expiration-of-expanded-tax-credit

Tatar, M., Shoorekchali, J. M., Faraji, M. R., Seyyedkolaee, M. A., Pagán, J. A., & Wilson, F. A. (2022). COVID-19 vaccine inequality: A global perspective. *Journal of Global Health*, *12*, 03072. https://doi.org/10.7189/jogh.12.03072

The Guardian. (2021, January 27). *Why the EU and AstraZeneca are stuck in a Covid vaccines row*. https://www.theguardian.com/business/2021/jan/27/eu-covid-vaccines-row-astrazeneca-boss-reveals-problems

The Lancet. (2021). Access to COVID-19 vaccines: Looking beyond COVAX. *The Lancet, 397*(10278), 941. https://doi.org/10.1016/S0140-6736(21)00617-6

U.S. Department of Health and Human Services. (2022). *Addressing health worker burnout.* https://www.hhs.gov/sites/default/files/health-worker-wellbeing-advisory.pdf

UNDP. (2021). *Global dashboard for vaccine equity.* United Nations Development Programme. https://data.undp.org/vaccine-equity/

UNICEF Supply Division. (2021, September 28). *The historic push to provide ultra-cold chain freezers around the world.* https://www.unicef.org/supply/stories/historic-push-provide-ultra-cold-chain-freezers-around-world

United Kingdom: Office for National Statistics (ONS). (2021). *Coronavirus (COVID-19) latest data and analysis.* Retrieved from https://www.ons.gov.uk/peoplepopulationandcommunity/healthandsocialcare/conditionsanddiseases

United Nations. (2021, February 17). *Secretary-General calls vaccine equity "biggest moral test" for global community, as Security Council considers equitable availability of doses.* United Nations Meetings Coverage SC/14438. https://press.un.org/en/2021/sc14438.doc.htm

Vosoughi, S., Roy, D., & Aral, S. (2018). The spread of true and false news online. *Science, 359*(6380), 1146–1151. https://doi.org/10.1126/science.aap9559

Wagner, C. E., Saad-Roy, C. M., Morris, S. E., Baker, R. E., Mina, M. J., Farrar, J., Holmes, E. C., Pybus, O. G., Graham, A. L., Emanuel, E. J., Levin, S. A., Metcalf, C. J. E., & Grenfell, B. T. (2021). Vaccine nationalism and the dynamics and control of SARS-CoV-2. *Science, 373*(6562), eabj7364. https://doi.org/10.1126/science.abj7364

Wang, Z., Duan, Y., Jin, Y., & Zheng, Z.-J. (2020). Coronavirus disease 2019 (COVID-19) pandemic: How countries should build more resilient health systems for preparedness and response. *Global Health Journal, 4*(4), 139–145. https://doi.org/10.1016/j.glohj.2020.12.001

WHO Africa. (2020). *COVID-19 response in Rwanda: Use of drones in community awareness.* World Health Organization Regional Office for Africa. https://www.afro.who.int/news/covid-19-response-rwanda-use-drones-community-awareness

Wilkinson, E., Giovanetti, M., Tegally, H., San, J. E., Lessells, R., Cuadros, D., Martin, D. P., Rasmussen, D. A., Zekri, A. R. N., Sangare, A. K., Ouedraogo, A. S., Sesay, A. K., Priscilla, A., Kemi, A. S., Olubusuyi, A. M., Oluwapelumi, A. O. O., Hammami, A., Amuri, A. A., Sayed, A., … de Oliveira, T. (2021). A year of genomic surveillance reveals how the SARS-CoV-2 pandemic unfolded in Africa. *Science, 374*(6566), 423–431. https://doi.org/10.1126/science.abj4336

World Bank. (2021). *World Development Indicators.* Retrieved from https://data.worldbank.org/indicator

World Bank. (2022). *Access to electricity (% of population) – Sub-Saharan Africa.* World Bank Data.

World Health Organization (WHO). (2020, August 25). *Immunizing the public against misinformation (WHO news feature).* Retrieved from https://www.who.int/news-room/feature-stories/detail/immunizing-the-public-against-misinformation

World Health Organization (WHO). (2021a). *Training on handling, storing and transporting Pfizer-BioNTech vaccine.* World Health Organization. https://www.who.int/docs/default-source/coronaviruse/act-accelerator/covax/training-on-pfizer-vaccine-management.pdf

World Health Organization (WHO). (2021b). Challenges in ensuring global access to COVID-19 vaccines. *The Lancet, 397*(10278), 1006–1008. https://doi.org/10.1016/S0140-6736(21)00306-8

World Health Organization (WHO). (2021c, April). *Director-General's opening remarks at the media briefing on COVID-19 – 9 April 2021.* https://www.who.int/director-general/speeches/detail/director-general-s-opening-remarks-at-the-media-briefing-on-covid-19-9-april-2021

World Health Organization (WHO). (2021d, December 23). *Achieving 70% COVID-19 immunization coverage by mid-2022*. World Health Organization. https://www.who.int/news/item/23-12-2021-achieving-70-covid-19-immunization-coverage-by-mid-2022

World Health Organization (WHO). (2021e). *WHO public health research agenda for managing infodemics*. World Health Organization. https://www.who.int/publications/i/item/9789240019508

World Health Organization (WHO). (2022a). *Vaccine equity*. World Health Organization. https://www.who.int/campaigns/vaccine-equity

World Health Organization (WHO). (2022b, January 16). *COVAX delivers its 1 billionth COVID-19 vaccine dose*. World Health Organization. https://www.who.int/news/item/16-01-2022-covax-delivers-its-1-billionth-covid-19-vaccine-dose

World Health Organization (WHO). (2024). *COVID-19 epidemiological update – 24 December 2024*. https://www.who.int/publications/m/item/covid-19-epidemiological-update---24-december-2024#:~:text=Using%20the%20new%20monitoring%20approach,Global%20overview%20since%20the%20pandemic

World Trade Organization. (2020, October 2). *Members continue discussion on proposal for temporary IP waiver in response to COVID-19*. https://www.wto.org/english/news_e/news20_e/trip_10dec20_e.htm

Wouters, O. J., Shadlen, K. C., Salcher-Konrad, M., Pollard, A. J., Larson, H. J., Teerawattananon, Y., & Jit, M. (2021). Challenges in ensuring global access to COVID-19 vaccines: Production, affordability, allocation, and deployment. *The Lancet*, *397*(10278), 1023–1034. https://www.thelancet.com/journals/lancet/article/PIIS0140-6736(21)00306-8/fulltext

Wright, L., Fortune, S., & Nayamuth, V. (2021). Challenges of ultra-cold supply chain for COVID-19 vaccine distribution in low-income countries. *Journal of Global Health*, *11*, 16010.

Xue, H., Gong, X., & Stevens, H. (2022). COVID-19 vaccine fact-checking posts on facebook: Observational study. *Journal of Medical Internet Research*, *24*(6), e38423. https://doi.org/10.2196/38423

Zarocostas, J. (2020). How to fight an infodemic. *The Lancet*, *395*(10225), 676. https://doi.org/10.1016/S0140-6736(20)30461-X

Zhou, A., Liu, W., & Yang, A. (2023). Politicization of science in COVID-19 vaccine communication: Comparing US politicians, medical experts, and government agencies. *Political Communication*, *41*(4), 649–671. https://doi.org/10.1080/10584609.2023.2201184

11 Into the Abyss

How Core Mental Models Influenced Global Pandemic Thinking

At the deepest level of our pandemic analysis lie the mental models—our fundamental frameworks for understanding reality—that shaped public responses to the health emergency (Figure 11.1). Like the dark depths beneath an iceberg where water pressure shapes ice formation, these deep-seated cognitive and cultural frameworks ultimately determined how populations interpreted and responded to the crisis. At the individual level, these frameworks manifested through what we observe as biases, determining how people process risk and uncertainty. These individual frameworks operated within broader cultural mental models that influenced whether populations viewed crisis response through collective or individualistic lenses. How different societies conceptualized institutional authority and expertise further shaped their responses, with some mental models facilitating trust while others triggered skepticism. As the crisis extended, these frameworks underwent significant adaptation, revealing how populations process and adjust to prolonged emergency situations.

The interaction of these various mental models—individual, cultural, institutional, and temporal—ultimately determined how different populations interpreted information, processed fear, and responded to public health measures. Understanding these fundamental frameworks, rather than just their surface

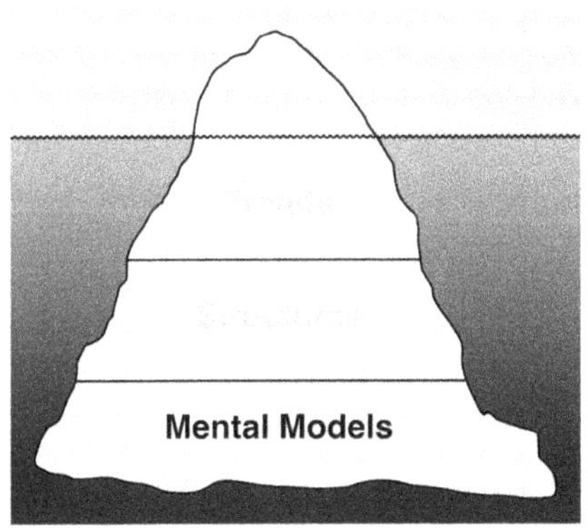

Figure 11.1 Iceberg Model—Mental Models.

DOI: 10.4324/9781003595564-14

manifestations, proves crucial for developing more effective approaches to future crisis management.

The following analysis examines each level of these mental models:

- ***Individual Mental Models: How Personal Cognition Shapes Crisis Response***
- ***Collective Mental Models: How Culture Shapes Shared Crisis Understanding***
- ***Institutional Mental Models: How Trust and Authority Guide Response Frameworks***
- ***Temporal Mental Models: How Crisis Duration Shapes Adherence and Adaptation***
- ***Fear and Uncertainty: How Threat Perception Distorts Information and Risk***

Individual Mental Models: How Cognitive Frameworks Shape Crisis Response

The COVID-19 pandemic revealed how individual mental models—our fundamental frameworks for processing reality—shape personal responses to crisis. What we observe as cognitive biases represents deeper frameworks through which individuals make sense of threat, uncertainty, and collective challenges. Understanding these core mental models provides insight into why individuals interpret and respond to a crisis in fundamentally different ways, even within the same cultural or institutional context.

Understanding Mental Models Through Cognitive Biases

When faced with a crisis like COVID-19, why do people react in such different ways, even when given the same information? The answer lies in our mental models—the deep-seated frameworks through which we understand and interpret reality. While we can't observe these mental models directly, we can understand them by examining cognitive biases—the consistent patterns in how people process information and make decisions during crises.

Think of cognitive biases (Table 11.1) as the visible tips of much deeper icebergs. When we see someone consistently downplaying their personal risk during a pandemic, or firmly believing things will quickly return to normal despite evidence to the contrary, we're witnessing these biases in action. But beneath these visible behaviors lie deeper frameworks that shape how people fundamentally understand reality, risk, and change. As Johnson-Laird (2010) explains, mental models are the cognitive structures that allow humans to make sense of new situations by drawing on existing knowledge and experience. These models guide reasoning processes, even when we're unaware of their influence.

Mental Model Formation and Individual Differences

How do these individual mental models form in the first place? According to Morgan et al. (2001), people construct mental models through a combination of prior experiences, education, and information sources. In the context of COVID-19, individuals often analogized the coronavirus to past disease outbreaks (like the seasonal flu or SARS) to form an initial understanding. However, these models varied significantly even among people within the same communities due to individual differences in risk perception and information processing.

Research by Van Bavel et al. (2020) found that factors such as scientific literacy, previous experience with disease outbreaks, and personal vulnerability all influenced how individuals constructed their mental models of the pandemic. For example, healthcare workers with direct exposure to infectious diseases typically built more accurate mental models of COVID-19 transmission compared to those without such experience. Similarly, those with higher scientific literacy were better able to grasp concepts like exponential growth, which many found difficult to understand. In one study cited by Van Bavel et al. (2020), simply explaining the concept of exponential disease spread significantly improved the accuracy of risk assessments and support for preventive measures.

These individual differences help explain why simply providing identical information to everyone produces such varied responses. As Jones et al. (2011) note,

Table 11.1 Cognitive Biases and Their Underlying Mental Models in COVID-19 Response

Cognitive Bias	*Observable Behavior During COVID-19*	*Underlying Mental Model*
Optimism Bias	Downplaying personal risk due to age or health status	Belief in personal exceptionalism and control over health vulnerabilities
Normalcy Bias	Assuming disruptions are short-lived and life will quickly return to normal	Expectation that stability is the default state and crises are brief interruptions
Confirmation Bias	Seeking out only information that supports pre-existing views on health measures	Filtering reality through alignment with prior beliefs
Availability Heuristic	Judging threat level based on media coverage or visible outbreaks	Understanding risk through vivid storytelling rather than data or statistics
Anchoring Bias	Comparing COVID-19 to familiar illnesses like the seasonal flu	Interpreting new risks using initial reference points or familiar comparisons
Worst-Case Bias	Hoarding supplies, believing extreme rumors, experiencing heightened anxiety	Resolving uncertainty toward maximum threat potential rather than likely outcomes
Bias Interaction	Combined resistance to guidelines due to multiple reinforcing biases	Overlapping mental models reinforcing skepticism and fragmented understanding

Sources: Dolinski et al. (2020), Sharot (2011) (Optimism Bias); Raude et al. (2020) (Normalcy Bias); Nickerson (1998), Van Bavel et al. (2020) (Confirmation Bias); Tversky and Kahneman (1974) (Availability Heuristic, Anchoring Bias); Pakpour and Griffiths (2020) (Worst-Case Bias); Halpern et al. (2020) (Bias Interaction).

mental models are not just cognitive structures but complex interdisciplinary constructs that integrate personal experiences, emotions, and social context—creating significant individual variations even within shared cultural settings.

Established theoretical frameworks like the *Health Belief Model* (Rosenstock, 1974) and *Protection Motivation Theory* (Rogers, 1975) provide additional insight into how these mental models connect to behavior. These frameworks, developed through decades of health behavior research, demonstrate that individuals who perceive a higher personal risk are more likely to adopt protective behaviors (van der Pligt, 1996). Consistent with these models, nationwide surveys early in the pandemic confirmed that individuals who believed they were likely to catch COVID-19 were significantly more likely to engage in health-protective actions, such as hand washing and social distancing (Garfin et al., 2021). These theoretical approaches highlight how mental models of risk aren't just abstract cognitive constructs, but directly shape behavioral responses during crises.

Optimism Bias: Mental Models of Personal Risk and Control

The tendency to underestimate personal risk—known as optimism bias—reveals a deeper mental framework about vulnerability and control. This mental model positions the self as inherently more capable and less vulnerable than others, reflecting deep-seated beliefs about personal exceptionalism and control over fate.

During the pandemic's early stages, this framework manifested powerfully among young adults. Research by Dolinski et al. (2020) found that a majority of respondents, especially young adults, rated their own infection risk as lower than their peers', even as cases rose dramatically. Many processed COVID-19 risks through a mental model that positioned youth as an inherently protective shield—viewing it as a core element of identity that conferred immunity to harm. Even as hospitals reported increasing cases among younger populations, many maintained beliefs about their personal invulnerability, explaining their behavior through frameworks of exceptional circumstance: "*I'm young and healthy*" or "*I have a strong immune system.*"

The emotional dimension of optimism bias is significant. Sharot (2011) demonstrates that this bias isn't merely a cognitive error but serves an emotional function—maintaining psychological well-being by creating a sense of control in threatening situations. This helps explain why optimism bias proved particularly resistant to correction through mere information provision. When public health messages emphasized vulnerability across all age groups, many young adults maintained optimistic assessments of their personal risk, as acknowledging vulnerability threatened not just cognitive beliefs, but emotional security.

A nationwide U.S. survey in March 2020 quantified this pattern: individuals who perceived themselves as having low personal risk were significantly less likely to adopt protective behaviors like handwashing and social distancing compared to those with higher risk perceptions (Garfin et al., 2021). This pattern wasn't universal, however. As Calvillo et al. (2020) documented, individual differences in scientific literacy, risk sensitivity, and trust in institutions created significant variations in how optimism bias manifested—some individuals maintained realistic risk assessments from the beginning, while others developed extreme optimism that resisted correction despite mounting evidence.

Normalcy Bias: Mental Models of Stability and Change

While optimism bias shapes how individuals process personal risk, another fundamental framework influences how we process change itself. Normalcy bias—the tendency to minimize the likelihood of disaster—stems from a deeper framework for understanding stability and disruption. This mental model positions stability as the natural state of existence and dramatic change as a temporary deviation, reflecting core beliefs about the predictability and controllability of our environment.

This mental model profoundly shapes how people conceive of crisis situations. Rather than processing new information objectively, individuals filter emerging threats through a framework that automatically categorizes major disruptions as temporary aberrations from an inevitable return to normal. Surveys conducted in February 2020 revealed that large majorities in several European countries believed their personal chance of contracting COVID-19 was only around 1%—a dramatic underestimation that exemplified this bias (Raude et al., 2020).

During the COVID-19 pandemic, many individuals held firmly to the belief that life would "*go back to normal*" within weeks or months, despite mounting evidence suggesting long-term impacts on social, economic, and healthcare systems. This belief represented a fundamental way of maintaining cognitive coherence in the face of vast, sudden, and unprecedented change.

In this scenario, normalcy bias wasn't merely a cognitive miscalculation, but reflected deeper mental models about how the world operates. For many, the framework of "temporary disruption" made the crisis psychologically manageable by providing a mental timeline for endurance. This partly explains why, as the pandemic continued, many resisted accepting extended mitigation measures—their mental models hadn't prepared them for sustained adaptation rather than a quick return to pre-pandemic conditions.

This bias was particularly evident in behavioral patterns documented by Halpern et al. (2020): people continued routine activities like traveling and socializing even as case numbers rose, indicating a mental model that couldn't properly incorporate the possibility of prolonged disruption. The psychological need for normalcy created powerful resistance to evidence suggesting fundamental changes to daily life would be necessary for an extended period.

Confirmation Bias: Mental Models of Truth and Knowledge

As individuals process both personal risk and societal change, they engage with information through specific frameworks for determining truth. Confirmation bias—the tendency to seek information that confirms existing beliefs—reveals deep-seated mental models about the nature of truth and knowledge. This mental model positions personal intuition and existing beliefs as primary filters for truth, reflecting core assumptions about how knowledge is constructed and validated.

The pandemic provided clear examples of these frameworks in action. When presented with data about mask effectiveness, individuals often sought sources that aligned with their pre-existing views. Those skeptical of masks frequently cited studies questioning their effectiveness while dismissing larger bodies of research supporting mask use. Those favoring masks similarly gravitated toward confirming evidence while overlooking legitimate questions about optimal use scenarios. Van Bavel et al. (2020) documented how this bias fed the spread of misinformation on social media, with people sharing dubious claims that aligned with their narrative while ignoring reputable information that challenged their viewpoint.

Confirmation bias proved particularly powerful during the pandemic because of how deeply it connects to identity and worldview. Calvillo et al. (2020) found that in the United States, political ideology became a powerful predictor of COVID-19 risk perception, with conservatives consistently perceiving lower threat levels than liberals. This wasn't simply about different information sources—when presented with identical data, individuals interpreted it through their already existing belief frameworks.

The information environment exacerbated these tendencies. Social media algorithms reinforced confirmation bias by creating what Van Bavel et al. (2020) termed "epistemic bubbles"—information ecosystems where users primarily encountered content supporting their existing views. By mid-2020, these bubbles had solidified to the point that public health communication faced significant challenges: the same message would be interpreted entirely differently based on the receiver's pre-existing mental framework.

The psychological mechanism behind confirmation bias isn't simply borne from innate stubbornness, but reflects how humans construct knowledge. Nickerson (1998) explains that we seek cognitive coherence—when new information threatens our existing mental frameworks, the psychological discomfort (cognitive dissonance) drives us to reject contradictory evidence rather than restructure our entire belief system. During COVID-19, this meant that initial impressions about the virus became remarkably resistant to change, even as scientific understanding evolved rapidly.

Availability Heuristic: Mental Models of Threat Recognition

The availability heuristic—our tendency to assess risk based on easily recalled examples—reveals a fundamental framework for threat assessment and pattern recognition. During the pandemic, this mental model shaped how people conceived of threat proximity and severity, creating distinct frameworks for processing risk based on personally witnessed or vividly reported experiences.

This model illustrates how humans understand the world primarily through stories and immediate examples rather than statistics and abstract probabilities. When early pandemic coverage focused on specific hotspots like Wuhan or Northern Italy, people operated within mental frameworks that processed the proximity of threat through narrative and visible evidence. Research has shown that many individuals struggle to grasp the concept of exponential growth; however, even simple explanations or small nudges significantly improved their risk assessment and compliance behaviors (Banerjee et al., 2021).

The availability heuristic created deep variations in risk perception based on geographic and media exposure. In areas with visible outbreaks, individuals demonstrated heightened risk perception and compliance with protective measures. Conversely, in regions with few early cases, many struggled to process the threat as real despite statistical warnings—the lack of immediately available examples made the danger seem abstract rather than concrete. As documented by Morgan et al. (2001), this heuristic explains why vivid stories of individual COVID-19 cases often proved more persuasive in changing behavior than statistical reports of rising case numbers. Effective public health communication needed to recognize this mental model by providing concrete examples that made abstract risks mentally "available" to the public.

Anchoring Bias: Mental Models of Initial Understanding

Our initial reference points create powerful frameworks for understanding new phenomena. During the pandemic, early comparisons to familiar diseases like the flu established fundamental frameworks through which people processed all future COVID-19 information. Studies found that Americans who regularly got flu shots were more likely to later say they would get a COVID-19 vaccine, suggesting they framed COVID-19 in reference to flu risks (Southwell et al., 2020).

When COVID-19 emerged, populations automatically processed it through existing mental models of previously familiar diseases. Humans create foundational frameworks for understanding novel phenomena by anchoring them to prior known experiences. These initial frameworks persisted even as evidence showed COVID-19's unique characteristics, demonstrating how deeply these anchor points connect to our fundamental ways of processing new information.

The persistence of these initial anchors proved remarkably difficult to overcome. Describing COVID-19 as "similar to the flu" in early 2020 set a reassuring initial mental reference point for many. Tversky and Kahneman (1974) demonstrated how first impressions create powerful baseline expectations that resist adjustment, even when substantial contradictory evidence emerges. Even after scientific updates revealed COVID-19's higher fatality rate and evidence of asymptomatic transmission, many people adjusted their mental models insufficiently—the early "it's like the flu" anchor continued to influence risk assessment and behavior. Public health experts noted that had COVID-19 initially been framed as akin to a more deadly disease, risk perceptions might have been higher and responses more urgent from the beginning.

Worst-Case Bias: When Mental Models Catastrophize

While much of this chapter has focused on biases that lead to risk underestimation, a significant subset of individuals exhibited the opposite tendency—worst-case bias, or catastrophic thinking. This represents another mental model framework that filters reality through expectations of extreme negative outcomes. During COVID-19, individuals with this bias often hoarded supplies, believed unverified rumors of extreme dangers, and experienced high anxiety even in relatively low-risk situations.

The psychological mechanism behind catastrophic thinking involves a mental model that emphasizes maximum threat potential rather than most likely outcomes. For these "over-reactors," any rise in cases became evidence of societal collapse, and uncertainty was always resolved toward worst-case interpretations. Pakpour and Griffiths (2020) found that individuals with pre-existing anxiety disorders were particularly susceptible to this bias, as their mental models were already primed to anticipate and react to threat. While appropriate caution was prudent during the pandemic, excessive pessimism proved counterproductive—people overwhelmed by fear became more susceptible to sensational misinformation that magnified their dread, creating cycles of escalating anxiety that impaired rational decision-making.

This illustrates that mental models can distort risk perception in both directions—underestimation through optimism bias or overestimation through catastrophic thinking—highlighting the challenge of fostering balanced, evidence-based frameworks during crisis situations (Kreps & Kriner, 2020).

Interactive Cognitive Biases: How Mental Models Work Together

Mental models rarely operate in isolation. Instead, they interact to create comprehensive ways of understanding and responding to crises. When faced with a novel threat like COVID-19, individuals process information through multiple, interconnected frameworks simultaneously. Understanding these interactions explains why changing behavior often requires more than addressing a single bias or providing new information.

During the pandemic, these mental models worked together to shape individual responses: anchoring to familiar diseases (*"It's like the flu"*), optimism in personal risk assessment (*"I rarely get sick"*), desire for normalcy (*"Things will go back to normal"*), confirmation bias in information seeking (*"These experts agree with me"*), and threat perception shaped by immediate experiences (*"No one I know is sick"*). Conversely, those susceptible to worst-case bias typically experienced interactions between catastrophic thinking, availability heuristic (focusing on worst outcomes), and confirmation bias toward alarming information.

The same interplay of mental models influenced institutional decision-making, leading healthcare organizations to delay new protocols, underestimate resource needs, rely too heavily on existing systems, and maintain business-as-usual approaches for too long.

Mental Model Updating and Adaptation

While biases often hampered effective responses, some individuals demonstrated a remarkable ability to update their mental models as new information emerged.

What distinguished those who successfully adapted their understanding from those who rigidly maintained initial frameworks? Southwell et al. (2020) found that effective mental model updating typically involved what they termed "bridging experiences"—events that connected abstract risks to concrete personal reality.

For example, some individuals who initially downplayed COVID-19 risks dramatically revised their mental models after a friend or family member became seriously ill. These experiences created cognitive dissonance that couldn't be easily dismissed, forcing recalibration of underlying mental frameworks. Others updated their models through exposure to trusted sources that carefully explained why initial comparisons (like seasonal flu) were inadequate. As Betsch et al. (2020a, 2020b) documented, effective communication that acknowledged existing mental models before introducing new information proved more successful at facilitating updates than approaches that ignored or dismissed prior beliefs.

The challenge of updating public mental models during crises has been long recognized in risk communication research. Reynolds and Seeger (2005) developed an integrative model of crisis and emergency risk communication that emphasized the need to address pre-existing beliefs and emotional reactions rather than simply providing facts. Their framework highlighted how effective crisis messaging must first acknowledge current mental models before attempting to modify them—a principle that proved crucial during the rapidly evolving COVID-19 situation.

Pakpour and Griffiths (2020) identified emotional responses as crucial components in mental model adaptation. Their research found that appropriate levels of fear served as motivational drivers for model updating—too little fear maintained complacency, while excessive fear could trigger defensive denial or catastrophic thinking. This highlights how emotional and cognitive elements work together in mental model formation and revision. The most adaptable individuals maintained what Halpern et al. (2020) described as "flexible skepticism"—willingness to revise beliefs when presented with new evidence while avoiding both rigid denial and uncritical acceptance of all information.

Cognitive Biases Across Cultures

While these mental models operate at individual and institutional levels, they exist within broader cultural frameworks that shape their expression. Different societies revealed distinct patterns in how these cognitive frameworks manifested during the pandemic, pointing to deeper, culturally shaped mental models.

South Korea's response revealed mental models shaped by previous epidemic experiences. Rather than anchoring to seasonal flu, their mental models referenced recent SARS and MERS outbreaks, creating frameworks that balanced confidence with preparedness. This approach reflected a culturally influenced understanding of viral threats as concrete rather than abstract possibilities. COVID-19 mortality data showed South Korea maintaining extremely low death rates throughout 2020—under 1,000 deaths in a population of 51 million.

In contrast, many Western nations demonstrated mental models that positioned pandemics as historical or distant threats. Strong anchoring to flu experiences and overconfidence in healthcare systems created frameworks that struggled to process immediate viral danger. These societies needed to reconstruct their fundamental ways of categorizing threats as the crisis unfolded.

The United States' emphasis on individualism amplified optimism bias and confirmation bias, while institutional overconfidence led to delayed preparation. Americans often interpreted the pandemic through mental models that framed personal liberty as paramount, creating unique challenges for public health strategies. Surveys by Van Bavel et al. (2020) found that by mid-2020, Democrats consistently perceived COVID-19 as a greater risk and reported higher mask-wearing than Republicans, reflecting differing mental models shaped by partisan narratives.

Cultural psychologists have characterized the United States as a relatively "loose" culture, meaning social norms are more relaxed and rule-breaking is more tolerated (Gelfand et al., 2021). This cultural backdrop created an environment where optimism and normalcy biases flourished, reinforced by polarized information sources. By mid-2020, this cultural looseness manifested in concrete outcomes: Americans showed significantly lower compliance with health measures compared to "tighter" cultures, with mask usage varying from 40 to 95% depending on region and political affiliation. Gelfand et al. (2021) found that "loose" countries like the United States suffered significantly higher case and death rates—on the order of five to eight times more—compared to culturally "tight" countries, after controlling for other factors.

Germany demonstrated a cultural predisposition toward structure and institutional trust. While normalcy bias influenced public perception, it operated within frameworks that assumed collective action could manage disruptions. Their institutional confidence balanced systematic preparation rather than overconfidence. Comparative studies by Schmidt-Petri et al. (2022) found that Germans exceeded Japanese in certain protective actions during 2020—a higher proportion reported avoiding crowds, handshaking, and public transport.

Germany's culture lies between the United States and East Asia in terms of norm adherence; it is often characterized as orderly and rule-following, yet with an emphasis on individual reasoning. A strong societal norm of "Ordnung" (order) and past experiences (e.g., memories of disease outbreaks) fostered vigilance. The COVID-19 Snapshot Monitoring project (COSMO Germany) tracked public perceptions and behaviors throughout the pandemic, finding that risk perception in Germany remained relatively stable and high compared to other European countries, with corresponding consistency in preventive behaviors (Betsch et al., 2020a, 2020b). However, cultural individualism in Germany (though lower than in the United States) meant that variation between subgroups was greater than in more collective societies like Japan. By late 2020, Germany saw the emergence of the "Querdenker" (contrarian) movement, where thousands protested mask mandates and lockdowns, exemplifying how even in relatively tight cultures, pockets of resistance can emerge based on confirmation bias and overconfidence bias (Schmidt-Petri et al., 2022).

Japan's response highlighted how collective norms can override individual biases. Mask usage reached over 95% compliance without mandates, reflecting cultural mental models that prioritize group welfare over individual preferences. By mid-2020, about 70% of Japanese respondents reported being very afraid of contracting COVID-19, compared to only 49% in the United States (Gelfand et al., 2021).

Japan exemplifies a "tight" culture with strict social norms and a high emphasis on collective harmony. Even before the pandemic, mask-wearing during illness was a common courtesy, reflecting pre-existing mental models of disease as a collective concern. What's particularly notable is that Japan imposed fewer government lockdowns and restrictions than many Western countries, yet maintained lower infection rates through much of 2020. The homogeneity of response across different ages and regions was striking—there were no large subgroups defying recommendations as seen in looser cultures. By the end of 2020, Japan (population 126 million) recorded under 4,000 COVID-19 deaths, compared to tens of thousands in each major Western nation. The Japanese concept of "jishuku" (自粛, self-restraint) guided behavior: individuals curbed social activities not because they thought themselves invulnerable (optimism bias was minimal), but out of a sense of collective responsibility.

These cross-cultural variations (Table 11.2) highlight how individual cognitive biases don't exist in isolation but are instead shaped by broader cultural frameworks that determine their expression and impact during crisis situations.

Table 11.2 Cognitive Cultural Variations in COVID-19 Mental Models

Example Country	*Dominant Mental Models*	*Key Manifestations*	*Cultural Influences*
South Korea	**Concrete threat framework**	Proactive testing; contact tracing	Previous epidemic experience; collective responsibility values
United States	**Individual liberty framework**	Resistance to mandates; varied compliance	Strong individualism; decentralized governance; distrust in authority
Germany	**Structured response framework**	High compliance with formal guidelines	Cultural value of order; trust in institutional expertise
United Kingdom	**Historical resilience framework**	Initial downplaying of threat; "keep calm" approach	Cultural narratives of stoicism; historical reference to endurance
Japan	**Social harmony framework**	Voluntary compliance; peer-influenced behaviors	Cultural emphasis on avoiding social disruption; group conformity

Sources: Gelfand et al. (2021) (Cultural tightness-looseness analysis); Schmidt-Petri et al. (2022) (Germany-Japan comparison); Calvillo et al. (2020) (U.S. response patterns); Van Bavel et al. (2020) (Cross-cultural behavioral evidence).

From Cognitive Biases to Mental Models

The COVID-19 pandemic revealed how cognitive biases reflect deeper mental models that shape our understanding of reality. These frameworks—whether processing personal risk, validating information, or assessing threat—operate at individual, institutional, and even cultural levels. They represent fundamental ways of making sense of crisis situations and determine how people respond to public health measures.

Recognizing these mental models helps explain why simply providing new information often fails to change behavior. People don't just need facts; they need frameworks that help them process those facts in meaningful ways. Research by Halpern et al. (2020) demonstrated that effective public health messaging must address these underlying mental models, not just surface-level behaviors. As Jones et al. (2011) emphasize, mental models are interdisciplinary constructs that bridge cognitive, social, and cultural domains—making them particularly valuable for understanding complex crisis responses. The interaction between these individual mental models and broader cultural frameworks creates complex patterns of response that vary significantly across different populations and contexts, which we will explore further in the next section.

Collective Mental Models: Cultural Frameworks for Crisis Understanding

The COVID-19 pandemic revealed how deeply embedded mental models—our fundamental ways of understanding ourselves, society, and crisis—shaped public responses to the health emergency. Different societies' core beliefs about identity, responsibility, and the relationship between individual and community profoundly influenced how populations interpreted and responded to public health measures. While systemic structures provided the framework for pandemic response, it was these underlying mental models that determined how people made sense of the crisis and chose to act. These collective mental models represent shared cognitive frameworks through which communities interpret and respond to threats. They function as cultural lenses that filter information, shape risk perception, and guide behavioral responses during crises.

Mental Models of Collective Identity and Social Harmony

In many East Asian societies, deeply embedded mental models emphasize the interconnected nature of human existence and frame individual identity as inherently tied to collective welfare. These mental models manifest in fundamental beliefs like "jeong" (정, Korean understanding of emotional connection and responsibility to others), "giri" (義理, Japanese conception of duty to community), and "wa" (和, Japanese value of social harmony and group cohesion). Such core assumptions about human nature and social organization created natural cognitive frameworks for processing public health measures as expressions of collective care rather than impositions on individual liberty (Markus & Kitayama, 1991; Song & Choi, 2023).

These collective frameworks were reinforced by historical experiences with previous epidemics. East Asian societies like South Korea, Taiwan, Japan, and Singapore had confronted SARS (2003), H1N1 (2009), and MERS (2015) outbreaks in recent memory, creating established mental templates for pandemic response. These historical encounters helped shape population-level mental models that recognized infectious disease as a concrete, recurring threat requiring collective action rather than a distant, abstract possibility (Schmidt-Petri et al., 2022). When COVID-19 emerged, these societies had both institutional preparedness and psychological readiness—their populations could draw on mental models shaped by recent epidemic experiences rather than having to construct entirely new frameworks for understanding the threat. Maaravi et al. (2021) found that countries with a history of previous epidemic outbreaks generally responded more effectively to COVID-19, particularly when their cultural orientation emphasized collectivist values over individualist ones.

Research in cultural psychology has long noted that East Asian cultures promote interdependent conceptions of the self, linking personal well-being to group welfare (Markus & Kitayama, 1991). During COVID-19, this translated into a distinctive way of processing threat and safety: personal protective actions were naturally interpreted as expressions of social responsibility rather than individual choice (Leong et al., 2022; Song & Choi, 2023). For example, South Korea's communal values of solidarity (jeong) helped the public readily conform to mask-wearing and social distancing, perceiving these as altruistic acts for the common good rather than impositions (Song & Choi, 2023). Likewise, in Japan, cultural principles of giri and wa fostered a sense that individual sacrifices were moral obligations to protect the community (Lu et al., 2021). This deep-seated belief that safeguarding community health inherently safeguards individual well-being was reflected in high compliance rates: empirical studies found that individuals with stronger collectivistic orientations were significantly more likely to comply with health interventions, even at personal cost (Leong et al., 2022). Survey data showed citizens in collectivist societies emphasizing communal benefits over personal inconvenience, with those expressing greater trust in government significantly more likely to follow recommended preventive measures (Gotanda et al., 2021). As Jones et al. (2011) explain, these mental models function as interdisciplinary constructs that integrate cultural traditions, shared beliefs, and social context to create powerful frameworks for collective action. Beyond compliance, Xiao (2021) found that collectivist orientation was strongly correlated with more adaptive psychological responses during the pandemic, suggesting these mental models provided psychological resources for coping with crisis restrictions. In collectivist frameworks, protective behaviors are internalized as normative obligations rather than externally forced rules (Lu et al., 2021).

Beyond specific behaviors, these mental models provide comprehensive frameworks for making sense of crisis situations. They offer built-in cognitive pathways for processing uncertainty through collective action, understanding personal sacrifice as a form of social contribution, and viewing compliance with health measures as an expression of cultural values rather than submission to authority

(Southwell et al., 2020). For example, prioritizing the group's well-being can help normalize rapidly changing guidelines: populations grounded in these views were more willing to tolerate scientific uncertainty or evolving recommendations if such changes were communicated as necessary to protect the community (Han et al., 2021a; Leong et al., 2022).

Mental Models of Individual Autonomy and Personal Rights

In Western societies, such as in the United States and parts of Europe, dominant mental models center on the individual as the primary unit of social meaning. These deeply held frameworks conceptualize personal autonomy not merely as a right but as a fundamental truth about human nature (Song & Choi, 2023; Triandis, 1995). Decades of cross-cultural research have characterized Western cultures as more individualistic, prioritizing personal freedom and self-determination over collective obligations (Triandis, 1995). Such mental models shape how people instinctively process any collective action requirements—viewing them first through the lens of individual rights rather than community benefit (Bazzi et al., 2021; Song & Choi, 2023). For instance, a comparative analysis noted that Americans, reflecting an individualistic culture, were more likely to resist government policies that restricted personal freedom, perceiving such measures as infringements on individual rights (Song & Choi, 2023). This outlook stands in contrast to the East Asian patterns: in the United States, personal liberty was often treated as paramount even amid a public health emergency (Bazzi et al., 2021).

However, important variations existed within these broad cultural categories. Nordic countries like Denmark and Sweden, while sharing Western individualist values, demonstrated more nuanced collective mental models that balanced individual autonomy with high institutional trust and social solidarity. These societies maintained relatively high compliance with voluntary guidelines rather than strict mandates, revealing mental frameworks that processed public health recommendations through strong social trust rather than legal obligation (Van Bavel et al., 2020). Kaasa and Andriani (2022) found that institutional trust is deeply embedded in cultural contexts, with Nordic countries showing consistently higher levels of trust in government institutions compared to other Western nations, which explained some of their distinctive pandemic response patterns despite sharing individualist values with countries like the United States. Similarly, within East Asia, significant differences emerged between countries like South Korea, which leveraged technology-driven approaches and extensive testing, and Japan, which relied more heavily on social conformity with less testing but high voluntary mask compliance (Schmidt-Petri et al., 2022).

These individualistic mental models create specific ways of understanding causality and responsibility in public health. When faced with health threats, people operating within these frameworks naturally process decisions through questions of personal risk assessment and individual autonomy rather than collective impact (Bazzi et al., 2021; Leong et al., 2022; Song & Choi, 2023). The core assumption that individual judgment supersedes collective wisdom makes centralized health measures feel inherently suspect, triggering deep-seated resistance patterns rooted in fundamental beliefs about freedom and self-determination. This perspective aligns with known cognitive tendencies toward optimism bias, where individuals often underestimate their personal risk compared to others (Sharot, 2011). Bazzi et al. (2021) argued that regions with strong traditions of "rugged individualism" struggled to enact coordinated responses because many citizens were less inclined to follow directives for the common good. Blum et al. (2020) characterize this phenomenon as "Toxic Wild West Syndrome" in the United States—a combination of performative hyper-individualism and resistance to collective measures that manifested in visible protests against public health directives, often framed as patriotic defense of personal liberty.

The relationship between individualism-collectivism and COVID-19 outcomes has been quantitatively demonstrated. Jiang et al. (2022) analyzed data from 69 countries and found that a one-standard-deviation increase in individualism was associated with a 30% increase in the growth rate of confirmed cases during the early stage of the pandemic. Similarly, Rajkumar (2021) found significant positive correlations between individualism scores and COVID-19 case fatality rates across nations, even after controlling for potential confounding variables like healthcare quality, suggesting that cultural mental models directly influenced pandemic outcomes.

The COVID-19 pandemic highlighted how economic factors significantly interacted with cultural mental models to shape response patterns. Economic constraints often mediated how individuals and communities could operationalize their underlying mental frameworks. In collectivist societies, government support often aligns with cultural expectations of mutual care, enabling populations to actualize collective mental models through behaviors like staying home during outbreaks. For example, Japan's employment protection schemes and South Korea's robust financial support for quarantined individuals made it economically feasible to prioritize collective health needs over short-term individual economic interests (Gelfand et al., 2021).

In contrast, many individualist societies faced tensions between economic necessity and public health measures. The United States' patchwork system of financial support during lockdowns meant many workers faced difficult choices between income security and health safety, regardless of their personal risk assessment. These economic constraints sometimes reinforced individualist mental models by forcing personal cost-benefit calculations that pitted immediate financial survival against abstract collective benefit. Survey data showed that economic precarity was a significant predictor of non-compliance with health measures, independent of cultural or political factors (Van Bavel et al., 2020). Huang et al. (2022) presented compelling evidence that the relationship between individualism and COVID-19 outcomes was partly mediated by economic factors, finding that countries with both high individualism and limited economic safety nets experienced significantly worse health outcomes than those with stronger social support systems.

The COVID-19 vaccination rollout succinctly demonstrated these mental models in action. Across many Western societies, especially the United States, decisions to vaccinate were processed primarily as matters of personal choice rather than collective responsibility. When faced with vaccine mandates, individuals operating through these frameworks didn't simply question the policy—they experienced it as a fundamental challenge to their understanding of medical autonomy and personal freedom. This was evident in widespread public discourse opposing mandates as "government overreach" and in protests that evoked slogans of liberty and individual rights (Bazzi et al., 2021; Lazarus et al., 2021). Indeed, global surveys in 2020–2021 showed that English-speaking Western countries had among the highest levels of COVID-19 vaccine hesitancy in the developed world, often tied to these central concerns about personal freedom and distrust of authority (Carrieri et al., 2023; Lazarus et al., 2021). Another prominent example is Wang and Liu's (2022) systematic review of COVID-19 vaccine hesitancy that confirms these patterns, finding that right-wing political ideology and individualistic values predicted refusal of vaccination, with conservatives being two to three times more likely to reject vaccines than those with more communal orientations.

These individual-centered frameworks fundamentally shaped how people engaged with vaccination information. Even compelling data about community protection and herd immunity often failed to resonate because these concepts operated outside the dominant mental model of personal medical choice (Bazzi et al., 2021; Leong et al., 2022). The widespread resistance to vaccine requirements revealed a deep cultural framework where public health measures are invariably processed through a lens of individual liberty, even during global emergencies. For example, recent studies have found that U.S. counties with more individualistic cultural values had significantly lower COVID-19 vaccination rates, even when vaccines were widely available—due in part to a preference for personal risk assessment over collective responsibility and diminished responsiveness to public health messages framed around community protection (Fu et al., 2024; Vu, 2021). Research across Western societies found that messages emphasizing "protecting others" or "community immunity" were often less effective than those framed around personal choice or regaining individual freedoms. This pattern has been documented in COVID-19 vaccination studies (Callaghan et al., 2021; Kasting et al., 2022), pre-pandemic research on influenza vaccination (Quinn et al., 2017), and analysis of vaccine discourse in Canada (Griffith et al., 2021). While these response patterns are influenced by multiple factors beyond just cultural orientation, they consistently reflect how individualistic mental models create frameworks that prioritize personal over collective benefit when evaluating health interventions.

Mental Models of Authority and Expertise

How different societies conceptualize authority and expertise proved crucial during the pandemic. In some cultures, mental models frame expertise as a collective achievement, viewing scientific consensus as an expression of accumulated wisdom. These frameworks allow for a more fluid integration of expert guidance into individual decision-making, as following such guidance aligns with deep-seated views about knowledge and authority. For instance, populations with high trust in scientists and public institutions were more likely to comply with non-pharmaceutical interventions (NPIs), as they saw expert recommendations as credible and in the public's best interest. Cross-national research spanning 12 countries found that trust in scientific experts strongly predicted support for and compliance with COVID-19 measures, further emphasizing the impact of cultural models that elevate scientific authority (Algan et al., 2021; Leong et al., 2022; Marziali et al. 2024; Suhay et al. 2022; Troeger & Bollykyk, 2021).

In East Asian contexts, where respect for collective expertise and technocratic governance is often emphasized, people tended to accept health directives more readily as expressions of collective wisdom rather than as arbitrary rules. For example, epidemiologists' recommendations to close schools or implement lockdowns in South Korea or Japan were generally heeded by the public, reflecting a cultural inclination to trust experts and a belief that these authorities were guiding the nation safely. Survey evidence from Japan confirms that individuals with greater trust in government and health experts were significantly more likely to adhere to preventive measures, indicating that deference to expertise facilitated compliance (Gotanda et al., 2021; Song & Choi, 2023).

Contrasting mental models in other societies position expertise as potentially threatening to individual discernment. These frameworks process expert guidance through inherent skepticism, reflecting core beliefs about the primacy of personal judgment and deep-seated assumptions about institutional power (Bazzi et al., 2021; Pagliaro et al., 2021). In environments where skepticism of institutional authority runs high, even well-intended expert advice may be met with doubt or resistance. For example, in segments of the United States and United Kingdom, a notable portion of the public opted to "do their own research" via the internet or social networks rather than rely on official guidance, revealing a cultural undercurrent that external authorities must be personally verified or can be overridden by individual knowledge. This pattern aligns with the judgment under uncertainty frameworks described by Tversky and Kahneman (1974), where people rely on cognitive heuristics rather than expert assessments when facing complex risks.

Han et al. (2021a) found that across 23 countries, individuals' willingness to adopt COVID health behaviors was strongly tied to trust in government; thus, where trust was low, compliance suffered, presumably due to these skeptical mental models that favor personal interpretation of risk over expert directives. Pagliaro et al. (2021) found similar results, showing that trust was a key predictor of both prescribed and discretionary COVID-19 behaviors across different countries. Consistently, U.S. data show that trust in scientists and public health agencies declined through 2020, particularly among groups inclined to distrust centralized authority, leading to lower adherence to expert guidance (Pollard & Davis, 2022).

The response to school closures and lockdowns during the pandemic vividly illustrated these competing frameworks. In East Asian societies, decisions about both measures were largely processed through mental models that trusted expert assessment of public health risk. When epidemiologists in South Korea or Japan recommended closing schools or implementing lockdowns to prevent viral spread, these recommendations were generally accepted as expressions of collective wisdom rather than controversial impositions (Song & Choi, 2023).

In contrast, many Western societies processed both school closure and lockdown recommendations through more contested frameworks. In the United States, expert guidance often collided with mental models that prioritized individual or local judgment over centralized expertise. These decisions became battlegrounds between competing sources of authority—public health experts, state and local officials, parent groups, and political leaders. A cross-country study in Europe likewise noted that regions with higher trust in institutions had more uniform adherence to lockdown rules, whereas regions with distrust saw more varied compliance as people followed local leaders or personal beliefs instead (Bargain & Aminjonov, 2020).

Mental Models of Risk and Uncertainty

The pandemic highlighted fundamental differences in how societies conceptualize risk and process uncertainty. Some mental models embrace uncertainty as an inherent aspect of collective life, creating cognitive frameworks that can accommodate evolving scientific understanding and changing health guidance. These models view uncertainty not as a failure of expertise, but as an expected part of knowledge development, allowing populations to maintain trust in public health guidance even as recommendations evolved (Algan et al., 2021; Han et al., 2021a). Studies also found that risk perception itself was strongly associated with emotional responses, with different cultural contexts mediating how risk perceptions translated to psychological outcomes (Han et al., 2021b). For example, societies or groups with a comfort with uncertainty mindset were more accepting of the fact that scientific advice (like mask or quarantine guidelines) might change as new evidence emerged.

Comparative research between Japan and Germany demonstrated how different cultural approaches to uncertainty affected compliance with evolving guidelines. Schmidt-Petri et al. (2022) found that social norms in Japan tended to reinforce adaptation to changing information, while creating greater normative pressure for compliance with preventive measures. This cultural comfort with evolving situations helped maintain trust in public health authorities despite changing recommendations.

Digital contact tracing adoption provides a particularly clear example of how cultural mental models influenced specific technology responses during the pandemic. South Korea's rapid and widespread adoption of digital contact tracing applications reflected collective mental frameworks that prioritized community protection over individual privacy concerns. The population largely viewed privacy trade-offs as reasonable sacrifices for collective benefit, processing the technology through mental models that emphasized social responsibility (Leong et al., 2022). Park et al. (2020) documented South Korea's extensive contact tracing system that combined digital technology with traditional epidemiological investigation, finding remarkably high public compliance despite the significant privacy implications. By March 2020, South Korea had already traced 9,137 confirmed COVID-19 cases, identifying over 1,200 transmission events and effectively controlling early outbreaks through these collective-oriented technological approaches.

By contrast, in countries like the United States and parts of Europe, digital tracing applications faced significant resistance rooted in mental models that prioritized individual privacy rights and harbored deeper skepticism of government data collection. Even when applications were designed with strong privacy protections, adoption rates remained low in many Western countries, with fewer than 20% of citizens in some regions downloading available apps (Van Bavel et al., 2020). Maaravi et al. (2021) found that individualism scores were strongly associated with lower rates of contact tracing compliance and technology adoption, with citizens in highly individualistic countries expressing significantly greater concerns about government surveillance and data privacy than those in collectivist societies. This profound contrast points to fundamental differences in how populations conceptualized the balance between individual rights and collective welfare during a health emergency.

Taiwan and New Zealand can be seen as examples: both maintained public trust amid shifting recommendations by being transparent that policies would adjust with new data, and their populaces largely understood this adaptation as appropriate and necessary (Carrieri et al., 2023; Wilson, 2020). In Taiwan, prior experience with epidemics and a cultural emphasis on pragmatism meant that when mask guidelines or travel rules changed, the public incorporated these changes without a loss of faith in health officials. Similarly, New Zealand's leadership frequently acknowledged uncertainties and explained policy shifts (e.g., regarding lockdown timing or mask use) in a way that resonated with the public's understanding that uncertainty is a natural part of crisis management.

In contrast, mental models that demand certainty often struggle to process the pandemic's evolving nature. These frameworks seek fixed truths and clear answers, making it difficult to integrate new information or adapt to changing circumstances. In cultures or subcultures with discomfort with uncertainty, shifting public health messages were frequently interpreted as mistakes or deceit rather than as the product of new learning. Perhaps no single issue better illustrated this tension than the evolution of mask-wearing guidance.

Early in the pandemic, public health experts discouraged mask use among the general public, driven by concerns about supply shortages for healthcare workers and limited evidence of widespread community transmission. As understanding of SARS-CoV-2 transmission improved, including evidence of asymptomatic and aerosolized spread, recommendations shifted to advocate for universal masking as a critical tool in reducing transmission.

For those whose mental models relied on certainty, these changes appeared inconsistent or even contradictory. Rather than interpreting evolving guidance as the natural progression of a rapidly advancing body of knowledge, some viewed it as evidence of incompetence or dishonesty on the part of public health authorities. This perception eroded trust and created new avenues for misinformation and alternative narratives to gain traction (Carrieri et al., 2023; Zarocostas, 2020). In the United States, for example, the flip-flopping of mask guidelines was seized upon by skeptics and conspiracy theorists as "proof" that experts were clueless or lying—an accusation that gained currency in already-polarized communities predisposed to distrust government pronouncements.

This pattern of discomfort with scientific uncertainty manifested strongly in vaccination decisions as well. Gerretsen et al. (2021) found that "mistrust of vaccine benefit" was the principal determinant of COVID-19 vaccine hesitancy, explaining 38% of variance in vaccination intentions. Their research showed that individuals who demanded certainty in public health guidance were significantly more likely to refuse vaccination when confronted with evolving information about vaccine safety and efficacy. A cross-European analysis similarly found that a one-time policy reversal (such as the temporary suspension of the AstraZeneca vaccine in 2021) significantly increased vaccine hesitancy, especially among people with pre-existing low trust in science and institutions (Carrieri et al., 2023). These findings confirm how mental models that struggle with uncertainty directly shaped crucial health behaviors throughout the pandemic, creating cognitive barriers to accepting both evolving guidance and the interventions based on that guidance.

Table 11.3 Cultural Mental Models in Pandemic Response

Mental Model	*Core Belief*	*COVID-19 Response Pattern*	*Example Regions*
Collective Harmony	Individual well-being is connected to group welfare	High voluntary compliance; protective actions seen as civic or moral duties	*Japan, South Korea, Taiwan*
Individual Autonomy	Personal freedom is a foundational right	Resistance to mandates; framing of health decisions as matters of personal choice	*United States, parts of Europe*
Trust in Collective Expertise	Scientific consensus reflects accumulated wisdom	Deference to expert guidance; acceptance of evolving recommendations	*Germany, Scandinavia*
Skepticism of Institutional Authority	Personal judgment supersedes external authority	Questioning of guidance; preference for personal research over official sources	*United States, United Kingdom*
Comfort with Uncertainty	Evolving understanding is a natural part of science	Trust maintained amid shifting recommendations and evolving data	*Taiwan, New Zealand*
Discomfort with Uncertainty	Changes in guidance reflect incompetence or deceit	Loss of trust; belief that guidance should be fixed and unchanging	*Prevalent in polarized societies*

Sources: Adapted from cross-cultural analyses of pandemic responses (Algan et al., 2021; Bazzi et al., 2021; Carrieri et al., 2023; Han et al., 2021a, 2021b, 2023; Lu et al., 2021; Pagliaro et al., 2021; Song & Choi, 2023).

Mental Models as Foundations for Public Health Response

The pandemic revealed that effective public health responses require engaging with underlying mental models that shape how societies process and respond to crises (Table 11.3). These fundamental frameworks proved more influential than specific policies or communication strategies in determining public response. Countries where pandemic measures resonated with prevailing cultural models generally saw higher compliance and better health outcomes, as people made sense of the crisis in ways congruent with their existing worldview. By contrast, where there was a clash between public health directives and the population's default mental models, responses were often fraught with confusion, contestation, or non-compliance (Han et al. 2023).

Successful public health communication during the pandemic didn't just rely on clear messaging—it required alignment with existing mental models. Messages resonated when they worked within, rather than against, established frameworks (Gursoy et al., 2022). Countries that achieved high compliance with health measures often succeeded not because they had better information, but because they presented that information in ways that aligned with their population's fundamental ways of understanding reality. For example, in collectivist contexts, officials appealed to values of community and mutual care (e.g., presenting mask-wearing as protecting one's family and nation), whereas in more individualistic contexts, some successful campaigns linked health behaviors to personal freedom (e.g., "Mask up so we can open up"—implying that individual action would restore individual liberties).

Airhihenbuwa et al. (2020) argue that culture serves as the central organizing principle for health behaviors in any community, and therefore, pandemic communication strategies must be deeply informed by cultural frameworks. Their analysis of COVID-19 communication across Africa, the United States, and Europe highlighted how ignoring cultural mental models in health messaging significantly undermined response effectiveness, particularly in culturally diverse societies. They propose that cultural framework models should be foundational in designing public health interventions that engage with—rather than override—existing community mental models. As Basabe and Ros (2005) have established in their comprehensive review of cultural dimensions, individualism-collectivism and power distance fundamentally shape how societies respond to authority and group norms, making cultural adaptation of health measures a critical component of effective pandemic management.

While cultural mental models provide powerful explanatory frameworks for pandemic responses, it's important to acknowledge their limitations too. These collective frameworks interact with numerous other factors—including institutional quality, economic resources, demographic variables, and healthcare infrastructure—that together determine pandemic outcomes. The most effective approaches recognize both the influence of cultural mental models and the complex systems in which they operate.

Looking forward, improving pandemic preparedness requires understanding and working with these deep-seated mental models. Rather than attempting to impose uniform approaches, public health strategies must recognize and adapt to different ways of conceptualizing identity, responsibility, and social relationships (Van Bavel et al., 2020). For example, future public health messaging might present vaccination both as an expression of community protection in collectivist societies and as a means of preserving individual freedom of movement and activity in individualist societies. Both ultimately achieve the same outcome through different mental model frameworks. By crafting interventions that "speak" to a population's prevailing mental models—be it collective harmony, personal liberty, trust in expertise, or comfort with uncertainty—public health officials can foster greater trust and compliance. This approach aligns with established frameworks for crisis and emergency risk communication that emphasize the need for culturally tailored messaging (Reynolds & Seeger, 2005).

While these collective cultural frameworks played a crucial role in shaping pandemic responses, they did not operate in isolation. As we will explore in the next section, institutional mental models further mediated how populations interpreted and responded to public health guidance, creating another layer of influence on pandemic outcomes.

Institutional Mental Models: Frameworks of Trust and Authority

The pandemic revealed how deeply embedded mental models about trust, authority, and collective action shaped public responses to health measures. While social trust is often measured through compliance behaviors, these visible patterns reflect deeper frameworks through which people conceptualize and process institutional authority, scientific expertise, and collective action. Understanding these underlying mental models provides insight into why different populations interpreted and responded to public health guidance in fundamentally different ways.

Table 11.4 outlines five core domains where institutional mental models shaped pandemic response. Each reflects a different way institutions conceptualized their role, interpreted uncertainty, and interacted with the public.

Mental Models Within Public Health Institutions

The pandemic exposed how public health institutions themselves operate through distinct mental models that shape their approach to crisis. Some health agencies functioned through frameworks that positioned public health as primarily a technical, expert-driven domain. Within this mental model, institutional responses focused on scientific consensus and standardized protocols, sometimes struggling to adapt when faced with novel challenges that didn't fit established or predefined patterns (Bargain & Aminjonov, 2020; Brauner et al., 2021).

Other health institutions operated through mental models that viewed public health as a dynamic interface between scientific knowledge and social context.

Table 11.4 Key Domains of Institutional Mental Models in Pandemic Response

Domain	*What It Reflects*	*Why It Matters in a Pandemic*
Public Health Role	How institutions define the purpose and scope of public health	Shapes whether health is treated as purely technical or socially embedded
Authority and Legitimacy	How institutions are granted and maintain public trust	Determines whether populations follow guidance or resist it
Agency Coordination	How institutions relate to one another	Affects the speed and coherence of policy response
Evidence Use	How institutions gather and interpret data	Influences the precision and flexibility of interventions
Communication	How institutions engage with the public	Impacts compliance, trust, and message adaptation

Sources: Institutional response domains synthesized from pandemic analyses (Algan et al., 2021; Bargain & Aminjonov, 2020; Halpern et al., 2020; Van Bavel et al., 2020).

These frameworks allowed for more adaptive responses, recognizing that pandemic management requires both technical expertise and contextual understanding of how populations process health guidance. For example, Singapore's public health institutions demonstrated this framework by rapidly developing culturally tailored communication strategies when initial technical approaches proved insufficient for reaching migrant worker communities (Yip et al., 2021).

The contrast became evident in how different health institutions approached uncertainty. Those with rigid technical frameworks often struggled when faced with evolving evidence, sometimes delaying action until definitive data emerged (Xiao, 2021). The initial response in Sweden exemplifies this challenge, where health authorities maintained standard protocols despite emerging evidence about asymptomatic transmission, resulting in delayed preventive measures and higher excess mortality compared to neighboring countries (Brusselaers et al., 2022). Similarly, during the pandemic, the United Kingdom initially employed a one-way transmission approach. Sanders (2020) analyzed how U.K. government institutions conceptualized their communication role during COVID-19, finding that they operated through mental models that positioned communication primarily as information transfer—experts providing guidance to a receiving public—rather than as a collaborative process of meaning-making. This institutional framework focused on clarity and accuracy but often failed to engage with how different populations would process and respond to the information, contributing to declining adherence over time. Williams et al. (2021) documented how this institutional communication model led to what they termed "alert fatigue," where the public's responsiveness to guidance diminished due to the overwhelming volume of messages from authorities. Institutions with more adaptive frameworks acknowledged uncertainty as an inevitable aspect of novel disease response, implementing precautionary measures while clearly communicating the evolving nature of their understanding (Wilson, 2020). As Wilson (2020) noted, leaders in New Zealand acted decisively ahead of definitive evidence—rapidly closing borders and implementing lockdowns when case numbers were still low—explicitly to "go hard and go early" in the face of uncertainty.

A global study published in *Science* (Brauner et al., 2021) found that in combination, NPIs reduced the virus reproduction rate (Rt) by 77%, with the mean Rt without any NPIs being 3.3. However, the effectiveness varied dramatically based on how institutions implemented and coordinated these measures. Haug et al. (2020) further analyzed the relative effectiveness of different interventions, finding that the most effective measures were those targeting small gathering cancellations, closure of educational institutions, and border restrictions, while less disruptive measures like governmental support to vulnerable populations and risk communication strategies also showed significant benefits. Generally speaking, countries with more integrated, adaptive institutional approaches achieved higher compliance rates and better outcomes.

Mental Models of Institutional Authority and Legitimacy

Public perceptions of institutional legitimacy revealed underlying mental models about authority. Beyond notions of trust or distrust, these frameworks determine how people fundamentally process institutional guidance. In some contexts, legitimacy is primarily processed through technical credentials and expertise. When operating within this framework, populations evaluate institutions based on demonstrated competence and specialized knowledge (Van Bavel et al., 2020).

Alternative mental models position legitimacy primarily through relational and value-based frameworks. Here, institutional authority is processed through perceived alignment with community values and priorities (Vu, 2021). When the Centers for Disease Control and Prevention (CDC) in the United States initially recommended against mask-wearing, many evaluated this guidance not only through its technical merits but through frameworks that questioned whether the institution was prioritizing public welfare over other considerations.

This distinction explains why technically sound guidance sometimes failed to gain a strong foothold. When institutional communications didn't engage with the legitimacy frameworks through which populations processed authority, even scientifically accurate information struggled to influence public behavior (Mace, 2020). Brazil's response during the early pandemic illustrates this challenge, where presidential dismissal of scientific guidance created legitimacy conflicts between federal and local authorities, undermining trust in health institutions and contributing to low compliance with preventive measures (Ortega & Orsini, 2020). Conversely, when South Korea's health authorities framed guidance in ways that acknowledged both technical expertise and community values, their recommendations achieved higher compliance.

Research has also shown that cultural factors influenced compliance during the pandemic. Communities with more collectivist orientations, which emphasize shared values and group welfare, exhibited higher compliance when health measures were framed as protecting the community (Xiao, 2021). By contrast, in settings where there was a mismatch between public health policies and the community's core values—such as a legacy of distrust in government or strong leanings toward individual liberties—compliance was much more tentative.

The impact of these legitimacy models is reflected in concrete metrics. A global analysis published in *Scientific Reports* found that compliance with public health measures dropped dramatically over time, "from over 85% in the first half of 2020 to less than 40% at the start of 2021" (Agyapon-Ntra & McSharry, 2023). This decline represents not only "pandemic fatigue," but the failure of institutional frameworks to maintain legitimacy as the crisis evolved.

Interagency Mental Models of Coordination

The pandemic revealed how government agencies conceptualize their relationships with other institutions. Some operated through mental models of institutional sovereignty, where agencies viewed themselves as distinct entities with clearly bounded responsibilities. Within this framework, coordination occurred through formal channels and predefined protocols. This approach created stability, but sometimes impeded rapid adaptation when novel scenarios required unconventional collaboration.

Contrasting mental models framed interagency relationships through frameworks of shared mission and flexible boundaries. Agencies operating within these mental models could more readily form ad hoc partnerships and adapt roles when faced with emerging challenges. Taiwan's successful pandemic response demonstrated this framework quite well, with public health agencies, technology ministries, and economic departments rapidly creating novel collaborative structures that transcended traditional institutional boundaries.

These interagency mental models became particularly evident in border control and travel restriction decisions. Countries where agencies operated through rigid sovereignty frameworks often implemented inconsistent measures, with immigration authorities, public health institutions, and transportation ministries applying disconnected approaches. Italy's early pandemic response exemplifies these challenges, where disconnects between regional and national authorities created delays in implementing coordinated lockdown measures, contributing to the virus's rapid spread across northern regions (Capano, 2020). Conversely, countries where agencies shared mental models of flexible collaboration implemented more coherent, comprehensive travel policies.

Research on interagency coordination during crises has found that countries with layered mechanisms—spanning strategic, operational, and tactical levels—implemented before or immediately after the first reported cases achieved measurably better outcomes (Ngoy et al., 2022). In particular, decentralized but well-coordinated frameworks allowed nations to maintain essential services while adapting rapidly to evolving conditions, whereas countries with fragmented or overlapping authority structures experienced significant delays in responding to emerging threats (Sachs, 2021; Turner et al., 2022; Wolbers et al., 2018). These coordination challenges became especially apparent during the pandemic, where fragmented systems struggled to implement comprehensive surveillance and emergency response measures in a timely manner.

Mental Models of Data and Evidence

Institutional approaches to data collection and interpretation revealed underlying mental models about evidence. Some health agencies, such as the World Health Organization (WHO), operated within frameworks that viewed data primarily through quantitative, standardized metrics. This mental model prioritized consistency and comparability, but sometimes struggled to capture complex social realities that affected pandemic spread and intervention effectiveness.

Alternative frameworks positioned evidence as inherently multidimensional, integrating quantitative metrics with qualitative understanding of local contexts. Institutions operating within these mental models developed more nuanced approaches to pandemic monitoring, recognizing that effective response required understanding not just the raw case numbers, but the social patterns and behavioral factors that influenced transmission.

Germany's health institutes demonstrated this more integrated approach by complementing standard epidemiological data with detailed investigation of social transmission contexts and behavioral patterns. This mental model allowed for more targeted interventions that addressed the underlying social dimensions beyond the numerical reality of the pandemic. In contrast, India's initial COVID-19 data collection focused predominantly on case counting without capturing important contextual factors, leading to challenges in identifying and protecting vulnerable populations in densely populated areas (Choutagunta et al., 2021).

The importance of such adaptive responses becomes even more evident when considering that the reliability of pandemic data itself varied dramatically across countries. Farhadi and Lahooti (2021) identified significant discrepancies in data transparency, finding that only 27 countries (15.3%) consistently provided highly reliable COVID-19 data, including the United Kingdom, Australia, Spain, Israel, and Germany. Meanwhile, another 26 nations published significantly less reliable data—often due to limited infrastructure, testing capacity, or inconsistent reporting—creating barriers to effective cross-border coordination and evidence-based policy (Calgua, 2022; Rotulo et al., 2023). These data gaps ultimately shaped how institutions communicated with the public and determined which interventions were prioritized.

Mental Models of Public Communication

How institutions communicated with the public revealed fundamental frameworks for understanding the relationship between expertise and society. Some operated through mental models that positioned communication primarily as information transfer—experts providing guidance to a receiving public. This framework focused on clarity and accuracy, but sometimes failed to engage with how different populations would process and respond to the information (Zarocostas, 2020). During the pandemic, the United Kingdom initially employed this one-way transmission approach, with health authorities announcing restrictions and guidelines without sufficiently addressing public concerns, contributing to confusion and declining adherence to measures over time (Hyland-Wood et al., 2021; Sanders, 2020).

Other institutions functioned through mental models that framed communication as meaning-making—a collaborative process between authorities and communities. Within this framework, effective communication requires understanding the mental models through which different populations would interpret information. New Zealand's approach exemplified this mental model quite well, with health authorities actively engaging with diverse communities to understand how messages would be received and adapted, particularly among the culturally distinct Māori and Pacific populations (Wilson, 2020).

The contrast became evident in messaging about uncertainty. Institutions operating through information transfer models often struggled when communicating evolving guidance, as this framework provided limited tools for maintaining authority while acknowledging uncertainty. Those working within meaning-making frameworks more successfully navigated changing recommendations by engaging transparently with the process of scientific discovery rather than focusing solely on current conclusions.

Porat et al. (2020) quantified the impact of different communication approaches, finding that strategies balancing autonomy and guidance achieved higher sustained compliance rates. The study highlighted that communication strategies emphasizing collaborative approaches and trust-building were particularly effective in contexts with diverse populations, reducing disparities in health outcomes compared to top-down information dissemination approaches. As Demirtaş-Madran (2021) noted, communication strategies based on "essential principles of human rights, including autonomy, equality, dignity, and privacy" were more effective than fear-based messaging.

Mental Models as Foundations of Institutional Response

The pandemic revealed that institutional effectiveness depended not just on resources or formal structures, but on the underlying mental models through which institutions conceptualized their role, relationships, and responsibilities. These foundational frameworks—whether positioning public health as purely technical or socio-technical, viewing institutional boundaries as rigid or flexible, approaching evidence as standardized or contextual—shaped how organizations responded to the crisis.

For example, the U.S. CDC initially relied on rigid protocols that struggled to address the specific needs of vulnerable populations such as migrant workers. Clark et al. (2020) examined how health institutions operated through mental models that viewed public health primarily as a technical, expert-driven domain rather than as a socio-technical interface. Their analysis showed that these institutional frameworks led agencies to develop standardized approaches that failed to account for the unique circumstances of immigrant communities, creating significant gaps in pandemic response for these populations. In contrast, Singapore adapted its communication strategies to reflect cultural and contextual understanding, leading to more effective outreach (Yip et al., 2021). Similarly, the CDC's early stance on masking—framed narrowly as a clinical intervention—conflicted with public values and created confusion. By contrast, South Korea framed masking as a collective, communal act, aligning guidance with societal norms and trust. You (2020) analyzed how South Korean institutions operated through mental models that positioned public health as inherently both technical and social. Korean public health agencies constructed their pandemic guidance through frameworks that recognized the importance of public perception and social context, not just scientific evidence. This institutional approach allowed them to develop mask-wearing policies that were presented not merely as technical interventions but as expressions of collective responsibility.

Fragmented coordination across U.S. agencies also slowed critical responses due to rigid role definitions and a lack of integrated structures. Taiwan, however, demonstrated effective interagency collaboration through a shared mission and flexible role distribution. In terms of evidence use, institutions like the WHO often focused on standardized case counts, missing key social dynamics. Germany's response, in contrast, incorporated behavioral context and localized data to shape interventions. Lastly, U.S. briefings tended to emphasize one-way information delivery, which eroded public trust during uncertain phases of the pandemic. Meanwhile, New Zealand engaged the public through transparent, evolving communication strategies that fostered shared understanding (Wilson, 2020).

Van Bavel et al. (2020) yielded a striking finding: combinations of less disruptive and costly policy measures could be as effective as more intrusive actions when properly coordinated across institutions. Analysis of over 6,000 hierarchically coded non-pharmaceutical interventions across 79 territories by Haug et al. (2020) supported this, revealing that strategically combined less intrusive measures reduced transmission rates comparable to national lockdowns. Research from Wang et al. (2022a) later reported that the pandemic's true impact was substantially greater than officially reported, with an estimated 18.2 million excess deaths globally (compared to the approximately 5.9 million reported deaths at the time of their publication). Their research indicated that many of these deaths could have been prevented had institutions overcome rigid mental models to enable more effective cooperation from local to international levels. This highlights how institutional frameworks that allowed for flexible, more coordinated approaches often achieved better outcomes than those relying on singular, dogmatic interventions.

Building institutional resilience requires examining and potentially evolving these mental models (Table 11.5). Institutions with rigid technical frameworks may need to develop more integrated approaches that recognize public health's social dimensions. Those with strong sovereignty models might benefit from collaborative frameworks that enable adaptive coordination across traditional boundaries. These adjustments would enable the institutional agility needed for future emergencies, where complexity and uncertainty are inherent features rather than anomalies. Ultimately, the lessons from COVID-19 suggest that institutional preparation for future pandemics must transcend protocols and resources to address the deeper mental models shaping how organizations process information, make decisions, and engage with the public during health emergencies.

Table 11.5 Institutional Mental Models—Rigid vs. Adaptive Models

Domain	*Rigid Model*	*Observed Impact (Rigid)*	*Adaptive Model*	*Observed Impact (Adaptive)*
Public Health Role	Technical, expert-driven	Struggled with novel or local challenges	Socio-technical, context-aware	Better alignment with community needs and complex realities
Authority and Legitimacy	Based on credentials and expertise	Evidence-based advice ignored if misaligned with public values	Based on shared values and trust	Increased uptake of guidance and public cooperation
Agency Coordination	Fixed roles, formal protocols	Delays and fragmentation when agencies failed to coordinate	Shared mission, flexible roles	Faster, more cohesive decision-making
Evidence Use	Standardized, quantitative metrics	Missed key behavioral and social dynamics	Integrated with social context	Interventions adapted more successfully to local conditions
Communication	One-way information transfer	Trust eroded under unidirectional messaging during uncertainty	Collaborative meaning-making	Sustained public trust and more effective behavior change

Sources: Adapted from multi-country pandemic analyses of institutional responses (Algan et al., 2021; Bargain & Aminjonov, 2020; Brauner et al., 2021; Halpern et al., 2020; Van Bavel et al., 2020; Wilson, 2020).

As we will explore in the next section, these institutional mental models operate within specific temporal contexts, with the duration of a crisis creating additional challenges for how populations sustain response efforts and adapt to prolonged emergency situations.

Temporal Mental Models: Processing Extended Crisis and Adaptation

The COVID-19 pandemic revealed fundamental frameworks through which humans process and respond to prolonged crisis situations. What we observe as "pandemic fatigue" reflects deeper mental models about time, endurance, and adaptation during extended emergencies. These temporal mental models—our internal timelines for crisis duration, adaptation thresholds, and recovery trajectories—shaped how different populations conceptualized and navigated the prolonged nature of the crisis. While measurable behaviors like compliance patterns

provided visible indicators, these observable trends stemmed from profound frameworks governing how people process time itself during extended threats, influencing both individual resilience and collective endurance across cultural and institutional contexts.

Implicit and Explicit Temporality in Crisis

Just as mental models shape how people interpret risk, authority, and responsibility, they also influence how we experience time during a crisis. Temporal mental models refer to our internal expectations for how crises unfold, resolve, or persist—and how we adapt when those expectations are disrupted.

One useful lens comes from Fuchs (2013), who distinguishes between implicit temporality—the automatic, taken-for-granted flow of time that structures daily life—and explicit temporality, which arises when that flow is interrupted, and time becomes fragmented into uncertain futures or suspended presents, which can trigger disorientation, anxiety, or a sense of unreality.

The COVID-19 pandemic triggered this shift at a global scale. As routines collapsed and uncertainty expanded, individuals were forced into heightened temporal awareness. Normal time markers—work, school, weekends, holidays—lost consistency, contributing to widespread temporal disorientation. Velasco et al. (2021) describe this breakdown as a loss of "temporal scaffolding," with many reporting that time felt frozen, accelerated, or surreal.

These disruptions prompted the emergence of new temporal frameworks for processing risk, duration, and adaptation. As Fuchs notes, our experience of time is shaped not only cognitively, but also socially and biologically. When bodily rhythms and shared schedules are destabilized, so too is our sense of coherence—and our capacity to endure prolonged uncertainty. These shifts help explain the emergence of widespread temporal disorientation and offer insight into how populations began recalibrating their sense of risk, trust, and resilience over the course of the pandemic.

Mental Models of Crisis Duration and Endurance

The psychological strain of pandemic fatigue reveals deep-seated mental models about how crises should unfold. The dominant framework in many societies positions crisis as inherently temporary – a model that assumes emergencies should have clear beginnings and endings. When confronted with a prolonged pandemic that defied this mental model, people experienced cognitive strain not just from the restrictions themselves, but from the fundamental challenge to their understanding of how a crisis should unfold over time (Masten & Motti-Stefanidi, 2020; Michie et al., 2020).

This mental model manifests in widespread emotional exhaustion. The cumulative stress of navigating COVID-19 risks—whether due to fear of infection, financial instability, or disruptions to daily life—challenged basic assumptions about human endurance. People found it increasingly difficult to sustain protective behaviors as their mental models of "emergency response" collided with the

Table 11.6 Temporal Mental Models and Responses Across the COVID-19 Pandemic

Pandemic Phase	*Temporal Model*	*Behavioral Pattern*	*Psychological Impact*
Early 2020 *(Initial Outbreak)*	**Acute Crisis**	High compliance; rapid lifestyle shifts	Acute anxiety; hypervigilance
Mid 2020 *(First Wave)*	**Extended Emergency**	Sustained compliance with strain manifesting	Persistent stress; early fatigue
Late 2020 *(Multiple Waves)*	**Chronic Disruption**	Selective compliance; risk parsing begins	Fatigue; social friction; cognitive dissonance
Early 2021 *(Vaccine Rollout)*	**Transitional Resolution**	Mixed adherence based on vaccine status	Cautious optimism amid chronic strain
2022–2023 *(Early Endemicity)*	**New Normal**	Partial return to routine; residual precautions	Endemic caution; emotional burnout
2023–Present *(Post-Pandemic)*	**Transformed Risk**	Personalized long-term risk strategies	Lingering fatigue; recalibrated vigilance

Sources: Table synthesized from findings in Daly et al. (2022); Du et al. (2022); Giuntella et al. (2021); Kim et al. (2023); Leung et al. (2022); Pierce et al. (2020); Santomauro et al., 2021; Trabelsi et al. (2021); Wang et al. (2022b).

pandemic's indefinite timeline characterized by recurring waves of infection and restriction (Gassen et al., 2022; Trabelsi et al., 2021).

Table 11.6 integrates findings from global pandemic monitoring studies and psychological research to illustrate the evolving relationship between mental models, behavior, and psychological, fatigue-related impact during COVID-19.

Over time, this framework began to shift as people processed risk differently. Early in the pandemic, the threat of COVID-19 felt immediate and severe, aligning with mental models of acute crisis. However, as people's frameworks adapted to living with the virus, their fundamental way of processing the threat evolved. This transformation represented a core change in mental models about risk and normalcy (Gassen et al., 2022; Wang et al., 2022b).

Longitudinal research by Gassen et al. (2022) provides quantitative evidence of this pattern. Their study examined changes in COVID-19 concern over time, identifying distinct classes of individuals with varying levels of initial concern. Despite these differences, all groups showed decreasing levels of concern over time, even when infection risks remained stable or increased—a pattern researchers identified as "pandemic fatigue." This study found these declines in concern were reflected in physiological measures like reduced heart rate and blood pressure, suggesting genuine adaptation rather than merely reported differences (Gassen et al., 2022). Importantly, this adaptation occurred in predictable temporal phases, with most participants showing a threshold effect around 8–12 weeks after initial exposure to pandemic stressors, when baseline concern levels began to decrease regardless of actual risk levels.

Cultural Mental Models of Prolonged Crisis

Different societies revealed distinct mental models for processing extended emergencies, particularly evident in collectivist versus individualist cultures. These differences represented fundamental frameworks for understanding collective endurance and adaptation.

In collectivist societies, pre-existing mental models often positioned extended hardship as a shared experience requiring collective endurance. Japan's sustained compliance with health measures reflected a deeper framework where individual exhaustion was processed through models of collective responsibility (Guan et al., 2020). The cultural value of "meiwaku" (迷惑; avoiding causing inconvenience to others) represented a fundamental way of conceptualizing one's communal role during a prolonged crisis (Yamawaki, 2012). These collectivist temporal models featured notably different adaptation timelines, with greater persistence of protective behaviors over extended periods compared to individualist societies (Atalay & Solmazer, 2021; Wang et al., 2022c).

In contrast, individualist societies often operated through mental models that positioned personal endurance as separate from collective endurance. As pandemic fatigue began to set in, these frameworks interpreted ongoing restrictions as increasingly unsustainable impositions on individual freedom and autonomy. This perspective emerged from fundamental models about the limits of collective sacrifice versus personal choice during an extended crisis (Huynh, 2020; Wang et al., 2022c). Research has identified temporal patterns in compliance with protective measures, with notable decreases often occurring between months 3 and 6 of restrictions, a finding observed more prominently in societies with stronger individualist orientations (Atalay & Solmazer, 2021; Tran, 2022).

In the United States, the complex mix of responses reflected competing mental models about individual versus collective endurance during crisis. The fragmentation stemmed from fundamentally different frameworks for processing the relationship between personal and collective endurance during extended emergencies. Some populations operated through mental models that viewed extended compliance as an expression of community resilience, while others understood it through frameworks of unsustainable restriction (Guan et al., 2020; Huynh, 2020). These differences in temporal framing were not static but evolved over distinct phases of the pandemic, with Daly and Robinson (2021) documenting a pronounced threshold effect in U.S. populations around eight to ten weeks (approximately month two to three) of restrictions, after which mental health impacts began to diminish regardless of ongoing pandemic threats.

Research supports these cross-cultural differences. A population-based study by Leung et al. (2022) conducted in Hong Kong found that 43.7% of participants reported high pandemic fatigue, with significant variations across demographic groups. Younger adults (18–24) showed higher levels of pandemic fatigue compared to older adults (55+ years), with those aged 65+ being 67% less likely to report high fatigue. This age-related pattern suggests that mental models for processing prolonged crisis may vary both across and within cultures, with older individuals potentially drawing on different temporal frameworks shaped by previous life experiences (Leung et al., 2022). The study further identified critical temporal thresholds when pandemic fatigue intensified: around 4–6 months into the pandemic for younger adults, 8–10 months for middle-aged adults, and much later (12+ months) or not at all for older adults—revealing how age influences the timeline of adaptation to prolonged crisis (Leung et al., 2022).

Best et al. (2023) further explored these age-related differences in their 29-wave longitudinal study covering 16 months of the pandemic. They found that while younger adults consistently experienced greater psychological distress throughout the pandemic, these age-related differences narrowed over time—highlighting stable but temporally modulated age effects. Their study revealed that the gap between younger and older adults' distress levels decreased in later phases, though younger adults maintained consistently higher levels of distress throughout the entire period.

Mental Models of Adaptation and Normalcy

As the pandemic stretched on, people's mental models of "normal life" underwent a significant transformation. The phenomenon of "behavioral drift" reveals how mental frameworks gradually adjust to incorporate new realities while attempting to maintain existing models of normal social function. This manifests through cognitive dissonance—the psychological tension that emerged between understanding the pandemic's severity and the desire to return to normalcy—prompting people to justify selective compliance with public health measures as an adaptive strategy (Festinger, 1957; Harmon-Jones & Mills, 2019). These justifications represent deeper attempts to reconcile conflicting models of reality (Michie et al., 2020; Tang et al., 2021). Simultaneously, risk recalibration occurred as the pandemic unfolded, with people developing evolving mental models to gauge threat levels, creating new frameworks to decide which activities felt "safe enough" or "worth the risk." This recalibration reflected fundamental shifts in how people conceptualized and processed risk itself (Gassen et al., 2022; Kim et al., 2023).

A large-scale longitudinal study by Giuntella et al. (2021) quantified these adaptive changes, tracking university students before and during the pandemic. The research found dramatic behavioral shifts as mental models adapted: average daily steps declined from approximately 10,000 to 4,600, sleep increased by 25–30 minutes per night, social time declined by over half to less than 30 minutes daily, while screen time more than doubled to over 5 hours per day. These behavioral adaptations occurred alongside significant mental health impacts as well, with depression rates increasing by up to 90% compared to pre-pandemic levels (Giuntella et al., 2021; Luong et al., 2024). This data revealed how fundamentally mental models of "normalcy" had to shift to accommodate a prolonged crisis reality.

Significant to the temporal dimension, Giuntella et al. (2021) also documented that these behavioral adaptations followed distinct temporal patterns. Initial abrupt changes (0–6 weeks) were followed by periods of partial rebound (7–16 weeks) and finally stabilization at a "new normal" that remained significantly different from pre-pandemic patterns even 10–12 months into the pandemic. This temporal trajectory of behavioral adaptation demonstrates how mental models gradually recalibrate over time in response to extended crisis (Giuntella et al., 2021).

Temporal Disorientation and Uncertainty

The pandemic created profound temporal disorientation that shaped behavioral responses over time. Velasco et al. (2022) identified six distinct forms of temporal disorientation during COVID-19: temporal rift (disconnection from normal time), temporal vertigo (loss of temporal stability), impoverished time (reduced temporal variation), tunnel vision (narrow temporal focus), weakened social scaffolding of time, and suspended time (the feeling that normal time has stopped). This multifaceted disorientation fundamentally shaped how people processed the ongoing crisis. Their research distinguishes between "episodic" disorientation (temporary confusion) and "existential" disorientation (fundamental disruption of temporal frameworks), with COVID-19 producing the more profound existential form they termed "suspended time"—a state where normal temporal progression feels halted despite chronological time continuing (Velasco et al., 2022).

This temporal disorientation directly influenced decision-making processes. Wu et al. (2022) demonstrated through a series of experiments that pandemic-induced uncertainty significantly altered intertemporal choice—the trade-offs people make between present and future benefits. Their research showed that participants experiencing greater uncertainty related to COVID-19 displayed stronger preferences for smaller, immediate rewards over larger, delayed ones. Critically, they identified future orientation as the mediating factor, with pandemic uncertainty reducing people's ability to maintain future-oriented thinking. This empirical evidence helps explain why maintaining protective behaviors became increasingly difficult over time, as prolonged uncertainty eroded the future orientation necessary for compliance with preventative measures that involve immediate costs for future benefits (Wu et al., 2022, 2024).

Physiological manifestations of these temporal disruptions appeared as pandemic fatigue, a measurable phenomenon validated by the development of specific assessment tools (Rodríguez-Blázquez et al., 2022). This fatigue was more than just psychological, however, and manifested in physical symptoms that continued even after infection risk decreased, with research showing a 68% higher risk of fatigue-related illness post-COVID (Vu et al., 2024). The persistence of these symptoms illustrates how temporal disorientation impacts biological as well as psychological functioning.

Mental Models of Institutional Endurance and Trust

How different populations processed extended government interventions revealed underlying mental models about institutional authority. The sustainability of public health measures depended on how people's mental frameworks interpreted prolonged institutional guidance.

In countries where governments maintained transparent, empathetic communication, like New Zealand and Australia, this aligned with mental models that viewed institutional authority as a sustained partner in crisis response. This approach resonated with frameworks that positioned government communication as an ongoing dialogue rather than a series of directives (Wang et al., 2022c). Daly et al. (2022) documented that these positive mental models of institutional endurance exhibited distinct temporal advantages, maintaining public compliance for three to four months longer than in countries where institutional trust deteriorated rapidly.

Conversely, in regions where leadership was inconsistent or dismissive, this challenged mental models about institutional reliability during crisis. Brazil's experience demonstrated how conflicting messages disrupted fundamental frameworks for processing institutional guidance, leading many to develop alternative mental models for assessing risk and making decisions (Huynh, 2020). Research on public trust during the pandemic has shown that inconsistent messaging significantly impacted compliance with health measures, with trust deteriorating most rapidly during the first two to three months of conflicting guidance (Huang et al., 2023).

Institutional Construction and Modulation of Temporal Urgency

The effectiveness of institutional responses depended not only on trust but on how organizations communicated urgency over extended periods. Skade et al. (2025) examined this dynamic through their study of Germany's Robert Koch Institute (RKI), the central organization for disease control during the pandemic. Their research revealed how organizations actively construct and modulate temporal urgency during prolonged crises rather than simply responding to external timeframes. Through a process they call "modulating urgency," the RKI translated temporal cues of the crisis by strategically escalating, pausing, or modulating activities and communications to maintain appropriate levels of public response over an extended period.

This research identified multiple forms of urgency beyond the simple "act now" messaging common in acute emergencies. Organizations employed different temporal strategies at different pandemic phases for internal institutional coordination, focusing on how to effectively manage ongoing operations during extended crisis conditions. Importantly, Skade et al. (2025) found that effective crisis communication required adapting temporal messaging to match the evolving mental models of the population. When institutional temporal frames conflicted with public temporal experience, communication effectiveness declined sharply, highlighting how closely entwined institutional trust and shared temporal frameworks become during extended crises.

Daly et al. (2022) documented how mental health impacts evolved over time as mental models adapted to the crisis through their U.K. Household Longitudinal

Study. The prevalence of mental health problems increased by 13.5 percentage points from 24.3% pre-pandemic to 37.8% in April 2020, then showed evidence of adjustment as the rate declined to 31.9% by June 2020 (Daly et al., 2022). This pattern of initial deterioration followed by partial recovery demonstrates how mental models for processing institutional responses evolved over time, with different population subgroups showing varying trajectories of adaptation.

Building on this, Pierce et al. (2021) identified five distinct temporal trajectories of mental health response during the pandemic using latent class analysis: resilient (58.4% of participants), showing minimal mental health disruption throughout; improving (2.0%), showing initial distress but rapid recovery; deteriorating (7.0%), showing progressive worsening; fluctuating (8.2%), showing oscillating patterns mirroring lockdown phases; and consistently poor (12.3%), showing sustained distress. These trajectories illustrate how temporal mental models influence crisis adaptation at the individual level, with clear temporal thresholds of change occurring at predictable intervals (Pierce et al., 2021).

Interactive Mental Models in Long-Term Crisis Response

These various mental models interacted to create comprehensive frameworks for processing prolonged crises. Models of crisis duration interacted with models of institutional trust, frameworks for personal endurance influenced models of collective responsibility, and mental models of risk adaptation shaped frameworks for social interaction. For example, when individuals justified gathering with friends despite outbreaks of high case numbers, they were operating through multiple, interconnected mental models: processing the crisis timeline through frameworks of "new normal," understanding risk through evolved models of threat assessment, and balancing social needs through frameworks of acceptable risk (Du et al., 2022; Gassen et al., 2022).

Kim et al. (2023) documented these interaction effects through a longitudinal study that followed participants through the pandemic in Hong Kong, a city with previous pandemic experience. The research found significant temporal variations in behavioral and mental health responses, with patterns of adherence to protective measures changing over time. The study found behavioral "fatigue" in social distancing increased over time even as mask wearing remained high, showing how interconnected mental models created distinct trajectories during different phases of the pandemic (Kim et al., 2023).

The interactive nature of these mental models is further illustrated in research on long-term crisis processing, which suggests a temporal progression in how people adapt to extended crises. This progression typically involves several phases: an initial acute response characterized by high compliance but mounting stress; followed by a period of adaptation and recalibration when new mental frameworks develop to accommodate ongoing stressors; then a phase of integration and resolution when adapted mental models stabilize; and finally a long-term assimilation when transformed risk perceptions are fully incorporated into everyday mental models. This temporal progression reflects not just linear change, but complex interactions between personal, social, and institutional mental frameworks throughout the crisis lifecycle (Schäfer et al., 2020, 2022).

Kim et al. (2023) conducted a longitudinal study tracking mental and behavioral responses across five waves during the pandemic, finding that mental stress declined over time in correlation with actual risk of infection. However, even at the final observation point, when outbreak numbers had dropped significantly, 58.8% of respondents still reported high stress levels—considerably higher than pre-pandemic baselines of 44.5%. This pattern illustrates how mental models for processing prolonged crisis evolve and maintain alterations even when objective conditions improve (Kim et al., 2023).

Importantly, research by Daly and Robinson (2021) documented temporal patterns in psychological adaptation during the pandemic. Their study of U.S. adults showed that after around eight to ten weeks of pandemic exposure, psychological distress began declining on average, suggesting a predictable temporal adaptation pattern in mental models of crisis. This adaptation pattern was observed across age groups and demographic factors, though the timeline varied, with younger adults taking two to four weeks longer to exhibit psychological adaptation than older adults. The study also found that across the full course of the pandemic, these adaptation patterns were influenced by multiple factors, though certain consistent trajectories emerged regardless of varying environmental conditions (Daly & Robinson, 2021).

From Crisis Temporality to Adaptive Models

The pandemic revealed that our capacity to sustain emergency responses stems from fundamental mental models about crisis duration and human adaptation. These frameworks—whether processing extended emergencies as collective or individual challenges, viewing institutional guidance as dialogue or imposition, understanding adaptation as compromise or failure—shaped how populations navigated the prolonged crisis.

Building resilience for future extended crises requires understanding how people fundamentally think about and process prolonged emergency situations. This means engaging with temporal mental models rather than simply addressing visible fatigue. It also means recognizing how different populations fundamentally conceptualize extended crisis situations. Resistance to prolonged measures often stems from an asymmetry in established mental models rather than exhaustion itself. Effective long-term crisis response must work within or carefully evolve existing frameworks for emergency duration and adaptation.

By addressing these deeper frameworks, we can better prepare populations for the psychological demands of sustained emergency response while fostering more resilient approaches to prolonged crisis management (Masten & Motti-Stefanidi, 2020; World Health Organization (WHO), Regional Office for Europe, 2020). Significantly, research on resilience trajectories by Schäfer et al. (2020) suggests that mental adaptability to extended crisis follows predictable temporal patterns that can be anticipated and supported through targeted interventions aligned with each phase of crisis response. Understanding these temporal thresholds—when public compliance naturally wanes, when mental health impacts begin to stabilize, when new risk frameworks become established—allows for more effective crisis communication and support strategies that acknowledge the natural evolution of temporal mental models rather than fighting against them.

Understanding how people adapted to the prolonged timeline of the COVID-19 crisis provides critical insight into behavioral fatigue and compliance trajectories. But temporality alone cannot fully explain the complexity of human responses. Equally important were the emotional forces—particularly fear and uncertainty—that shaped how individuals processed information and navigated evolving risks. As we turn to the next section, we examine how these emotional dimensions activated distinct mental models of threat, trust, and meaning-making, profoundly influencing both individual and societal outcomes.

Fear and Uncertainty: Mental Models of Threat and Information

The psychological toll of the COVID-19 pandemic was immense, with fear and uncertainty playing central roles in shaping public responses. According to the WHO, global rates of anxiety and depression increased by roughly one-quarter during 2020. As the SARS-CoV-2 virus spread, emotions like fear influenced behaviors in both positive and negative ways. On one hand, fear motivated many people to comply with health measures (e.g., mask-wearing, hygiene practices) as a protective response; on the other hand, excessive or mismanaged fear led some to panic, freeze into inaction, or even react defiantly against public health advice. In societies where trust in institutions was strong, fear could be channeled constructively through psychological frameworks that helped individuals process uncertainty. However, in contexts where this foundation was weaker, the emotional burden of the pandemic often gave rise to distinctive patterns of information-processing that undermined effective response. Studies consistently find that high institutional trust generally correlates with acceptance of scientific guidance and higher compliance, whereas low trust—often polarized along political lines—is associated with lower compliance and poorer health outcomes.

The Multidimensional Impact of Fear

COVID-19 triggered widespread fear: fear of infection, fear of death, and fear of the unknown. Unlike some previous disease outbreaks, this pandemic created a prolonged state of uncertainty operating across multiple interconnected levels. This multilayered experience of fear stretched beyond individual psychology to reshape community dynamics and institutional responses (Van Bavel et al., 2020). At the individual level, fear often manifests in heightened stress, disrupted sleep patterns, and persistent anxiety about potential exposure (Luong et al., 2024; Santomauro et al., 2021; Taylor et al., 2020; Trabelsi et al., 2021; WHO, 2022b).

Many people developed new routines and even ritualistic behaviors to regain a sense of control over their environment—constant disinfecting of surfaces, compulsive news-checking, and elaborate personal protection rituals became common coping mechanisms (Taylor et al., 2020).

These individual experiences were amplified by collective fear dynamics. Social media and 24/7 news coverage created feedback loops of anxiety, as people were bombarded with alarming information in real time. Communities grappled with hyper-vigilance and sometimes stigmatization of those perceived as high-risk or non-compliant. Fear-based stigma became a concern: for example, unfounded assumptions about contagion risk led to people avoiding or ostracizing healthcare workers, COVID-19 survivors, and others (Earnshaw, 2020). Such stigma is a well-recognized consequence of pandemic fear and can undermine social cohesion and effective response (WHO, Regional Office for Europe, 2020; WHO, UNICEF, & IFRC, 2020).

The effectiveness of institutional responses in managing public fear largely depended on credibility and communication. Institutions that maintained clear, consistent messaging while openly acknowledging uncertainty tended to preserve public trust most effectively (Hatton et al., 2022; Kreps & Kriner, 2020). Regular updates based on emerging evidence—combined with accessible mental health support and community engagement—helped populations cope with ongoing stress (Harper et al., 2021; Van Bavel et al., 2020). Conversely, authorities that issued contradictory guidance or allowed health measures to become politicized often saw an erosion of trust and increased psychological distress. Research by Hatton et al. (2022) found deep partisan divides in the United States: when official guidance changed or became entangled in political controversy, confidence in public health agencies declined sharply, with trust in institutions like the CDC splitting along entrenched party lines. This loss of trust had tangible effects, as segments of the public became less willing to follow health recommendations, compounding the pandemic's impact (Hatton et al., 2022; Kreps & Kriner, 2020).

Research published during the pandemic also highlighted how an intolerance of uncertainty can exacerbate fear in an information-rich environment. In one study, individuals with high intolerance of uncertainty experienced significantly more fear when compulsively searching for COVID-19 information online, compared to those more comfortable with ambiguity (Baerg & Bruchmann, 2022). This "information overload" effect created a vicious cycle: those most disturbed by uncertainty tended to seek more information in an attempt to quell their fears, but excessive media consumption often increased rather than decreased their anxiety (McLaughlin et al., 2023). For people high in uncertainty-intolerance, each additional hour spent reading pandemic news was linked to a measurable uptick in anxiety (Baerg & Bruchmann, 2022). In other words, the people least equipped to handle uncertainty were paradoxically the most likely to overdose on information, heightening their fear. This phenomenon, sometimes dubbed "doomscrolling," became a common maladaptive response during COVID-19 (McLaughlin et al., 2023).

Mental Models of Information Processing During Crisis

Beyond these general trends, individuals differed markedly in how they interpreted pandemic information and uncertainty. Drawing from psychology, communication, and behavioral science research, we unpack five primary mental models of information-processing that emerged as lenses through which people navigated the crisis. These models are supported by converging evidence across multiple studies and literature in Table 11.7 (Agley & Xiao, 2021; Allington et al., 2021; Bridgman et al., 2020; Cinelli et al., 2020; Festinger, 1957; Fletcher et al., 2020; Freeman et al., 2022; Golman et al., 2017; Hatton et al., 2022; Hornik et al., 2021; Imhoff & Lamberty, 2020; Kreps & Kriner, 2020; Kunda, 1990; Mace, 2020; Mills & St. Clair, 2023; Nichols, 2024; Nielsen et al., 2020; Pagliaro et al., 2021; Pennycook et al., 2020; Romer & Jamieson, 2020; Van Bavel et al., 2020).

The "Scientific Consensus" model positioned peer-reviewed research and expert consensus as the primary validators of truth, viewing scientific uncertainty as a normal, expected part of the evolution of knowledge. In contrast, the "Personal Experience" framework privileged direct observation and trusted social networks over institutional expertise—adherents of this model often interpreted evolving official guidance as evidence of incompetence or inconsistency rather than as adaptive learning. The "Conspiracy Belief" model rejected official narratives entirely, embracing alternative explanations that attribute nefarious or malicious intent to authorities (Allington et al., 2021; Romer & Jamieson, 2020). The "Information Avoidance" approach manifested as deliberate disengagement from pandemic news to reduce stress, resulting in minimal awareness and inconsistent protective behaviors (Fletcher et al., 2020). Finally, the "Social Media–Dependent" model reflected a heavy reliance on algorithm-driven online information (e.g., Facebook or YouTube) and peer sharing; this often led to emotionally charged, polarized viewpoints and increased exposure to misinformation (Adebesin et al., 2023; Allington et al., 2021; Cascini et al. 2022; Ferreira Caceres et al., 2022; Kim et al., 2022; Rodrigues et al., 2024; Skafle et al., 2022).

These mental models are not merely academic constructs, but powerful determinants of behavior. Studies demonstrated that individuals operating within different interpretive frameworks could encounter the same facts yet reach dramatically different conclusions about appropriate actions or attribution to basic foundations of reality (Imhoff & Lamberty, 2020). This helps explain why seemingly straightforward public health recommendations often produce wildly divergent behavioral responses and beliefs among the public.

The psychological foundations of these mental models were often established long before the pandemic. Pre-existing trust in institutions served as a critical mediating factor: higher institutional trust correlated strongly with acceptance of the "Scientific Consensus" approach, whereas low trust predisposed individuals to adopt the "Personal Experience" or conspiracy-driven models (Hatton et al., 2022). Surveys in Western countries during 2020–2021 indicated that roughly half or more of the public maintained strong trust in scientific authorities and adherence to official guidance, with approximately 72% of U.K. respondents classified

Table 11.7 Information Processing Models During Public Health Emergencies

Framework/Model	*Core Processing Pattern*	*Emotional Response*	*Behavioral Outcome*	*Estimated Prevalence*
Scientific Consensus	Evaluates claims against established evidence; sees uncertainty as normal in science	Managed anxiety; cautious but rational concern	Follows public health guidance; takes appropriate precautions	46–51% in Western populations
Personal Experience	Trusts direct observation and close social circles over government/public institutions	Anxiety varies with context	Selective compliance based on perceived risk	24% of general population
Conspiracy Belief	Interprets events through a lens of hidden agendas, nefarious motivations, and manipulation	Heightened fear, distrust	Rejects official guidance; embraces false or "alternative" narratives	20–40% depending on region
Information Avoidance	Avoids news and information to reduce stress	Reduced short-term anxiety; long-term confusion	Inconsistent engagement; minimal protective action	22% regularly avoided COVID news
Social Media—Dependent	Relies on algorithm-curated online info (e.g., Facebook, X/Twitter)	Emotionally reactive; echo chamber exposure	Heavily influenced by peers; often misinformed or polarized	53% misinformation traced to Facebook alone

Sources: This original framework synthesizes patterns observed across multiple research sources, including studies from Pew Research Center, Nature Human Behaviour, Reuters Institute, YouGov-Cambridge Globalism Project, and Center for Countering Digital Hate (2020–2021).

as psychologically resilient and accepting of expert advice in mid-2020. Research by Pagliaro et al. (2021) showed that trust levels strongly predicted compliance with both prescribed and discretionary COVID-19 preventive behaviors across 23 countries.

Longitudinal research tracking information-processing patterns found that these mental frameworks remained remarkably stable throughout the pandemic, suggesting they reflected deeper cognitive mindsets rather than momentary reactions to news. By 2022–2023, polarization was so extreme in some societies that nearly 70% of likely right-leaning voters in the United States said they trust "the common sense of ordinary people" over "the knowledge of trained experts" on COVID, compared to 72% of left-leaning voters who believed public health officials had done a good job (Mills & St. Clair, 2023; Nichols, 2024).

The Role of Conspiracy Theories in Shaping Mental Models

During the pandemic, conspiracy theories—problematic for unified public health messaging—nevertheless served important psychological functions amid extreme uncertainty and threat. Psychological research shows that conspiratorial thinking can fulfill basic cognitive and emotional needs. By recasting ambiguous dangers into narratives with clear villains and plots, conspiracy beliefs offer people a sense of understanding, control, and meaning when the world feels chaotic (Douglas et al., 2017). Indeed, crises tend to fuel conspiracy thinking: such theories reliably surge during societal upheavals as individuals grasp for patterns and explanations in the face of fear. Embracing a COVID-19 conspiracy often became a coping mechanism to regain clarity and agency amid chaos, rather than a simple act of ignorance.

Research indicates that endorsing conspiracy theories can temporarily alleviate anxiety by providing an illusion of certainty or someone to blame (Douglas, 2021). For example, people who feel powerless or anxious are more drawn to conspiratorial narratives as a way to make sense of events and restore a feeling of security and a sense of "knowing." In this way, conspiracy beliefs can yield a kind of emotional "reward," similar to superstitious or religious beliefs, by delivering comfort through sense-making and clear causation (Cardi et al., 2021).

Unsurprisingly, the appeal of COVID-19 conspiracy frameworks cut across demographics and political lines, revealing near-universal psychological vulnerabilities. Faced with an overwhelming and existential threat, many minds instinctively sought patterns and agents to blame—even at the expense of factual accuracy. Global surveys found that 20–40% of people in many countries endorsed some form of COVID-19 conspiracy at the pandemic's height (Henley & McIntyre, 2020). For instance, the October 2020 YouGov-Cambridge Globalism Project (25 countries, ~26,000 people) found that 38% of Americans, 30% of Italians, and 28% of Germans believed the deadliness of COVID-19 was being exaggerated—with over 40% in countries like South Africa, Poland, and Greece sharing that belief. Similarly, nearly 60% of respondents in Nigeria agreed that the pandemic's dangers were grossly overstated (Henley & McIntyre, 2020). Such findings reveal that a substantial minority worldwide embraced "alternative" narratives (e.g., that the virus was a hoax or deliberate bioweapon) during peak uncertainty.

Cognitive scientists note that conspiracy narratives often exploit pattern-seeking tendencies: people who more readily perceive meaningful patterns in randomness are more susceptible to both conspiracy and supernatural beliefs. In neural terms, repeatedly finding "hidden truth" in conspiracies may even engage reward pathways tied to the satisfaction of solving puzzles or confirming biases – reinforcing the behavior.

An intriguing phenomenon was the prevalence of "mixed mental models," where individuals simultaneously held contradictory beliefs about the pandemic. Agley and Xiao (2021), using latent profile analysis in their *BMC Public Health* study, identified sizable segments of the public who simultaneously accepted both scientific explanations and certain conspiracy claims. Their U.S. survey revealed that while 70% of respondents belonged to a profile rejecting misinformation and endorsing scientific consensus (e.g., that COVID-19 has a natural origin), the remaining 30% showed blended belief profiles—they did not wholly reject mainstream views but simultaneously believed in one or more misinformation narratives. In other words, believing the "official" story did not preclude many from also believing conspiratorial narratives. For example, a person might diligently follow health guidelines like masking and handwashing while subscribing to theories about a "plandemic" or lab-created bioweapon virus. Such compartmentalization suggests these frameworks operate less like rigid ideologies and more like flexible psychological toolkits deployed to manage stress and uncertainty.

Crucially, this understanding helps explain why traditional fact-checking or debunking often proved frustratingly ineffective against certain false beliefs. When a conspiracy framework is serving a psychological need—quelling anxiety or affirming one's world-view—simply providing corrective facts seldom succeeds. Studies have found that once conspiracy beliefs take hold, direct counter-arguments or fact-checks rarely change the believer's mind in meaningful ways (O'Mahony et al., 2023). A systematic review of interventions concluded that "traditional fact-checking and counterarguments are the least effective means of combating conspiracy beliefs," especially if applied after the person is already exposed to the conspiracy claim. In contrast, approaches that preemptively inoculate people (for example, by fostering critical thinking habits or forewarning about common misinformation tactics) show more promise (Basol et al., 2020; O'Mahony et al., 2023). This implies that unless the underlying anxieties and needs driving conspiracy adoption are addressed, pure information correction is unlikely to penetrate.

In practice, effective debunking during COVID-19 often had to pair myth-busting with empathy and psychological support. For instance, communicators found more success when they not only disproved a false claim, but also acknowledged the audience's fears and offered an alternative source of meaning or control (e.g., emphasizing constructive actions people could take). Recent research by Costello et al. (2024) has shown that artificial intelligence (AI)–based dialogue approaches that focus on empathetic reasoning can effectively reduce conspiracy beliefs over time, offering a promising new intervention method. Their study in *Science* used the large language model GPT-4 Turbo to engage participants in personalized, multi-round conversations about their conspiracy beliefs. This AI–driven approach reduced belief in these theories by 20% on average. Remarkably, this reduction persisted undiminished for at least two months after the intervention, with no evidence of decay in effectiveness over this period. The study found consistent results across a wide range of conspiracy theories, from classic conspiracies to those related to COVID-19 and recent political events, even affecting deeply entrenched beliefs. Such findings challenge the notion that conspiracy believers are inherently resistant to evidence-based persuasion.

By late 2021, the real public-health consequences of these conspiracy-driven mental models were evident: surges in vaccine hesitancy, organized anti-lockdown protests, and even violence against 5G infrastructure. Research documented how a small core of online misinformation "superspreaders" —dubbed the "Disinformation Dozen"—produced up to 65% of anti-vaccine content on major social media platforms, greatly amplifying conspiracy-fueled fears (Center for Countering Digital Hate, 2021; see also Coaston, 2020; Romano, 2020; Rogers de Waal, 2020). In sum, conspiracy theories during COVID-19 were more than just fringe ideas; they actively shaped many individuals' mental models of the crisis, with significant implications for behavior and policy compliance. They offered psychological solace and narrative simplicity, but at the cost of undermining consensus and fracturing the public response.

Fear-Based Messaging: The Psychology of Threat Response

The COVID-19 crisis provided unique insights into how threat-related emotions influence decision-making under prolonged uncertainty. Public health authorities had to strike a delicate balance in leveraging fear as a motivator without inducing despair or burnout. From an evolutionary perspective, the human threat response system evolved to handle immediate, acute dangers (e.g., a predator) more so than diffuse, long-term threats like a multi-year pandemic. Research in health psychology shows that fear appeals can be effective motivators only under specific conditions —essentially, when people perceive a threat as severe but also actionable, when clear protective actions are known, and when individuals feel a sense of personal efficacy in carrying them out (Tannenbaum et al., 2015). If those conditions are met, moderate fear can galvanize preventive behavior; if not—for example, if the danger seems hopeless or instructions confusing—fear can backfire, leading to paralysis or avoidance.

During COVID-19, these parameters varied dramatically across populations and over time, yielding very different psychological responses to the same risk messages. In early 2020, images of overflowing hospitals and exponential death curves created a high perceived severity, and officials issued simple, efficacy-based instructions ("Wear a mask; stay home to save lives"). In many places, this combination successfully spurred the public to take precautions. A meta-analysis of 127 studies confirms that fear-based messages paired with efficacy information significantly improve adherence to health guidance, compared to either element alone (Tannenbaum et al., 2015). Messages that instilled appropriate concern about COVID while also empowering people with concrete steps (handwashing, distancing, etc.) generally led to greater compliance with those behaviors (Pagliaro et al., 2021). By contrast, where official messages either downplayed the threat or overwhelmed people with dread without solutions, many individuals reacted with denial, fatalism, or tuning out the information.

Individual differences in tolerance for uncertainty emerged as a critical factor shaping pandemic responses. An intolerance of uncertainty—a dispositional inability to handle the unknown – was associated with higher anxiety and, often, information avoidance during COVID-19. In one U.K. survey, 22% of respondents said they "often or always" actively tried to avoid COVID-19 news in spring 2020, and nearly 60% admitted to at least sometimes avoiding pandemic news (Fletcher et al., 2020). This spike in news avoidance was linked largely to people's worries about the impact of constant bad news on their mental health. Those with lower tolerance for uncertainty and higher baseline anxiety were more prone to cope by tuning out—even though doing so left them less informed about safety guidance. By contrast, people more comfortable with uncertainty or ambiguity tended to adapt more calmly to evolving guidelines and shifting risk estimates (Baerg & Bruchmann, 2022; Brenning et al., 2023). For example, longitudinal studies found that individuals high in cognitive flexibility (ability to adjust thinking in the face of change) maintained steadier adherence to precautions despite the whiplash of changing rules (Bennett et al., 2023; Lo Coco et al., 2023). This suggests that beyond the content of the message, the audience's mindset—anxious or resilient, avoidant or analytical—influenced whether fear-based messaging led to constructive action or disengagement (Cardi et al., 2021; Seaborn et al., 2022).

When heightened fear was sustained for long periods without relief, distinct psychological patterns emerged. Initial vigilance and alarm in early 2020 often gave way, after months of stress, to a phenomenon psychologists label "threat habituation" (Taylor et al., 2020; Veronese et al., 2023). This is the natural process by which constant exposure to a threat stimulus gradually dampens the emotional response, even if the objective danger remains. Essentially, people get used to living with a risk. By mid-2020 and especially into 2021, many individuals reported feeling numb or "worn out" by COVID warnings that once provoked fear (Fancourt et al., 2021; McLaughlin et al., 2023). This habituation likely contributed to the declining adherence to safety measures observed in later pandemic phases—not necessarily outright denial of COVID's reality, but a predictable psychological fatigue with maintaining high alert (WHO, Regional Office for Europe, 2020).

As previously discussed in Section 2.5.4 about temporal mental models, the WHO formally recognized this as "pandemic fatigue" in late 2020, defining it as a gradual demotivation to follow recommended protective behaviors, brought on by persistent stress and burnout (WHO, Regional Office for Europe, 2020). Surveys across Europe at that time found sizable portions of the public were less vigilant than earlier, not because they believed the threat was gone, but because they were emotionally exhausted (WHO, Regional Office for Europe, 2020). In practical terms, policies like lockdowns and mask mandates that were largely accepted in spring 2020 met more resistance by late 2020–2021, as people's capacity to tolerate disruption dwindled. Public health officials noted this fatigue in explaining why a "second wave" of cases often wasn't met with the same level of collective urgency as the first.

The most effective public health messaging acknowledged and adapted to these psychological dynamics over time. Early in the pandemic, strong fear-based communications (e.g., dire warnings from leaders and media showing overflowing ICUs) successfully grabbed attention and galvanized protective behaviors by emphasizing the severe consequences of unchecked spread. However, as the crisis wore on, a shift in tone became necessary for maintaining compliance. By late 2020, many health campaigns transitioned toward more sustainable motivational frameworks—highlighting efficacy, collective responsibility, hope, and progress—rather than relying on constant fear appeals. For example, messaging in 2021 tended to stress how individual actions were making a difference ("Your masking and distancing saved X lives") and promoted positive community norms ("Most people in your town are doing the right thing"). This strategy tapped into empowerment and solidarity rather than fear.

Research on risk communication finds that messages combining realistic acknowledgment of ongoing risk with hope and efficacy can sustain engagement far better than apocalyptic warnings alone (Tannenbaum et al., 2015). Accordingly, many COVID campaigns began featuring stories of recovery, resilience, or vaccine success to balance the grim statistics. Such approaches were intended to replenish the public's emotional energy and trust: reminding people that their sacrifices were yielding results and that there was light at the end of the tunnel. In contrast, messaging that tried to keep the public in a prolonged state of high fear eventually lost impact or even backfired—breeding cynicism, hopelessness, and greater defiance of guidelines (O'Mahony et al., 2023).

In sum, the psychology of threat response during COVID-19 emphasizes a classic principle of health communication: fear can spur action, but only if coupled with efficacy and only for so long. Overuse of fear risks numbness and backlash, whereas a calibrated approach that evolves with the audience's emotional state is crucial for long-term crises.

Building Mental Resilience Through Literacy

A key lesson from COVID-19 is that effective crisis management requires not just robust healthcare systems and information channels, but also psychologically literate populations. In other words, communities need cognitive and emotional tools to process complex, evolving information under uncertainty. Psychological resilience within the populace became as important as medical resources in determining pandemic outcomes.

The pandemic illustrated how profoundly our mental frameworks influence our ability to navigate complex threats. Across diverse populations, certain psychological factors—such as tolerance for uncertainty, cognitive flexibility, critical thinking ability, and emotional regulation skills—proved more predictive of adaptive responses than many demographic variables like age or income (Lo Coco et al., 2023; Pagliaro et al., 2021). For example, a cross-national study found that people's trust in science and willingness to accept new evidence predicted compliance with COVID precautions more strongly than their gender or education level (Pagliaro et al., 2021). Similarly, longitudinal data from Italy (nearly 4,000 adults) identified clear mental health trajectories during 2020–2021: about 54% of individuals demonstrated a resilient trajectory—maintaining stable or even improved mental well-being through the crisis—while the remaining subgroups showed more vulnerable trajectories with rising depression, anxiety, and stress over time (Lo Coco et al., 2023).

Notably, these resilience vs. distress outcomes correlated less with socio-economic status than with psychological habits and coping styles. Statistical modeling in the Italian study pinpointed certain cognitive-emotional patterns as risk factors for poor adaptation: namely, high expressive suppression (tendency to bottle up emotions) and high intolerance of uncertainty were strongly associated with the vulnerable mental health trajectories (Lo Coco et al., 2023). Individuals who chronically avoided confronting uncertain situations or suppressed their fears were more likely to spiral into distress as the pandemic wore on.

Conversely, one mental skill consistently emerged as a powerful protective factor: cognitive reappraisal, the ability to reframe a threatening situation in a more positive or neutral light. This concept, while implicitly present throughout much of the resilience literature but not always labeled consistently, refers to the cognitive process of deliberately changing how one interprets an emotional stimulus. People who habitually used cognitive reappraisal to regulate their emotions showed significantly greater resilience and less anxiety during COVID-19, as documented in both cross-sectional and longitudinal studies (Brenning et al., 2023; Cardi et al., 2021). In the Italian four-wave panel, those with higher self-reported use of cognitive reappraisal were substantially less likely to fall into the "chronically distressed" classes, even after controlling for other variables (Lo Coco et al., 2023). Likewise, an independent study in the United Kingdom found that greater use of cognitive reappraisal was linked to higher feelings of hope, resourcefulness, and proactive coping during lockdown—essentially a buffer against pandemic stress (Bennett et al., 2023; Cardi et al., 2021).

Taken together, these findings suggest that psychological resilience in crises is not a fixed trait one simply has or lacks, but a set of skills and mindsets that can vary—and crucially, that can be developed. If certain mental habits predict who thrives versus who struggles in a global emergency, it follows that building population-wide psychological resilience should become a public health priority, on par with promoting physical health (Choukou et al., 2022; Kaye-Kauderer et al., 2021; Seaborn et al., 2022). Experts have called for educational and community interventions that cultivate the kinds of cognitive skills associated with better coping (Chen et al., 2025; Pasha et al., 2025). Promising approaches include programs to foster tolerance for ambiguity, cognitive flexibility, and emotion-regulation techniques in the general public. For instance, teaching people strategies to manage anxiety about the unknown—rather than defaulting to denial or conspiracy—could blunt the impact of future uncertainty.

Interventions that improve these skills have shown real benefits. A 2023 review of methods to counteract conspiracy beliefs found that a 3-month course on distinguishing scientific evidence from pseudoscience led to significant reductions in conspiratorial thinking (O'Mahony et al., 2023). Similarly, inoculation games and media literacy training have been shown to increase the public's resistance to misinformation by 20–30%, by exposing participants to weakened doses of fake news techniques (Basol et al., 2020; Roozenbeek et al., 2020). These examples point to the value of proactively enhancing the public's "mental toolkit."

In the context of public health, this could mean incorporating basic training in media literacy, risk assessment, and stress management into educational curricula or community workshops. Such training helps people interpret evolving scientific news more calmly and accurately, without resorting to panic or dismissal. Even brief exercises in analytical thinking—for example, prompting individuals to pause and consider evidence quality—have been shown to reduce susceptibility to false claims (Pennycook et al., 2020).

By enabling individuals to better self-regulate their information-processing and emotions, we make society more psychologically "fit" to handle a crisis. Building these mental frameworks requires going beyond simply providing factual information during emergencies. It calls for weaving insights from psychology into public communication and education. One important concept is cultivating metacognitive awareness—helping people recognize how their own thinking is influenced by emotions or biases. For example, a public campaign might encourage individuals to notice when fear or anger is driving them to share unverified rumors, and to take a moment to double-check facts. Teaching citizens about common biases (like confirmation bias, which leads us to believe information that confirms our pre-existing views) can empower them to approach sensational claims more critically. Likewise, disseminating knowledge about how misinformation spreads (for instance, the tactics used in doctored headlines or social media bots) can make the public less likely to be fooled (Bridgman et al., 2020; Cha et al., 2021; Mace, 2020).

Several countries have started initiatives along these lines, such as Finland's national curriculum on information literacy, which aims to vaccinate students against fake news. Additionally, promoting emotional resilience skills—like mindfulness techniques, healthy coping outlets, and community support networks—can improve collective mental endurance in a protracted crisis. The WHO has advocated for "psychosocial preparedness" as part of pandemic planning, emphasizing that mental health support and trust-building are as vital as logistical readiness (WHO, 2022a).

This emerging focus on the "psychology of uncertainty" represents a promising frontier in public health preparedness. By strengthening the mental and emotional toolkit of populations, we can transform how communities respond to complex threats in an increasingly uncertain world. Recent long-term studies from Pew Research Center (Tyson et al., 2025) show that five years after the pandemic, most

Americans believe COVID-19 drove the country apart rather than together, highlighting the critical importance of trust-building and psychological resilience for future crises. Additional Pew surveys (Kennedy & Tyson, 2023; Tyson & Kennedy 2024) have documented a continued decline in Americans' trust in scientists and science generally, with these divisions occurring predominantly along established political lines. This widening partisan gap in institutional trust highlights the continuing challenge of developing shared confidence in scientific expertise and evidence-based approaches to public health emergencies, both in the United States and globally.

In short, COVID-19 taught us that bolstering mental resilience and literacy may be as crucial to saving lives as vaccines, treatments, or ventilators. A population that can stay informed without succumbing to panic, that can adapt its behavior based on evidence, and that can resist the allure of false but comforting narratives—such a population is far better equipped to weather the next global emergency. Building that psychological resilience is a collective task: it means infusing our public discourse, education systems, and community practices with the understanding that how people think and cope in a crisis profoundly shapes what ultimately happens. If we take those lessons to heart, we can begin to inoculate society not just against viruses, but against the fear, confusion, and disinformation that accompany them.

In Part III, we will build on these insights as we examine current best practices for pandemic prevention, using the mental models framework developed here to inform more effective, practical, and sustainable approaches to future health emergencies.

References

Adebesin, F., Smuts, H., Mawela, T., Maramba, G., & Hattingh, M. (2023). The role of social media in health misinformation and disinformation during the COVID-19 pandemic: Bibliometric analysis. *JMIR Infodemiology, 3*, e48620. https://doi.org/10.2196/48620

Agley, J., & Xiao, Y. (2021). Misinformation about COVID-19: Evidence for differential latent profiles and a strong association with trust in science. *BMC Public Health, 21*(89), 1–12. https://doi.org/10.1186/s12889-020-10103-x

Agyapon-Ntra, K., & McSharry, P. E. (2023). A global analysis of the effectiveness of policy responses to COVID-19. *Scientific Reports, 13*, 5629. https://doi.org/10.1038/s41598-023-31709-2

Airhihenbuwa, C. O., Iwelunmor, J., Munodawafa, D., Ford, C. L., Oni, T., Agyemang, C., Mota, C., Ikuomola, O. B., Simbayi, L., Fallah, M. P., Qian, Z., Makinwa, B., Niang, C., & Okosun, I. (2020). Culture matters in communicating the global response to COVID-19. *Preventing Chronic Disease, 17*, E60. https://doi.org/10.5888/pcd17.200245

Algan, Y., Cohen, D., Davoine, E., Foucault, M., & Stantcheva, S. (2021). Trust in scientists in times of pandemic: Panel evidence from 12 countries. *Proceedings of the National Academy of Sciences, 118*(40), e2108576118. https://doi.org/10.1073/pnas.2108576118

Allington, D., Duffy, B., Wessely, S., Dhavan, N., & Rubin, J. (2021). Health-protective behaviour, social media usage and conspiracy belief during the COVID-19 public health emergency. *Psychological Medicine, 51*(10), 1763–1769. https://doi.org/10.1017/S003329172000224X

Atalay, A., & Solmazer, G. (2021). Cultural orientation and behavioral changes during the COVID-19 pandemic: A cross-country analysis. *Frontiers in Psychology, 12*, 578190. https://doi.org/10.3389/fpsyg.2021.578190

Baerg, L., & Bruchmann, K. (2022). COVID-19 information overload: Intolerance of uncertainty moderates the relationship between frequency of internet searching and fear of COVID-19. *Acta Psychologica, 224*, 103534. https://doi.org/10.1016/j.actpsy.2022.103534

Banerjee, R., Bhattacharya, J., & Majumdar, P. (2021). Exponential-growth prediction bias and compliance with safety measures related to COVID-19. *Social Science & Medicine, 268*, 113473. https://doi.org/10.1016/j.socscimed.2020.113473

Bargain, O., & Aminjonov, U. (2020). Trust and compliance to public health policies in times of COVID-19. *Journal of Public Economics, 192*, 104316. https://doi.org/10.1016/j.jpubeco.2020.104316

Basabe, N., & Ros, M. (2005). Cultural dimensions and social behavior correlates: Individualism-collectivism and power distance. *International Review of Social Psychology, 18*(1), 189–225.

Basol, M., Roozenbeek, J., & van der Linden, S. (2020). Good news about bad news: Gamified inoculation boosts confidence and cognitive immunity against fake news. *Journal of Cognition, 3*(1), 2. https://doi.org/10.5334/joc.91

Bazzi, S., Fiszbein, M., & Gebresilasse, M. (2021). "Rugged individualism" and collective (in)action during the COVID-19 pandemic. *Journal of Public Economics, 195*, 104357. https://doi.org/10.1016/j.jpubeco.2020.104357

Bennett, K. M., Panzeri, A., Derrer-Merk, E., Butter, S., Hartman, T. K., Mason, L., …, & Gibson-Miller, J. (2023). Predicting resilience during the COVID-19 pandemic in the United Kingdom: Cross-sectional and longitudinal results. *PLoS One, 18*(5), e0283254. https://doi.org/10.1371/journal.pone.0283254

Best, R., Strough, J., & Bruine de Bruin, W. (2023). Age differences in psychological distress during the COVID-19 pandemic: March 2020–June 2021. *Frontiers in Psychology, 14*, 1101353. https://doi.org/10.3389/fpsyg.2023.1101353

Betsch, C., Wieler, L. H., Bosnjak, M., Ramharter, M., Stollorz, V., Omer, S. B., Korn, L., Sprengholz, P., Felgendreff, L., Eitze, S., & Schmid, P. (2020a). *Germany COVID-19 Snapshot Monitoring (COSMO Germany): Monitoring knowledge, risk perceptions, preventive behaviours, and public trust in the current coronavirus outbreak in Germany*. PsychArchives. https://doi.org/10.23668/psycharchives.2776

Betsch, C., Wieler, L. H., & Habersaat, K., & COSMO Group. (2020b). Monitoring behavioural insights related to COVID-19. *The Lancet, 395*(10232), 1255–1256. https://doi.org/10.1016/S0140-6736(20)30729-7

Blum, D., Smith, S., & Sanford, A. (2020). Chapter 13: Toxic Wild West Syndrome: Individual rights vs. community needs. In D. Blum, S. Smith, & A. Sanford (Eds.), *COVID-19 in the global south: Impacts and responses*. Routledge. https://doi.org/10.4324/9781003142065-13

Brauner, J. M., Mindermann, S., Sharma, M., Johnston, D., Salvatier, J., Gavenčiak, T., …, & Teh, Y. W. (2021). Inferring the effectiveness of government interventions against COVID-19. *Science, 371*(6531), eabd9338. https://doi.org/10.1126/science.abd9338

Brenning, K., Waterschoot, J., Dieleman, L., Morbée, S., Vermote, B., Soenens, B., Van der Kaap-Deeder, J., van den Bogaard, D., & Vansteenkiste, M. (2023). The role of emotion regulation in mental health during the COVID-19 outbreak: A 10-wave longitudinal study. *Stress and Health: Journal of the International Society for the Investigation of Stress, 39*(3), 562–575. https://doi.org/10.1002/smi.3204

Bridgman, A., Merkley, E., Loewen, P. J., Owen, T., Ruths, D., Teichmann, L., & Zhilin, O. (2020). The causes and consequences of COVID-19 misperceptions: Understanding the role of news and social media. *Harvard Kennedy School (HKS) Misinformation Review*. https://doi.org/10.37016/mr-2020-028

Brusselaers, N., Steadson, D., Bjorklund, K., Breland, S., Stilhoff Sörensen, J., Ewing, A., Bergmann, S., & Steineck, G. (2022). Evaluation of science advice during the COVID-19 pandemic in Sweden. *Humanities and Social Sciences Communications*, *9*, 91. https://doi.org/10.1057/s41599-022-01097-5

Calgua, E. (2022). COVID-19: Data collection and transparency among countries. *COVID-19 Pandemic* (pp. 163–172). https://doi.org/10.1016/B978-0-323-82860-4.00020-3

Callaghan, T., Moghtaderi, A., Lueck, J. A., Hotez, P., Strych, U., Dor, A., Fowler, E. F., & Motta, M. (2021). Correlates and disparities of intention to vaccinate against COVID-19. *Social Science & Medicine* (1982), *272*, 113638. https://doi.org/10.1016/j.socscimed.2020.113638

Calvillo, D. P., Ross, B. J., Garcia, R. J., Smelter, T. J., & Rutchick, A. M. (2020). Political ideology predicts perceptions of the threat of COVID-19 (and susceptibility to fake news about it). *Social Psychological and Personality Science*, *11*(8), 1119–1128. https://doi.org/10.1177/1948550620940539

Capano, G. (2020). Policy design and state capacity in the COVID-19 emergency in Italy: If you are not prepared for the (un)expected, you can be only what you already are. *Policy and Society*, *39*(3), 326–344. https://doi.org/10.1080/14494035.2020.1783790

Cardi, V., Albano, G., Gentili, C., & Sudulich, L. (2021). The impact of emotion regulation and mental health difficulties on health behaviours during COVID-19. *Journal of Psychiatric Research*, *143*, 409–415. https://doi.org/10.1016/j.jpsychires.2021.10.001

Carrieri, V., Guthmuller, S., & Wübker, A. (2023). Trust and COVID-19 vaccine hesitancy. *Scientific Reports*, *13*(9245). https://doi.org/10.1038/s41598-023-35974-z

Cascini, F., Pantovic, A., Al-Ajlouni, Y. A., Failla, G., Puleo, V., Melnyk, A., Lontano, A., & Ricciardi, W. (2022). Social media and attitudes towards a COVID-19 vaccination: A systematic review of the literature. *eClinicalMedicine*, *48*, 101454. https://doi.org/10.1016/j.eclinm.2022.101454

Center for Countering Digital Hate. (2021, March 24). *The Disinformation Dozen: Why platforms must act on twelve leading online anti-vaxxers*. https://counterhate.com/research/the-disinformation-dozen/

Cha, M., Cha, C., Singh, K., Lima, G., Ahn, Y. Y., Kulshrestha, J., & Varol, O. (2021). Prevalence of misinformation and factchecks on the COVID-19 pandemic in 35 countries: Observational infodemiology study. *JMIR Human Factors*, *8*(1), e23279. https://doi.org/10.2196/23279

Chen, S., Cheung, M. W.-L., & Cheng, C. (2025). Flexibility in coping deployment and psychological adjustment during COVID-19: A three-level meta-analysis across 33 countries. *Social Science & Medicine*, *318*, 118229. https://doi.org/10.1016/j.socscimed.2025.118229

Choukou, M. A., Sanchez-Ramirez, D. C., Pol, M., Uddin, M., Monnin, C., & Syed-Abdul, S. (2022). COVID-19 infodemic and digital health literacy in vulnerable populations: A scoping review. *Digital Health*, *8*, 20552076221076927. https://doi.org/10.1177/20552076221076927

Choutagunta, A., Manish, G. P., & Rajagopalan, S. (2021). Battling COVID-19 with dysfunctional federalism: Lessons from India. *Southern Economic Journal*, *87*(4), 1267–1299. https://doi.org/10.1002/soej.12501

Cinelli, M., Quattrociocchi, W., Galeazzi, A., Valensise, C. M., Brugnoli, E., Schmidt, A. L., Zola, P., Zollo, F., & Scala, A. (2020). The COVID-19 social media infodemic. *Scientific Reports*, *10*(1), 16598. https://doi.org/10.1038/s41598-020-73510-5

Clark, E., Fredricks, K., Woc-Colburn, L., Bottazzi, M. E., & Weatherhead, J. (2020). Disproportionate impact of the COVID-19 pandemic on immigrant communities in the United States. *PLOS Neglected Tropical Diseases*, *14*(7), e0008484. https://doi.org/10.1371/journal.pntd.0008484

Coaston, J. (2020, April 13). *Why coronavirus conspiracy theories have spread so quickly*. *Vox*. https://www.vox.com/2020/4/13/21205833/coronavirus-pandemic-conspiracy-theories

Costello, T. H., Pennycook, G., & Rand, D. G. (2024). Durably reducing conspiracy beliefs through dialogues with AI. *Science*, *385*(6714), eadq1814. https://doi.org/10.1126/science.adq1814

Daly, M., & Robinson, E. (2021). Psychological distress and adaptation to the COVID-19 crisis in the United States. *Journal of Psychiatric Research*, *136*, 603–609. https://doi.org/10.1016/j.jpsychires.2020.10.035

Daly, M., Sutin, A. R., & Robinson, E. (2022). Longitudinal changes in mental health and the COVID-19 pandemic: Evidence from the UK Household Longitudinal Study. *Psychological Medicine*, *52*(13), 2549–2558. https://doi.org/10.1017/S0033291720004432

Demirtaş-Madran, H. A. (2021). Accepting restrictions and compliance with recommended preventive behaviors for COVID-19: A discussion based on the key approaches and current research on fear appeals. *Frontiers in Psychology*, *12*, 558437. https://doi.org/10.3389/fpsyg.2021.558437

Dolinski, D., Dolinska, B., Zmaczynska-Witek, B., Banach, M., & Kulesza, W. (2020). Unrealistic optimism in the time of coronavirus pandemic: May it help to kill, if so—Whom: Disease or the person? *Journal of Clinical Medicine*, *9*(5), 1464. https://doi.org/10.3390/jcm9051464

Douglas, K. M. (2021). Are conspiracy theories harmless? *Spanish Journal of Psychology*, *24*, Article e13. https://doi.org/10.1017/SJP.2021.10

Douglas, K. M., Sutton, R. M., & Cichocka, A. (2017). The psychology of conspiracy theories. *Current Directions in Psychological Science*, *26*(6), 538–542. https://doi.org/10.1177/0963721417718261

Du, Z., Wang, L., Shan, S., Lam, D., Tsang, T. K., Xiao, J., Gao, H., Yang, B., Ali, S. T., Pei, S., Fung, I. C. H., Lau, E. H. Y., Liao, Q., Wu, P., Meyers, L. A., Leung, G. M., & Cowling, B. J. (2022). Pandemic fatigue impedes mitigation of COVID-19 in Hong Kong. *Proceedings of the National Academy of Sciences*, *119*(48), e2213313119. https://doi.org/10.1073/pnas.2213313119

Earnshaw, V. A. (2020, April 6). Don't let fear of COVID-19 turn into stigma. *Harvard Business Review*. https://hbr.org/2020/04/dont-let-fear-of-covid-19-turn-into-stigma

Fancourt, D., Steptoe, A., & Bu, F. (2021). Trajectories of anxiety and depressive symptoms during enforced isolation due to COVID-19 in England: A longitudinal observational study. *The Lancet Psychiatry*, *8*(2), 141–149. https://doi.org/10.1016/S2215-0366(20)30482-X

Farhadi, A., & Lahooti, M. (2021). Are COVID-19 data reliable? A quantitative analysis of pandemic data from 182 countries. *COVID*, *1*(1), 137–152. https://doi.org/10.3390/covid1010013

Ferreira Caceres, M. M., Sosa, J. P., Lawrence, J. A., Sestacovschi, C., Tidd-Johnson, A., Rasool, M. H. U., Gadamidi, V. K., Ozair, S., Pandav, K., Cuevas-Lou, C., Parrish, M., Rodriguez, I., & Fernandez, J. P. (2022). The impact of misinformation on the COVID-19 pandemic. *AIMS Public Health*, *9*(2), 262–277. https://doi.org/10.3934/publichealth.2022018

Festinger, L. (1957). *A theory of cognitive dissonance*. Stanford University Press.

Fletcher, R., Kalogeropoulos, A., Simon, F., & Nielsen, R. K. (2020). *Information inequality in the UK coronavirus communications crisis*. Reuters Institute for the Study of Journalism. https://reutersinstitute.politics.ox.ac.uk/information-inequality-uk-coronavirus-communications-crisis

Freeman, D., Waite, F., Rosebrock, L., Petit, A., Causier, C., East, A., Jenner, L., Teale, A. L., Carr, L., Mulhall, S., Bold, E., & Lambe, S. (2022). Coronavirus conspiracy beliefs, mistrust, and compliance with government guidelines in England. *Psychological Medicine*, *52*(2), 251–263. https://doi.org/10.1017/S0033291720001890

Fu, W., Wang, L.-S., & Chou, S.-Y. (2024). A single dose for me, a wealth of protection for us: The public health cost of individualism in the rollout of COVID-19 vaccine. *Social Science & Medicine*, *348*, 116849. https://doi.org/10.1016/j.socscimed.2024.116849

Fuchs, T. (2013). Temporality and psychopathology. *Phenomenology and the Cognitive Sciences*, *12*(1), 75–104. https://doi.org/10.1007/s11097-010-9189-4

Garfin, D. R., Fischhoff, B., Holman, E. A., & Silver, R. C. (2021). Risk perceptions and health behaviors as COVID-19 emerged in the United States: Results from a probability-based nationally representative sample. *Journal of Experimental Psychology: Applied*, *27*(4), 584–598. https://doi.org/10.1037/xap0000374

Gassen, J., Nowak, T. J., Henderson, A. D., Weaver, S. P., Baker, E. J., & Muehlenbein, M. P. (2022). Longitudinal changes in COVID-19 concern and stress: Pandemic fatigue overrides individual differences in caution. *Journal of Public Health Research*, *11*, 22799036221119011. https://doi.org/10.1177/22799036221119011

Gelfand, M. J., Jackson, J. C., Pan, X., Nau, D., Pieper, D., Denison, E., Dagher, M., Van Lange, P. A. M., Chiu, C. Y., & Wang, M. (2021). The relationship between cultural tightness–looseness and COVID-19 cases and deaths: A global analysis. *The Lancet Planetary Health*, *5*(3), e135–e144. https://doi.org/10.1016/S2542-5196(20)30301-6

Gerretsen, P., Kim, J., Caravaggio, F., Quilty, L., Sanches, M., Wells, S., Brown, E. E., Agic, B., Pollock, B. G., & Graff-Guerrero, A. (2021). Individual determinants of COVID-19 vaccine hesitancy. *PLoS One*, *16*(11), e0258462. https://doi.org/10.1371/journal.pone.0258462

Giuntella, O., Hyde, K., Saccardo, S., & Sadoff, S. (2021). Lifestyle and mental health disruptions during COVID-19. *Proceedings of the National Academy of Sciences*, *118*(9), e2016632118. https://doi.org/10.1073/pnas.2016632118

Golman, R., Hagmann, D., & Loewenstein, G. (2017). Information avoidance. *Journal of Economic Literature*, *55*(1), 96–135. https://doi.org/10.1257/jel.20151245

Gotanda, H., Miyawaki, A., Tabuchi, T., & Tsugawa, Y. (2021). Association between trust in government and practice of preventive measures during the COVID-19 pandemic in Japan. *Journal of General Internal Medicine*, *36*(10), 3471–3477. https://doi.org/10.1007/s11606-021-06959-3

Griffith, J., Marani, H., & Monkman, H. (2021). COVID-19 vaccine hesitancy in Canada: Content analysis of tweets using the theoretical domains framework. *Journal of Medical Internet Research*, *23*(4), e26874. https://doi.org/10.2196/26874

Guan, Y., Deng, H., & Zhou, X. (2020). Understanding the impact of the COVID-19 pandemic on career development: Insights from cultural psychology. *Journal of Vocational Behavior*, *119*, 103438. https://doi.org/10.1016/j.jvb.2020.103438

Gursoy, D., Ekinci, Y., Can, A. S., & Murray, J. C. (2022). Effectiveness of message framing in changing COVID-19 vaccination intentions: Moderating role of travel desire. *Tourism Management*, *90*, 104468. https://doi.org/10.1016/j.tourman.2021.104468

Halpern, S. D., Truog, R. D., & Miller, F. G. (2020). Cognitive bias and public health policy during the COVID-19 pandemic. *JAMA*, *324*(4), 337–338. https://doi.org/10.1001/jama.2020.11623

Han, Q., Zheng, B., Agostini, M., Bélanger, J. J., Gützkow, B., Kreienkamp, J., Reitsema, A. M., & van Breen, J. A., & PsyCorona Collaboration. (2021a). Trust in government regarding COVID-19 and its associations with preventive health behavior and prosocial behavior during the pandemic: A cross-sectional and longitudinal study. *Psychological Medicine*. Advance online publication. https://doi.org/10.1017/S0033291721001306

Han, Q., Zheng, B., Agostini, M., Bélanger, J. J., Gützkow, B., Kreienkamp, J., Reitsema, A. M., van Breen, J. A., Collaboration, P., Leander, N. P. & PsyCorona Collaboration. (2021b). Associations of risk perception of COVID-19 with emotion and mental health during the pandemic. *Journal of Affective Disorders*, *284*, 247–255. https://doi.org/10.1016/j.jad.2021.01.049

Han, Q., Zheng, B., Cristea, M., Agostini, M., Bélanger, J. J., Gützkow, B., Kreienkamp, J., PsyCorona Collaboration, & Leander, N. P. (2023). Trust in government regarding COVID-19 and its associations with preventive health behaviour and prosocial behaviour during the pandemic: A cross-sectional and longitudinal study. *Psychological Medicine*, *53*(1), 149–159. https://doi.org/10.1017/S0033291721001306

Harmon-Jones, E., & Mills, J. (2019). An introduction to cognitive dissonance theory and an overview of current perspectives on the theory. In E. Harmon-Jones (Ed.), *Cognitive dissonance* (2nd ed., pp. 3–24). APA. https://doi.org/10.1037/0000135-001

Harper, C. A., Satchell, L. P., Fido, D., & Latzman, R. D. (2021). Functional fear predicts public health compliance in the COVID-19 pandemic. *International Journal of Mental Health and Addiction*, *19*(5), 1875–1888. https://doi.org/10.1007/s11469-020-00281-5

Hatton, C. R., Barry, C. L., Levine, A. S., McGinty, E. E., & Han, H. (2022). American trust in science and institutions in the time of COVID-19. *Daedalus*, *151*(4), 83–97. https://doi.org/10.1162/daed_a_01945

Haug, N., Geyrhofer, L., Londei, A., Dervic, E., Desvars-Larrive, A., Loreto, V., Pinior, B., Thurner, S., & Klimek, P. (2020). Ranking the effectiveness of worldwide COVID-19 government interventions. *Nature Human Behaviour*, *4*, 1303–1312. https://doi.org/10.1038/s41562-020-01009-0

Henley, J., & McIntyre, N. (2020, October 26). Survey uncovers widespread belief in 'dangerous' Covid conspiracy theories. *The Guardian*. https://www.theguardian.com/world/2020/oct/26/survey-uncovers-widespread-belief-dangerous-covid-conspiracy-theories

Hornik, R., Kikut, A., Jesch, E., Woko, C., Siegel, L., & Kim, K. (2021). Association of COVID-19 misinformation with face mask wearing and social distancing in a nationally representative US sample. *Health Communication*, *36*(1), 6–14. https://doi.org/10.1080/10410236.2020.1847437

Huang, L., Li, O. Z., Wang, B., & Zhou, J. (2022). Individualism and the fight against COVID-19. *Humanities and Social Sciences Communications*, *9*, 120. https://doi.org/10.1057/s41599-022-01124-5

Huang, Y., Zhang, H., Peng, Z., & Fang, M. (2023). Public trust and policy compliance during the COVID-19 pandemic: The role of professional trust. *BMC Public Health*, *23*(1), 751. https://doi.org/10.1186/s12889-023-15643-6

Huynh, T. L. D. (2020). Does culture matter social distancing under the COVID-19 pandemic? *Safety Science*, *130*, 104872. https://doi.org/10.1016/j.ssci.2020.104872

Hyland-Wood, B., Gardner, J., Leask, J., & Ecker, U. K. H. (2021). Toward effective government communication strategies in the era of COVID-19. *Humanities and Social Sciences Communications*, *8*, 30. https://doi.org/10.1057/s41599-020-00701-w

Imhoff, R., & Lamberty, P. (2020). A bioweapon or a hoax? The link between distinct conspiracy beliefs about the coronavirus disease (COVID-19) outbreak and pandemic behavior. *Social Psychological and Personality Science*, *11*(8), 1110–1118. https://doi.org/10.1177/1948550620934692

Jiang, S., Wei, Q., & Zhang, L. (2022). Individualism versus collectivism and the early-stage transmission of COVID-19. *Social Indicators Research*, *164*, 791–821. https://doi.org/10.1007/s11205-022-02972-z

Johnson-Laird, P. N. (2010). Mental models and human reasoning. *Proceedings of the National Academy of Sciences*, *107*(43), 18243–18250. https://doi.org/10.1073/pnas.1012933107

Jones, N. A., Ross, H., Lynam, T., Perez, P., & Leitch, A. (2011). Mental models: An interdisciplinary synthesis of theory and methods. *Ecology and Society*, *16*(1), 46. http://www.jstor.org/stable/26268859

Kaasa, A., & Andriani, L. (2022). Determinants of institutional trust: The role of cultural context. *Journal of Institutional Economics*, *18*(1), 45–65. https://doi.org/10.1017/S1744137421000199

Kasting, M., Macy, J., Grannis, S., Wiensch, A., Lavista Ferres, J., & Dixon, B. (2022). Factors associated with the intention to receive the COVID-19 vaccine: Cross-sectional national study. *JMIR Public Health and Surveillance*, *8*(11), e37203. https://doi.org/10.2196/37203

Kaye-Kauderer, H., Feingold, J. H., Feder, A., Southwick, S., & Charney, D. (2021). Resilience in the age of COVID-19. *BJPsych Advances*, 1–13. https://doi.org/10.1192/bja.2021.5

Kennedy, B., & Tyson, A. (2023, November 14). *Americans' trust in scientists, positive views of science continue to decline: Among both democrats and republicans, trust in scientists is lower than before the pandemic.* Pew Research Center. https://www.pewresearch.org/science/2023/11/14/americans-trust-in-scientists-positive-views-of-science-continue-to-decline/

Kim, J. H., Kwok, K. O., Huang, Z., Chan, E. Y. Y., Lo, E. S., Wong, S. Y. S., & Chan, H. (2023). A longitudinal study of COVID-19 preventive behavior fatigue in Hong Kong: A city with previous pandemic experience. *BMC Public Health, 23*(1), 618. https://doi.org/10.1186/s12889-023-15257-y

Kim, S., Capasso, A., Ali, S. H., Lopez, L. R., & Vu, T. H. (2022). What predicts people's belief in COVID-19 misinformation? A retrospective study using a nationwide online survey among adults residing in the United States. *BMC Public Health, 22*, 2114. https://doi.org/10.1186/s12889-022-14431-y

Kreps, S. E., & Kriner, D. L. (2020). Model uncertainty, political contestation, and public trust in science: Evidence from the COVID-19 pandemic. *Science Advances, 6*(43), eabd4563. https://doi.org/10.1126/sciadv.abd4563

Kunda, Z. (1990). The case for motivated reasoning. *Psychological Bulletin, 108*(3), 480–498. https://doi.org/10.1037/0033-2909.108.3.480

Lazarus, J. V., Ratzan, S. C., Palayew, A., et al. (2021). A global survey of potential acceptance of a COVID-19 vaccine. *Nature Medicine, 27*(2), 225–228. https://doi.org/10.1038/s41591-020-1124-9

Leong, S., Eom, K., Ishii, K., Aichberger, M. C., Fetz, K., Müller, T. S., …, & Sherman, D. K. (2022). Individual costs and community benefits: Collectivism and individuals' compliance with public health interventions. *PLoS One, 17*(11), e0275388. https://doi.org/10.1371/journal.pone.0275388

Leung, H. T., Gong, W. J., Sit, S. M. M., Ho, S. Y., Deng, Y., Wang, M. P., Lam, T. H., & Fielding, R. (2022). COVID-19 pandemic fatigue and its sociodemographic and psychobehavioral correlates: A population-based cross-sectional study in Hong Kong. *Scientific Reports, 12*(1), 16114. https://doi.org/10.1038/s41598-022-19692-6

Lo Coco, G., Salerno, L., Albano, G., Pazzagli, C., Lagetto, G., Mancinelli, E., Freda, M. F., Bassi, G., Giordano, C., Gullo, S., & Di Blasi, M. (2023). Psychosocial predictors of trajectories of mental health distress during the COVID-19 pandemic: A four-wave panel study. *Psychiatry Research, 326*, 115262. https://doi.org/10.1016/j.psychres.2023.115262

Lu, J. G., Jin, P., & English, A. S. (2021). Collectivism predicts mask use during COVID-19. *Proceedings of the National Academy of Sciences, 118*(23), e2021793118. https://doi.org/10.1073/pnas.2021793118

Luong, N., Mark, G., Kulshrestha, J., & Aledavood, T. (2024). Sleep during the COVID-19 pandemic: Longitudinal observational study combining multisensor data with questionnaires. *JMIR mHealth and uHealth, 12*(1), e53389. https://doi.org/10.2196/53389

Maaravi, Y., Levy, A., Gur, T., Confino, D., & Segal, S. (2021). The tragedy of the commons: How individualism and collectivism affected the spread of the COVID-19 pandemic. *Frontiers in Public Health, 9*, 627559. https://doi.org/10.3389/fpubh.2021.627559

Mace, C. (2020). *Impact of communication on public trust in institutions during the COVID-19 pandemic.* Clemson University Open Textbooks. https://opentextbooks.clemson.edu/stswu1010fall2020/chapter/impact-of-communication-on-public-trust-during-the-covid-19-pandemic/

Markus, H. R., & Kitayama, S. (1991). Culture and the self: Implications for cognition, emotion, and motivation. *Psychological Review, 98*(2), 224–253. https://doi.org/10.1037/0033-295X.98.2.224

Marziali, M. E., Hogg, R. S., Hu, A., & Card, K. G. (2024). Social trust and COVID-19 mortality in the United States: Lessons in planning for future pandemics using data from the general social survey. *BMC Public Health*, *24*(1), 2323. https://doi.org/10.1186/s12889-024-19805-y

Masten, A. S., & Motti-Stefanidi, F. (2020). Multisystem resilience for children and youth in disaster: Reflections in the context of COVID-19. *Adversity and Resilience Science*, *1*, 95–106. https://doi.org/10.1007/s42844-020-00010-w

McLaughlin, B., Gotlieb, A., & Mills, A. (2023). Caught in a dangerous world: Problematic news consumption and its relationship to mental and physical ill-being. *Health Communication*, *38*(12), 2687–2697. https://doi.org/10.1080/10410236.2022.2106086

Michie, S., West, R., & Harvey, N. (2020). The concept of "fatigue" in tackling covid-19. *BMJ*, *371*, m4171. https://doi.org/10.1136/bmj.m4171

Mills, M. A., & St. Clair, P. (2023, March 9). The strange new politics of science. *Issues in Science and Technology*. https://issues.org/new-politics-science-mills-st-clair/

Morgan, M. G., Fischhoff, B., Bostrom, A., & Atman, C. J. (2001). *Risk communication: A mental models approach*. Cambridge University Press.

Ngoy, N., Oyugi, B., Ouma, P. O., Conteh, I. N., Woldetsadik, S. F., Nanyunja, M., Okeibunor, J. C., Yoti, Z., & Gueye, A. S. (2022). Coordination mechanisms for COVID-19 in the WHO regional office for Africa. *BMC Health Services Research*, *22*(1), 711. https://doi.org/10.1186/s12913-022-08035-w

Nichols, T. (2024, March 22). When experts fail: They saved us from disaster during the pandemic—But they also made costly errors. *The Atlantic*. https://www.theatlantic.com/ideas/archive/2024/03/experts-failure-covid-19-pandemic/677816/

Nickerson, R. S. (1998). Confirmation bias: A ubiquitous phenomenon in many guises. *Review of General Psychology*, *2*(2), 175–220. https://doi.org/10.1037/1089-2680.2.2.175

Nielsen, R. K., Fletcher, R., Newman, N., Brennen, J. S., & Howard, P. N. (2020, April 15). *Navigating the 'infodemic': How people in six countries access and rate news and information about coronavirus*. Reuters Institute for the Study of Journalism, University of Oxford. https://reutersinstitute.politics.ox.ac.uk/infodemic-how-people-six-countries-access-and-rate-news-and-information-about-coronavirus

O'Mahony, C., Brassil, M., Murphy, G., & Linehan, C. (2023). The efficacy of interventions in reducing belief in conspiracy theories: A systematic review. *PLoS One*, *18*(4), e0280902. https://doi.org/10.1371/journal.pone.0280902

Ortega, F., & Orsini, M. (2020). Governing COVID-19 without government in Brazil: Ignorance, neoliberal authoritarianism, and the collapse of public health leadership. *Global Public Health*, *15*(9), 1257–1277. https://doi.org/10.1080/17441692.2020.1795223

Pagliaro, S., Sacchi, S., Pacilli, M. G., Brambilla, M., Lionetti, F., Bettache, K., …, & Zubieta, E. (2021). Trust predicts COVID-19 prescribed and discretionary behavioral intentions in 23 countries. *PLoS One*, *16*(3), e0248334. https://doi.org/10.1371/journal.pone.0248334

Pakpour, A. H., & Griffiths, M. D. (2020). The fear of COVID-19 and its role in preventive behaviors. *Journal of Concurrent Disorders*, *2*(1), 58–63. https://doi.org/10.54127/WCIC8036

Park, Y., Choe, Y., Park, O., Park, S., Kim, Y., Kim, J., & Jeong, E. (2020). Contact tracing during coronavirus disease outbreak, South Korea, 2020. *Emerging Infectious Diseases*, *26*(10), 2465–2468. https://doi.org/10.3201/eid2610.201315

Pasha, A., Inusah, A. H., Nayem, J., Li, X., & Qiao, S. (2025). A systematic review of psychological resilience in the COVID-19 responses: Current research and future directions. *medRxiv: The preprint server for health sciences*, 2025.02.15.25322337. https://doi.org/10.1101/2025.02.15.25322337

Pennycook, G., McPhetres, J., Zhang, Y., Lu, J. G., & Rand, D. G. (2020). Fighting COVID-19 misinformation on social media: Experimental evidence for a scalable accuracy-nudge intervention. *Psychological Science*, *31*(7), 770–780. https://doi.org/10.1177/0956797620939054

Pierce, M., Hope, H., Ford, T., Hatch, S., Hotopf, M., John, A., Kontopantelis, E., Webb, R., Wessely, S., McManus, S., & Abel, K. M. (2020). Mental health before and during the COVID-19 pandemic: A longitudinal probability sample survey of the UK population. *The Lancet Psychiatry*, *7*(10), 883–892. https://doi.org/10.1016/S2215-0366(20)30308-4

Pierce, M., McManus, S., Hope, H., Hotopf, M., Ford, T., Hatch, S. L., John, A., Kontopantelis, E., Webb, R. T., Wessely, S., & Abel, K. M. (2021). Mental health responses to the COVID-19 pandemic: A latent class trajectory analysis using longitudinal UK data. *The Lancet Psychiatry*, *8*(7), 610–619. https://doi.org/10.1016/S2215-0366(21)00151-6

Pollard, M. S., & Davis, L. M. (2022). Decline in trust in the centers for disease control and prevention during the COVID-19 pandemic. *Rand Health Quarterly*, *9*(3), 23.

Porat, T., Nyrup, R., Calvo, R. A., Paudyal, P., & Ford, E. (2020). Public health and risk communication during COVID-19—Enhancing psychological needs to promote sustainable behavior change. *Frontiers in Public Health*, *8*, 573397. https://doi.org/10.3389/fpubh.2020.573397

Quinn, S. C., Jamison, A., Freimuth, V. S., An, J., Hancock, G. R., & Musa, D. (2017). Exploring racial influences on flu vaccine attitudes and behavior: Results of a national survey of White and African American adults. *Vaccine*, *35*(8), 1167–1174. https://doi.org/10.1016/j.vaccine.2016.12.046

Rajkumar, R. P. (2021). The relationship between measures of individualism and collectivism and the impact of COVID-19 across nations. *Public Health in Practice*, *2*, 100143. https://doi.org/10.1016/j.puhip.2021.100143

Raude, J., McColl, K., Flamand, C., & Apostolidis, T. (2020). Understanding health behaviour changes in response to outbreaks: Findings from a longitudinal study of a large epidemic of mosquito-borne disease. *Social Science & Medicine*, *230*, 233–241. https://doi.org/10.1016/j.socscimed.2019.04.009

Reynolds, B., & Seeger, M. W. (2005). Crisis and emergency risk communication as an integrative model. *Journal of Health Communication*, *10*(1), 43–55. https://doi.org/10.1080/10810730590904571

Rodríguez-Blázquez, C., Romay-Barja, M., Falcón, M., Ayala, A., & Forjaz, M. J. (2022). Psychometric properties of the COVID-19 Pandemic Fatigue Scale: Cross-sectional online survey study. *JMIR Public Health and Surveillance*, *8*(9), e34675. https://doi.org/10.2196/34675

Rodrigues, F., Newell, R., Babu, G. R., Chatterjee, T., Sandhu, N. K., & Gupta, L. (2024). The social media infodemic of health-related misinformation and technical solutions. *Health Policy and Technology*, *13*(2), 100846. https://doi.org/10.1016/j.hlpt.2024.100846

Rogers, R. W. (1975). A protection motivation theory of fear appeals and attitude change. *The Journal of Psychology*, *91*(1), 93–114. https://doi.org/10.1080/00223980.1975.9915803

Rogers de Waal, J. (2020, November 10). Globalism Project 2020: Populist beliefs down but conspiracy beliefs up? *YouGov*. https://business.yougov.com/content/32973-globalism-project-2020-populist-beliefs-down-consp-1

Romano, A. (2020, November 18). Conspiracy theories, explained: Americans are embracing dangerous conspiratorial beliefs, from QAnon to coronavirus denial. *Vox*. https://www.vox.com/21558524/conspiracy-theories-2020-qanon-covid-conspiracies-why

Romer, D., & Jamieson, K. H. (2020). Conspiracy theories as barriers to controlling the spread of COVID-19 in the U.S. *Social Science & Medicine* (1982), *263*, 113356. https://doi.org/10.1016/j.socscimed.2020.113356

Roozenbeek, J., Schneider, C. R., Dryhurst, S., Kerr, J., Freeman, A. L. J., Recchia, G., van der Bles, A. M., & van der Linden, S. (2020). Susceptibility to misinformation about COVID-19 around the world. *Royal Society Open Science*, *7*(10), 201199. https://doi.org/10.1098/rsos.201199

Rosenstock, I. M. (1974). Historical origins of the health belief model. *Health Education Monographs*, *2*(4), 328–335. https://doi.org/10.1177/109019817400200403

Rotulo, A., Kondilis, E., Thwe, T., Gautam, S., Torcu, Ö., Vera-Montoya, M., Marjan, S., Gazi, M. I., Putri, A. S., Hasan, R. B., Mone, F. H., Rodríguez-Castillo, K., Tabassum, A., Parcharidi, Z., Sharma, B., Islam, F., Amoo, B., Lemke, L., & Gallo, V. (2023). Mind the gap: Data availability, accessibility, transparency, and credibility during the COVID-19 pandemic, an international comparative appraisal. *PLOS Global Public Health*, *3*(4), e0001148. https://doi.org/10.1371/journal.pgph.0001148

Sachs, R. (2021). Encouraging interagency collaboration: Learning from COVID-19. *Journal of Law & Innovation*. https://ssrn.com/abstract=3853425

Sanders, K. B. (2020). British government communication during the 2020 COVID-19 pandemic: Learning from high reliability organizations. *Church, Communication and Culture*, *5*(3), 356–377. https://doi.org/10.1080/23753234.2020.1824582

Santomauro, D. F., Herrera, A. M. M., Shadid, J., Zheng, P., Ashbaugh, C., Pigott, D. M., …, & Ferrari, A. J. (2021). Global prevalence and burden of depressive and anxiety disorders in 204 countries and territories in 2020 due to the COVID-19 pandemic. *The Lancet*, *398*(10312), 1700–1712. https://doi.org/10.1016/S0140-6736(21)02143-7

Schäfer, S. K., Kunzler, A. M., Kalisch, R., Tüscher, O., & Lieb, K. (2022). Trajectories of resilience and mental distress to global major disruptions. *Trends in Cognitive Sciences*, *26*(12), 1171–1189. https://doi.org/10.1016/j.tics.2022.09.017

Schäfer, S. K., Sopp, M. R., Schanz, C. G., Staginnus, M., Göritz, A. S., & Michael, T. (2020). Impact of COVID-19 on public mental health and the buffering effect of a sense of coherence. *Psychotherapy and Psychosomatics*, *89*(6), 386–392. https://doi.org/10.1159/000510752

Schmidt-Petri, C., Schröder, C., Okubo, T., Graeber, D., & Rieger, T. (2022). Social norms and preventive behaviors in Japan and Germany during the COVID-19 pandemic. *Frontiers in Public Health*, *10*, 842177. https://doi.org/10.3389/fpubh.2022.842177

Seaborn, K., Henderson, K., Gwizdka, J., Mokrosinska, M., Bartolomé Peral, E., & Pennycook, G. (2022). A meta-review of psychological resilience during COVID-19. *npj Mental Health Research*, *1*, 5. https://doi.org/10.1038/s44184-022-00005-8

Sharot, T. (2011). The optimism bias. *Current Biology*, *21*(23), R941–R945. https://doi.org/10.1016/j.cub.2011.10.030

Skade, L., Lehrer, E., Hamdali, Y., & Koch, J. (2025). The temporality of crisis and the crisis of temporality: On the construction and modulation of urgency during prolonged crises. *Journal of Management Studies*, *62*, 1087–1120. https://doi.org/10.1111/joms.13124

Skafle, I., Nordahl-Hansen, A., Quintana, D. S., Wynn, R., & Gabarron, E. (2022). Misinformation about COVID-19 vaccines on social media: Rapid review. *Journal of Medical Internet Research*, *24*(8), e37367. https://doi.org/10.2196/37367

Song, S., & Choi, Y. (2023). Differences in the COVID-19 pandemic response between South Korea and the United States: A comparative analysis of culture and policies. *Journal of Asian and African Studies*, *58*(2), 196–213. https://doi.org/10.1177/00219096221137655

Southwell, B. G., Kelly, B. J., Bann, C. M., Squiers, L. B., Ray, S. E., & McCormack, L. A. (2020). Mental models of infectious diseases and public understanding of COVID-19 prevention. *Health Communication*, *35*(14), 1707–1710. https://doi.org/10.1080/10410236.2020.1837462

Suhay, E., Soni, A., Persico, C., & Marcotte, D. E. (2022). Americans' trust in government and health behaviors during the COVID-19 pandemic. *RSF: The Russell Sage Foundation Journal of the Social Sciences*, *8*(8), 221–244. https://doi.org/10.7758/RSF.2022.8.8.10

Tang, D., Wang, F., & Xu, S. (2021). Impact of pandemic fatigue on the spread of COVID-19: A mathematical modelling study. *arXiv*. https://arxiv.org/abs/2104.04235

Tannenbaum, M. B., Hepler, J., Zimmerman, R. S., Saul, L., Jacobs, S., Wilson, K., …, & Albarracín, D. (2015). Appealing to fear: A meta-analysis of fear appeal effectiveness and theories. *Psychological Bulletin*, *141*(6), 1178–1204. https://doi.org/10.1037/a0039729

Taylor, S., Landry, C. A., Paluszek, M. M., Rachor, G. S., Asmundson, A. J., & Asmundson, G. J. (2020). Development and initial validation of the COVID Stress Scales. *Journal of Anxiety Disorders*, *72*, 102232. https://doi.org/10.1016/j.janxdis.2020.102232

Trabelsi, K., Ammar, A., Masmoudi, L., Boukhris, O., Chtourou, H., Bouaziz, B., Brach, M., Bentlage, E., How, D., Ahmed, M., Müller, P., Müller, N., Aloui, A., Hammouda, O., Paineiras-Domingos, L. L., Braakman-jansen, A., Wrede, C., Bastoni, S., Pernambuco, C. S., …, Hoekelmann, A. (2021). Globally altered sleep patterns and physical activity levels by confinement in 5056 individuals: ECLB COVID-19 international online survey. *Biology of Sport*, *38*(4), 495–506. https://doi.org/10.5114/biolsport.2021.101605

Tran, C. (2022). *Effects of cultural orientation and privacy perspectives on trust in public health officials during COVID-19* [Master's thesis, UC San Diego]. https://escholarship.org/uc/item/8mv128f6

Triandis, H. C. (1995). *Individualism and collectivism* (1st ed.). Routledge. https://doi.org/10.4324/9780429499845

Troeger, C., & Bollyky, T. J. (2021, November 30). *Ending the COVID-19 pandemic hinges on trust: Science alone won't pull us out of the pandemic*. Think Global Health. https://www.thinkglobalhealth.org/article/ending-covid-19-pandemic-hinges-trust

Turner, S., Segura, C., & Niño, N. (2022). Implementing COVID-19 surveillance through inter-organizational coordination: A qualitative study of three cities in Colombia. *Health Policy and Planning*, *37*(2), 232–242. https://doi.org/10.1093/heapol/czab145

Tversky, A., & Kahneman, D. (1974). Judgment under uncertainty: Heuristics and biases. *Science*, *185*(4157), 1124–1131. https://doi.org/10.1126/science.185.4157.1124

Tyson, A., & Kennedy, B. (2024, November 14). *Public trust in scientists and views on their role in policymaking: Trust moves slightly higher but remains lower than before the pandemic*. Pew Research Center. https://www.pewresearch.org/science/2024/11/14/public-trust-in-scientists-and-views-on-their-role-in-policymaking/

Tyson, A., Lipka, M., & Deane, C. (2025, February 12). *5 years later: America looks back at the impact of COVID-19—Most Americans say the pandemic drove the country apart*. Pew Research Center. https://www.pewresearch.org/politics/2025/02/12/5-years-later-america-looks-back-at-the-impact-of-covid-19/

Van Bavel, J. J., Baicker, K., Boggio, P. S., Capraro, V., Cichocka, A., Cikara, M., …, & Willer, R. (2020). Using social and behavioural science to support COVID-19 pandemic response. *Nature Human Behaviour*, *4*(5), 460–471. https://doi.org/10.1038/s41562-020-0884-z

van der Pligt, J. (1996). Risk perception and self-protective behavior. *European Psychologist*, *1*(1), 34–43. https://doi.org/10.1027/1016-9040.1.1.34

Velasco, P. F., Perroy, B., & Casati, R. (2021). The collective disorientation of the COVID-19 crisis. *Global Discourse*, *11*(3), 441–462. https://doi.org/10.1332/204378921X16146158263164

Velasco, P. F., Perroy, B., Gurchani, U. et al. (2022). Lost in pandemic time: A phenomenological analysis of temporal disorientation during the Covid-19 crisis. *Phenomenology and the Cognitive Sciences*, *22*, 1121–1144 (2023). https://doi.org/10.1007/s11097-022-09847-1

Veronese, G., Cavazzoni, F., & Pepe, A. (2023). Trajectories of quality of life and mental health during the Covid-19 lockdown and six months after in Italy. A longitudinal exploration. *Zeitschrift fur Gesundheitswissenschaften = Journal of Public Health*, 1–11. Advance online publication. https://doi.org/10.1007/s10389-023-01913-5

Vu, Q. M., Takahashi, S. M., Tupper, P., Muirhead, N., Morshed, M., Mackay, M., Fraser, M., Deans, G., Patrick, D., & Dawar, M. (2024). Estimates of incidence and predictors of fatiguing illness after SARS-CoV-2 infection. *Emerging Infectious Diseases*, *30*(3), 539–547. https://doi.org/10.3201/eid3003.231194

Vu, T. V. (2021). *Long-term cultural barriers to sustaining collective effort in vaccination against COVID-19*. SSRN. https://doi.org/10.2139/ssrn.3943011

Wang, H., Paulson, K. R., Pease, S. A., Watson, S., Comfort, H., Zheng, P., . . . , & Murray, C. J. L. (2022a). Estimating excess mortality due to the COVID-19 pandemic: A systematic analysis of COVID-19-related mortality, 2020–21. *The Lancet*, *399*(10334), 1513–1536. https://doi.org/10.1016/S0140-6736(21)02796-3

Wang, Y. Y., Luk, T. T., Ho, S. Y., Viswanath, K., Chan, S. S. C., Mak, Y. W., Lei, B., Fong, D. Y. T., Wang, M. P., Lam, T. H., & Fielding, R. (2022b). COVID-19 pandemic fatigue and its sociodemographic and psycho-behavioral correlates: A population-based cross-sectional study in Hong Kong. *Scientific Reports*, *12*(1), 16114. https://doi.org/10.1038/s41598-022-19692-6

Wang, Y., & Liu, Y. (2022). Multilevel determinants of COVID-19 vaccination hesitancy in the United States: A rapid systematic review. *Preventive Medicine Reports*, *25*, 101673. https://doi.org/10.1016/j.pmedr.2021.101673

Wang, Z., Li, Y., Xu, R., & Yang, H. (2022c). How culture orientation influences the COVID-19 pandemic: An empirical analysis. *Frontiers in Psychology*, *13*, 899730. https://doi.org/10.3389/fpsyg.2022.899730

Williams, S. N., Armitage, C. J., Tampe, T., & Dienes, K. A. (2021). Public perceptions of non-adherence to pandemic protection measures by self and others: A study of COVID-19 in the United Kingdom. *PLoS One*, *16*(10), e0258781. https://doi.org/10.1371/journal.pone.0258781

Wilson, S. (2020). Pandemic leadership: Lessons from New Zealand's approach to COVID-19. *Leadership*, *16*(3), 279–293. https://doi.org/10.1177/1742715020929151

Wolbers, J., Boersma, K., & Groenewegen, P. (2018). Introducing a fragmentation perspective on coordination in crisis management. *Organization Studies*, *39*(11), 1521–1546. https://doi.org/10.1177/0170840617717095

World Health Organization (WHO). (2022a, March 2). COVID-19 pandemic triggers 25% increase in prevalence of anxiety and depression worldwide [News release]. https://www.who.int/news/item/02-03-2022-covid-19-pandemic-triggers-25-increase-in-prevalence-of-anxiety-and-depression-worldwide

World Health Organization (WHO). (2022b, March 2). Mental health and COVID-19: Early evidence of the pandemic's impact [Scientific brief]. https://www.who.int/publications/i/item/WHO-2019-nCoV-Sci_Brief-Mental_health-2022.1

World Health Organization (WHO) Regional Office for Europe. (2020a, November). *Pandemic fatigue: Reinvigorating the public to prevent COVID-19*. https://www.who.int/europe/publications/i/item/WHO-EURO-2020-1573-41324-56242

World Health Organization (WHO), Regional Office for Europe. (2020b). *Pandemic fatigue – Reinvigorating the public to prevent COVID-19: Policy framework for supporting pandemic prevention and management*. World Health Organization, Regional Office for Europe. https://iris.who.int/handle/10665/335820

World Health Organization (WHO), United Nations Children's Fund (UNICEF), & International Federation of Red Cross and Red Crescent Societies (IFRC). (2020, February 24). *Social stigma associated with COVID-19: A guide to preventing and addressing social stigma*. https://www.who.int/publications/i/item/social-stigma-associated-with-covid-19

Wu, Q., Xu, Q., Zhu, X., Yan, J., Zhang, L., Wang, Y., & Shi, L. (2024). Pandemic fatigue and depressive symptoms among college students in the COVID-19 context. *BMC Psychology*, *12*, 21. https://doi.org/10.1186/s40359-024-01521-2

Wu, X., Li, J., & Li, Y. (2022). The impact of uncertainty induced by the COVID-19 pandemic on intertemporal choice. *Journal of Experimental Social Psychology*, *103*, 104397. https://doi.org/10.1016/j.jesp.2022.104397

Xiao, W. S. (2021). The role of collectivism–individualism in attitudes toward compliance and psychological responses during the COVID-19 pandemic. *Frontiers in Psychology*, *12*, 600826. https://doi.org/10.3389/fpsyg.2021.600826

Yamawaki, N. (2012). Within-culture variations of collectivism in Japan. *Journal of Cross-Cultural Psychology*, *43*(8), 1191–1204. https://doi.org/10.1177/0022022111428171

Yip, W., Ge, L., Ho, A. H. Y., Heng, B. H., & Tan, W. S. (2021). Building community resilience beyond COVID-19: The Singapore way. *The Lancet Regional Health – Western Pacific*, *7*, 100091. https://doi.org/10.1016/j.lanwpc.2020.100091

You, J. (2020). Lessons from South Korea's Covid-19 policy response. *The American Review of Public Administration*, *50*(6–7), 801–808. https://doi.org/10.1177/0275074020943708

Zarocostas, J. (2020). How to fight an infodemic. *The Lancet*, *395*(10225), 676. https://doi.org/10.1016/S0140-6736(20)30461-X

Part III

Pandemic-Proofing the World

Current Best Practices for Prevention

12 Non-Pharmaceutical Interventions

The First Line of Defense

Non-pharmaceutical interventions (NPIs) such as masking, social distancing, hand hygiene, school and business closures, lockdowns, travel bans, and contact tracing and quarantining are crucial for slowing the spread of pandemics. These simple measures play a significant role in protecting individuals and communities, even when virus mutations outpace vaccines. This section explores the evolution of these interventions in the United States and compares them to other global strategies. Understanding these shifts offers critical insights into how public health measures can be scaled, sustained, or modified in future pandemics based on cultural norms, political dynamics, and evolving scientific knowledge.

Masking

Masking emerged as a key NPI during the COVID-19 pandemic, aimed at reducing the transmission of respiratory droplets that carry the virus. Widespread mask use, particularly in indoor and crowded settings, proved effective in lowering infection rates, especially when combined with other measures like physical distancing and ventilation. As a low-cost and accessible strategy, masking played a vital role in protecting both individuals and communities, especially before vaccines were widely available. Over time, it evolved from a public health mandate to a voluntary practice based on personal risk and situational awareness.

Masking Policies in the United States (2020–2025)

2020 From Confusion to Mandates: In the early stages of the COVID-19 pandemic, the Centers for Disease Control and Prevention (CDC) did not recommend masking for the general public, aiming to preserve limited supplies for healthcare workers. However, in April 2020, the CDC shifted its guidance to recommend cloth face coverings in public settings, especially where social distancing was difficult to maintain. This led to a wave of state-level mandates, with states like California and New York implementing broad masking requirements. Despite these efforts, masking quickly became a politically divisive issue, with significant resistance and inconsistent adherence across the country (CDC, 2024c).

DOI: 10.4324/9781003595564-16

2021 Vaccine Rollout and Policy Shifts: Following the initial vaccine rollout, the CDC announced in May 2021 that fully vaccinated individuals could forgo masks indoors. This abrupt change led to confusion and uneven implementation across states and businesses. By mid-summer, with the rise of the Delta variant, many jurisdictions reinstated indoor masking recommendations or mandates. Mask policies became highly regionalized, reflecting differing political climates and public health strategies (CDC, 2024c).

2022 Omicron and a Decentralized Approach: The emergence of the Omicron variant led to renewed calls for masking, particularly in crowded or indoor settings. However, federal mandates waned, and in April 2022, a court ruling struck down the federal mask requirement on public transportation. Masking decisions became largely decentralized, left to local governments, private businesses, and individuals. Public health agencies emphasized personal risk assessment over mandates (CDC, 2024c).

2023–2025 Seasonal and Situational Use: Mask mandates have been lifted in nearly all public spaces. In the current phase, masking in the United States has become a voluntary and situational practice. Individuals choose to wear masks primarily during respiratory virus season, in healthcare settings, or if they are at high risk of severe illness. Masking is now viewed as a personal health behavior, much like hand hygiene, available as a protective tool, but no longer mandated (CDC, 2024b).

Global Masking Approaches

While masking in the United States followed a trajectory shaped by evolving public health guidance, political dynamics, and individual decision-making, global approaches varied significantly. Many countries adopted distinct strategies based on cultural norms, governmental structures, and levels of public trust. Table 12.1 provides a comparative overview of masking policies across select countries from 2020 to 2025, illustrating both similarities and differences in pandemic response and policy evolution.

Lessons Learned

Masking practices during the COVID-19 pandemic varied significantly across regions, influenced by cultural norms, political climate, and levels of public trust. Many Asian countries saw higher voluntary compliance with mask-wearing, even in the absence of formal mandates, reflecting strong social norms around collective responsibility and public health. In contrast, Western countries, where individual freedom was often prioritized, tended to lift mask mandates earlier and saw more resistance to prolonged policies. Today, masking has transitioned from a government-enforced rule to a seasonal or situational preventive tool, used voluntarily based on personal risk and setting.

Social Distancing

Social distancing is a core NPI used to reduce the spread of infectious diseases by minimizing close contact between individuals. During the COVID-19 pandemic, it

Table 12.1 Masking Approaches of Select Regions (2020–2025)

Region	*2020*	*2021*	*2022*	*2023–2025*
Japan	Strongly encouraged (not mandated)	High compliance	Continued compliance	Official guidance removed in 2023
South Korea	Strict mandates with penalties	Maintained during Delta/ Omicron	No longer mandatory outdoors	Gradual rollback in 2023
The United Kingdom	Mandatory in public transport and shops	Mandatory during Omicron	Voluntary	Little official guidance remains
Germany	Mandatory; fines imposed in some states	Medical-grade masks mandated	Mandatory healthcare settings and long-distance travel	Mandates terminated in March 2023
Sweden	No mask mandates	Recommended use on public transit	Recommended use on public transit	None
Taiwan	Mandated in all public spaces	Adjusted with each wave	Mask needed if symptoms present	Recommended in select settings

Sources: Adapted from: Lai et al. (2020), Penn (2021), Seoul Metropolitan Government (2022), Suzuki et al. (2024), Lim & Sohn (2022), Deutsche Welle (2021), Hobbs & Bunn (2020), Bundesministerium für Gesundheit (n.d.), Kim & Choi (2023), CNN, E. M. (2021), Norberg (2023), Schmitz (2020), Otte (2021), Taiwan Ministry of Health and Welfare (2020), Taiwan Centers for Disease and Control (2022).

played a vital role in slowing transmission, protecting vulnerable populations, and preventing healthcare system overload—especially before vaccines were widely available. Measures included maintaining physical distance, limiting gatherings, closing high-risk venues, and shifting to remote work and schooling. Though highly effective in early phases, social distancing strategies evolved over time, eventually becoming more targeted and voluntary as population immunity increased and other protective tools became available.

Social Distancing Policy in the United States (2020–2025)

2020 Strict Nationwide Recommendations: In March 2020, the CDC launched the "15 Days to Slow the Spread" campaign, later extended to "30 Days," urging Americans to stay 6 feet apart and avoid gatherings of more than ten people. These guidelines led to widespread closures of schools, restaurants, gyms, theaters, and other public spaces. Most states imposed strict gathering limits and capacity restrictions in businesses and places of worship. Remote work and virtual schooling became the norm as social distancing became the centerpiece of the national response (Feuer & Higgins-Dunn, 2021).

2021 Easing and Reinstating with Variants: With the introduction of COVID-19 vaccines in early 2021, many areas began relaxing distancing measures.

However, the emergence of the Delta variant in mid-2021 caused several regions to reintroduce restrictions, particularly in indoor settings. Social distancing policies became increasingly varied across the country, largely influenced by local case rates and vaccination coverage (CDC, 2024c).

2022 Shift toward Personal Responsibility: By 2022, the CDC eased formal distancing recommendations, citing widespread population immunity and the milder nature of the Omicron variant. Most states and localities dropped remaining mandates, including for schools, workplaces, and public events. Instead, strategies like hybrid work models, improved ventilation, and targeted protective measures started replacing rigid distancing rules (CDC, 2024c).

2023–2025 Distancing as a Recommendation, Not Rule: In the current phase, social distancing is no longer mandated at the federal or state level. It has become a voluntary measure, particularly encouraged in crowded or poorly ventilated environments, and remains in use in high-risk settings like hospitals and eldercare facilities. Public health messaging now emphasizes personal distancing when sick from respiratory viruses, regardless of the virus (CDC, 2024a, 2024b).

Global Social Distancing Strategies

While social distancing in the United States followed a phased approach shaped by evolving epidemiological trends and public policy, other countries adopted a range of strategies based on cultural attitudes, legal frameworks, and public health capacities. Table 12.2 presents a comparative overview of social distancing measures in selected countries from 2020 to 2025, highlighting variations in enforcement, public compliance, and the pace at which restrictions were lifted.

Lessons Learned

From 2020 to 2021, social distancing was a central strategy in global pandemic control, especially before the availability of vaccines. Countries differed in their approaches—some, like Germany and South Korea, implemented legally enforced distancing mandates, while others, such as Sweden and Japan, relied more on public recommendations and voluntary compliance. By 2022–2023, most nations phased out formal distancing rules, shifting the responsibility to individuals to assess and manage their own risk. Today, social distancing remains a non-pharmaceutical option primarily used in high-risk environments like hospitals and nursing homes, during outbreaks or seasonal surges, and by vulnerable individuals as a personal preventive measure.

Hand Hygiene

Hand hygiene policies became one of the most essential NPIs during the COVID-19 pandemic. Regular handwashing with soap and water, along with the use of hand sanitizers, was widely promoted to reduce the transmission of the virus, as it can spread through contact with contaminated surfaces. These practices were integral

Table 12.2 Social Distancing Strategies of Select Regions (2020–2025)

Region	*2020*	*2021*	*2022*	*2023–2025*
The United Kingdom	2 meter distancing rule; "Rule of Six"	All distancing laws removed in July 2021	No distancing mandates; personal choice	No distancing mandates
Germany	1.5 meter distancing; closures of public venues	Gradual regional lifting	1.5 meter distancing in workplace recommended	Normalized life; distancing not required
Japan	Avoiding the "Three Cs"	Government urges social distancing	Guidance remained but voluntary	High self-regulation
Taiwan	1.5 meter distancing indoors; 1 meter distancing outdoors	Taiwan Social Distancing App	Optimized Taiwan Social Distancing App	Focus on self-management
South Korea	3-level system; two-arms-length distance	Gradual easing of restrictions for vaccinated	Restrictions lifted in April	Seasonal reminders; not mandatory
Sweden	Banned crowding indoors; distancing in restaurants	Remote work and distance schooling encouraged	Restrictions lifted	Normalized life

Sources: Adapted from: Institute for Government (n.d.), GOV.UK (2020), Morton (2021), Heath (2022), Kim et al. (n.d), Simmons & Simmons (2022), Penn (2021), U.S. Embassy & Consulates in Japan (2021), Taiwan Ministry of Health and Welfare (2020), Taiwan Centers for Disease and Control (2022), Seoul Metropolitan Government (2022), European Chamber of Commerce in Korea (2022), Claeson & Hanson (2021), Rajapaksa & Alvarez (2023).

to controlling outbreaks, especially in settings like healthcare facilities, schools, and workplaces. While simple and cost-effective, hand hygiene policies required consistent public adherence and widespread educational efforts. The success of these measures underscores the importance of hygiene in preventing the spread of infectious diseases and provides insights for managing future global health threats.

Hand Hygiene Policies in the United States (2020–2025)

2020 – Foundational Public Health Message: Hand hygiene was a core early preventive measure. The CDC promoted frequent handwashing with soap and water for at least 20 seconds and encouraged alcohol-based hand sanitizers (≥60% alcohol) when soap wasn't available. Public campaigns like "Clean Hands Save Lives" were widely adopted, and sanitizer stations became standard in public spaces (CDC, 2024c).

2021 – Continued Emphasis with Evolving Guidance: Hand hygiene remained part of layered prevention efforts alongside masking and distancing. While the CDC clarified that surface (fomite) transmission was less common than airborne spread, handwashing was still recommended, particularly after public exposure or respiratory symptoms (CDC, 2024c).

2022 – Reduced Focus, Targeted Use: As messaging shifted toward airborne transmission and respiratory protections, hand hygiene received less emphasis in public campaigns. However, it remained important in healthcare, food service, and other high-risk environments (CDC, 2024c).

2023–2025 – Routine Practice, Not Pandemic-Specific: Hand hygiene returned to routine public health guidance. Sanitizer access remains common in public spaces, but without formal monitoring. Messaging now centers on respiratory etiquette, with handwashing promoted as part of general hygiene rather than a primary COVID-specific measure (CDC, 2024b).

Global Hand Hygiene Policies

Although hand hygiene was universally recognized as a critical NPI during the early stages of the COVID-19 pandemic, countries implemented and emphasized these measures in varying ways. Cultural norms, previous public health experiences, and infrastructure influenced the extent and duration of hand hygiene promotion. Table 12.3 outlines how selected countries approached hand hygiene policies and public messaging from 2020 through 2025, reflecting both initial urgency and the gradual normalization of hygiene practices.

Lessons Learned

In 2020–2021, hand hygiene was a foundational and widely adopted public health measure, with most countries rapidly installing sanitizer stations in public spaces. From 2022 onward, as focus shifted to airborne transmission, hand hygiene messaging was scaled back. By 2023–2025, handwashing became part of routine hygiene rather than a pandemic-specific intervention. While sanitizer infrastructure remains common, actual use now varies based on cultural norms and individual habits.

School and Business Closures

The COVID-19 pandemic led to unprecedented disruptions across the United States, with widespread school and business closures in 2020 as part of the effort to contain the virus. These closures, along with the shift to remote learning and work, marked a significant change in daily life and public health strategies. Over the following years, as vaccines were rolled out and the virus became more manageable, policies shifted toward a gradual reopening, with localized restrictions and a focus on maintaining public health protocols. By 2023, closures were no longer a standard strategy, and the focus shifted to individual risk management and flexibility in

Table 12.3 Hand Hygiene Policies of Select Regions (2020–2025)

Region	*2020*	*2021*	*2022*	*2023–2025*
The United Kingdom	National campaigns ("Hands. Face. Space.")	Continued focus, especially in schools	Emphasized for protection against all respiratory illnesses	Hygiene normalized; no formal campaigns
Germany	Strong hygiene culture; public notices displayed	Recommended, but more emphasis on vaccinations	Phased out public messaging	Routine hygiene
Japan	High baseline hygiene culture; widespread sanitizer use	Hand hygiene strongly encouraged	Continued public compliance voluntarily	Normal behavior; not policy-driven
South Korea	Aggressive campaigns and public hand hygiene stations	Still widely practiced and encouraged	Recommended	Cultural norm; hygiene stations remain
Taiwan	Strong public compliance from SARS-era habits	Hand sanitizer in all public venues	Remains standard, especially during flu/ COVID season	Part of seasonal health promotion, not enforced
Australia	"Wash your hands" emphasized early on	Continued public reminders in transport and healthcare	Recommended messaging	Hygiene routine; emphasis on respiratory hygiene
Sweden	Recommended but not heavily promoted	Focused more on distancing and symptom awareness	Minimal government messaging	Returned to pre-pandemic norms

Sources: Adapted from: Read et al. (2022), UK Health Security Agency (2022), Wiemann (2020), Bundesministerium für Gesundheit (n.d.), Takebayashi et al. (2023), Seoul Metropolitan Government (2022), Taiwan Ministry of Health and Welfare (2020), Taiwan Centers for Disease Control (2022), Australian Commission on Safety and Quality in Healthcare (2019).

work and education settings. This timeline outlines the progression of school and business closures in the United States and the transition toward reopening and adaptation in response to the evolving pandemic.

School and Business Closures in the United States (2020–2025)

2020 Widespread Closures: In March 2020, the COVID-19 pandemic prompted nearly all K–12 schools, colleges, and universities to close or transition to online learning. Most non-essential businesses, including restaurants, gyms, entertainment venues, and retail stores, were ordered to close by state governments. Essential services such as healthcare, grocery stores, and logistics continued to operate with additional precautions. Remote work and online learning became the new norm across the country (CDC, 2024c).

2021 Gradual Reopening with Caution: As vaccines became available in early 2021, schools began reopening with hybrid models that combined in-person and online learning. Businesses also started reopening, but with capacity limits, masking, and social distancing measures in place. The Delta variant surge in mid-2021 led some areas to re-tighten restrictions, although closures were more localized. Emphasis shifted to enhancing ventilation, testing, and vaccination efforts to ensure institutions could remain open (CDC, 2024c).

2022 Omicron and Return to Normal Operations: Despite the Omicron wave, widespread reopening continued into 2022. While temporary disruptions occurred due to staffing shortages and local outbreaks, no large-scale or national closures took place. Schools implemented masking and testing protocols to maintain in-person learning, and businesses adapted to fluctuating case rates with flexible policies (CDC, 2024c).

2023–2025 Closure No Longer a Strategy: By 2023, school and business closures were no longer part of the pandemic response strategy. Schools and businesses remained open without federal or state mandates, with a focus on individual risk management, remote work flexibility, and enhanced sick leave support. Closures were only considered in extreme cases of localized outbreaks (such as measles or RSV), not for COVID-19 (CDC, 2024b).

Global Approaches to School and Business Closures

As the United States navigated widespread closures and phased reopenings during the COVID-19 pandemic, countries around the world implemented their own strategies, shaped by local epidemiology, public health infrastructure, and societal values. While some nations imposed strict national lockdowns with prolonged disruptions, others maintained greater continuity through targeted interventions and public compliance. Table 12.4 compares school and business closure policies across selected countries from 2020 to 2025, highlighting key differences in duration, implementation, and long-term adaptation.

Lessons Learned

In 2020, universal school and business closures were widely adopted globally to curb COVID-19 transmission. By 2021, phased and localized reopenings began, with many schools implementing hybrid models and businesses operating under restrictions. From 2022 to 2025, a global shift toward permanent reopening took place, even during surges. COVID-19 management increasingly relied on vaccination, testing, and workplace flexibility rather than closures. Remote infrastructure, including platforms like Zoom, e-learning, and telework, became long-term assets in maintaining operational continuity.

Table 12.4 School and Business Closures of Select Regions (2020–2025)

Region	*2020*	*2021*	*2022*	*2023–2025*
The United Kingdom	School and business closures; phased reopening mid-2020 in England	Primary and secondary schools open	Fully open; remote work optional	Normal operations; remote work common
Germany	Schools closures in May; strict business closures	Gradual reopening of schools and businesses	No further school closures or lockdowns in August	Fully open; no mandated closures
Japan	Schools closed Feb–March; businesses not legally mandated to close	Minimal closures, strong guidance	Remained open with masking and distancing	All operations normal; cultural caution remains
South Korea	Schools closed briefly; strict measures	Schools returned with precautions	Fully reopened with testing and apps	Regular operations; tech integration continues
Taiwan	Schools and businesses remained open	School and some business closures mid-2021	Very limited disruption	Fully operational; high public trust
Australia	Closure of non-essential businesses; remote schooling	Pattern of closing and reopening	Sporadic closures	Remote options preserved; no closures
Sweden	Schools for <16 stayed open; businesses advised but not forced to close	Very limited school/ business closures	Adult remote learning lifted	Normal life, closure not part of strategy

Sources: Adapted from: Institute for Government (n.d.), Bundesministerium für Gesundheit (n.d.), Ministry of Education, Culture, Sports, Science and Technology of Japan (n.d.), Kim et al. (n.d.), Wieler et al. (n.d.), Taiwan Ministry of Health and Welfare (2020), Reserve Bank of Australia (n.d.), Kavaliunas et al. (2020), Rajapaksa & Alvarez (2023).

Lockdown Policies

Lockdowns are one of the most stringent NPIs used to control the spread of infectious diseases. During the COVID-19 pandemic, lockdowns were implemented to restrict movement, limit gatherings, and temporarily close schools and businesses. Their primary goal was to reduce transmission rates, protect healthcare capacity, and buy time for the development and distribution of medical countermeasures such as vaccines. While effective in the early stages, lockdowns also carried significant social, economic, and psychological costs, leading to ongoing debate about their role in future public health responses.

Lockdown Policies in the United States (2020–2025)

2020 Widespread and Disorganized Lockdowns: In response to the rapid spread of COVID-19, a national emergency was declared in March 2020. While the federal government did not issue a nationwide lockdown, most states independently implemented stay-at-home orders and closures of schools and non-essential businesses. Lockdowns were strictest in states like California and New York, while some southern states adopted more lenient approaches. These measures aimed to "flatten the curve" and prevent healthcare system overload, but they also led to significant economic disruption and mental health challenges (CDC, 2024c).

2021 Localized Restrictions and Reopenings: As vaccines became available in late 2020, many states eased lockdowns, transitioning to tiered systems with targeted capacity limits and restrictions. However, the emergence of the Delta variant in mid-2021 prompted some regions to reinstate partial restrictions. There was no return to nationwide lockdowns, and public sentiment grew increasingly divided, reflecting deepening political polarization over pandemic policies (CDC, 2024c).

2022 Post-Omicron Shift: With the arrival of the highly transmissible but generally milder Omicron variant, lockdowns fell out of favor both politically and practically. The United States shifted to a "living with COVID" model, emphasizing vaccination, personal responsibility, and healthcare system resilience. Even during surges, full-scale lockdowns, school closures, and business shutdowns were no longer utilized (CDC, 2024c).

2023–2025 Lockdowns Off the Table: By this period, lockdowns had effectively disappeared from U.S. pandemic response. Public health efforts focused instead on voluntary isolation, protecting vulnerable populations, and integrating COVID-19 management into broader health infrastructure. The legacy of lockdowns continues to influence public discourse, but their use as a primary control measure has been firmly set aside (CDC, 2024b).

Global Lockdown Policies

Globally, countries adopted a wide range of lockdown strategies during the COVID-19 pandemic, reflecting differences in governance, healthcare capacity, and risk tolerance. While some nations pursued aggressive elimination strategies involving repeated city-wide or national lockdowns, others relied more heavily on public guidance, testing, and targeted restrictions. Table 12.5 summarizes lockdown policies across selected countries from 2020 to 2025, illustrating how approaches evolved in response to emerging variants, vaccine availability, and shifting public attitudes.

Table 12.5 Lockdown Policies of Select Regions (2020–2025)

Region	*2020*	*2021*	*2022*	*2023–2025*
China	Strict national lockdowns (e.g., Wuhan)	"Zero-COVID" with rolling city-wide lockdowns	Major lockdowns (e.g., Shanghai in spring); mass testing	Policy abandoned in Dec 2022; shift to endemic strategy
New Zealand	Early, aggressive national lockdown	National and regional lockdowns	Most restrictions lifted end of 2022	Living with COVID; no lockdown use
Australia	Nationwide lockdowns	Delta drove strict state-level lockdowns	Phased reopening late 2022	No lockdowns, "living with the virus"
The United Kingdom	3 national lockdowns in 2020–2021	Gradual reopening in stages	No new lockdowns despite Omicron	Normalized COVID response; no return to lockdowns
Taiwan	No full lockdown, but strict border control and contact tracing	Short "soft lockdown" in mid-2021	Avoided lockdowns during Omicron	Focused on vaccination and risk communication
Sweden	No formal lockdowns	Maintained voluntary distancing	Criticized early; later aligned with EU strategies	Pandemic integrated into routine healthcare

Sources: Adapted from: Ba et al. (2023), Morton (2021), Song et al. (2023), NZ Royal Commission (2024), Reserve Bank of Australia (n.d.), Australian Government (n.d.), Australian Government Department of the Prime Minister and Cabinet (2024), Institute for Government (n.d.), Taiwan Ministry of Health and Welfare (2020), Rajapaksa & Alvarez (2023).

Lessons Learned

Early lockdowns played a critical role in slowing the initial spread of COVID-19 and buying time to prepare healthcare systems. However, they came with significant social and economic costs, including job losses, educational disruption, and mental health strain. As the pandemic evolved, most governments shifted away from broad lockdowns, turning instead to vaccination campaigns, risk-based policies, and strengthening public health infrastructure. Growing public fatigue and political resistance further reduced the feasibility of prolonged or repeated lockdowns. Today, lockdowns are viewed as a last-resort, short-term measure reserved for extreme public health emergencies—not a standard pandemic response.

Travel Bans

The COVID-19 pandemic led to the widespread use of NPIs, including travel bans, to limit the spread of the virus. By restricting international and domestic movement, governments aimed to prevent the importation of cases, control outbreaks, and protect public health systems from being overwhelmed. While these measures were effective in slowing transmission, they also had significant economic and social consequences. Understanding the role of travel bans as an NPI helps policymakers balance public health priorities with economic stability and personal freedoms in future global health crises.

Travel Ban Policies in the United States (2020–2025)

2020 Strict and Expanding Bans: In response to the COVID-19 outbreak, the United States imposed its first travel restriction on January 31, 2020, targeting travelers from China. Over the following months, bans extended to Iran, the Schengen Area, the United Kingdom, Ireland, and others. By March, nonessential travel across U.S. borders with Canada and Mexico was halted. Air traffic declined sharply, and several states implemented quarantine mandates for incoming travelers. While no national domestic travel ban was issued, interstate travel advisories were common (CDC, 2024c).

2021 Variant-Driven Adjustments: In early 2021, all international travelers were required to present a negative COVID-19 test. As new variants emerged, such as Delta, regional bans were reinstated. In November, the United States reopened to fully vaccinated travelers from 33 countries. However, the Omicron variant led to brief renewed restrictions on southern African nations (CDC, 2024c).

2022 Transition to Risk Mitigation: The United States phased out travel bans in favor of vaccination and testing requirements. By mid-2022, the testing mandate for international air travel was dropped, and land borders with Canada and Mexico were fully reopened (CDC, 2024c).

2023–2025 Normalization of Travel: By 2023, all COVID-specific travel restrictions, including vaccination and testing requirements, were lifted. The United States resumed standard border and visa protocols, shifting its focus to general health screening and voluntary travel guidance (CDC, 2024b, 2025).

Global Approaches to Travel Bans

Around the world, travel bans emerged as one of the first defensive measures against COVID-19, particularly during the early stages of the pandemic. Countries varied significantly in their implementation—some enacted full border closures, while others used selective entry bans, quarantine protocols, or vaccine requirements. As the pandemic evolved and community transmission became widespread, the utility of travel bans diminished, and most nations shifted toward risk mitigation strategies. Table 12.6 outlines the progression of travel-ban policies across selected countries from 2020 to 2025, offering insight into how national responses adapted to changing epidemiological and political contexts.

Table 12.6 Travel Restrictions of Select Regions (2020–2025)

Region	*2020*	*2021*	*2022*	*2023–2025*
China	Full border closure to foreigners; some exceptions	Vaccination and 2 tests required	Lifting of "Zero COVID" in Dec	Fully reopened with minimal restrictions
New Zealand	Border closure to non-citizens	Full vaccination for non-citizens	Borders reopened	Travel fully normalized
Australia	Strict restrictions for foreigners; 14-day quarantine	Reopened for vaccinated visa holders	Reopened for all visa holders	Open borders
The United Kingdom	Bans on select regions; full lockdowns	Traffic light system; restrictions based upon country's "color"	Restrictions lifted; testing required for travelers from China	Fully reopened, no COVID travel rules
Europe (Schengen)	Borders closed internally and externally	Reopened with EU digital COVID certificate	All intra-EU travel restrictions lifted	Standard visa and travel rules resumed
Taiwan	Early and strict border control; near full closure	Strict border control measures remain	Gradual easing of border controls and shortened quarantine periods	Normal entry resumed with no COVID restrictions
Japan	Banned nearly all foreign travelers	Gradual easing, but reversed due to Omicron	Opened to tourists in late 2022 with certain restrictions	Travel fully restored, no COVID bans

Sources: Adapted from: Huld (2022), NZ Royal Commission (2024), Ministry of Business, Innovation and Employment of New Zealand (2023), Parliament of Australia (2023), UK Government (2020), European Commission (n.d.), European Union (2020), Taiwan Ministry of Health and Welfare (2020), Ministry of Foreign Affairs of Japan (2020), Consulate-General of Japan in Seattle (2022), Ministry of Health, Labour and Welfare of Japan (n.d.), McElhinney (2020).

Lessons Learned

Travel restrictions can delay viral entry and buy time early in a pandemic, but they are not effective long-term once community transmission is widespread. They are best seen as temporary tools rather than sustained containment strategies, particularly given their global economic and diplomatic impacts.

Contact Tracing and Quarantine

Contact tracing and quarantining emerged as critical NPIs during the COVID-19 pandemic. Contact tracing involves identifying and notifying individuals who may have been exposed to the virus, while quarantining isolates potentially infected individuals to prevent further transmission. These strategies helped break the chain of viral spread, especially in the early stages of the pandemic, and were key to managing localized outbreaks. However, they also posed logistical challenges and required significant resources. Understanding the role of these NPIs highlights the balance between effective disease control and societal impact, providing valuable lessons for future global health emergencies.

Contact Tracing and Quarantine Policies in the United States (2020–2025)

2020 Rapid Scaling, Uneven Implementation: In the early months of the pandemic, the CDC and state health departments rapidly launched manual contact tracing programs. Thousands of contact tracers were hired across the United States, aiming to identify and isolate potential exposures. Quarantine protocols required close contacts to quarantine for 14 days, and infected individuals to isolate for 10–14 days, regardless of symptoms. However, these efforts faced major limitations due to asymptomatic transmission, testing delays, and public skepticism. The United States did not adopt a national digital contact tracing app, as privacy concerns limited the use and effectiveness of digital tools (CDC, 2024c).

2021 Fatigue and Focused Response: As vaccines became widely available, quarantine and isolation guidelines evolved. Fully vaccinated individuals were exempt from quarantine after exposure unless symptomatic. The CDC shortened recommended isolation to five days followed by five days of masking. With widespread community transmission and new variants, contact tracing was gradually scaled back, especially outside of high-risk settings (CDC, 2024c).

2022 De-Prioritization of Contact Tracing: During the Omicron wave, the CDC and many jurisdictions acknowledged that traditional contact tracing was no longer effective given the variant's high transmissibility and short incubation period. The focus shifted to protecting vulnerable environments like healthcare and long-term care facilities. For the general public, quarantine was no longer required for most exposures, with guidance emphasizing self-monitoring and masking (CDC, 2024c).

2023–2025 Voluntary and Situational Practices: By 2023, formal contact tracing programs had ended. Isolation was only recommended for those who tested positive or showed symptoms. Public health strategy transitioned toward personal responsibility, with institutions such as schools and workplaces setting their own exposure protocols. National policy emphasized flexibility, individual judgment, and risk-based decision-making (CDC, 2024b).

Global Approaches to Contact Tracing and Quarantine Policies

Throughout the COVID-19 pandemic, countries around the world adopted varying approaches to contact tracing and quarantine, reflecting differences in public health infrastructure, digital privacy norms, and levels of community transmission. Nations with strong central coordination and public trust implemented aggressive tracing and

Table 12.7 Contact Tracing and Quarantining Policies of Select Regions (2020–2025)

Region	*2020*	*2021*	*2022*	*2023–2025*
South Korea	Data collected from credit cards, hospital logs, cell phone, and CCTV; KI-Pass	14-day quarantine strictly enforced; fines for violation	Eased to 7-day, then removed in 2022	Shift to an "endemic" approach
The United Kingdom	NHS COVID-19 app; phone and manual tracing	"Pingdemic" led to mass 10-day quarantines	Quarantine rules removed early 2022	No contact tracing or quarantine
Germany	Corona Warn App launched	Digital pass used for entry	Tracing and quarantine phased out mid-2022	No national policy; self-monitoring only
Australia	Phone interviews and COVIDSafe app used	Case-initiated contact tracing method adopted	Quarantine measures removed	Normalized; no tracing/ quarantine
New Zealand	Swift contact tracing using app; MIQ launched	MIQ extends facilities	MIQ ended in mid-2022	No tracing/ quarantine policies now
Sweden	Minimal tracing; voluntary reporting	No mandatory quarantine	Continued light-touch approach	No policies in place
Taiwan	Advanced digital tracing; QR-code check-ins	1922 SMS contact tracing system	Eased quarantine in late 2022	No quarantine; digital tracing retired

Sources: Adapted from: Kim et al. (n.d.), Wieler et al. (n.d.), The Korea Times (2024), BBC (2020, 2021), UK Government (2020), Deutsche Welle (20222), Bundesministerium für Gesundheit (n.d.), Thurau (2020), Australian Government (n.d.), Shearer et al. (2024), Victoria Department of Health (2022), NZ Royal Commission (2024), Ministry of Business, Innovation and Employment of New Zealand (2023), Claeson & Hanson (2021), Travel Bans (2024), Taipei Times (2021), Taiwan Republic of China (2022), Taiwan Ministry of Health and Welfare (2020).

centralized quarantine measures, while others relied on voluntary compliance or phased out efforts as the pandemic evolved. Table 12.7 outlines contact tracing and quarantine strategies across selected countries from 2020 to 2025, highlighting key shifts from intensive early interventions to individualized risk management.

Lessons Learned

Contact tracing and quarantine were vital early tools, especially in low-transmission settings. Over time, guidelines became shorter and more targeted.

By 2022, high case volumes made broad contact tracing and quarantine impractical. From 2023 onward, these measures became voluntary and focused on high-risk settings. The United States and other countries shifted toward personal responsibility of symptom monitoring, testing, and risk-based decisions, highlighting the limits of tracing and quarantine once widespread transmission is established.

Conclusion

The implementation of NPIs, including masking, social distancing, hand hygiene, closures, quarantining, and contact tracing played a critical role in controlling the spread of COVID-19, especially in the early stages of the pandemic when pharmaceutical interventions were not yet available. These strategies, while varying in effectiveness and public acceptance across regions, collectively helped reduce transmission, protect vulnerable populations, and buy time for medical advancements. In the following section, we discuss the various vaccines and treatments developed throughout the pandemic.

References

Australian Commission on Safety and Quality in Health Care. (2019). *National hand hygiene initiative*. Australian Commission on Safety and Quality in Health Care. https://www.safetyandquality.gov.au/our-work/infection-prevention-and-control/national-hand-hygiene-initiative

Australian Government. (n.d.). *COVIDSafe legislation*. Australian Government. https://www.ag.gov.au/rights-and-protections/privacy/covidsafe-legislation

Australian Government Department of the Prime Minister and Cabinet. (2024). COVID-19 Response Inquiry Summary Report: Lessons for the next crisis. In *Australian Government Department of the Prime Minister and Cabinet*. https://www.pmc.gov.au/resources/covid-19-response-inquiry-summary-report-lessons-next-crisis/introduction#the-transition-recovery-phase-december-2021-to-the-present-day

Ba, Z., Li, Y., Ma, J., Qin, Y., Tian, J., Meng, Y., Yi, J., Zhang, Y., & Chen, F. (2023). Reflections on the dynamic zero-COVID policy in China. *Preventive Medicine Reports*, *36*(102466), 102466–102466. https://doi.org/10.1016/j.pmedr.2023.102466

BBC. (2020, September 24). *Coronavirus: NHS contact tracing app available in England and Wales*. BBC Newsround. https://www.bbc.co.uk/newsround/54116886

BBC. (2021, July 26). *What is the "pingdemic" and why does it mean empty shelves in the supermarkets?* BBC. https://www.bbc.co.uk/newsround/57926014

Bundesministerium fur Gesundheit. (n.d.). *Coronavirus pandemic: What happened when?* Bundesgesundheitsministerium.de. https://www.bundesgesundheitsministerium.de/coronavirus/chronik-coronavirus.html

CDC. (2024a, March 1). *Background for CDC's updated respiratory virus guidance*. Cdc.gov. https://www.cdc.gov/respiratory-viruses/guidance/background.html

CDC. (2024b, March 1). *CDC updates and simplifies respiratory virus recommendations*. CDC. https://www.cdc.gov/media/releases/2024/p0301-respiratory-virus.html

CDC. (2024c, March 1). *Respiratory virus guidance*. CDC. https://www.cdc.gov/respiratory-viruses/guidance/?CDC_AAref_Val=https://www.cdc.gov/respiratory-viruses/guidance/respiratory-virus-guidance.html

CDC. (2024d, July 8). *CDC Museum COVID-19 timeline*. CDC. https://www.cdc.gov/museum/timeline/covid19.html#Early-2021

CDC. (2025, April 18). *Air travel*. CDC. https://www.cdc.gov/yellow-book/hcp/travel-air-sea/air-travel.html

Claeson, M., & Hanson, S. (2021). COVID-19 and the Swedish enigma. *The Lancet*, *397*(10271). https://doi.org/10.1016/s0140-6736(20)32750-1

CNN, E. M. (2021, January 22). *European countries mandate medical-grade masks over cloth face coverings*. CNN. https://www.cnn.com/2021/01/22/europe/europe-covid-medical-masks-intl/index.html

Consulate-General of Japan in Seattle. (2022, May 26). *Reviewed requirements of on-arrival COVID-19 testing and quarantine period after entry to Japan (new border measures (28)) | Consulate-general of Japan in Seattle*. Consulate-General of Japan in Seattle. https://www.seattle.us.emb-japan.go.jp/itpr_en/20220526_border28.html

Deutsche Welle. (2022, October 1). *New German COVID rules come into force*. Dw.com; Deutsche Welle. https://www.dw.com/en/new-german-covid-19-rules-come-into-force-as-infections-rise-in-colder-months/a-63305695

European Chamber of Commerce in Korea. (2022, April 15). *COVID-19 update (April 15, 2022)*. European Chamber of Commerce in Korea. https://ecck.or.kr/covid-19-update-april-15-2022/

European Commission. (n.d.). *Travel during the Coronavirus pandemic*. European Commission. https://commission.europa.eu/strategy-and-policy/coronavirus-response/travel-during-coronavirus-pandemic_en

European Union. (2020, March 16). *COVID-19: Temporary restriction on non-essential travel to the EU*. European Union. https://eur-lex.europa.eu/legal-content/EN/TXT/?uri=CELEX%3A52020DC0115

Feuer, W., & Higgins-Dunn, N. (2021, March 16). *A year later, Trump's '15 days to slow the spread' campaign shows how little we knew about Covid*. CNBC. https://www.cnbc.com/2021/03/16/covid-a-year-later-trumps-15-days-to-slow-the-spread-pledge-shows-how-little-we-knew.html

GOV.UK. (2020, June 26). *Review of two metre social distancing guidance*. GOV.UK. https://www.gov.uk/government/publications/review-of-two-metre-social-distancing-guidance/review-of-two-metre-social-distancing-guidance

Heath, S. (2022, August 3). *What are the current Covid rules in England?* Covid Aid Charity. https://covidaidcharity.org/advice-and-information/current-covid-rules-england

Hobbs, A., & Bunn, S. (2020). COVID-19: July update on face masks and face coverings for the general public. *UK Parliament*. https://post.parliament.uk/covid-19-july-update-on-face-masks-and-face-coverings-for-the-general-public/

Huld, A. (2022, December 22). *China travel restrictions 2021/22 – latest travel and entry requirements*. China Briefing News. https://www.china-briefing.com/news/china-travel-restrictions-2021-2022-an-explainer-updated/

Institute for Government. (n.d.). *Timeline of UK government Coronavirus lockdowns and measures, March 2020 to December 2021*.

Kavaliunas, A., Ocaya, P., Mumper, J., Lindfeldt, I., & Kyhlstedt, M. (2020). Swedish policy analysis for Covid-19. *Health Policy and Technology*, *9*(4). https://doi.org/10.1016/j.hlpt.2020.08.009

Kim, H., & Choi, S.-H. (2023, January 30). South Korea drops indoor anti-COVID mask mandate, infection fears linger. *Reuters*. https://www.reuters.com/world/asia-pacific/south-korea-drops-indoor-anti-covid-mask-mandate-infection-fears-linger-2023-01-30/

Kim, J.-H., Ah-Reum An, J., Oh, S. J., Oh, J., & Lee, J.-K. (n.d.). *Emerging COVID-19 success story: South Korea learned the lessons of MERS*. Exemplars.health. https://www.exemplars.health/emerging-topics/epidemic-preparedness-and-response/covid-19/south-korea

Lai, C.-C., Yen, M.-Y., Lee, P.-I., & Hsueh, P.-R. (2020). How to keep COVID-19 at Bay: A Taiwanese perspective. *Journal of Epidemiology and Global Health*, *11*(1). https://doi.org/10.2991/jegh.k.201028.001

Lim, S., & Sohn, M. (2022). How to cope with emerging viral diseases: Lessons from South Korea's strategy for COVID-19, and collateral damage to cardiometabolic health. *The Lancet Regional Health – Western Pacific*, *30*(100581), 100581. https://doi.org/10.1016/j.lanwpc.2022.100581

McElhinney, D. (2021, December 2). *Japan's travel ban spells anguish for foreigners, businesses*. Aljazeera. https://www.aljazeera.com/economy/2021/12/2/japans-travel-ban-spells-anguish-for-foreign-community

Ministry of Business, Innovation and Employment of New Zealand. (2023, June). *MIQ timeline | Ministry of business, innovation & employment*. Govt.nz. https://www.mbie.govt.nz/immigration-and-tourism/isolation-and-quarantine/managed-isolation-and-quarantine/about-miq/miq-timeline

Ministry of Education, Culture, Sports, Science and Technology – Japan. (n.d.). *Information on MEXT's measures against COVID-19*. MEXT. https://www.mext.go.jp/en/mext_00006.html

Ministry of Foreign Affairs of Japan. (2020, March 18). *Strengthening border measures related to novel Coronavirus (COVID-19): Visa restrictions*. Ministry of Foreign Affairs of Japan. https://www.mofa.go.jp/ca/fna/page6e_000199.html

Ministry of Health, Labour and Welfare of Japan. (n.d.). *COVID-19: Current Japanese border measures*. Ministry of Health, Labour and Welfare of Japan. https://www.mhlw.go.jp/stf/covid-19/bordercontrol.html

Morton, B. (2021, July 12). Covid: England lockdown rules to end on 19 July, PM confirms. *BBC News*. https://www.bbc.com/news/uk-57809691

Norberg, J. (2023, August 29). *Sweden during the pandemic*. Cato.org. https://www.cato.org/policy-analysis/sweden-during-pandemic#

NZ Royal Commission. (2024). Whītiki Aotearoa: Lessons from COVID-19 to prepare Aotearoa New Zealand for a future pandemic. In *NZ Royal Commission*. https://www.covid19lessons.royalcommission.nz/reports-lessons-learned/main-report/part-two/1-1-timeline-of-key-events/

Otte, J. (2021, November 29). Covid: As rules on mask wearing in England return, what exactly is the law? *The Guardian*. https://www.theguardian.com/world/2021/nov/29/covid-as-rules-on-mask-wearing-in-england-return-what-exactly-is-the-law

Parliament of Australia. (2023). Report 494: Inquiry into the Department of Foreign Affairs and Trade's crisis management arrangements. In *Parliament of Australia* (pp. 35–26). https://www.aph.gov.au/Parliamentary_Business/Committees/Joint/Public_Accounts_and_Audit/DFATcrisismanagement/Report_494_Inquiry_into_the_Department_of_Foreign_Affairs_and_Trades_crisis_management_arrangem/C_Timeline_of_key_events?utm_source=chatgpt.com

Penn, M. (2021, April 5). *Working timeline of Covid-19 in Japan*. SNA Japan. https://shingetsunewsagency.com/2021/04/05/working-timeline-of-covid-19-in-japan/

Rajapaksa, S., & Alvarez, E. (2023). *Sweden physical distancing policies and epidemiology from January 2020 – August 2022: A case report. Policy Frameworks and Epidemiology of COVID-19 Working Group*. https://covid19-policies.healthsci.mcmaster.ca/wp-content/uploads/2023/10/Sweden-physical-distancing-policies-and-epidemiology-from-January-2020-August-2022-A-case-report.pdf

Read, B., McNulty, C. A. M., Verlander, N. Q., Moss, N., & Lecky, D. M. (2022). Comparing public knowledge around value of hand and respiratory hygiene, vaccination, and pre- and post-national COVID-19 lockdown in England. *Public Health*, *212*, 76–83. https://doi.org/10.1016/j.puhe.2022.08.015

Reserve Bank of Australia. (n.d.). *The COVID-19 Pandemic: 2020 to 2021*. https://www.rba.gov.au/education/resources/explainers/pdf/the-covid-19-pandemic-2020-to-2021.pdf

Schmitz, R. (2020, April 27). *Masks become compulsory in Germany as lockdown restrictions slowly ease*. NPR. https://www.npr.org/sections/coronavirus-live-updates/2020/04/27/845535990/masks-become-compulsory-in-germany-as-lockdown-restrictions-slowly-ease

Seoul Metropolitan Government. (2022, May 4). *Masks no longer mandatory outdoors starting May 2, 2022 (exceptions apply) -*. Seoul Metropolitan Government. https://english.seoul.go.kr/masks-no-longer-mandatory-outdoors-starting-may-2-2022-exceptions-apply/

Shearer, F. M., McCaw, J. M., Ryan, G. E., Hao, T., Tierney, N. J., Lydeamore, M. J., Wu, L., Ward, K., Ellis, S., Wood, J., McVernon, J., & Golding, N. (2024). Estimating the impact of test–trace–isolate–quarantine systems on SARS-CoV-2 transmission in Australia. *Epidemics*, *47*, 100764–100764. https://doi.org/10.1016/j.epidem.2024.100764

Simmons & Simmons. (2022, April 12). *COVID-19: New occupational health and safety regulation for Germany*. Simmons-Simmons.com. https://www.simmons-simmons.com/en/publications/ckh1rs2cv0vmc0931oa7w6y9h/covid-19-update-on-lockdown-measures-in-germany

Song, W., Horton, J., & Howell, J. (2023, January 16). *China Covid: How many cases and deaths are there?* BBC. https://www.bbc.com/news/59882774

Suzuki, R., Iizuka, Y., Sugawara, H., & Lefor, A. K.. (2024). Wearing masks is easy but taking them off is difficult – A situation in Japan during COVID-19 pandemic and after. *Dialogues in Health*, *4*, 100172–100172. https://doi.org/10.1016/j.dialog.2024.100172

Taipei Times. (2021, May 24). COVID-19: SMS registration used for tracing "confirmed cases." *Taipei Times*. https://www.taipeitimes.com/News/taiwan/archives/2021/05/24/2003757951

Taiwan Centers for Disease and Control. (2022, November 28). *Taiwan To ease current mask mandate and related epidemic prevention measures starting December 1*. Cdc.gov.tw. https://www.cdc.gov.tw/En/Bulletin/Detail/VRVYABkMZ3OLkKDMQk1RFQ?typeid=158

Taiwan Ministry of Health and Welfare. (2020, May 14). *Crucial Policy for Combating COVID-19*. Ministry of Health and Welfare. https://covid19.mohw.gov.tw/en/sp-timeline0-206.html

Taiwan Republic of China. (2022, July 5). *Entry restrictions for foreigners to Taiwan in response to COVID-19 outbreak*. https://www.taiwanembassy.org/va_en/post/4343.html

Takebayashi, M., Kaneda, Y., Namba, M., Yamashiro, A., & Takebayashi, K.. (2023). Assessing hand sanitizer usage in Japanese elderly day care centers: An observational and interventional study. *Cureus*, *15*(10). https://doi.org/10.7759/cureus.46834

The Korea Times. (2024, April 19). Korea to fully shift to "endemic" from COVID-19 pandemic starting next month. *The Korea Times*. https://www.koreatimes.co.kr/southkorea/society/20240419/korea-to-fully-shift-to-endemic-from-covid-19-pandemic-starting-next-month

Thurau, J. (2020, October 23). *Germany's Coronavirus app gets a boost*. Deutsche Welle. https://www.dw.com/en/germanys-coronavirus-app-goes-international-and-gets-a-boost/a-55363937

Travel Bans. (2024). *Sweden – Quarantine, travel regulations, Coronavirus regulations, travel bans – travelbans*. Travel Bans. https://travelbans.org/en/europe/sweden/quarantine#content

U.S. Embassy & Consulates in Japan. (2021, April 26). *Health alert – U.S. Embassy Tokyo (April 26, 2021)*. U.S. Embassy & Consulates in Japan. https://jp.usembassy.gov/health-alert-u-s-embassy-tokyo-april-26-2021/

UK Government. (2020, March 12). *COVID-19: Guidance for households with possible Coronavirus infection*. GOV.UK. https://www.gov.uk/government/publications/covid-19-stay-at-home-guidance#full-publication-update-history

UK Government. (2021a, April 9). *Global travel taskforce sets out framework to safely reopen international travel*. GOV.UK; Johnson Conservative Government. https://www.gov.uk/government/news/global-travel-taskforce-sets-out-framework-to-safely-reopen-international-travel

UK Government. (2021b, June 22). *Travel to England from another country during Coronavirus (COVID-19)*. GOV.UK. https://www.gov.uk/guidance/travel-to-england-from-another-country-during-coronavirus-covid-19#full-publication-update-history

UK Health Security Agency. (2022, April 1). *Living safely with respiratory infections, including COVID-19*. GOV.UK. https://www.gov.uk/guidance/living-safely-with-respiratory-infections-including-covid-19

Victoria Department of Health. (2022). *Quarantine isolation and testing order*. Vic.gov.au. https://www.health.vic.gov.au/covid-19/quarantine-isolation-and-testing-order

Wieler, L., Rexroth, U., & Gottschalk, R. (n.d.). *Emerging COVID-19 success story: The challenge of maintaining progress*. Exemplars. https://www.exemplars.health/emerging-topics/epidemic-preparedness-and-response/covid-19/germany

Wiemann, T. (2020, October 15). *Global Handwashing Day 2020*. News.ophardt.com. https://news.ophardt.com/en/global-handwashing-day-2020-handhygiene

World Health Organization. (2020). Calibrating long-term non-pharmaceutical interventions for COVID-19. Principles and facilitation tools. In *who.int*. https://iris.who.int/bitstream/handle/10665/332099/WPR-DSE-2020-018-eng.pdf?sequence=8

13 Vaccines and Treatments

Core Pillars of Pandemic Control

The global response to COVID-19 led to the rapid development of vaccines and treatments that dramatically reduced severe illness and mortality. Over 14 countries produced vaccines using diverse technologies: mRNA, protein subunit, inactivated virus, and viral vector, with varying efficacy. Treatment strategies evolved from repurposed drugs to targeted antivirals and monoclonal antibodies, adapting to emerging variants. While high-income countries achieved broad vaccine coverage, disparities remain, especially in low-income regions. However, countries like Nicaragua demonstrated how strong public health infrastructure and community-based approaches can overcome these gaps. Continued innovation and equitable access remain crucial as the world transitions from emergency response to long-term management.

COVID-19 Vaccines: Types Available Globally and Their Efficacy

The development of COVID-19 vaccines was a remarkable global effort in mitigating the impact caused by the pandemic, with 14 countries leading the charge in creating and distributing vaccines. These vaccines utilized a range of technologies, and their efficacy varied across regions and against different variants of the virus. Table 13.1 outlines the manufacturer, origin, type, and initial efficacy of various COVID-19 vaccines.

COVID-19 Treatments: A Chronological Timeline

The development of treatments for COVID-19 progressed rapidly as the global medical community raced to combat a novel and highly infectious virus. Early in the pandemic, much of the focus was on repurposing existing drugs in a bid to offer immediate solutions, while researchers simultaneously explored targeted therapies. Over time, the approach evolved, with treatments becoming more sophisticated and variant-specific as new challenges emerged. This timeline highlights key stages in the evolving COVID-19 treatment strategy.

DOI: 10.4324/9781003595564-17

Table 13.1 Manufacturer, Origin, Type, and Initial Efficacy of COVID-19 Vaccines

Vaccine	*Manufacturer*	*Origin*	*Type*	*Clinical Efficacy (%)*
Comirnaty	Pfizer/BioNTech	Germany, the United States	mRNA	**95**
Spikevax	Moderna	The United States	mRNA	**94.1**
Soberana Plus (FINLAY-FR-1A)	Finlay Institute	Cuba	Protein subunit	**92.40**
CIGB-66	Abdala	Cuba	Protein subunit	**92.28**
Sputnik V	The Gamaleya Center	Russia	Viral vector	**91.6**
MVC-COV1901	Medigen Biologics Corporation	Taiwan	Protein subunit	**91**
Nuvaxoid	Novavax	The United States	Protein subunit	**90**
COVIran Barekat (BIV1-CovIran)	Shifa Pharmed	Iran	Inactivated virus	**83.1**
QazVac (QazCovid-in)	Scientific Research Institute for Biological Safety Problems of the Republic of Kazakhstan	Kazakhstan	Inactivated virus	**82**
FakhraVac	Iran Ministry of Defense	Iran	Inactivated virus	**81.5**
ZF2001	Anhui Zhifei Longcom	China	Protein subunit	**81.4**
Sputnik Light	The Gamaleya Center	Russia	Viral vector	**78.6**
BBIBP-CorV	Sinopharm	China	Inactivated virus	**78.1**
Covaxin	Bharat Biotech	India	Inactivated virus	**77.8**
Vaxzevria	AstraZeneca	The United Kingdom	Viral vector	**73.7**
Covifenz	Medicago/GSK	Canada	Plant-based virus-like particle (VLP)	**71**
Soberana 02 (FINLAY-FR-2)	Finlay Institute	Cuba	Protein subunit	**71**
CoronaVac	Sinovac	China	Inactivated virus	**67.7**
ZyCoV-D	Zydus Cadila	India	DNA-based	**66.6**
Janssen	Johnson & Johnson	The United States	Viral vector	**66**
Convidecia	CanSino	China	Viral vector	**57.5**

(*Continued*)

Table 13.1 (Continued)

Vaccine	*Manufacturer*	*Origin*	*Type*	*Clinical Efficacy (%)*
Kostaive (ARCT-154)	Arcturus Therapeutics/ Meiji Saika Pharma	Japan	Self-amplifying mRNA (sa-mRNA)	**56.6**
Corbevax	Biological E. Limited	India	Protein subunit	**N/A**
EpiVacCorona	Vector Institute	Russia	Peptide-based	**N/A**
CoviVac	Chumakov Center	Russia	Inactivated virus	**N/A**
SKYCovione	SK Bioscience	South Korea	Recombinant protein subunit	**N/A**
Razi Cov Pars (RCP)	Razi Vaccine and Serum Research Institute, Iran	Iran	Recombinant protein subunit	**N/A**

Sources: Pfizer (2020), Czarska-Thorley (2021), Novavax (2022), Toledo-Romaní et al. (2021), Martínez (2021), Halperin et al. (2022), CDC (2022), Lee et al. (2024), WHO (2022), Mohraz et al. (2023), Beigel et al. (2020), The Gamaleya Institute (2021), Pramod et al. (2022), Lairun et al. (2022), Gavi (2021), Government of Canada (n.d.), AstraZeneca (n.d.), Farida et al. (2022), Dai et al. (2022), Hồ et al., (2024), Khairullin et al. (2022), Logunov et al. (2021), Solaymani-dodaran et al. (2022).

2020: Early Discoveries and Treatment Development

Initial efforts repurposed existing drugs like hydroxychloroquine, lopinavir/ritonavir, and convalescent plasma, but these showed little to no benefit in large trials. The first major breakthrough came mid-2020 with dexamethasone, a low-cost, widely available corticosteroid. The U.K.-based RECOVERY trial found dexamethasone reduced mortality by one-third in ventilated patients and one-fifth in those receiving oxygen only (The RECOVERY Collaborative Group, 2021). Within weeks of the RECOVERY trial's publication, health agencies worldwide, including the WHO and National Institutes of Health (NIH), endorsed its use. It quickly became the standard of care globally for hospitalized patients requiring respiratory support, though it showed no benefit in early disease stages.

Around the same time, remdesivir emerged as one of the first promising antiviral treatments. Originally developed for hepatitis C and Ebola, remdesivir works by inhibiting viral RNA replication. The NIH-sponsored Adaptive COVID-19 Treatment Trial (ACTT-1) demonstrated that patients receiving remdesivir recovered four days faster than those given placebo (Beigel et al., 2020). While the drug demonstrated clear benefits in reducing hospital stays, it did not significantly impact overall mortality rates. Its primary value lay in treating patients early in the disease course, before progression to critical stages requiring mechanical ventilation.

Late 2020: Monoclonal Antibody Therapies

As COVID-19 cases surged in late 2020, therapeutic options expanded to include treatments targeting early infection in high-risk outpatients. Monoclonal antibodies like bamlanivimab and REGEN-COV (casirivimab and imdevimab) were authorized for non-hospitalized patients at high risk for severe outcomes, blocking the virus's spike protein to prevent disease progression (Copin et al., 2021). These were most effective early in infection and faced logistical challenges that limited their widespread implementation. The requirement for intravenous administration in clinical settings created access barriers, particularly for those in remote areas. Limited supply amid high demand further restricted availability, and the lack of long-term data on efficacy raised questions about their sustained utility. Nevertheless, these therapies provided critical outpatient solutions at a time when vaccines were not yet widely available, offering a lifeline for those at highest risk for severe COVID-19 outcomes.

2021: Rise of Variants and Oral Antivirals

The Delta variant, first detected in India in October 2020 and spreading globally by spring 2021, represented a significant shift in the pandemic landscape. The WHO classified it as a "Variant of Concern" due to its 60% higher transmissibility compared to the Alpha variant. The variant's nine spike protein mutations contributed to its rapid spread and partial resistance to neutralizing antibodies (McCrone et al., 2022). Most monoclonal antibodies, including etesevimab, casirivimab, and imdevimab retained their effectiveness against Delta; however, bamlanivimab lost antiviral activity against this variant (Institut Pasteur, 2024).

By autumn 2021, the Omicron variant emerged with over 30 spike protein mutations. These extensive mutations enhanced Omicron's ability to evade immune responses generated by both vaccines and monoclonal antibodies. Approximately two-thirds of monoclonal antibodies in use or development lost their antiviral activity against Omicron (Institut Pasteur, 2024). However, AstraZeneca's Evusheld, a dual monoclonal antibody therapy for pre-exposure prevention of COVID-19, retained neutralizing activity against Omicron and was authorized for immunocompromised individuals or those unable to receive COVID-19 vaccines (AstraZeneca, 2021).

The development of oral antiviral treatments marked a significant milestone in the fight against COVID-19, particularly as more transmissible variants emerged. Molnupiravir became the first approved oral antiviral for SARS-CoV-2, inhibiting viral replication through viral error induction. By November 2021, the United Kingdom became the first country to approve molnupiravir for emergency use, providing a critical tool for managing COVID-19 in outpatient settings (Syed, 2022).

During this time, Pfizer was also developing its own oral antiviral treatment, Paxlovid, which soon emerged as a more effective option. Clinical trials demonstrated Paxlovid's impressive efficacy, reducing the risk of hospitalization or death by approximately 89% for unvaccinated, high-risk patients (Pfizer, 2021). Paxlovid combines two components: nirmatrelvir, which inhibits a key viral protease essential for replication, and ritonavir, which slows the breakdown of nirmatrelvir in the body to maintain effective drug levels. By December 2021, the U.S. FDA issued an EUA for Paxlovid, making it the first oral antiviral approved in the United States for treating COVID-19 (Pfizer, 2023).

2022: Clinical Implementation

Clinical adoption of Paxlovid faced significant challenges that limited its optimal utilization. Physician hesitancy in prescribing Paxlovid stemmed from multiple concerns, including potential rebound effects, high costs, and difficulties in accurately identifying high-risk individuals who would benefit most from treatment. Drug interaction concerns presented another major barrier, with studies indicating nearly half of potential patients were taking medications potentially contraindicated with Paxlovid. To expand access, the U.S. FDA expanded prescribing authority to pharmacists in July 2022. However, strict requirements, including the need to verify renal and hepatic function through recent health records, limited pharmacists's practical ability to provide prescriptions (Adams & Eid, 2023).

Clinical effectiveness questions also emerged as more data became available. While Pfizer's 2022 clinical trials demonstrated clear benefits for unvaccinated middle-aged adults, subsequent trials challenged assumptions about Paxlovid's effectiveness in certain populations (Hammond et al., 2024). A natural experiment in Ontario, where Paxlovid access was restricted to those 70 and older from April to November 2022, provided particularly compelling data. Despite a 118% increase in prescriptions for patients at age 70, researchers observed no corresponding reduction in COVID-19-related hospitalizations, overall hospitalizations, or mortality raising important questions about optimal targeting of this therapy (Mafi et al., 2025).

2023–2024: Regulatory Transitions and Innovation

In May 2023, the WHO declared an end to the COVID-19 pandemic as a global health emergency, marking a shift in the response to the virus. However, the need for effective prevention and treatment continues, especially for vulnerable populations. Authorization of Pemgarda, a specially engineered monoclonal antibody designed to prevent severe illness in high-risk populations, established itself as the sole COVID-19 pre-exposure prophylaxis available, addressing a critical need in preventive care for vulnerable populations. This authorization came as the U.S. FDA simultaneously revoked authorizations for four previously prominent monoclonal antibodies—Lilly's bebtelovimab, AstraZeneca's Evusheld, GSK's sotrovimab, and Regeneron's REGEN-COV—due to their reduced effectiveness against evolving variants (Food and Drug Administration, 2025).

The ongoing search for a broadly protective "pan-coronavirus" vaccine remains a priority. Promising candidates include nanoSTING, a nasal spray that can prevent various respiratory infections, and Duke University's combination COVID vaccine, designed to target multiple strains. Government initiatives such as Project NextGen are also dedicated to developing the next generation of COVID-19 vaccines and therapeutics (Fickman, 2024; Graff, 2024).

An Exploration of Global COVID-19 Vaccination Rates

Vaccination Rates by Region

Vaccination coverage across continents presents another insight into global immunization efforts. Regional disparities, shaped by healthcare capacity, vaccine access, and logistical constraints, remain evident. Table 13.2 outlines initial COVID-19 vaccination protocol completion by region, featuring countries with some of the highest and lowest vaccination rates within their region.

Vaccination Rates by Income

Vaccination rates are closely tied to national income levels. High-income and upper-middle-income countries report much higher COVID-19 vaccination coverage, compared to lower-middle-income and low-income countries. As of April

Table 13.2 Vaccination of Rates by Continent with Select Regions

Region	*Average Rate (%)*	*High Coverage Areas*	*Low Coverage Areas*
Europe	67	Portugal (85.5), Spain (85.2), Italy (83.0), Ireland (79.6), Germany (75.6), The United Kingdom (74.4)	Romania (42.3), Serbia (48.3), Ukraine (38.3), Bosnia and Herzegovina (26.4)
Asia	73.6	UAE (95.6), Singapore (92.9), China (90.1), Taiwan (88.8), South Korea (85.6), Japan (82.8), Saudi Arabia (79.0)	Afghanistan (45.3), Georgia (33.6), Iraq (18.0), Syria (10.5), Yemen (2.1)
North America	65.7	Nicaragua (91.0), Cuba (90.9), Costa Rica (86.0), Canada (81.8)	Guatemala (40.0), Bahamas (42.0), Jamaica (26.8), Haiti (3.2)
South America	78.4	Chile (90.5), Peru (85.8), Uruguay (85.6), Brazil (83.8), Ecuador (79.9), Argentina (76.9)	Venezuela (53.0), Bolivia (51.0), Paraguay (52.5), Guyana (46.8), Suriname (38.2)
Africa	32.1	Rwanda (76.2), Morocco (63.0)	Nigeria (42.0), Ethiopia (41.9), Algeria (14.3), DRC (14.1), Cameroon (11.6), Congo (10.8), Madagascar (8.6)
Oceania	63	New Zealand (83.6), Australia (82.6), Fiji (69.7)	Solomon Islands (32.6), Papua New Guinea (3.1)

Source: Mathieu et al. (2020).

2024, 70.6% of the global population had received at least one dose; however, only 32.7% of people living in low-income countries have received one dose (Minges, 2024). This disparity is further reflected in the number of doses administered per 100 people across income groups. As of August 2024, high-income countries administered 233.77 doses per 100 people, upper-middle-income countries administered 210.33 doses, lower-middle-income countries administered 140.93 doses, and low-income countries administered just 45.70 doses (Mathieu et al., 2020).

Table 13.2 reflects this general trend. For example, Africa, with many low-income countries, has an average vaccination rate of 32.1%, while Asia, home to several high-income countries, averages 73.6%. Similarly, within regions, high-income countries like Portugal (85.5%) or the UAE (95.6%) far outpace lower-income counterparts like Haiti (3.2%) or Yemen (2.1%).

Impact of Economic Factors and Vaccine Hesitancy

While national income plays a significant role in vaccination uptake, vaccine hesitancy is just as critical. A cross-sectional analysis explored vaccination rates across 145 countries at four time intervals, 6, 12, 18, and 24 months, following the global rollout of COVID-19 vaccinations. The analysis focused on two primary factors: GDP per capita (a proxy for national income) and vaccine hesitancy (defined as the percentage of individuals that strongly disagree that vaccines are safe). In six months, countries in the top 20% GDP per capita achieved vaccination rates 22% higher than those in the bottom 20%. The disparity widened to 38% by 12 months. The effect of vaccine distrust became significant at 12 months and increased at 24 months, particularly in lower-income countries. By 24 months, countries with high levels of vaccination distrust had 17% lower vaccination rates than countries with low distrust (Moradpour et al., 2023).

Nicaragua's Success in Overcoming Vaccine Inequity

Generally, lower-income countries have lower vaccination rates; however, Nicaragua, one of the poorest countries in North America, exceeded most high-income countries in vaccination coverage. Nicaragua managed to increase its vaccine coverage through a combination of strong government commitment, strategic planning, community engagement, and international support. Since 2007, Nicaragua has been making significant investments in strengthening their public health services, increasing their number of doctors and building new hospitals and health facilities. Their long-term focus on public health greatly benefited their preparedness and response to the pandemic. In January 2020, a special commission was created to tackle the virus threat before the country detected its first case. The following month, a joint protocol with the Pan-American Health Organization was created. The government prioritized vaccination efforts, allocating resources and securing doses through global initiatives like COVAX. A community-based approach was used, where community health teams visited approximately 5 million house visits to educate people, identify possible COVID-19 cases, and counteract misinformation.

A cornerstone of their success was the *Corta el Contagio* ("Cut the Transmission") campaign, a comprehensive multi-ethnic health initiative implemented by the Ministry of Health and supported by UNICEF. This campaign addressed the significant challenge of vaccine hesitancy through culturally adapted communication strategies. The program utilized community leaders and volunteers to disseminate information, supported by educational kits containing detailed materials on prevention protocols, patient care guidelines, and vaccination importance. The cultural sensitivity of this approach proved crucial in effectively reaching Nicaragua's diverse population (Pan American Health Organization, 2021; Perry, 2020; UNICEF, 2022).

Conclusion

The global response to COVID-19 showcased an unprecedented collaboration in science, public health, and policy. The rapid development and distribution of vaccines, spanning diverse technologies and global origins, significantly reduced severe disease and death. Simultaneously, treatment strategies evolved from repurposed drugs to advanced antivirals and monoclonal antibodies, adapting to new variants and shifting clinical needs. Although disparities in vaccine access and uptake exist, success stories like Nicaragua's highlight the impact of strong public health infrastructure and community engagement. While advancements provided protection to the broader population, vulnerable groups continued to face severe outcomes and barriers to care. The following chapter examines the disproportionate impact of COVID-19 on high-risk groups, including those with chronic illnesses, obesity, immunodeficiencies, and older adults.

References

Adams, A. J., & Eid, D. D. (2023). Federal pharmacist Paxlovid prescribing authority: A model policy or impediment to optimal care? *Exploratory Research in Clinical and Social Pharmacy*, *9*, 100244. https://doi.org/10.1016/j.rcsop.2023.100244

AstraZeneca. (n.d.). *Annex I: Summary of product characteristics*. https://www.ema.europa.eu/en/documents/product-information/vaxzevria-epar-product-information_en.pdf

AstraZeneca. (2021, December 8). *Evusheld (formerly AZD7442) long-acting antibody combination authorised for emergency use in the US for pre-exposure prophylaxis (prevention) of COVID-19*. AstraZeneca. https://www.astrazeneca.com/media-centre/press-releases/2021/evusheld-long-acting-antibody-combination-authorised-for-emergency-use-in-the-us-for-pre-exposure-prophylaxis-prevention-of-covid-19.html#

Beigel, J. H., Tomashek, K. M., Dodd, L. E., Mehta, A. K., Zingman, B. S., Kalil, A. C., Hohmann, E., Chu, H. Y., Luetkemeyer, A., Kline, S., Lopez de Castilla, D., Finberg, R. W., Dierberg, K., Tapson, V., Hsieh, L., Patterson, T. F., Paredes, R., Sweeney, D. A., Short, W. R., & Touloumi, G. (2020). Remdesivir for the treatment of Covid-19—Final report. *New England Journal of Medicine*, *383*(19), 1813–1826. https://doi.org/10.1056/nejmoa2007764

CDC. (2022, August 22). *Grading of recommendations, assessment, development, and evaluation (GRADE): Janssen COVID-19 vaccine*. Advisory Committee on Immunization Practices (ACIP); CDC. https://www.cdc.gov/acip/grade/covid-19-janssen-vaccine.html

Copin, R., Baum, A., Wloga, E., Pascal, K. E., Giordano, S., Fulton, B. O., Zhou, A., Negron, N., Lanza, K., Chan, N., Coppola, A., Chiu, J., Ni, M., Wei, Y., Atwal, G. S., Hernandez, A. R., Saotome, K., Zhou, Y., Franklin, M. C., & Hooper, A. T. (2021). The monoclonal antibody combination REGEN-COV protects against SARS-CoV-2 mutational escape in preclinical and human studies. *Cell*, *184*(15), 3949–3961.e11. https://doi.org/10.1016/j.cell.2021.06.002

Czarska-Thorley, D. (2021). *Spikevax (previously COVID-19 vaccine moderna)*. European Medicines Agency. https://www.ema.europa.eu/en/medicines/human/EPAR/spikevax

Dai, L., Gao, L., Tao, L., Hadinegoro, S. R., Erkin, M., Ying, Z., He, P., Girsang, R. T., Vergara, H., Akram, J., Satari, H. I., Khaliq, T., Sughra, U., Celi, A. P., Li, F., Li, Y., Jiang, Z., Dalimova, D., Tuychiev, J., & Turdikulova, S. (2022). Efficacy and safety of the RBD-dimer–based Covid-19 vaccine ZF2001 in adults. *New England Journal of Medicine*, *386*(22), 2097–2111. https://doi.org/10.1056/nejmoa2202261

Fickman, L. (2024, August 6). *University of Houston researchers create new treatment and vaccine for flu and various coronaviruses*. Uh.edu; University of Houston. https://www.uh.edu/news-events/stories/2024/august/08062024-varadarajan-nanosting-rx-and-vaccine.php

Farida, I. A., Stanciole, E., Aden, B., Timoshkin, A., Najim, O., Zaher, A., Fatima, A. A., Mazrouie, A., Rizvi, T. A., & Mustafa, F. (2022). Impact of the Sinopharm's BBIBP-CorV vaccine in preventing hospital admissions and death in infected vaccinees: Results from a retrospective study in the emirate of Abu Dhabi, United Arab Emirates (UAE). *Vaccine*, *40*(13), 2003–2010. https://doi.org/10.1016/j.vaccine.2022.02.039

Gavi. (2021, July 6). *India's "Covaxin" vaccine shows high efficacy against COVID-19 infections in phase 3 trial*. Gavi. https://www.gavi.org/vaccineswork/indias-covaxin-vaccine-shows-high-efficacy-against-covid-19-infections-phase-3

Government of Canada. (n.d.). *Medicago Covifenz COVID-19 vaccine*. Canada. https://www.canada.ca/en/health-canada/services/drugs-health-products/covid19-industry/drugs-vaccines-treatments/vaccines/medicago.html

Graff, F. (2024, February 22). *Human trials start this year on Duke's combo coronavirus vaccine*. PBS North Carolina. https://www.pbsnc.org/blogs/science/human-trials-start-this-year-on-dukes-combo-coronavirus-vaccine/

Halperin, S. A., Ye, L., MacKinnonCameron, D., Smith, B., Cahn, P. E., RuizPalacios, G. M., Ikram, A., Lanas, F., Guerrero, L., Raúl, S., Sued, O., Lioznov, Dmitry, A., Dzutseva, V., Parveen, G., Zhu, F., Leppan, L., Langley, J. M., Barreto, L., Gou, J., & Zhu, T. (2022). Final efficacy analysis, interim safety analysis, and immunogenicity of a single dose of recombinant novel coronavirus vaccine (adenovirus type 5 vector) in adults 18 years and older: An international, multicentre, randomised, doubleblinded, placebocontrolled phase 3 trial. *The Lancet*, *399*(10321), 237–248. https://doi.org/10.1016/S0140-6736(21)02753-7

Hammond, J., Fountaine, R. J., Yunis, C., Fleishaker, D., Almas, M., Bao, W., Wisemandle, W., Baniecki, M. L., Hendrick, V. M., Kalfov, V., Simón-Campos, J. A., Pypstra, R., & Rusnak, J. M. (2024). Nirmatrelvir for vaccinated or unvaccinated adult outpatients with Covid-19. *New England Journal of Medicine*, *390*(13), 1186–1195. https://doi.org/10.1056/nejmoa2309003

Hồ, N. T., Hughes, S. G., Ta, V. T., Phan, L. T., Đỗ, Q., Nguyễn, T. V., Thị, A., Mai, Nguyễn, L. V., Vinh, T. Q., Phạm, H. N., Chử, M. V., Nguyễn, T. T., Lương, Q. C., Vy, L., Nguyễn, T. V., Trần, L., Van, T., Nguyen, A. N., & Nguyen, N. (2024). Safety, immunogenicity and efficacy of the selfamplifying mRNA ARCT-154 COVID-19 vaccine: Pooled phase 1, 2, 3a and 3b randomized, controlled trials. *Nature Communications*, *15*(1), 4081. https://doi.org/10.1038/s41467-024-47905-1

Institut Pasteur. (2024, March 11). *COVID-19: Which monoclonal antibodies should be used for vulnerable individuals?* Institut Pasteur. https://www.pasteur.fr/en/research-journal/reports/covid-19-which-monoclonal-antibodies-should-be-used-vulnerable-individuals

Khairullin, B., Zakarya, K., Orynbayev, M., Abduraimov, Y., Kassenov, M., Sarsenbayeva, G., Sultankulova, K., Chervyakova, O., Myrzakhmetova, B., Nakhanov, A., Nurpeisova, A., Zhugunissov, K., Assanzhanova, N., Nurabayev, S., Kerimbayev, A., Yershebulov, Z., Burashev, Y., Kulmagambetov, I., Davlyatshin, T., & Sergeeva, M. (2022). Efficacy and safety of an inactivated wholevirion vaccine against COVID-19, QazCovid-in®, in healthy adults: A multicentre, randomised, single-blind, placebo-controlled phase 3 clinical trial with a 6-month follow-up. *eClinicalMedicine*, *50*. https://doi.org/10.1016/j.eclinm.2022.101526

Lairun, J., Li, Z., Zhang, X., Li, J., & Zhu, F. (2022). CoronaVac: A review of efficacy, safety, and immunogenicity of the inactivated vaccine against SARS-CoV-2. *Human Vaccines & Immunotherapeutics*, *18*(6), 2096970. https://doi.org/10.1080/21645515.2022.2096970

Lee, C.-Y., Kuo, H.-W., Liu, Y.-L., Chuang, J.-H., & Chou, J.-H. (2024, March). Population-based evaluation of vaccine effectiveness against SARS-CoV-2 infection, severe illness, and death, Taiwan. *Emerging Infectious Diseases Journal – CDC*, 30(3). wwwnc.cdc.gov, https://doi.org/10.3201/eid3003.230893

Logunov, D. Y., Dolzhikova, I. V., Shcheblyakov, D. V., Tukhvatulin, A. I., Zubkova, O. V., Dzharullaeva, A. S., Kovyrshina, A. V., Lubenets, N. L., Grousova, D. M., Erokhova, A. S., Botikov, A. G., Izhaeva, F. M., Popova, O., Ozharovskaya, T. A., Esmagambetov, I. B., Favorskaya, I. A., Zrelkin, D. I., Voronina, D. V., Shcherbinin, Dmitry, N., & Semikhin, A. S. (2021). Safety and efficacy of an rAd26 and rAd5 vector-based heterologous prime-boost COVID-19 vaccine: An interim analysis of a randomised controlled phase 3 trial in Russia. *The Lancet*, *397*(10275), 671–681. https://doi.org/10.1016/S0140-6736(21)00234-8

Mafi, J. N., Vangala, S., Kapral, M. K., Wu, P. E., Cui, M., Romanov, A., & Kahn, K. L. (2025). Hospitalizations and mortality among older adults with and without restricted access to Nirmatrelvir-Ritonavir. *JAMA*, *333*(13), 1172–1175. https://doi.org/10.1001/jama.2024.28099

Martínez, L. (2021, June 22). *Abdala, with three doses, demonstrates 92.28% efficacy*. Granma.cu. https://en.granma.cu/cuba/2021-06-22/abdala-with-three-doses-demonstrates-9228-efficacy

Mathieu, E., Ritchie, H., Rodés-Guirao, L., Appel, C., Gavrilov, D., Giattino, C., Hasell, J., Macdonald, B., Dattani, S., Beltekian, D., Ortiz-Ospina, E., & Roser, M. (2020). *Coronavirus (COVID-19) vaccinations*. Our World in Data. https://ourworldindata.org/covid-vaccinations

McCrone, J. T., Hill, V., Bajaj, S., Pena, R. E., Lambert, B. C., Inward, R., Bhatt, S., Volz, E., Ruis, C., Dellicour, S., Baele, G., Zarebski, A. E., Sadilek, A., Wu, N., Schneider, A., Ji, X., Raghwani, J., Jackson, B., Colquhoun, R., & O'Toole, Á. (2022). Context-specific emergence and growth of the SARS-CoV-2 delta variant. *Nature*, *610*(7930), 154–160. https://doi.org/10.1038/s41586-022-05200-3

Minges, M. (2024, April 24). *Q&A: Current global access to the COVID-19 vaccine*. American University. https://www.american.edu/alumni/news/q-a-with-public-health-expert.cfm

Mohraz, M., Vahdat, K., Ghamari, S., AbbasiKangevari, M., Ghasemi, E., Ghabdian, Y., Rezaei, N., Pouya, M. A., Abdoli, A., Malekpour, M., Koohgir, K., Moghaddam, S., Tabarsi, P., Moghadami, M., Khorvash, F., Khodashahi, R., Salehi, M., & Hosseini, H. (2023). Efficacy and safety of an inactivated virus-particle vaccine for SARS-CoV-2, BIV1-CovIran: Randomised, placebo controlled, double blind, multicentre, phase 3 clinical trial. *BMJ*, *382*, e070464. https://doi.org/10.1136/bmj-2023-070464

Moradpour, J., Shajarizadeh, A., Carter, J., Chit, A., & Grootendorst, P. (2023). The impact of national income and vaccine hesitancy on countrylevel COVID19 vaccine uptake. *PLoS ONE*, *18*(11), e0293184. https://doi.org/10.1371/journal.pone.0293184

Novavax. (2022). *Novavax and Serum Institute of India announce first emergency use authorization of Novavax' COVID-19 vaccine in adolescents ≥12 to <18 in India*. Novavax. https://ir.novavax.com/press-releases/2022-03-22-Novavax-and-Serum-Institute-of-India-Announce-First-Emergency-Use-Authorization-of-Novavax-COVID-19-Vaccine-in-Adolescents-12-to-18-in-India

Our World in Data. (2024). *Coronavirus (COVID-19) vaccinations – Statistics and research*. Our World in Data. https://ourworldindata.org/covid-vaccinations

Pan American Health Organization. (2021, March 16). *Nicaragua receives its first COVID-19 vaccines through the COVAX facility*. PAHO; World Health Organization. https://www.paho.org/en/news/16-3-2021-nicaragua-receives-its-first-covid-19-vaccines-through-covax-facility

Perry, J. (2020, May 30). *Nicaragua battles COVID-19 and a disinformation campaign*. Council on Hemispheric Affairs. https://coha.org/nicaragua-battles-covid-19-and-a-disinformation-campaign/

Pfizer. (2020, November 18). *Pfizer and BioNTech conclude phase 3 study of COVID-19 vaccine candidate, meeting all primary efficacy endpoints*. Pfizer. https://www.pfizer.com/news/press-release/press-release-detail/pfizer-and-biontech-conclude-phase-3-study-covid-19-vaccine

Pfizer. (2021, November 5). *Pfizer's novel COVID-19 oral antiviral treatment candidate reduced risk of hospitalization or death by 89% in interim analysis of phase 2/3 EPIC-HR study*. Pfizer. https://www.pfizer.com/news/press-release/press-release-detail/pfizers-novel-covid-19-oral-antiviral-treatment-candidate

Pfizer. (2023, May 25). *Pfizer's PAXLOVID™ receives FDA approval for adult patients at high risk of progression to severe COVID-19*. Pfizer. https://www.pfizer.com/news/press-release/press-release-detail/pfizers-paxlovidtm-receives-fda-approval-adult-patients

Pramod, S., Govindan, D., Ramasubramani, P., Kar, S. S., Aggarwal, R., Manoharan, N., Chinnakali, P., Thulasingam, M., Sarkar, S., & Thabah, M. M. (2022). Effectiveness of Covishield vaccine in preventing Covid19 – A testnegative casecontrol study. *Vaccine*, *40*(24), 3294–3297. https://doi.org/10.1016/j.vaccine.2022.02.014

Solaymani-dodaran, M., Basiri, P., Moradi, M., Gohari, K., Sheidaei, A., Ahi, M., Ansarifar, A., Rahimi, Z., Gholami, F., karimi Rahjerdi, A., Farahani, R. H., Naderi saffar, K., Ghasemi, S., Shooshtari, A., Honari, M., Mozafari, A., Khodaverdloo, S., & Forooghizadeh, M. (2022). Safety and efficacy of the FAKHRAVAC compared with BBIBP-Corv2 against SARS-CoV-2 in adults: A non-inferiority multi-center trial. *SSRN Electronic Journal*. https://doi.org/10.2139/ssrn.4249796

Syed, Y. Y. (2022). Molnupiravir: First approval. *Drugs*, *82*(4), 455–460. https://doi.org/10.1007/s40265-022-01684-5

The Gamaleya Center. (2021, June 2). *Sputnik light vaccine (the first component of Sputnik V vaccine) demonstrates 78.6–83.7% efficacy among the elderly in Argentina*. Sputnikvaccine. https://sputnikvaccine.com/newsroom/pressreleases/sputnik-light-vaccine-the-first-component-of-sputnik-v-vaccine-demonstrates-78-6-83-7-efficacy-among/

The RECOVERY Collaborative Group. (2021). Dexamethasone in hospitalized patients with Covid-19. *New England Journal of Medicine*, *384*(8), 693–704. https://doi.org/10.1056/nejmoa2021436

Toledo-Romaní, M. E., GarcíaCarmenate, M., ValenzuelaSilva, C., BaldoquínRodríguez, W., MartínezPérez, M., RodríguezGonzález, M., ParedesMoreno, B., MendozaHernández, I., Romero, G., SamónTabio, O., VelazcoVillares, P., BacallaoCastillo, J. P., LiceaMartín, E., RodríguezOrtega, M., HerreraMarrero, N., CaballeroGonzález, E., EgüesTorres, L., DuartesGonzález, R., GarcíaBlanco, S., & PérezCabrera, S. (2023). Safety and efficacy of the two doses conjugated protein based SOBERANA-02 COVID-19 vaccine and of a heterologous three-dose combination with SOBERANA-Plus: A double-blind, randomised, placebo-controlled phase 3 clinical trial. *The Lancet Regional Health – Americas, 18*. https://doi.org/10.1016/j.lana.2022.100423

U.S. Food and Drug Administration. (2025). *EUA archive*. U.S. Food and Drug Administration. https://www.fda.gov/emergency-preparedness-and-response/mcm-legal-regulatory-and-policy-framework/emergency-use-authorization-archived-information?utm_medium=email&utm_source=govdelivery#covid19

UNICEF. (2022, September 26). *Cut the transmission, the multi-ethnic health campaign that promoted vaccination*. UNICEF. https://www.unicef.org/nicaragua/en/stories/cut-transmission-multi-ethnic-health-campaign-promoted-vaccination

WHO. (2022, September 28). *The Novavax vaccine against COVID-19: What you need to know*. WHO. https://www.who.int/news-room/feature-stories/detail/the-novavax-vaccine-against-covid-19-what-you-need-to-know

14 High-Risk Factors

Understanding Vulnerable Groups in the Pandemic

The differential impact of COVID-19 on individuals can be attributed to varying levels of health resilience, influenced by factors such as chronic diseases, obesity, immunodeficiency, and age. These factors increase susceptibility to severe outcomes from the virus, potentially leading to serious complications or longer recovery times. The pandemic has highlighted the critical role of these factors in determining the severity of illness and has emphasized the need for tailored public health strategies to mitigate their effects.

Chronic Diseases

Chronic diseases, also known as noncommunicable diseases, are defined as conditions that last for a year or more and require long-term medical care or directly or indirectly affect daily life (Centers for Disease Control and Prevention (CDC), n.d.). Chronic diseases such as heart disease, cancer, and diabetes killed at least 43 million people in 2021. Of the 43 million deaths, an estimated 18 million deaths occurred in those before the age of 70 (World Health Organization (WHO), 2024a). Approximately 73% of all chronic disease deaths occur in low- and middle-income countries, and by 2030, chronic disease costs are expected to reach $47 trillion (Hacker, 2024).

Impact of the Pandemic

Individuals with chronic diseases often exhibit impaired immune function, which can affect their ability to effectively combat viral infections such as COVID-19. As a result, they are at heightened risk for developing severe illness, including increased likelihood of hospitalization, intensive care unit (ICU) admission, and mechanical ventilation, and experience higher health and economic burdens. Moreover, the presence of chronic conditions may diminish vaccine efficacy, potentially leading to reduced immunological protection following vaccination.

Hypertension and lipid metabolism disorders are the most common comorbidities, while obesity, diabetes complications, and anxiety disorders are considered the strongest risk factors for severe COVID-19 disease. Using data from over 800 U.S. hospitals, a Centers for Disease Control and Prevention (CDC) study

DOI: 10.4324/9781003595564-18

found that the most common chronic comorbid conditions among hospitalized COVID-19 patients aged 18 years or older were primary hypertension (50.4%), lipid metabolism disorders (49.4%), obesity (33.0%), diabetes complications (31.8%), and coronary atherosclerosis and other heart diseases (24.9%) (Kompaniyets et al., 2021).

Common chronic diseases have varying degrees of impact on the risk of death in COVID-19 patients. A retrospective study published in *Nature* investigated the relationship between comorbidities and COVID-19 in-hospital mortality using a cohort of 6,036 patients. Higher odds of mortality was observed in patients with the following conditions: lymphoma (OR 2.78), metastatic cancer (OR 2.17), solid tumor without metastasis (OR 1.67), liver disease (OR 2.50), congestive heart failure (OR 1.69), chronic obstructive pulmonary disease (OR 1.43), obesity (OR 5.28), renal disease (OR 1.81), and dementia (OR 1.44). Notably, asthma (OR 0.60) was associated with a 40% lower odds of mortality compared to non-asthma patients. Patients with two comorbidities (OR 1.79) and those with three or more comorbidities (OR 1.80) had higher odds of mortality, emphasizing the impact of multimorbidity on COVID-19 outcomes (Bucholc et al., 2022).

Obesity

The WHO defines overweight as a body mass index (BMI) of 25 kg/m^2 or higher and obesity as a BMI of 30 kg/m^2 or higher. Overweight is characterized by excessive fat accumulation, while obesity is a chronic disease involving significant fat deposits that can impair health. Obesity is linked to numerous health complications affecting nearly every system in the body, including heart disease, stroke, sleep apnea, gallbladder disease, osteoarthritis, infertility, increased cancer risk, and cognitive decline (World Health Organization (WHO), 2024b).

Data from 2022 indicates that approximately one in eight people worldwide are obese, with adult obesity rates doubling since 1990 and childhood obesity rates quadrupling. Pacific Island nations have some of the highest obesity rates, accounting for nine out of the ten most obese countries globally (World Health Organization (WHO), 2024b). Obesity rates have risen most rapidly in North Africa and the Middle East, tripling in men and doubling in women. By 2050, over half of the world's adults (around 3.8 billion) are expected to be overweight or obese. While China, India, and the United States will continue to have the largest numbers, sub-Saharan Africa is projected to see a growth of 254.8%, with Nigeria expected to rank fourth globally with 141 million affected adults (Ng et al., 2025).

Impact of the Pandemic

Obesity was already a major public health concern before the COVID-19 pandemic, with rising prevalence worldwide due to poor lifestyle behaviors. The pandemic further exacerbated this issue, leading to significant increases in obesity rates across various populations. A *BMC Public Health* review investigated global obesity rates before and after the pandemic. Obesity rates before the pandemic were approximately 11% for men and 15% for women. After the pandemic obesity rose to 25.3% in men and 42.4% in women. Multiple factors contributed to this surge.

The most common determinants identified included physical inactivity, increasing sedentary behavior, and consuming unhealthy foods. Additionally, other contributing factors included age, gender, ethnic minority, increased hunger, overeating, low-quality or unbalanced diets, excessive consumption of sweet beverages, snacks, salty foods, and soda, binge eating, and reduced water intake. Furthermore, fear of COVID-19, anxiety, stress, and low mood during lockdowns contributed to emotional eating and reduced motivation for physical activity. Increased screen time due to internet or social media addiction, prolonged sitting hours, and substance abuse were also associated with weight gain during this period (Nour & Altintaş, 2023).

COVID-19 Severity Linked to Obesity

In addition to the aforementioned health risks associated with obesity, multiple studies have found obesity is a strong predictor of severe COVID-19 outcomes. Obese individuals are more likely to contract COVID-19 after exposure and experience reduced vaccine effectiveness (Hajifathalian et al., 2020).

A meta-analysis quantified the association between overweight and obesity and adverse COVID-19 outcomes, including hospitalizations and mortality, using data from 208 studies. The analysis revealed that overweight individuals had 19% increased odds of COVID-19-related hospitalization and 2% increased odds of mortality. In comparison, individuals with obesity exhibited 72% increased odds of hospitalization and 25% increased odds of mortality, with those categorized as having extreme obesity facing the highest risks—153% increased odds of hospitalization and 106% increased odds of mortality (Sawadogo et al., 2022).

A study led by investigators from Mass General Brigham revealed that obesity may serve as a major risk factor for contracting COVID-19. Their research, published in *PNAS Nexus*, analyzed electronic health records from Mass General Brigham and found that individuals with obesity had 34% higher odds of testing positive for COVID-19 after reported exposure compared to those without obesity. These findings suggest that obesity, which is already recognized as a risk factor for more severe COVID-19 outcomes, may also increase the risk of initial infection (Matamalas et al., 2024).

An additional meta-analysis concluded that obese individuals face more severe health risks after contracting COVID-19. Researchers found the odds of poorer COVID-19 outcomes are 1.68 times greater, the odds of severe illness are 4.17 times greater, the odds of ICU care are 1.57 times greater, the odds of requiring invasive ventilator support are 2.13 greater, and the odds of disease progression are 1.41 times greater compared to non-obese individuals. (Chu et al., 2020). These findings not only emphasize the threat of COVID-19 to obese individuals but also highlight the potential for more severe consequences during the course of the disease.

Furthermore, obesity not only negatively impacts immunity but also reduces the effectiveness of vaccines. A study in the United Kingdom found that individuals who are underweight or obese are still at a significantly higher risk of hospitalization or death from COVID-19, even after completing the second dose of vaccination, compared to those with normal (Piernas et al., 2022).

Immunodeficiency

Immunodeficiency refers to a problem with various components of the immune system, such as lymphocytes, phagocytes, and the complement system, which leads to their dysfunction or absence. Immunodeficiency status encompasses a diverse population, and this defect can be caused by congenital (primary) or acquired (secondary) factors. Primary immunodeficiency mainly includes defects in T cells, B cells, or both T and B cells, as well as deficiencies in different types of complement, phagocytes, and immunoglobulin A. Secondary immunodeficiency can be caused by the use of steroids, malnutrition, obesity, acquired immunodeficiency syndrome (such as AIDS), or other viral infections. Due to immune system dysfunction, these individuals are more susceptible to various infections and require attention to their immune status when facing diseases and treatments to ensure appropriate protection and medical measures (Vaillant & Qurie, 2023).

Relationship Between Immunodeficiency and COVID-19

Individuals with immunodeficiencies, including organ transplant patients, blood cancer patients, individuals with congenital immunodeficiency, HIV-infected patients, and patients receiving immunosuppressants, chemotherapy, or radiotherapy, face a higher risk of contracting COVID-19 and undergoing severe COVID-19 outcomes. Although these populations are generally considered a priority for vaccination and are actively encouraged to receive new vaccines, relying on COVID-19 vaccine protection alone may not be sufficient.

A study published in *Clinical Infectious Diseases* emphasized the need for personalized preventive strategies beyond vaccination for individuals with immune deficiencies. The study noted that different populations have varying effective antibody responses after vaccination. Researchers found that 92.4% of non-immunocompromised individuals were seropositive, compared to 78.7% of those with solid tumors, 79.8% with HIV, 50% with hematological malignancies, and only 30.7% among organ transplant recipients (Haidar et al., 2022).

The INFORM study (Evans et al., 2023) utilized a representative sample of electronic healthcare records to evaluate the burden and risk of severe COVID-19 outcomes among immunocompromised individuals in England during 2022. During this period, COVID-19 vaccination programs were well established. Immunocompromised status included individuals with conditions such as malignancy, solid organ transplantation, or autoimmune disorders that compromise immune function. Despite comprising only 3.9% of the total population, immunocompromised individuals accounted for 22% of COVID-19-related hospitalizations, 28% of ICU admissions, and 24% of deaths, indicating a markedly disproportionate impact.

Notably, over 80% of this population had received at least three doses of a COVID-19 vaccine, highlighting the aforementioned study's findings that current vaccination strategies may not provide sufficient protection for those with impaired immunity. After adjusting for age, sex, and other comorbidities, the relative risk of hospitalization and death among immunocompromised individuals remained significantly elevated, ranging from 1.3- to 13.1-fold for hospitalization and 1.3- to 19.9-fold for mortality, compared to the non-immunocompromised population. Among these groups, solid organ transplant recipients exhibited the highest risk for both hospitalization and death. Given these findings, medical institutions should provide closer monitoring and support for immunocompromised individuals to ensure timely and effective COVID-19 treatment and management (Evans et al., 2023).

Aging

Aging is an inevitable physiological process characterized by gradual changes in the structure and function of organisms over time. The causes of aging are multifaceted, including genetic factors, environmental influences, lifestyle choices, and overall health status. The possibility of accelerated aging during the COVID-19 pandemic is attributed to factors such as disease infection, social isolation, and chronic stress.

Age Vulnerability and Immune Challenges of COVID-19

Aging is marked by inflammaging, a chronic, low-grade inflammatory state driven by cellular senescence, physiological stress, and environmental factors. This persistent inflammation underlies many age-related conditions, including cardiovascular disease, diabetes, sarcopenia, and neurodegeneration, and creates an immune landscape that is particularly vulnerable to infections like COVID-19. The virus exacerbates this pro-inflammatory state by activating immune receptors through pathogen and damage-associated molecular patterns, triggering cytokine release and intensifying disease severity. Elevated inflammatory markers, such as IL-6, in older adults are linked to frailty, reduced mobility, and greater disability, making them especially susceptible to poor outcomes, prolonged recovery, and functional decline following infection (Bektas et al., 2020).

Inflammaging is often a consequence of immunosenescence, the gradual decline in immune function with aging (Ajoolabady et al., 2024). This process is partly due to decreased production of immune cells from the bone marrow and thymus, which results in reduced immune responses. Immunosenescence also contributes to diminished vaccine efficacy, highlighting the importance of monitoring and optimizing vaccine effectiveness in older populations (Allen et al., 2020).

This heightened vulnerability is reflected in mortality data. According to a report by the U.S. CDC, 81% of COVID-19-related deaths in 2020 occurred among

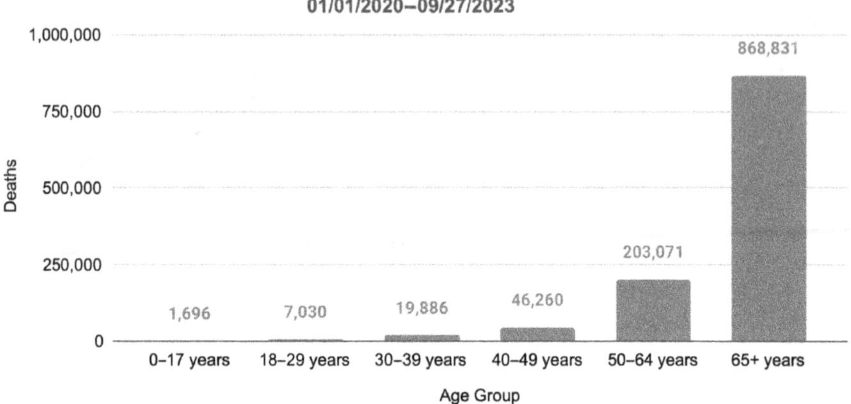

Figure 14.1 U.S. COVID-19 Deaths by Age Group (01/01/2020–09/27/2023).
Source: CDC (n.d.).

individuals aged 65 and older (Tejada-Vera & Kramarow, 2022). Subsequent data through late September 2023 showed that older adults continued to account for over 77% of COVID-19 deaths in the United States (Figure 14.1). Similarly, Eurostat data indicates that Europe experienced comparable trends, with the majority of COVID-19 fatalities occurring among those aged 65 and above (Figure 14.2), reflecting a global pattern of elevated mortality risk in aging populations.

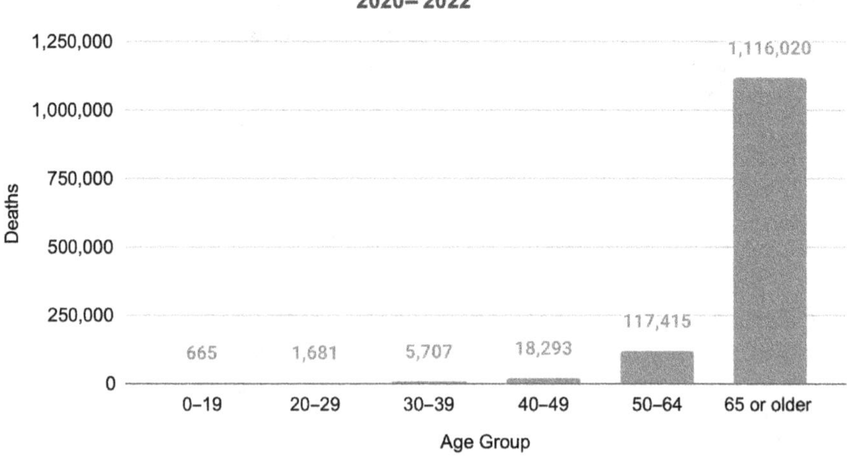

Figure 14.2 Europe COVID-19 Deaths by Age Group (2020–2022).
Source: Eurostat (2025).

Social and Healthcare Marginalization

Social isolation refers to the lack of meaningful relationships with others, characterized by limited social support and contact. During the pandemic, many elderly individuals experienced prolonged isolation, negatively impacting their mental and physical well-being. Nearly one-quarter of adults aged 65 and older experience social isolation, which has been linked to a 50% increased risk of dementia, a 29% higher probability of heart disease, and a 32% elevated risk of stroke (National Academies of Sciences, Engineering, and Medicine (NASEM), 2020).

Equally concerning is the systematic exclusion of older adults from clinical research. Despite their high vulnerability, older adults have historically been excluded from clinical trials, a pattern that persisted during the pandemic. Although they represent 9% of the global population, they accounted for 30–40% of cases and more than 80% of COVID-19 deaths. A review of 847 COVID-19 treatment and vaccine trials found that older adults are likely to be excluded from over 50% of clinical trials, and 100% of vaccine trials (Helfand et al., 2020).

Furthermore, older adults may experience decreased antibody responses to vaccines. Studies suggest that higher antigen levels, adjuvants, or repeated dosing may improve immune responses in the elderly. Without their inclusion in trials, the necessary adjustments to improve vaccine effectiveness for this group cannot be made. Some have argued that vaccinating younger populations alone would be sufficient to achieve herd immunity, but this ignores the unique risks faced by older adults, particularly in high-density settings such as nursing homes. Ensuring that COVID-19 clinical trials are both relevant and inclusive is critical for effective public health interventions and equitable treatment access (Helfand et al., 2020).

Conclusion

Chronic diseases, obesity, immune deficiencies, and aging all play a crucial role in the severity of COVID-19 outcomes. Individuals with these underlying conditions are at increased risk of hospitalization, ICU admission, and mortality, and may also exhibit reduced vaccine responsiveness. As we move forward, it is essential to address these health vulnerabilities through targeted prevention, early intervention, and effective treatment strategies. The following chapter explores the impact of healthy lifestyle behaviors, such as balanced diet, exercise, sleep, stress management, social connections, and abstinence from substance use, as a potential protective factor against the virus.

References

Ajoolabady, A., Pratico, D., Tang, D., Zhou, S., Franceschi, C., & Ren, J. (2024). Immunosenescence and inflammaging: Mechanisms and role in diseases. *Ageing Research Reviews*, *101*, 102540. https://doi.org/10.1016/j.arr.2024.102540

Allen, J. C., Toapanta, F. R., Chen, W., & Tennant, S. M. (2020). Understanding immunosenescence and its impact on vaccination of older adults. *Vaccine*, *38*(52), 8264–8272. https://doi.org/10.1016/j.vaccine.2020.11.002

Bektas, A., Schurman, S. H., Franceschi, C., *et al.* (2020. A public health perspective of aging: Do hyper-inflammatory syndromes such as COVID-19, SARS, ARDS, cytokine storm syndrome, and post-ICU syndrome accelerate short- and long-term inflammaging?. *Immunity & Ageing*, *17*, 23. https://doi.org/10.1186/s12979-020-00196-8

Bucholc, M., Bradley, D., & Bennett, D. *et al.* (2022). Identifying pre-existing conditions and multimorbidity patterns associated with in-hospital mortality in patients with COVID-19. *Scientific Reports*, *12*, 17313. https://doi.org/10.1038/s41598-022-20176-w

Centers for Disease Control and Prevention (CDC). (n.d.). *Provisional COVID-19 deaths by sex and age* [Dataset]. U.S. Department of Health & Human Services. https://data.cdc.gov/widgets/9bhg-hcku

Chu, Y., Yang, J., Shi, J., Zhang, P., & Wang, X. (2020). Obesity is associated with increased severity of disease in COVID-19 pneumonia: A systematic review and meta-analysis. *European Journal of Medical Research*, *25*(1), 64. https://doi.org/10.1186/s40001-020-00464-9

Eurostat. (2025). *Causes of death – Deaths by country of residence and occurrence –* [Dataset]. European Commission. https://data.europa.eu/doi/10.2908/hlth_cd_aro

Evans, R. A., Dube, S., Lu, Y., Yates, M., Arnetorp, S., Barnes, E., Bell, S., Carty, L., Evans, K., Graham, S., Justo, N., Moss, P., Venkatesan, S., Yokota, R., Ferreira, C., McNulty, R., Taylor, S., & Quint, J. K. (2023). Impact of COVID-19 on immunocompromised populations during the Omicron era: Insights from the observational population-based INFORM study. *The Lancet Regional Health – Europe*, *35*. https://doi.org/10.1016/j.lanepe.2023.100747

Hacker, K. (2024). The burden of chronic disease. *Mayo Clinic Proceedings: Innovations, Quality & Outcomes*, *8*(1), 112–119. https://doi.org/10.1016/j.mayocpiqo.2023.08.005

Haidar, G., Agha, M., Bilderback, A., Lukanski, A., Linstrum, K., Troyan, R., Rothenberger, S., McMahon, D. K., Crandall, M. D., Sobolewksi, M. D., Enick, N., Jacobs, J. L., Collins, K., Klamar-Blain, C., Macatangay, B. J. C., Parikh, U. M., Heaps, A., Coughenour, L., Schwartz, M. B., & Dueker, J. M. (2022). Prospective evaluation of Coronavirus disease 2019 (COVID-19) vaccine responses across a broad spectrum of immunocompromising conditions: The COVID-19 vaccination in the immunocompromised study (COVICS). *Clinical Infectious Diseases*, *75*(1), e630–e644. https://doi.org/10.1093/cid/ciac103

Hajifathalian, K., Kumar, S., Newberry, C., Shah, S., Fortune, B., Krisko, T., Ortiz-Pujols, S., Zhou, X. K., Dannenberg, A. J., Kumar, R., & Sharaiha, R. Z. (2020). Obesity is associated with worse outcomes in COVID-19: Analysis of early data from New York City. *Obesity (Silver Spring, Md.)*, *28*(9), 1606–1612.

Helfand, B. K. I., Webb, M., Gartaganis, S. L., Fuller, L., Kwon, C.-S., & Inouye, S. K. (2020). The exclusion of older persons from vaccine and treatment trials for coronavirus disease 2019—Missing the target. *JAMA Internal Medicine*, *180*(11), 1546–1549. https://doi.org/10.1001/jamainternmed.2020.5084

Kompaniyets, L., Pennington, A. F., Goodman, A. B., Rosenblum, H. G., Belay, B., Ko, J. Y., et al. (2021). Underlying medical conditions and severe illness among 540,667 adults hospitalized with COVID-19, March 2020–March 2021. *Preventing Chronic Disease*, *18*, 210123. https://doi.org/10.5888/pcd18.210123

Matamalas, J. T., Chelvanambi, S., Decano, J. L., França, R. F., Halu, A., SantinelliPestana, D. V., Aikawa, E., Malhotra, R., & Aikawa, M. (2024). Obesity and age are transmission risk factors for SARS-CoV-2 infection among exposed individuals. *PNAS Nexus*, *3*(8), 294. https://doi.org/10.1093/pnasnexus/pgae294

National Academies of Sciences, Engineering, and Medicine (NASEM). 2020. *Social isolation and loneliness in older adults: Opportunities for the health care system*. The National Academies Press. https://doi.org/10.17226/25663.

Ng, M., Gakidou, E., Lo, J., Abate, Y. H., Abbafati, C., Abbas, N., Abbasian, M., Abd El-Hafeez, S., Abdel-Rahman, W. M., Abd-Elsalam, S., Abdollahi, A., Abdoun, M., Abdulah, D. M., Abdulkader, R. S., Abdullahi, A., Abedi, A., Abeywickrama, H. M., Abie, A.,

Aboagye, R. G., & Abohashem, S. (2025). Global, regional, and national prevalence of adult overweight and obesity, 1990–2021, with forecasts to 2050: A forecasting study for the global burden of disease study 2021. *The Lancet*, *405*(10481). https://doi.org/10.1016/s0140-6736(25)00355-1

Nour, T. Y., & Altintaş, K. H. (2023). Effect of the COVID-19 pandemic on obesity and it is risk factors: A systematic review. *BMC Public Health*, *23*(1), 1018. https://doi.org/10.1186/s12889-023-15833-2

Piernas, C., Patone, M., Astbury, N. M., Gao, M., Sheikh, A., Khunti, K., ShankarHari, M., Dixon, S., Coupland, C., Aveyard, P., HippisleyCox, J., & Jebb, S. A. (2022). Associations of BMI with COVID-19 vaccine uptake, vaccine effectiveness, and risk of severe COVID-19 outcomes after vaccination in England: A population-based cohort study. *The Lancet Diabetes & Endocrinology*, *10*(8), 571–580. https://doi.org/10.1016/S2213-8587(22)00158-9

Sawadogo, W., Tsegaye, M., Gizaw, A., & Adera, T. (2022). Overweight and obesity as risk factors for COVID-19-associated hospitalisations and death: Systematic review and meta-analysis. *BMJ Nutrition, Prevention & Health*, e000375. https://doi.org/10.1136/bmjnph-2021-000375

Tejada-Vera, B., & Kramarow, E. A.. *COVID-19 mortality in adults aged 65 and over: United States, 2020. NCHS Data Brief, no 446*. National Center for Health Statistics. 2022. https://dx.doi.org/10.15620/cdc:121320

Vaillant, A. A. J., & Qurie, A. (2023, June 26). *Immunodeficiency*. PubMed; StatPearls Publishing. https://www.ncbi.nlm.nih.gov/books/NBK500027/

World Health Organization (WHO). (2024a, December 23). *Noncommunicable diseases*. World Health Organization. https://www.who.int/news-room/fact-sheets/detail/noncommunicable-diseases

World Health Organization (WHO). (2024b, March 1). *Obesity and overweight*. World Health Organization. https://www.who.int/news-room/fact-sheets/detail/obesity-and-overweight

15 Lifestyle as a Shield

Health Behaviors and Pandemic Resilience

The COVID-19 pandemic has emphasized the critical importance of holistic health in building resilience against infectious diseases. While vaccines and medical interventions remain essential, a growing body of research reveals that everyday lifestyle choices: diet, exercise, sleep, stress management, social connection, and substance use, profoundly influence vulnerability to illness and recovery outcomes. This section explores the intersection of these foundational elements with immune health and COVID-19, drawing on scientific evidence to illuminate how personal health behaviors can either protect or predispose individuals to severe disease. By understanding the biological and behavioral mechanisms that link these factors to immunity, we gain powerful tools for fostering both personal and public health resilience during pandemics and beyond.

This chapter reviews the protective benefits of a healthy lifestyle as a preventative measure against COVID-19:

- *Balanced Diets: A Potential Protective Factor Against COVID-19*
- *Exercise: Strengthening the Body's Defenses Against Infection*
- *Sleep and Circadian Rhythms: Foundation of Immune Strength*
- *Stress Management: Nurturing Mental Health During Challenging Times*
- *Social Connections: The Importance of Relationships for Overall Well-Being*
- *Substance Abuse: Health Risks and Consequences During a Pandemic*

Balanced Diets: A Potential Protective Factor Against COVID-19

Numerous studies have unveiled the transformative powers of a nutritious diet, highlighting its role in strengthening the immune system and enhancing our general well-being. Remarkably, such a diet has been shown to slash the risk of developing severe COVID-19 infection by a staggering 41%. To optimize health, focus on: a balanced diet (predominantly a plant-based or Mediterranean diet), sufficient intake of vitamins A, B, C, D, E, key trace elements (zinc, copper, selenium, iron), and proper hydration.

Given the importance of nutrition for overall health, particularly the immune system, it is crucial to focus on sustaining a strong immune response. A

DOI: 10.4324/9781003595564-19

Table 15.1 Impact of Diet on COVID-19 Outcomes

Diet Type/Focus	*Sample*	*Key Findings*	*Study*
Plant-based diet (fruits and vegetables)	592,571	• 9% lower risk of contracting COVID-19 • 41% lower risk of severe illness requiring hospitalization	Merino et al. (2021)
Plant-based and pescatarian diets	2884	• 73% lower odds of moderate-to-severe COVID-19 (plant-based) • 59% lower odds of moderate-to-severe COVID-19 (pescatarian)	Kim et al. (2021)
High fruit, vegetable, and fiber intake	250	• Lower severity, shorter hospital stays, and reduced risk of COVID-19 symptoms	Tadbir Vajargah et al. (2022)
Malnutrition	581	• Underweight patients are 10× more likely to have ICU admission • Overweight patients are 7× more likely ICU admission • Well-nourished patients are 94% more likely to survive	Jima et al. (2024)

well-functioning immune system enables the body to fight off infections and diseases. By integrating essential nutrients through a balanced diet, the immune system receives the necessary resources to function at its best.

To further explore the link between diet and immune health, several studies have investigated the effects of diet on COVID-19 outcomes. Key findings are outlined in Table 15.1.

Nutrition and Immunity: Exploring the Dietary Foundations of Immune Health

Consumption of a nutrient-dense diet is essential for a healthy immune system. Deficiencies in key vitamins and minerals can increase a person's susceptibility to viral infection and cause more severe symptoms (Rust & Ekmekcioglu, 2023). The COVID-19 pandemic initiated a heightened interest in foods purported to boost the immune system. Despite extensive research, the question of whether specific foods provide definitive protection against illness continues to be a subject of debate. The inherent complexities of controlling all variables within dietary studies can obscure the attainment of conclusive findings. Nevertheless, a thorough examination of the research can yield valuable insights.

Balanced Diet: A well-balanced diet is the foundation of a robust immune system. The International Society for Immunonutrition and the WHO emphasize the consumption of a variety of food groups, including whole grains, dairy, meat or alternatives, vegetables, fruits, oils, and nuts, to reduce the risk of chronic and infectious diseases (World Health Organization (WHO), n.d.).

High-Quality Protein: Protein is an essential nutrient in fueling bodily function and transporting oxygen throughout the body. It helps create antibodies to ward off illnesses and infections, as well as maintains and creates new cells (Cooper, 2024).

Adequate Vitamin Intake: Adequate intake of vitamins is crucial for the proper functioning of immune cells like B, T, and natural killer (NK) cells. Deficiencies can compromise immunity, while supplementation may enhance defense mechanisms. Table 15.2 summarizes vitamins and trace elements' role in supporting immune function and their potential effects on COVID-19.

Table 15.2 The Role of Vitamins and Trace Elements in Immunity and COVID-19 Outcomes

Vitamin/Trace Element	*Role in Immunity and COVID-19*	*Source*
Vitamin A	• Enhances immune function, strengthens defense against infectious diseases, restores epithelial mucosa, and modulates immune response. • Lower levels are found in infected COVID-19 individuals compared to healthy individuals.	Huang et al. (2018). Carvalho et al. (2023)
Vitamin B	• Supports immune function, metabolism, and cellular maintenance. • Emerging research suggests benefits in managing COVID-19 symptoms.	Shakoor et al. (2021)
Vitamin B1 (Thiamine)	• Supports immune function. • Deficiency increases inflammation, weakens immunity, and may lead to severe COVID-19 symptoms.	Shakoor et al. (2021)
Vitamin B2 (Riboflavin)	• Combined with UV light, it damages nucleic acids to prevent replication of viruses. • Reduces SARS-CoV-2 infectious titers in blood products.	Shakoor et al. (2021)
Vitamin B3 (Niacin)	• Reduces pro-inflammatory cytokines, neutrophil infiltration, and lung injury. • Prevents viral replication and lung tissue damage.	Shakoor et al. (2021)
Vitamin B5 (Pantothenic Acid)	• Supports red blood cells, hormone production, and metabolism. • One study found a 47% reduction in COVID-19 infection with higher intake.	Mount Sinai (n.d.) Darand et al. (2023)
Vitamin B6	• Regulates immune responses, reduces inflammation, preserves endothelial integrity, and prevents hypercoagulability in COVID-19 patients.	Shakoor et al. (2021)
Vitamin B7 (Biotin)	• Supports nervous system, liver, and skin functions. • Limited studies on COVID-19, but high intake linked to reduced infection odds in men.	Darand et al. (2023)

(*Continued*)

Table 15.2 (Continued)

Vitamin/Trace Element	*Role in Immunity and COVID-19*	*Source*
Vitamin B9 (Folate)	• Inhibits furin enzyme to prevent COVID-19 spike protein entry. • Molecular docking studies suggest potential as a COVID-19 treatment.	Shakoor et al. (2021)
Vitamin B12	• Supports red blood cell synthesis and nervous system health. • Deficiencies linked to inflammation and COVID-like complications. • Supplementation may reduce organ damage.	Shakoor et al. (2021)
Vitamin C	• Boosts innate and adaptive immunity. • High-dose vitamin C reduced COVID-19 mortality and severity, but did not significantly affect hospital stay.	Bhowmik et al. (2022)
Vitamin D	• Supports immune function. • Protects against respiratory infections.	Martineau et al. (2017)
Vitamin E	• Antioxidant that enhances immune function. • Reduces inflammation and oxidative stress in COVID-19 pneumonia patients when combined with pentoxifylline.	National Institutes of Health (NIH) (2024)
Zinc	• Supports cellular metabolism, immune function, antiviral, and anti-inflammatory defenses. • Deficiency increases susceptibility to infections. • When combined with treatments like vitamin C, it can reduce COVID-19 symptoms.	Jin et al. (2024)
Copper	• Essential for immune cell function. • Inactivates COVID-19 viral genomes and damages the virus's envelope and surface spikes.	Govind et al. (2021)
Selenium	• Enhances innate and adaptive immunity, reduces systemic inflammation and infection risk. • May reduce COVID-19 viral entry and replication, and alleviate inflammation and ARDS.	Alshammari et al. (2022)
Iron	• Involved in oxygen transport, cellular function, and growth. • Dysregulation is linked to long COVID symptoms like fatigue and brain fog. • Early treatment of iron imbalances may reduce the long COVID impact.	NIH (2024) Hanson et al. (2024)

While all vitamins and trace elements are essential in a healthy immune system, supplementation of selective nutrients such as zinc and vitamins D, C, and A is especially emphasized for at-risk populations and those with nutritional deficiencies.

Adequate Hydration: The human body comprises 50–70% water. Even a minor reduction of 1–2% in water intake can affect the proper functioning of the body. Dehydration can predispose individuals to infection and worsen disease severity.

Studies suggest that adequate hydration supports immune function, helps maintain mucosal barriers, and may limit viral spread, while fluid deficits can lead to complications like hypernatremia, which is associated with increased mortality. COVID-19 patients often experience fluid loss due to fever, insensible losses, and impaired kidney function, making hydration management essential yet challenging. Despite the complexities, maintaining proper hydration could improve patient outcomes and should be a key focus in clinical care (Healthcare Infection Society, 2021).

The Mediterranean Diet and COVID-19

Dietary choices significantly influence overall health, with one pattern consistently demonstrating notable benefits: the Mediterranean diet. The Mediterranean diet was first observed by Professor Ancel Keys, who noted the remarkable health of residents on the Greek island of Crete compared to other parts of the world. He attributed their longevity and lower rates of heart disease to their dietary patterns. The Mediterranean diet emphasizes fruits, vegetables, whole grains, legumes, nuts, seeds, fish, and poultry, with moderate consumption of dairy and red meat. Studies have shown that adherence to this diet significantly reduces deaths from cancer (6%), cardiovascular disease (13%), Alzheimer's disease (13%), and overall mortality (9%) (Sofi et al., 2008).

Immunologists and nutritionists suggest that the Mediterranean diet may enhance immune function and reduce the severity of COVID-19. One study analyzed 5194 university graduates from Seguimiento Universidad de Navarra (SUN) from February to December 2020. Dietary habits were assessed using a 136-item food frequency questionnaire and measured using the 0-to-9 Mediterranean Diet Score (MDS). Among the participants, 122 reported testing positive for COVID-19. The results indicated that moderate adherence to the Mediterranean diet ($3 < MDS \leq 6$) had significantly reduced odds of contracting COVID-19, and those with the strongest adherence ($MDS > 6$) displayed the lowest risk. Therefore, it is suggested that greater adherence to the Mediterranean diet may be linked to a substantially lower risk of COVID-19, with higher adherence associated with over a 60% reduction in risk (Perez-Araluce et al., 2022).

Conclusion

Substantial evidence supports the role of nutrition, particularly diets rich in fruits, vegetables, whole grains, legumes, healthy fats, and lean proteins, in enhancing immune function and reducing the severity of infectious diseases, including COVID-19. The Mediterranean diet, in particular, stands out for its association with lower risks of cardiovascular disease, cancer, cognitive decline, and severe COVID-19 outcomes. As the pandemic has highlighted the intersection between nutrition and immune resilience, prioritizing dietary improvements becomes not only a personal health strategy but a public health imperative. Building on the foundational role of diet, the following section examines another critical lifestyle factor, exercise, and its protective benefit against COVID-19.

Exercise: Strengthening the Body's Defenses Against Infection

Exercise is a cornerstone of physical and immune health. Regular physical activity not only reduces the risk of chronic diseases and premature death but also plays a critical role in strengthening the body's defenses against infections. During the pandemic, compelling evidence emerged linking consistent exercise to reduced infection rates, hospitalization, and mortality.

The Effects of Exercise on the Human Body

Exercise is a fundamental component of maintaining overall health and well-being. Regular physical activity, as outlined by the American College of Sports Medicine (ACSM), has been shown to significantly reduce the risk of mortality, enhance immune function, and mitigate inflammation. The ACSM recommends a minimum of 150 minutes of moderate-intensity exercise per week, coupled with at least two sessions of muscle-strengthening activities, to achieve these health benefits (American College of Sports Medicine, 2025).

A study published in the *Journal of the American Medical Association* (JAMA) involving 64,000 participants demonstrated that meeting weekly exercise recommendations was associated with a 30% reduction in mortality risk. However, it is crucial to approach exercise intensity with caution, as excessive physical exertion may temporarily suppress immune function. Moderate-intensity exercise remains the most effective and sustainable approach for promoting long-term health outcomes (O'Donovan et al., 2017).

Exercise Helps Combat COVID-19

During the COVID-19 pandemic, researchers discovered that regular exercise played a significant role in influencing the severity of COVID-19 outcomes. Physical activity offers immunoregulatory effects and protective benefits against respiratory infections, making it a valuable form of preventative medicine. Moreover, consistent physical activity is associated with reduced risk of comorbid conditions such as obesity and type 2 diabetes, both known to elevate the risk of severe COVID-19 complications.

The protective association between COVID-19 and physical activity is attributed to enhancements in immune function. These include increased NK cell activity and modulation of T-cell responses, which contribute to a lower risk of severe respiratory infection (Nieman & Wentz, 2019; Timmons & Cieslak, 2008). In addition, regular exercise has also been shown to reduce viral entry into cells and reduce inflammation. Improvements in pulmonary function, along with reductions in cardiovascular diseases, further contribute to the decreased susceptibility to severe COVID-19 outcomes among physically active individuals (Sittichai et al., 2022).

Large-scale evidence further reinforces these associations. A meta-analysis published in the *British Journal of Sports Medicine* found that those who engage in regular physical activity had an 11% lower risk of contracting COVID-19, a 36% lower risk of hospitalization, and a 43% lower risk of death related to COVID-19, compared to inactive individuals (Ezzatvar et al., 2022). A meta-analysis published in *Frontier* similarly showed that physically active individuals have 66% reduced odds of death and a lower likelihood of experiencing severe outcomes (Sittichai et al., 2022).

Further support is reflected in an additional *British Journal of Sports Medicine* study, which found that those who engaged in regular physical activity were 15% less likely to test positive for the virus, 58% less likely to experience severe outcomes, and 76% less likely to die from COVID-19. Notably, individuals who met the recommended guidelines for physical activity per week experienced the greatest protective benefits. In this group, the risk of infection was reduced by 22%, the risk of severe disease dropped by 38%, and the risk of death plummeted by 83% (Lee et al., 2022).

In contrast, studies focusing on physical inactivity highlighted significant risks. A retrospective cohort study found that individuals who were consistently inactive had more than twice the odds of hospitalization due to COVID-19. They also had 1.7 times higher odds of ICU admission and nearly 2.5 times higher odds of death compared to those who maintained regular physical activity (Sallis et al., 2021). Key findings from these studies are outlined in Table 15.3.

Table 15.3 Key Findings of Physical Activity and Inactivity on COVID-19 Outcomes

Focus	*Sample*	*Key Findings*	*Source*
Physical activity	1,853,610	Physically Active vs. Inactive: • 11% lower risk of COVID-19-related infection • 36% lower risk of hospitalization • 43% lower risk of COVID-19 related death	Ezzatvar et al. (2022)
Physical activity	1,618,680	Physically Active vs. Inactive: • 66% lower odds of death • 40% lower odds of severe outcomes	Sittichai et al. (2022)
Physical inactivity	48,440	Inactive vs. Physically Active: • 126% increased odds of hospitalization • 73% increased odds of ICU admission • 149% increased odds of death	Sallis et al. (2021)
Physical activity	76,395	Physically Active vs. Inactive • 15% less likely to test positive • 58% lower risk of severe outcomes • 76% lower risk of death **500–1000 MET min/week:** • 22% lower risk of infection • 38% lower risk of severe infection • 83% lower risk of death	Lee et al. (2022)

Note: Metabolic Equivalent Task (MET) is defined as the ratio of metabolic rate during physical activity relative to metabolic rate at rest. Levels of MET intensity include: Light < (3.0 METs), Moderate (3.0–6.0 METs), and Vigorous (> 6.0 METs). A minimum of 500 MET minutes per week is recommended (Roland, 2019).

Conclusion

Research has consistently demonstrated that exercise benefits physical health and enhances the immune system's capacity to combat viruses. Those who maintained consistent exercise routines experienced significantly reduced rates of infection, hospitalization, and mortality. These protective effects are attributed to improved immune function, cardiovascular health, pulmonary capacity, and metabolic resilience. In contrast, physical inactivity emerged as a major risk factor, associated with higher odds of ICU admission and death. In addition to exercise, sleep is essential for optimal immune function and disease resistance. The following section examines the powerful role of sleep in supporting immune health.

Sleep and Circadian Rhythms: Foundation of Immune Strength

Sleep is a critical, yet often overlooked, pillar of immune health. Extensive research reveals that insufficient or poor-quality sleep disrupts immune regulation, increases inflammation, and elevates the risk for a wide range of chronic and infectious diseases. These effects became especially salient during the pandemic, as studies linked sleep deprivation and disturbances to increased infection risk, hospitalization, and even mortality. Burnout and sleep disorders, particularly affecting healthcare workers, were also shown to exacerbate vulnerability. Furthermore, emerging evidence suggests circadian rhythms may influence vaccine effectiveness, highlighting the complex interplay between sleep, immunity, and pandemic outcomes.

The Relationship Between Sleep and the Immune System

Sleep plays a vital role in supporting immune function. Both experimental and epidemiological studies indicate that sleep, whether acute or chronic, can lead to immune dysregulation and increased susceptibility to a range of health conditions. Modern societal factors such as work demands, screen exposure, and lifestyle habits have contributed to widespread chronic sleep deprivation, which alters innate and adaptive immunity, elevates pro-inflammatory cytokines, and disrupts the balance of immune-signaling. This imbalance leads to chronic inflammation and increases the risks for various infectious, autoimmune, cardiovascular, neurodegenerative, and psychiatric diseases. Notably, sleep influences immunity not only through biochemical signaling, but also via neural communication pathways such as the vagus nerve, which connects the brain and immune system (Garbarino et al., 2021).

Supporting this connection, a study from *Sleep* demonstrated a clear relationship between sleep duration and susceptibility to illness. Researchers found that individuals who slept for more than 7 hours had a 17.2% chance of catching a cold, compared to 22.7% for those who slept 6–7 hours, 30% for 5–6 hours, and 45.2% for less than 5 hours. These findings highlight how even modest reductions in sleep can substantially impair immune defense (Potter & Weiler, 2015; Prather et al., 2015).

The Relationship Between Sleep and COVID-19

The relationship between sleep habits, burnout, and susceptibility to infectious diseases has garnered increasing attention, especially among healthcare workers exposed to high-risk environments. A *BMJ* study explored whether sleep habits and burnout were risk factors for COVID-19 among high-risk healthcare workers in six countries (France, Germany, Italy, Spain, the U.K., and the U.S.A.). Data on sleep duration, napping, sleep problems, burnout, and COVID-19 exposure was collected through a web-based survey from July to September 2020. The results showed that longer sleep duration, 1 hour more per night, was associated with 12% reduced odds of COVID-19. Those with three sleep problems had 88% greater odds of contracting COVID-19. Burnout, particularly reported every day, was strongly associated with higher odds of COVID-19, with more severe burnout linked to greater risk. These findings suggest that insufficient sleep and high burnout may increase COVID-19 risk in healthcare workers, highlighting the need for strategies to manage sleep and stress in high-exposure environments (Kim et al., 2021).

An additional Lancet study found that individuals with pre-existing sleep disturbances faced 12% higher odds of COVID-19 infection, 25% higher odds of hospitalization, 45% higher odds of mortality, and 36% higher odds of developing long COVID. Subgroup analyses also found that younger individuals with sleep disturbances were more likely to contract COVID-19 and require hospitalization, yet had a lower risk of mortality compared to older individuals. Males with sleep disturbances were found to have a higher risk of death from COVID-19. Further analysis of specific types of sleep disturbances demonstrated that obstructive sleep apnea (OSA), abnormal sleep duration, and night-shift work were associated with increased susceptibility to COVID-19 and a higher likelihood of hospitalization. Mortality was particularly linked to OSA, while the risk of developing long COVID was elevated in individuals with OSA, abnormal sleep duration, and insomnia (Zhou et al., 2024).

Recent research has also highlighted the role of timing COVID-19 vaccine administration, suggesting that the body's circadian rhythm may impact vaccine efficacy. A study published in *The Journal of Clinical Investigation* suggests that administering the COVID-19 mRNA vaccine around midday may improve its effectiveness in preventing infections, especially for children, teenagers, and adults over age 50. The study explored the potential impact of circadian rhythm on vaccine response. The researchers found that vaccines given between 10 a.m. and 2 p.m. showed an 8.6% to 25% increase in effectiveness compared to doses given in the evening. For high-risk groups such as the elderly and immunosuppressed individuals, evening vaccinations were associated with more hospitalizations. Although the exact biological mechanisms are not yet clear, researchers believe the immune system's day-night rhythms may play a role (Hazan et al., 2023). Key findings from these studies are outlined in Table 15.4.

Table 15.4 Table Summary: Key Findings of Sleep on COVID-19 Outcomes

Focus	*Sample*	*Key Findings*	*Source*
Sleep duration, sleep problems, burnout	2884	• Additional 1 hour of sleep/ night led to 12% lower odds of COVID-19 • 3 sleep problems led to 88% higher odds of COVID-19 • Daily burnout significantly increased COVID-19 risk	Kim et al. (2021).
Pre-existing sleep disturbances	8,664,026	Sleep disturbances increased odds of: • Infection by 12% • Hospitalization by 25% • Mortality by 45% • Long COVID by 36% • OSA, abnormal sleep, and night-shift work increased susceptibility and hospitalization • OSA increased mortality • OSA, insomnia, abnormal sleep increase long COVID risk	Zhou et al. (2024)
Vaccine timing	1,515,754	• Administration 10 a.m.–2 p.m. increased effectiveness from 8.6% to 25% • Evening doses led to more hospitalizations in the elderly and immunosuppressed	Hazan et al. (2023)

Note: OSA = Obstructive Sleep Apnea.

Conclusion

Sleep plays a vital role in maintaining a healthy immune system. Sleep deprivation disrupts the circadian rhythm, hindering the immune system's ability to fight infections and diseases. Studies demonstrate that insufficient sleep increases inflammation and reduces antibody production in response to vaccines. Conversely, adequate sleep (ideally more than 7 hours) strengthens the immune system, decreasing susceptibility to illnesses like colds and COVID-19. Interestingly, the time of day for vaccinations can also influence their effectiveness, further highlighting the complex interplay between sleep, circadian rhythms, and immunity. Sleep does not operate in isolation. It is closely intertwined with psychological stress, another major determinant of immune health. The following section explores how stress management can enhance immune resilience and protect health during pandemics and beyond.

Stress Management: Nurturing Mental Health During Challenging Times

The COVID-19 pandemic led to a global rise in psychological stress, which impaired immune function and worsened health outcomes. Evidence links higher

psychological distress to a greater risk of infection and illness severity. Women, youth, and frontline workers were especially affected, and significant increases in depression, anxiety, and distress were found in regions with greater inequality and poverty.

The Biological Pathway: Stress and the Immune System

The human stress response is a complex interaction between the nervous, endocrine, and immune systems. Activation of the hypothalamic-pituitary-adrenal (HPA) axis in response to stress leads to the release of glucocorticoids, primarily cortisol. While acute stress responses can enhance immune vigilance, chronic stress impairs immune function in several important ways.

Prolonged elevation of cortisol levels has been shown to suppress lymphocyte activity, including both T and B cell production. It also inhibits the function of NK cells, which play a key role in the early defense against viral infections. Additionally, chronic stress reduces cytokine signaling, which is crucial for coordinating effective antiviral responses. Simultaneously, it increases systemic inflammation, a condition that can exacerbate the pathology of viral infections such as COVID-19 (Chu et al., 2024).

Chronic psychological stress has well-documented effects on immune function, weakening both innate and adaptive immune responses and increasing vulnerability to infections. A meta-analysis published in the *Psychological Bulletin* found consistent evidence that prolonged stress is associated with immune dysregulation (Segerstrom & Miller, 2004). Building on this, researchers demonstrated that stress not only heightened susceptibility to respiratory viruses but also intensified the severity of resulting illnesses, even when controlling for other risk factors (Cohen, 2020). These physiological effects are particularly concerning in the context of COVID-19, where stress-induced immune alterations and systemic inflammation may contribute to worse outcomes. In addition, chronic stress is linked to reduced vaccine efficacy and a cascade of poor health behaviors, such as increased alcohol and substance use, unhealthy eating, disrupted sleep, and physical inactivity, that further impair immune defense and overall well-being (Alotiby, 2024).

The Global Surge in Psychological Stress

The COVID-19 pandemic triggered an unprecedented global increase in stress levels. Although the specific sources of stress varied across countries and communities, the psychological burden was nearly universal. Common stressors included lockdowns, economic uncertainty, fear of infection, social isolation, the loss of loved ones, and an overwhelming sense of uncertainty about the future.

In high-income countries, stress was frequently driven by job instability, disrupted daily routines, and reduced access to mental health services, which were overwhelmed by increased demand. In contrast, individuals living in low- and middle-income countries (LMICs) faced additional challenges, such as poverty, food insecurity, limited access to healthcare, and a lack of infrastructure to support remote work, education, or telehealth. For refugees and displaced populations, the pandemic layered new stressors onto pre-existing trauma, including crowded or unstable living conditions and inadequate access to even basic medical care.

A systematic review published in *The Lancet* found that global depression and anxiety increased significantly during the pandemic, with depression rates increasing 27.6% and anxiety increasing 25.6%. These increases, however, were not evenly distributed across populations. Women, young people, frontline healthcare workers, and those in economically or socially precarious situations were disproportionately affected. As a result, the pandemic not only magnified mental health needs globally but also deepened existing health inequities (COVID-19 Mental Disorders Collaborators, 2021).

A meta-analysis study published in *Nature Human Behaviour* reported similar rising levels of psychological distress across the globe. The pooled global prevalence during COVID-19 was estimated at 28% for depression, 26.9% for anxiety, 24.1% for post-traumatic stress symptoms, 36.5% for stress, 50% for psychological distress, and 27.6% for sleep problems. Findings also highlighted that equality and poverty were factors in the prevalence of mental health problems. For instance, higher prevalence of mental health issues was observed in countries with low-to-medium Human Development Index (HDI), regions with high gender inequality, and areas with lower counts of hospital beds (Nochaiwong et al., 2021).

The Impact of Stress on COVID-19 Outcomes

A study published in *Annals of Behavioral Medicine* examined how psychological factors influenced susceptibility to COVID-19 and symptom severity. In a longitudinal analysis of 1087 adults, researchers found that those with higher levels of psychological distress were more likely to report COVID-19 infection and experienced more severe symptoms (Ayling et al., 2022). Similarly, a study in *Maedica* explored the relationship between stress, symptom severity, and sleep quality in COVID-19 patients. Moderate stress levels were common, especially early in illness, often driven by fears of infecting loved ones. Hair loss was reported by 42.3% of patients, a symptom previously linked to high fever and illness severity. Over 80% of patients experienced sleep disturbances, such as delayed sleep onset, frequent awakenings, or nightmares. Higher stress levels were significantly associated with more severe respiratory, neurological, and gastrointestinal symptoms, as well as poorer sleep quality (Karimi et al., 2022). These results suggest a potential link between psychological well-being and vulnerability to COVID-19 and emphasize the need for further research into the underlying biological and behavioral mechanisms.

Conclusion

The COVID-19 pandemic accentuated the significant impact of psychological stress on immune function and disease outcomes. Chronic stress impairs both innate and adaptive immunity, increases systemic inflammation, and is linked to worse COVID-19 symptoms, reduced vaccine efficacy, and unhealthy behaviors. Globally, stress levels surged, with vulnerable populations, such as women, youth, and frontline workers, experiencing the greatest burden. Research consistently shows that higher psychological distress is associated with increased risk of infection and more severe illness. While stress management is vital in maintaining mental and physical health, meaningful connections with others have been recognized as an effective way to buffer stress and promote resilience. The following section examines how the presence, or absence, of social connections shaped psychological and immune outcomes during the pandemic.

Social Connections: The Importance of Relationships for Overall Well-Being

Human connection is a fundamental component of health. Strong social connections offer profound benefits for both mental and physical well-being, while social isolation and loneliness are recognized as significant risk factors for early mortality. The pandemic starkly highlighted this reality, as lockdown, quarantine, and distancing measures disrupted interpersonal bonds and exacerbated emotional distress.

Importance of Social Connections

The U.S. CDC defines social connection as "the size and diversity of one's social network and roles, the functions these relationships serve, and their positive or negative qualities" (CDC, 2024b). Maintaining strong social connections fosters a sense of belonging and reinforces feelings of being loved, cared for, and valued. These connections are essential for both mental and physical well-being, serving as a protective factor against serious illnesses and chronic diseases. Research consistently shows that individuals with robust social bonds are not only more likely to experience better health but also enjoy longer, more fulfilling lives. By staying connected, we nurture our overall resilience and enhance our quality of life.

Health Impacts of Social Isolation and Loneliness

While social connection supports well-being, its absence can be profoundly harmful. Social isolation (a lack of social contacts) and loneliness (the subjective feeling of being alone) are independent risk factors for numerous adverse health outcomes. These include: heart disease and stroke, type 2 diabetes, depression and anxiety, suicidality and self-harm, dementia, and premature death (CDC, 2024c).

A meta-analysis published in *Perspectives in Psychological Science* examined the impact of social isolation, loneliness, and living alone on early mortality and found that each of these factors significantly increased the risk of premature death.

Social isolation was associated with 29% greater odds, loneliness was associated with 26% greater odds, and living alone was associated with 32% greater odds. These increased odds were comparable in impact to other morality risk factors such as smoking or obesity. Notably, the study found no significant difference between objective and subjective isolation, meaning that both being alone and feeling alone are equally harmful. These results confirm that social connection is a critical factor in health. Just as poor diet or lack of exercise, lacking meaningful relations can increase the risk of premature death (Holt-Lunstad et al., 2015).

Social Connections and COVID-19

The COVID-19 pandemic drastically altered social dynamics, with quarantining and social distancing measures leading to significant disruptions in interpersonal relationships. While these public health interventions were necessary to curb the spread of the virus, they also had profound negative effects on social well-being. One of the most immediate consequences was widespread social isolation, particularly among those living alone or within high-risk groups. Prolonged isolation contributed to increased feelings of loneliness, which is recognized for its harmful effects on mental and physical health.

Social support, a known protective factor against psychological distress, played a critical role during the pandemic. A longitudinal study of 69,066 U.S. adults from the *All of Us* Research Program found that higher levels of social support had 55% lower odds of experiencing elevated depressive symptoms. The greatest protection was observed in those who perceived strong support across three areas: tangible support, emotional or informational support, and positive social interactions. They had an over six-fold reduction in the odds of depression compared to those with no support. Those who experienced strong emotional or informational support had the strongest individual effect. Notably, women, adults under 60 years old, those with a history of mood disorders, and those facing pandemic-related financial stress were at higher risk for depression, but experienced greater protective benefits from social support (Choi et al., 2023).

Additional longitudinal assessments revealed that social distancing policies changed the way people experience their relationships. Researchers compared data from 2018 and 2020 and found increases in emotional and instrumental support, but also a rise in loneliness and a decline in perceived friendship quality (Philpot et al., 2021). These findings suggest that while people may have leaned more heavily on support networks during the crisis, the physical restrictions limited casual social engagement, which is critical in maintaining a sense of companionship and shared joy.

The nature of face-to-face interaction was also fundamentally altered by the widespread use of face coverings. An online study found that despite masks obscuring lower facial expressions, people could still accurately perceive emotions. However, the emotional valence of interaction and the desire for physical and social proximity varied significantly by gender and mask type, with women more attuned to emotional cues and men more influenced by the type of face covering.

This reveals a more subtle, but important, way the pandemic reshaped human connection, not only through absence, but through altered presence (Calbi et al., 2021).

Conclusion

The COVID-19 pandemic revealed the critical role that social connections play in our overall health and well-being. As we emerge from the crisis, rebuilding and reinforcing these bonds is essential, not only to heal from the emotional toll of the pandemic but to safeguard public health in the long term. Prioritizing social connection, combating loneliness, and protecting vulnerable populations from isolation and abuse must become integral parts of health and social policy.

In the absence of healthy connections and coping strategies, some turned to maladaptive behaviors, such as excessive drinking, smoking, and other substances, as a means of managing stress and anxiety during the pandemic. The following section examines the repercussions of substance use on the immune system and COVID-19 outcomes.

Substance Use: Health Risks and Consequences During a Pandemic

Substance use, including tobacco, alcohol, and both legal and illegal drugs, poses significant threats to public health. These behaviors compromise immune function, aggravate existing chronic conditions, and compound vulnerability to severe illness. During the pandemic, health risks associated with substance use became more apparent, leading to higher rates of infection, hospitalization, and mortality.

The COVID-19 pandemic has had profound affects on global health, not only due to the virus itself but also through its impact on mental health, substance use, and addiction patterns. Lockdowns, social isolation, economic instability, and limited access to support services contributed to a significant shift in substance use behaviors. Table 15.5 highlights the notable increases in the use and misuse of various substances during the pandemic compared to pre-pandemic trends, stressing the urgency of addressing substance use as a parallel public health crisis.

Tobacco Use and COVID-19

According to the WHO, there are approximately 1.3 billion tobacco users worldwide, with tobacco use contributing to over 8 million deaths each year. Of these, more than 7 million are attributed to direct smoking, while 1.3 million result from secondhand exposure. Notably, 80% of tobacco users reside in low and middle-income countries, where the burden of tobacco-related illness is often compounded by limited healthcare resources (WHO, 2023). Tobacco use is the leading cause of chronic noncommunicable diseases, significantly increasing the risk of cancer, heart disease, stroke, lung diseases, diabetes, chronic obstructive pulmonary disease (COPD), tuberculosis, eye diseases, rheumatoid arthritis, and compromised immunity (CDC, 2022).

Table 15.5 Pre-Pandemic vs. Pandemic Trends: Alcohol, Opioid, Cannabis, Prescription Drug, and Illicit Drug

Substance Type	*Pre-Pandemic Trends*	*Pandemic Trends*
Alcohol	• Stable or slight decline in general use • ALD leading indicator of liver transplants	• 262% increase in online alcohol sales in the U.S. • Increase in heavy and binge drinking • 20% increase in ALD deaths
Opioids	• 80% of drug deaths related to opioids in 2019 • 1040% increase in synthetic opioid deaths from 2013 to 2019	• Increase in opioid-related overdoses • Increased use of synthetic opioids (fentanyl) • Increased use among 15–19 year olds
Cannabis	• Widespread use, legal in some areas • Increasing trends but moderate	• Higher daily use reported in young adults • Used as a coping mechanism for stress and anxiety
Prescription Drugs (e.g., benzodiazepines, stimulants)	• Moderate misuse rates • Ongoing concern in youth and adults	• Increased misuse, particularly of anti-anxiety meds • Telehealth access led to more prescriptions early in the pandemic
Illicit Drugs (e.g., cocaine, meth)	• Persistent concern	• Increase in use and overdose deaths • Supply chain disruptions led to dangerous substitutes

Sources: Adapted from Mattson et al. (2021), Pollard et al. (2020), Deutsch-Link et al. (2022), CDC (2022), WHO (2023), National Institute on Alcohol Abuse and Alcoholism (NIAAA) (2023), National Center for Drug Abuse Statistics (NCDAS) (2023), UNODC (2023), and NPR (2023).

Note: ALD = Alcohol-related liver disease

Smoking and vaping suppress the immune system and decrease lung capacity, amplifying the body's vulnerability to COVID-19. When inhaling cigarette smoke or nicotine, the lungs produce more ACE2 receptors/proteins, which create more accessibility for the virus to enter the body. A *Journal of Adolescent Health* study reports that e-cigarette users are five times more likely to be diagnosed with COVID-19, and those using both traditional and e-cigarettes are seven times more susceptible (Gaiha et al., 2020).

Excessive Alcohol Consumption and COVID-19

Excessive alcohol consumption includes binge drinking, heavy drinking, underage drinking, and drinking while pregnant. Excessive alcohol consumption is associated with chronic diseases such as high blood pressure, heart disease, stroke, liver disease, and digestive problems and increases cancer risk. Long-term, it weakens the immune system, making individuals more vulnerable to illness and potentially worsening mental health conditions, and can increase the risks of several types of cancers (CDC, 2024a).

A review published in *Digestive and Liver Disease* examined the impact of COVID-19 on individuals with alcohol use disorders and alcohol-associated liver disease (ALD). The study found that patients with ALD faced an increased risk of severe COVID-19 outcomes and higher mortality rates. Specifically, individuals with liver cirrhosis experienced a fatality rate of approximately 30%. The pandemic also disrupted access to care for those with ALD and individuals seeking treatment for alcohol use. Additionally, patients undergoing liver transplants were found to be at heightened risk for severe COVID-19 complications and mortality (Deutsch-Link et al., 2022).

The National Center for Drug Abuse Statistics reveals a significant COVID-19 pandemic impact on national alcohol consumption rates. Online alcohol sales in the U.S. surged by 262% year-over-year in the first three weeks of March 2020, alongside initial lockdown measures (NCDAS, 2023). In the U.S. alcohol-related deaths increased approximately 37.8% from 2019 to 2021, further highlighting the pandemic's detrimental influence on alcohol use (NIAAA, 2023).

Drug Use and COVID-19

The 2023 United Nations Office on Drugs and Crime report revealed that global drug use remains alarmingly high. In 2021, approximately 1 in 17 people worldwide had used drugs in the past 12 months, with the estimated number of users rising from 240 million in 2011 to 296 million in 2021, representing 5.8% of the global population aged 15–64 and a 23% increase, partly attributable to population growth. Additionally, an estimated 13.2 million people injected drugs in 2021, marking an 18% increase from 2020 (UNODC, 2023).

Drug use can exacerbate health complications from COVID-19. For instance, both COVID-19 and drug use can adversely affect cardiopulmonary function, amplifying the negative health effects. High doses of opioids can slow breathing and lead to lower oxygen levels in the blood, which can lead to complications in the heart, brain, and lungs. Since COVID-19 primarily affects the lungs, opioid users may be at risk for more severe illness if they become infected. Stimulants such as methamphetamine, cocaine, and amphetamines can constrict blood vessels, potentially increasing the risk of stroke, heart disease, arrhythmias, seizures, and other conditions that can lead to more severe heart or lung damage in individuals with COVID-19 (National Institute on Drug Abuse, 2023).

A large-scale analysis of electronic health records of over 73 million patients across 360 U.S. hospitals found that individuals with a recent diagnosis of a substance use disorder were at increased risk of contracting COVID-19. The risk was highest among individuals with opioid use disorders and tobacco use disorders. These elevated risks may be attributed not only to the direct physiological effects of substance use, but also to behavioral, environmental, and social factors that increase exposure and susceptibility to viral infection. Patients with substance use disorders also exhibited a significantly higher burden of comorbid conditions known to exacerbate COVID-19 outcomes, including chronic kidney, liver, and pulmonary diseases, cardiovascular diseases, type 2 diabetes, obesity, and cancer.

Table 15.6 Health Impacts and COVID-19 Outcomes of Substance Use

Category	*Health Impacts*	*COVID-19 Outcomes*
Tobacco Use (Smoking and E-cigarette)	• Increases expression of ACE2 receptors in the lungs • Suppresses the immune system • Decreases lung capacity	• E-cigarette users 5× more likely to contract COVID-19 • Dual users 7× more likely to contract COVID-19
Excessive Alcohol Consumption	• Worsens mental health and chronic diseases • Weakens the immune system over time • Increases vulnerability to infections • Increase the risk of liver diseases	• Patients with ALD increased risk of severe illness and death • Patients with liver cirrhosis had a 30% fatality rate
Substance Use Disorders (SUD)	• Increases risk of hepatitis C and HIV • Increase risk of cardio-vascular events • Impaired breathing and oxygen levels	• 1.5× more likely to contract COVID-19 • Increased hospitalization (41% vs. 30%) • Increased mortality (9.6% vs. 6.6%)

Sources: Adapted from Gaiha et al. (2020), Deutsch-Link et al. (2022), Wang et al. (2021), National Institute on Drug Abuse (2020; 2023).

Note: ALD = Alcohol-related liver disease

These comorbidities likely contribute to both increased infection risk and poorer clinical trajectories.

Notably, significant racial disparities were observed. African American patients with a recent substance use disorder diagnosis were more than twice as likely to contract COVID-19 compared to their Caucasian counterparts, with the disparity most pronounced among those with opioid use disorders. Furthermore, African Americans with both substance use disorders and COVID-19 experienced substantially worse outcomes, including higher rates of hospitalization (50.7% vs. 35.2%) and mortality (13.0% vs. 8.6%), compared to Caucasian patients with the same conditions. Overall, COVID-19 patients with substance use disorders, regardless of racial background, experienced poorer outcomes than COVID-19 patients without substance use disorders. Among the substance use disorder group, hospitalization and mortality rates were 41% and 9.6%, respectively, compared to 30.1% and 6.6% in the general COVID-19 population (Wang et al., 2021). Key findings from these studies are summarized in Table 15..

Conclusion

Tobacco use, excessive alcohol consumption, and drug use pose significant health risks, weakening the immune system and increasing susceptibility to infectious diseases like COVID-19. Smoking and vaping damage the lungs and suppress the body's defenses, making smokers and vapers more vulnerable to severe COVID-19 complications. Similarly, excessive alcohol and drug use can weaken the immune system, damage vital organs, and lead to comorbidities that worsen COVID-19 outcomes. The COVID-19 pandemic has further exacerbated these problems, with increased alcohol sales, rising drug-related deaths, and those with substance use disorders being disproportionately affected by the virus. Overall, drug use has severe repercussions on health, mental well-being, and social functioning.

Taken together, the lifestyle factors explored in this section—nutrition, physical activity, sleep, stress, social connection, and substance use—highlight the deep interconnection between daily behavior and pandemic resilience. These modifiable behaviors not only shape immune function and disease outcomes but also buffer against the mental health burdens and social dislocations that accompany prolonged public health crises.

When paired with vaccines, treatments, non-pharmaceutical interventions, and protections for vulnerable populations, lifestyle interventions offer a powerful, often overlooked, layer of defense. As we transition from crisis to recovery, the lessons of Part 3 remind us that resilience is not built solely in labs or hospitals—but also in homes, communities, and everyday habits. In Part 4, we look ahead to examine how COVID-19 is reshaping the landscape of future outbreaks, the threat of new and reemerging diseases, and the lasting imprint of this pandemic on global health systems.

References

Alotiby, A. (2024). Immunology of stress: A review article. *Journal of Clinical Medicine*, *13*(21). https://doi.org/10.3390/jcm13216394

Alshammari, M. K., Fatima, W., Ahmed, A. R., Alzahrani, K., Kamal, M., Saud, A. R., Alshammari, S. A., Alharbi, L. M., Alsubaie, N. S., Alosaimi, R. B., Basheeruddin, M., & Imran, M. (2022). Selenium and COVID-19: A spotlight on the clinical trials, inventive compositions, and patent literature. *Journal of Infection and Public Health*, *15*(11), 1225–1233. https://doi.org/10.1016/j.jiph.2022.09.011

American College of Sports Medicine. (2025). *Physical activity guidelines*. ACSM. https://acsm.org/education-resources/trending-topics-resources/physical-activity-guidelines/

Ayling, K., Jia, R., Coupland, C., Chalder, T., Massey, A., Broadbent, E., & Vedhara, K. (2022). Psychological predictors of self-reported COVID-19 outcomes: Results from a prospective cohort study. *Annals of Behavioral Medicine*, *56*(5), 484–497. https://doi.org/10.1093/abm/kaab106

Bhowmik, K. K., Barek, M. A., Aziz, M. A., & Islam, M. S. (2022). Impact of high-dose vitamin C on the mortality, severity, and duration of hospital stay in COVID-19 patients: A meta-analysis. *Health Science Reports*, *5*, e762. doi:10.1002/hsr2.762

Calbi, M., Langiulli, N., Ferroni, F., Montalti, M., Kolesnikov, A., Gallese, V., & Umiltà, M. A. (2021). The consequences of COVID-19 on social interactions: An online study on face covering. *Scientific Reports*, *11*(1), 2601. https://doi.org/10.1038/s41598-021-81780-w

CDC. (2022, May 11). *U.S. overdose deaths in 2021 increased half as much as in 2020 – But are still up 15%*. CDC. https://www.cdc.gov/nchs/pressroom/nchs_press_releases/2022/202205.htm

CDC. (2024a, October 11). *Facts about excessive drinking*. CDC. https://www.cdc.gov/drink-less-be-your-best/facts-about-excessive-drinking/index.html

CDC. (2024b). *Social connection.* Social Connection; CDC. https://www.cdc.gov/social-connectedness/about/index.html

CDC. (2024c, March 26). *Health effects of social isolation and loneliness.* Social Connection; CDC. https://www.cdc.gov/social-connectedness/risk-factors/index.html

Choi, K. W., Lee, Y. H., Liu, Z., Fatori, D., Bauermeister, J. R., Luh, R. A., Clark, C. R., Brunoni, A. R., Bauermeister, S., & Smoller, J. W. (2023). Social support and depression during a global crisis. *Nature Mental Health, 1*(6), 428–435. https://doi.org/10.1038/s44220-023-00078-0

Chu, B., Marwaha, K., Ayers, D., & Sanvictores, T. (2024). *Physiology, stress reaction.* PubMed; StatPearls Publishing. https://www.ncbi.nlm.nih.gov/books/NBK541120/

Cohen, S. (2020). Psychosocial vulnerabilities to upper respiratory infectious illness: Implications for susceptibility to coronavirus disease 2019 (COVID-19). *Perspectives on Psychological Science, 16*(1), 161–174. https://doi.org/10.1177/1745691620942516

Cooper, J. (2024, September 11). *Benefits of protein.* WebMD. https://www.webmd.com/diet/benefits-protein

da Cruz Carvalho, M. C., Araujo, J. K. C. P., da Silva, A. G. C. L., da Silva, N. S., de Araújo, N. K., Luchessi, A. D., da Silva Ribeiro, K. D., & Silbiger, V. N. (2023). Retinol levels and severity of patients with COVID-19. *Nutrients, 15*(21), 4642. https://doi.org/10.3390/nu15214642

Darand, M., Hassanizadeh, S., Martami, F., Shams, S., Mirzaei, M., & Hosseinzadeh, M. (2023). The association between B vitamins and the risk of COVID-19. *British Journal of Nutrition, 130*(1), 155–163. doi:10.1017/S0007114522003075

Deutsch-Link, S., Curtis, B., & Singal, A. K. (2022). Covid-19 and alcohol associated liver disease. *Digestive and Liver Disease: Official Journal of the Italian Society of Gastroenterology and the Italian Association for the Study of the Liver, 54*(11), 1459–1468. https://doi.org/10.1016/j.dld.2022.07.007

Ezzatvar, Y., RamírezVélez, R., Izquierdo, M., & GarciaHermoso, A. (2022). Physical activity and risk of infection, severity and mortality of COVID-19: A systematic review and nonlinear dose–response meta-analysis of data from 1 853 610 adults. *British Journal of Sports Medicine, 56*(20), 1188–1193. https://doi.org/10.1136/bjsports-2022-105733

Gaiha, S. M., Cheng, J., & Halpern-Felsher, B. (2020). Association between youth smoking, electronic cigarette use, and COVID-19. *Journal of Adolescent Health, 67*(4), 519–523. https://doi.org/10.1016/j.jadohealth.2020.07.002

Garbarino, S., Lanteri, P., Bragazzi, N. L., Magnavita, N., & Scoditti, E. (2021). Role of sleep deprivation in immune-related disease risk and outcomes. *Communications Biology, 4*(1), 1304. https://doi.org/10.1038/s42003-021-02825-4

Govind, V., Bharadwaj, S., Sai Ganesh, M. R., Vishnu, J., Shankar, K. V., Shankar, B., & Rajesh, R. (2021). Antiviral properties of copper and its alloys to inactivate Covid-19 virus: A review. *BioMetals, 34*(6), 1217–1235. https://doi.org/10.1007/s10534-021-00339-4

Hanson, A. L., Mulè, M. P., Ruffieux, H., Mescia, F., Bergamaschi, L., Pelly, V. S., Turner, L., Kotagiri, P., Cambridge Institute of Therapeutic Immunology and Infectious Disease-National Institute for Health Reasearch (CITIID-NIHR) COVID BioResource Collaboration, Göttgens, B., Hess, C., Gleadall, N., Bradley, J. R., Nathan, J. A., Lyons, P. A., Drakesmith, H., & Smith, K.. (2024). Iron dysregulation and inflammatory stress erythropoiesis associates with long-term outcome of COVID-19. *Nature Immunology, 25*(3), 471–482. https://doi.org/10.1038/s41590-024-01754-8

Hazan, G., Duek, O. A., Alapi, H., Mok, H., Ganninger, A., Ostendorf, E., Gierasch, C., Chodick, G., Greenberg, D., & Haspel, J. A. (2023). Biological rhythms in COVID-19 vaccine effectiveness in an observational cohort study of 1.5 million patients. *Journal of Clinical Investigation, 133*(11). https://doi.org/10.1172/JCI167339

Healthcare Infection Society. (2021, June 14). *The danger of dehydration: How can you spot it in COVID-19 patients.* Healthcare Infection Society. https://www.his.org.uk/news/2021/the-danger-of-dehydration-how-can-you-can-spot-it-in-covid-19-patients/

Holt-Lunstad, J., Smith, T. B., Baker, M., Harris, T., & Stephenson, D. (2015). Loneliness and social isolation as risk factors for mortality: A meta-analytic review. *Perspectives on Psychological Science*, *10*(2), 227–237. https://doi.org/10.1177/1745691614568352 (Original work published 2015)

Huang, Z., Liu, Y., Qi, G., Brand, D., & Zheng, S. G. (2018). Role of vitamin A in the immune system. *Journal of Clinical Medicine*, *7*(9), 258. https://doi.org/10.3390/jcm7090258

Jima, L. M., Atomsa, G. E., Allard, J. P., & Nigatu, Y. D. (2024). The effect of malnutrition on adult Covid-19 patient's ICU admission and mortality in Covid-19 isolation and treatment centers in Ethiopia: A prospective cohort study. *PLoS ONE*, *19*(3), e0298215. https://doi.org/10.1371/journal.pone.0298215

Jin, D., Wei, X., He, Y., Zhong, L., Lu, H., Lan, J., Wei, Y., Liu, Z., & Liu, H. (2024). The nutritional roles of zinc for immune system and COVID-19 patients. *Frontiers in Nutrition, 112024*. https://www.frontiersin.org/journals/nutrition/articles/10.3389/fnut.2024.1385591

Karimi, S., Derakhshan, M., & Tondro, A. (2022). Evaluation of the Relationship between Stress and Severity of Covid-19 Symptoms and Sleep Quality in Covid-19 Patients. *MAEDICA – A Journal of Clinical Medicine*, *17*(1). https://doi.org/10.26574/maedica.2022.17.1.129

Kim, H., Hegde, S., LaFiura, C., Raghavan, M., Luong, E., Cheng, S., Rebholz, C. M., & Seidelmann, S. B. (2021). COVID-19 illness in relation to sleep and burnout. *BMJ Nutrition, Prevention & Health*, *4*(1), null. https://doi.org/10.1136/bmjnph-2021-000228

Kim, H., Rebholz, C. M., Hegde, S., LaFiura, C., Raghavan, M., Lloyd, J. F., Cheng, S., & Seidelmann, S. B. (2021). Plant-based diets, pescatarian diets and COVID-19 severity: A population-based case-control study in six countries. *BMJ Nutrition, Prevention & Health*, *4*(1), null. https://doi.org/10.1136/bmjnph-2021-000272

Lee, S. W., Lee, J., Moon, S. Y., Jin, H. Y., Yang, J. M., Ogino, S., Song, M., Hong, S. H., Ramy, A. G., Kronbichler, A., Koyanagi, A., Jacob, L., Dragioti, E., Smith, L., Giovannucci, E., Lee, I., Lee, D. H., Lee, K. H., Shin, Y. H., & Kim, S. Y. (2022). Physical activity and the risk of SARS-CoV-2 infection, severe COVID-19 illness and COVID-19 related mortality in South Korea: A nationwide cohort study. *British Journal of Sports Medicine*, *56*(16), 901. https://doi.org/10.1136/bjsports-2021-104203

Mattson, C. L., Tanz, L. J., Quinn, K., Kariisa, M., Patel, P., & Davis, N. L. (2021). Trends and geographic patterns in drug and synthetic opioid overdose deaths—United States, 2013–2019. *MMWR. Morbidity and Mortality Weekly Report*, *70*(6), 202–207. https://doi.org/10.15585/mmwr.mm7006a4

Merino, J., Joshi, A. D., Nguyen, L. H., Leeming, E. R., Mazidi, M., Drew, D. A., Gibson, R., Graham, M. S., Lo, C., Capdevila, J., Murray, B., Hu, C., Selvachandran, S., Hammers, A., Bhupathiraju, S. N., Sharma, S. V., Sudre, C., Astley, C. M., Chavarro, J. E., & Kwon, S. (2021). Diet quality and risk and severity of COVID-19: A prospective cohort study. *Gut*, *70*(11), 2096. https://doi.org/10.1136/gutjnl-2021-325353

Mount Sinai. (n.d.). *Vitamin B5 (pantothenic acid)*. Mount Sinai Health System. https://www.mountsinai.org/health-library/supplement/vitamin-b5-pantothenic-acid

National Center for Drug Abuse Statistics (NCDAS). (2023). *Alcohol abuse statistics*. National Center for Drug Abuse Statistics. https://drugabusestatistics.org/alcohol-abuse-statistics/

National Institute on Alcohol Abuse and Alcoholism (NIAAA). (2023, April 12). *Alcohol-related deaths, which increased during the first year of the COVID-19 pandemic, continued to rise in 2021*. National Institute on Alcohol Abuse and Alcoholism. https://www.niaaa.nih.gov/news-events/research-update/alcohol-related-deaths-which-increased-during-first-year-covid-19-pandemic-continued-rise-2021

National Institute on Drug Abuse. (2020, July). *Addiction and health*. National Institute on Drug Abuse. https://nida.nih.gov/publications/drugs-brains-behavior-science-addiction/addiction-health

National Institute on Drug Abuse. (2023, November 20). *COVID-19 and substance use*. NIH National Institute on Drug Abuse; National Institutes of Health. https://nida.nih.gov/research-topics/covid-19-substance-use#health-outcomes

National Institutes of Health (NIH). (2024). *Office of dietary supplements – Dietary supplements in the time of COVID-19*. NIH. https://ods.od.nih.gov/factsheets/COVID19-HealthProfessional/#h41

Nieman, D. C., & Wentz, L. M. (2019). The compelling link between physical activity and the body's defense system. *Journal of Sport and Health Science*, *8*(3), 201–217. https://doi.org/10.1016/j.jshs.2018.09.009

Nochaiwong, S., Ruengorn, C., Thavorn, K., Hutton, B., Awiphan, R., Phosuya, C., Ruanta, Y., Wongpakaran, N., & Wongpakaran, T. (2021). Global prevalence of mental health issues among the general population during the coronavirus disease-2019 pandemic: A systematic review and meta-analysis. *Scientific Reports*, *11*(1), 10173. https://doi.org/10.1038/s41598-021-89700-8

NPR. (2023, May 10). *The pandemic-era rule that lets you get telehealth prescriptions just got extended*. NPR. https://www.npr.org/sections/health-shots/2023/05/10/1175272764/the-pandemic-era-rule-that-lets-you-get-telehealth-prescriptions-just-got-extend

O'Donovan, G., Lee, I., Hamer, M., & Stamatakis, E. (2017). Association of "weekend warrior" and other leisure time physical activity patterns with risks for all-cause, cardiovascular disease, and cancer mortality. *JAMA Internal Medicine*, *177*(3), 335–342. https://doi.org/10.1001/jamainternmed.2016.8014

Perez-Araluce, R., Martinez-Gonzalez, M. A., Fernández-Lázaro, C. I., Bes-Rastrollo, M., Gea, A., & Carlos, S. (2022). Mediterranean diet and the risk of COVID-19 in the "Seguimiento Universidad de Navarra" cohort. *Clinical Nutrition*, *41*(12), 3061–3068. https://doi.org/10.1016/j.clnu.2021.04.001

Philpot, L. M., Ramar, P., Roellinger, D. L., Barry, B. A., Sharma, P., & Ebbert, J. O. (2021). Changes in social relationships during an initial "stay-at-home" phase of the COVID-19 pandemic: A longitudinal survey study in the U.S. *Social Science & Medicine (1982)*, *274*, 113779. https://doi.org/10.1016/j.socscimed.2021.113779

Pollard, M. S., Tucker, J. S., & Green, H. D., Jr (2020). Changes in adult alcohol use and consequences during the COVID-19 pandemic in the US. *JAMA Network Open*, *3*(9), e2022942. https://doi.org/10.1001/jamanetworkopen.2020.22942

Potter, L. M., & Weiler, N. (2015, August 31). *Short sleepers are four times more likely to catch a cold*. UC San Francisco. https://www.ucsf.edu/news/2015/08/131411/short-sleepers-are-four-times-more-likely-catch-cold

Prather, A. A., Janicki-Deverts, D., Hall, M. H., & Cohen, S. (2015). Behaviorally assessed sleep and susceptibility to the common cold. *Sleep*, *38*(9), 1353–1359. https://doi.org/10.5665/sleep.4968

Roland, J. (2019, October 22). *What are METs, and how are they calculated?* Healthline. https://www.healthline.com/health/what-are-mets

Rust, P., & Ekmekcioglu, C. (2023). The role of diet and specific nutrients during the COVID-19 pandemic: What have we learned over the last three years? *International Journal of Environmental Research and Public Health*, *20*(7), 5400. https://doi.org/10.3390/ijerph20075400

Sallis, R., Young, D. R., Tartof, S. Y., Sallis, J. F., Sall, J., Li, Q., Smith, G. N., & Cohen, D. A. (2021). Physical inactivity is associated with a higher risk for severe COVID-19 outcomes: A study in 48 440 adult patients. *British Journal of Sports Medicine*, *55*(19), 1099. https://doi.org/10.1136/bjsports-2021-104080

COVID-19 Mental Disorders Collaborators (2021). Global prevalence and burden of depressive and anxiety disorders in 204 countries and territories in 2020 due to the COVID-19 pandemic. *The Lancet*, *398*(10312), 1700–1712. https://doi.org/10.1016/S0140-6736(21)02143-7

Segerstrom, S. C., & Miller, G. E. (2004). Psychological stress and the human immune system: A meta-analytic study of 30 years of inquiry. *Psychological Bulletin*, *130*(4), 601–630. https://doi.org/10.1037/0033-2909.130.4.601

Shakoor, H., Feehan, J., Mikkelsen, K., Dhaheri, A., Ali, H. I., Platat, C., Ismail, L. C., Stojanovska, L., & Apostolopoulos, V. (2021). Be well: A potential role for vitamin B in COVID-19. *Maturitas*, *144*, 108–111. https://doi.org/10.1016/j.maturitas.2020.08.007

Sittichai, N., Parasin, N., Saokaew, S., Kanchanasurakit, S., Kayod, N., Praikaew, K., Phisalprapa, P., & Prasannarong, M. (2022). Effects of physical activity on the severity of illness and mortality in COVID-19 patients: A systematic review and meta-analysis. *Frontiers in Physiology*, *132022*. https://doi.org/10.3389/fphys.2022.1030568

Sofi, F., Cesari, F., Abbate, R., Franco, G. G., & Casini, A. (2008). Adherence to Mediterranean diet and health status: Meta-analysis. *BMJ*, *337*, a1344. https://doi.org/10.1136/bmj.a1344

Tadbir Vajargah, K., Zargarzadeh, N., Ebrahimzadeh, A., Mousavi, S. M., Mobasheran, P., Mokhtari, P., Rahban, H., Găman, M.-A., Akhgarjand, C., Taghizadeh, M., & Milajerdi, A. (2022) Association of fruits, vegetables, and fiber intake with COVID-19 severity and symptoms in hospitalized patients: A cross-sectional study. *Frontiers in Nutrition* 9, 934568. doi: 10.3389/fnut.2022.934568

Timmons, B. W., & Cieslak, T. (2008). Human natural killer cell subsets and acute exercise: A brief review. *Exercise Immunology Review*, *14*, 8–23.

UNODC. (2023). *World Drug Report 2023*.United Nations Publication.

Wang, Q. Q., Kaelber, D. C., Xu, R., & Volkow, N. D. (2021). COVID-19 risk and outcomes in patients with substance use disorders: Analyses from electronic health records in the United States. *Molecular Psychiatry*, *26*(1), 30–39. https://doi.org/10.1038/s41380-020-00880-7

World Health Organization (WHO). (n.d.). *Nutrition advice for adults during the COVID-19 outbreak*. World Health Organization – Regional Office for the Eastern Mediterranean. https://www.emro.who.int/nutrition/covid-19/nutrition-advice-for-adults-during-the-covid-19-outbreak.html

World Health Organization (WHO). (2023, July 31). *Tobacco*. World Health Organization. https://www.who.int/news-room/fact-sheets/detail/tobacco

Zhou, J., Li, X., Zhang, T., Liu, Z., Li, P., Yu, N., & Wang, W. (2024). Preexisting sleep disturbances and risk of COVID-19: A meta-analysis. *eClinicalMedicine*, *74*. https://doi.org/10.1016/j.eclinm.2024.102719

Part IV

Beyond the Horizon

How COVID-19 Shapes the Next Pandemic Era

16 The Long Shadow

Six Enduring Impacts of the Pandemic

The COVID-19 pandemic cast a long shadow across global society, with effects that continue to reverberate years later. It reversed decades of progress in some areas (life expectancy, immunization, poverty), while accelerating transformations in others (digital work and schooling). By 2023–2025, some metrics rebounded to pre-pandemic levels (global life expectancy, jobs), whereas other impacts proved more persistent or worsening (mental health issues, learning deficits, trust in institutions). This section examines six enduring impacts that have not only altered our present circumstances but have fundamentally reshaped trajectories for individuals, communities, and nations indefinitely.

Global Impacts of COVID-19 (2019–2025): A Six-Dimensional Analysis

What started as a novel coronavirus outbreak evolved into a global crisis that would disrupt societies and have profound, historic impact that would go beyond the acute phase. This section provides a comprehensive analysis of six key dimensions of the pandemic's global effects from 2019 through early 2025: (1) Life Expectancy and Demographic Shifts, (2) Mortality Patterns and Indirect Health Outcomes, (3) Mental Health Fallout, (4) Workforce Transformation, (5) Educational Disruption, and (6) Institutional Trust. For each dimension, we examine initial shocks in 2020–2021 and subsequent trends (whether conditions have improved, worsened, or partially rebounded by 2023–2025), drawing on current statistics and expert insights. We highlight disparities between countries, regions, and demographics and discuss policy implications for recovery and resilience. Table 16.1 provides a broad overview of these global indicators across the pandemic's timeline.

Life Expectancy and Demographic Shifts

The COVID-19 pandemic delivered a sharp blow to global life expectancy, abruptly ending a decades-long upward trend. The world's average life expectancy at birth dropped by about 1.8 years between 2019 and 2021, falling from approximately 73.0 years to 71.2 years—essentially wiping out a decade of longevity gains in just two years (Our World in Data, 2023). Global healthy life expectancy also declined

DOI: 10.4324/9781003595564-21

Table 16.1 Selected Global Indicators Pre-Pandemic vs. During Pandemic and Beyond

Global Indicators	*Pre-COVID (2019)*	*Worst Point (2020–2021)*	*Recent (2023–2024)*
Life Expectancy at Birth	73.0 years	71.2 years (−1.8 years)	73.2 years (recovered)
Excess Mortality	(baseline)	+14.8 million deaths	±20 million; true toll uncertain
Routine Vaccine Coverage (diphtheria, tetanus, toxoid and pertussis)	86%	81% (30-year low)	84% (partial rebound)
Anxiety/Depression	10–15% prevalence	25–27% initial increase	Elevated globally
Unemployment Rate	5.4%	6.6%	Near pre-crisis (4.9–5.2%)
Education Disruption	(baseline)	1.6 billion learners affected; uneven gaps	Lasting learning loss; unequal recovery
Trust in Government	50%	Initial increase, followed by decline	39%; ongoing erosion

Sources: International Labour Organization (ILO) (2021a, 2021b, 2022, 2023, 2024), World Bank (2021a, 2021b, 2022, 2023), World Health Organization (WHO) (2022b, 2022c, 2024), Msemburi et al. (2023), Jones et al. (2024), Organisation for Economic Co-Operation and Development (OECD) (2023, 2024a, 2024b), Edelman Trust Institute (2023–2025), UNICEF (2021a, 2021b, 2021c, 2024), Our World in Data (2023), UNESCO (2021a, 2021b, 2023a, 2023b), COVID-19 Mental Disorders Collaborators (The Lancet) (2021), GBD 2021 Europe Life Expectancy Collaborators (2025).

by about 1.5 years over the same period. This setback is striking given that from 2000 to 2019, life expectancy had steadily increased worldwide.

The life expectancy shock varied dramatically across regions (Table 16.2), reflecting the uneven toll of the virus. According to Our World in Data estimates, the WHO regions of the Americas and South-East Asia were hit hardest, each experiencing declines of approximately 3.0 years between 2019 and 2021. In contrast, the Western Pacific region saw minimal disruption, with life expectancy falling by less than 0.2 years. Europe experienced an intermediate decline of about 1.8 years, while Africa saw a loss of approximately 1.5 years over the same period. Nationally, some countries endured historic setbacks. Peru—one of the worst affected—saw an extraordinary drop of about six to seven years during 2020–2021 (Pare, 2024). Other Latin American countries (such as Bolivia and Mexico) and parts of Eastern Europe similarly faced multi-year reversals. Meanwhile, several countries in East Asia and Oceania (including New Zealand, China, and Japan) experienced little to no decline, largely due to comprehensive containment measures or demographic advantages like younger population structures (United Nations, 2022).

Following the rollout of vaccines and improvements in treatment, COVID-19 mortality declined after 2021, allowing life expectancy to recover in many regions. Global life expectancy rebounded to roughly 72.6 years in 2022 and

Table 16.2 Global and Regional Life Expectancy Changes During the COVID-19 Pandemic (2019–2023)

Region	*Pre-Pandemic Life Expectancy (2019)*	*Pandemic Low (2021)*	*Net Change (2019–2021)*	*Recovery (2023)*	*Status vs. Pre-Pandemic*
Global Average	73.0 years	71.2 years	**−1.8 years**	73.2 years	Recovered
Europe	78.8 years	77.0 years	**−1.8 years**	79.1 years	Exceeded
Oceania	78.6 years	78.5 years	**−0.2 years**	79.2 years	Exceeded
Americas	76.9 years	73.9 years	**−3.0 years**	75.7 years	Partial Rec.
Asia	74.2 years	72.9 years	**−1.3 years**	74.1 years	Partial Rec.
E. Mediterranean	72.0 years	69.8 years	**−2.2 years**	71.2 years	Partial Rec.
South-East Asia	71.4 years	68.5 years	**−2.9 years**	71.1 years	Partial Rec.
Africa	64.5 years	63.0 years	**−1.5 years**	64.3 years	Partial Rec.

Sources: Our World in Data (2023), WHO (2024), Schöley et al. (2022), GBD 2021, Europe Life Expectancy Collaborators (2025).

climbed further to an estimated 73.2 years by 2023 (Our World in Data, 2023). This suggests that, at a global scale, the pre-pandemic longevity trend was fully regained by 2023, although some of the hardest-hit countries have yet to recover fully.

Beyond mortality, COVID-19 also influenced demographic dynamics through effects on fertility, migration, and population growth. Early in the pandemic, many countries experienced a "baby bust"—a short-term decline in birth rates amid economic uncertainty and lockdowns. For example, births in late 2020 to early 2021 fell sharply in the United States and parts of Europe, followed by a modest rebound later in 2021 (Kearney & Levine, 2022). However, this rebound was neither universal nor sustained. By 2022, fertility rates unexpectedly dropped again across many high-income countries, reaching record lows in some cases by 2022–2023 (United Nations, 2022).

Another tragic demographic fallout has been the surge in orphaned children. By mid-2022, an estimated 10.5 million children worldwide had lost a parent or primary caregiver due to COVID-19 (Centers for Disease Control and Prevention (CDC), 2022). This "hidden pandemic of orphanhood" carries long-term social repercussions, as these children face heightened risks of poverty, mental health challenges, and exploitation. A series of studies by Hillis et al. (2021, 2022a, 2022b) and collaborators used excess mortality models to identify how caregiver loss disproportionately affected children in low- and middle-income countries, with particularly severe rates in Latin America and sub-Saharan Africa. For instance, in Peru, about 1 in 100 children lost a caregiver. More recent data shows that the United States was also deeply affected: Villaveces et al. (2025) found that COVID-related caregiver loss in the United States fell disproportionately on Black, Hispanic, and Indigenous children, compounding pre-existing structural vulnerabilities.

Mortality Patterns and Indirect Health Outcomes

COVID-19 has directly caused millions of deaths, but its impact on mortality extends well beyond the virus itself. Understanding these broader mortality patterns is essential for gauging the pandemic's full toll. As of 2025, approximately 7.1 million deaths worldwide have been officially attributed to COVID-19. However, the true global death toll is likely much higher due to significant underreporting. A 2023 Nature analysis of WHO data estimated 14.8 million excess deaths occurred in 2020–2021 alone, which is 2.74 times the 5.4 million reported COVID-19 deaths during that period (Msemburi et al., 2023). Based on these trends, the cumulative global mortality from the pandemic may now exceed 20 million.

Mortality has been disproportionately concentrated among older adults and individuals with underlying health conditions. In many countries, people over 65 accounted for 70–80% of COVID-related deaths. Geographic disparities were also pronounced: countries that swiftly contained the virus experienced relatively low death rates, while others recorded some of the highest mortality levels in modern history. Peru's cumulative death rate, at over 600 per 100,000, remains the highest in the world, and severe mortality burdens were also observed in parts of Eastern Europe, Brazil, Mexico, South Africa, and other regions. Europe experienced diverging mortality outcomes, with some countries rebounding quickly, while others experienced prolonged stagnation. A regional analysis from the Global Burden of Disease Study found that these divergent trends were shaped not only by differences in COVID-related mortality but also by country-level patterns of cardiovascular disease (CVD), chronic illness, and socioeconomic inequality (GBD 2021 Europe Life Expectancy Collaborators, 2025).

Crucially, many of the excess deaths during the pandemic were not caused by COVID-19 infection itself but stemmed from indirect effects of the crisis (Table 16.3). Overstretched health systems, delayed treatments, economic

Table 16.3 Global Indirect Health Impacts of COVID-19

Health Category	*Estimated Global Impact*
Cancer Screenings	Screenings dropped 86–94% (U.S.) in 2020; cancer services disrupted by up to 50% globally.
Cardiovascular Disease	19M deaths in 2020 (32% of global total deaths); years of declining mortality reversed by pandemic.
Tuberculosis	Deaths rose from 1.4M (2019) to 1.6M (2021).
Malaria	Deaths increased from 568K (2019) to 625K (2020).
Childhood Vaccinations	23M children missed routine vaccines in 2020; highest decline since 2009.
Substance Use	600K global drug-related deaths in 2019; overdose risks worsened during pandemic.
Homicide	458K global homicides in 2021; rates rose in many regions post-2020.

Sources: Cancino et al. (2020); CDC (2022, 2023, 2024a, 2024b); Coronado et al. (2022); Vaduganathan et al. (2022), Jones et al. (2024); WHO (2022a, 2022b, 2022d, 2022e, 2022f); UNICEF (2021c); United Nations Office on Drugs and Crime (UNODC) (2023).

dislocation, and behavioral changes all contributed to rising mortality from other causes. In the United States, for example, excess deaths were recorded from heart disease, diabetes, hypertension, drug overdoses, homicides, and other non-COVID conditions. One study found that among younger adults in particular, indirect causes such as homicide and overdose contributed more to excess mortality than the virus itself during the 2020–2021 period.

Globally, several troubling reversals in health progress emerged. After more than a decade of decline, tuberculosis deaths rose from 1.4 million in 2019 to 1.6 million in 2021, driven by disruptions to diagnosis and treatment services (WHO, 2022d, 2022e). Malaria deaths also increased, climbing from 568,000 in 2019 to 625,000 in 2020 due to interruptions in control programs (WHO, 2022f). Recent estimates suggest that the global burden of malaria continued to worsen beyond 2020, with pandemic-related disruptions exacerbating conditions in high-transmission regions (Huang et al., 2025). These setbacks erased hard-won gains and highlighted the fragility of infectious disease infrastructure under global crisis conditions.

Childhood immunization programs were similarly impacted. In 2020, 23 million children worldwide missed basic routine vaccines—the highest number since 2009—largely due to clinic closures, supply chain challenges, and parental fears about exposure (UNICEF, 2021c; WHO, 2022b). DTP3 coverage dropped from 86% in 2019 to 81% in 2021, with only partial recovery in subsequent years. UNICEF warned that this backslide may heighten the risk of outbreaks from preventable diseases like measles and polio, particularly in low- and middle-income countries. By 2023, vaccination rates had stabilized but not fully recovered: over 14 million children still missed their first dose of Diphtheria, Tetanus, and Pertussis (DTP) vaccines, with nearly half living in fragile or conflict-affected settings—an alarming sign that routine immunization, one of global health's greatest success stories, remains on unsteady ground (Jones et al., 2024).

Cancer screenings experienced sharp reductions in the early phase of the pandemic, disrupting one of the most critical pathways for early detection and survivability. In the United States, screenings for breast, colorectal, and cervical cancer fell by 86–94% in early 2020, leading to a 19–78% drop in new diagnoses (Cancino et al., 2020). Globally, the WHO reported cancer services were disrupted by up to 50%—a particularly dire impact in regions with already limited access to early detection and treatment infrastructure (WHO, 2022a). Delays in diagnosis are now projected to lead to measurable increases in avoidable cancer deaths over the next decade, with disproportionate impacts in low-resource settings.

CVD, already the leading global cause of death, experienced a disturbing reversal of progress. Avoidable deaths surged as routine care collapsed—patients missed diagnoses, skipped procedures, or delayed seeking help due to fear of infection. Stress-related behaviors such as poor diet, inactivity, and substance use further compounded risk. In 2020, CVD accounted for over 19 million deaths, or roughly 32% of all global deaths (Roth et al., 2020; Vaduganathan et al., 2022). Several countries saw rising age-adjusted mortality for the first time in years, wiping out gains made through decades of prevention and treatment efforts.

Other shifts reflected wider social stressors. While early lockdowns briefly reduced traffic-related fatalities, they coincided with sharp rises in drug overdoses and violence. In the United States, over 100,000 overdose deaths occurred annually in 2020 and 2021, marking a grim national record. Globally, drug-related deaths likely increased, particularly in regions where addiction services were curtailed. Homicide rates also rose: the UN reported a sustained post-2020 increase in North America, reversing years of slow progress in reducing violent deaths (UNODC, 2023).

Taken together, these patterns suggest the pandemic's indirect death toll—through disrupted healthcare access, missed preventive care, and the amplification of structural vulnerabilities—may approach or even surpass the virus's direct toll in certain contexts. The pandemic did not merely expose existing health inequities; it actively widened them.

Mental Health Fallout

The COVID-19 pandemic triggered one of the most significant global mental health crises in modern history. Beyond its devastating physical health toll, the pandemic unleashed a wave of psychological distress that continues to affect millions worldwide (Table 16.4). In 2020, global prevalence of anxiety and depression increased by approximately 25%, according to the WHO and a major global study published in *The Lancet* by the COVID-19 Mental Disorders Collaborators (The Lancet) (2021), representing tens of millions of additional cases of mental disorders worldwide—all coinciding with pandemic-related stressors.

Even prior to the pandemic, the global burden of mental disorders was steadily rising, with the GBD 2019 Mental Disorders Collaborators (2022) documenting high and growing rates of anxiety, depression, and other conditions across nearly all world regions. While the pandemic did not create these challenges, it dramatically exacerbated them. Pandemic-related mental health stressors were complex and interconnected. Social isolation emerged as perhaps the most significant factor, with lockdowns and distancing measures severing people from support networks and daily routines. Many also faced pervasive uncertainty—fear of contracting a potentially deadly virus, concern for vulnerable loved ones, and doubt about when life might return to normal. Grief and trauma from widespread loss of life compounded these pressures. Frontline healthcare workers were particularly affected, reporting unprecedented levels of burnout, trauma, and even suicidal ideation from witnessing mass casualties while working under extreme pressure (CDC, 2023).

Mental health burdens during the pandemic have not been distributed evenly. Young people and women have consistently shown higher vulnerability. The WHO found the pandemic disproportionately affected young people's mental health, with youth experiencing elevated rates of anxiety, self-harm, and suicidal thoughts (WHO, 2022c). Recent U.S. CDC data shows that while there has been slight improvement, 40% of high school students still report feeling persistently sad or hopeless, down marginally from 42% in 2021 but still well above pre-pandemic levels (CDC, 2024a, 2024b). Women globally faced outsized mental health challenges as they shouldered greater caregiving responsibilities and experienced higher job losses in sectors like hospitality and retail. In the United States, the gender gap in mental health outcomes persists, with 36% of women reporting symptoms of anxiety/depression compared to 28% of men as of 2023 (Panchal et al., 2023). Certain vulnerable groups have also been at elevated risk: healthcare and essential workers experienced burnout and trauma at unprecedented levels; surveys in 2022 found that about 46% of health workers felt "often" burned out, up from one-third before the pandemic (CDC, 2023). Children and adolescents also faced increased mental health issues, from small children dealing with disrupted daily routines to teenagers grappling with missing formative social interactions and academic pressures. The UN's State of the World's Children 2021 report warned that young people could feel the mental health impacts for years to come (UNICEF, 2021a, 2021b).

Unlike the acute COVID infection waves which peaked and ebbed, the mental health fallout has proven far more persistent and less immediately visible. Even as

Table 16.4 Global Mental Health Impacts of the COVID-19 Pandemic (2019–2024)

Region/Group	*Pre-Pandemic Baseline*	*Pandemic Impact (2020–2021)*	*Current Status (2023–2024)*
Global Overview	10–15% prevalence of mental disorders	25–27% increase in anxiety and depression	Elevated prevalence: 28% depression, 27% anxiety
High Income Countries	Higher baseline access to mental healthcare	Significant declines observed	33–35% still experiencing distress in some countries
Low and Low-Middle Income Countries	82% of global mental health burden	Varied impact; limited system capacity	Some regions resilient; disparities persist
Youth/Young Adults	Rising concern pre-pandemic	Most severely affected group	40% of high school students report sadness
Women	Higher baseline prevalence than men	Disproportionate impact from caregiving, job loss	36% of women vs. 28% of men report symptoms
Healthcare Workers	32–33% reported burnout (2018)	46% reported burnout (2022)	Burnout and distress remain elevated
Mental Health Services	Significant treatment gaps	93% of countries reported disruptions	Access gaps and disruptions persist

Sources: WHO (2022c), Centers for Disease Control and Prevention (2022–2024), COVID-19 Mental Disorders Collaborators (The Lancet) (2021), GBD 2019 Mental Disorders Collaborators (The Lancet) (2022), Panchal et al. (2023), Sapien Labs (2025), National Alliance on Mental Illness (NAMI) (n.d.); SingleCare Team (2024); SingleCare Team (2025).

lockdowns eased and schools reopened in 2021–2022, demand for mental health services remained elevated. Many countries reported that rates of depression and anxiety had not returned to baseline. For instance, a U.K. study found that by mid-2021, rates of psychological distress were still markedly higher compared to 2019, despite improvements from the worst points of 2020 (Patel et al., 2022). Current U.S. CDC data indicates that approximately one in five American adults continue to experience symptoms of anxiety and depression, and nearly one in ten report experiencing depression (CDC, 2024a, 2024b). The mental health crisis has been further compounded by other societal challenges, with U.S. CDC data showing that deaths from drugs, alcohol, and suicide more than doubled between 2000 and 2017 and have continued increasing during and after the pandemic. In the United States, a survey found a record 17.8% of Americans currently have some form of depression, a continued rise over previous years's estimates (Goodwin et al., 2022).

It is worth noting that not all mental health outcomes during this period have been negative. Some communities have demonstrated remarkable resilience, and the crisis has spurred more open conversations about the importance of maintaining mental well-being. Telemedicine for therapy expanded dramatically during this period, potentially increasing access for previously underserved populations. Public health responses have evolved as well, with approximately 90% of countries surveyed by the WHO stating that they will include some form of mental health and psychosocial support in their COVID-19 and future pandemic response plans (Kestel, 2022). School districts across the United States have implemented new mental health resources and programs as well, with evidence suggesting these efforts may be contributing to the modest improvements observed in youth mental health indicators. However, despite these positive developments, the net impact has been a worsening of global mental health indicators overall, and an amplification of pre-existing gaps in mental healthcare access and delivery. The pandemic has laid bare the critical importance of mental health infrastructure and the need for continued investment in accessible, equitable mental healthcare systems worldwide.

Workforce Transformation

The COVID-19 era radically transformed the world of work. The crisis upended labor markets in 2020, causing both the sharpest employment shock since the Great Depression and catalyzing lasting changes in how and where people work. From mass layoffs and furloughs to the sudden shift to remote work, virtually all sectors experienced some form of disruption (Tables 16.5 and 16.6).

The initial lockdowns in Q2 2020 led to a worldwide contraction in economic activity. Global working hours in 2020 fell by an estimated 8.8% (equivalent to 255 million full-time jobs lost), according to the International Labour Organization (ILO) (ILO, 2020). Unemployment spiked in both advanced and developing countries. The global unemployment rate jumped from approximately 5.4% in 2019 to around 6.6% in 2020 (Reuters, 2023a, 2023b). In absolute terms, roughly 220 million people were unemployed in 2020–2021, up tens of millions from pre-pandemic levels. The worst impacts were felt in sectors requiring face-to-face interaction—such as hospitality, travel, retail, and entertainment—which suddenly shut down for weeks and even months in many regions.

Informal and gig economy workers, with little job security or social protection, were especially vulnerable. The World Bank estimated that COVID-19 pushed 97 million additional people into extreme poverty in 2020 due in part to lost income (World Bank, 2021a, 2021b). Women and youth bore a disproportionate share of early job losses. Women's employment fell by 4.2% globally in 2020 (54 million jobs lost), compared to a 3.0% decline for men (ILO, 2021a, 2021b). The gap widened existing disparities in workforce participation, setting back gender equality efforts by at least several years.

Government relief measures—such as wage subsidies, stimulus payments, and expanded unemployment benefits—helped cushion some of the early shock in many higher-income countries, but the level and duration of support varied. Overall, the pandemic-induced 2020 recession was the deepest and most damaging since World War II for the global economy (World Bank, 2020a, 2020b).

Amid economic doubt and uncertainty about the future, an unexpected phenomenon emerged in 2021: rather than immediately returning to their previous jobs, many workers quit or re-evaluated their careers altogether. Coined the "Great Resignation," this wave saw record numbers of workers voluntarily leaving jobs in the United States and beyond. Surveys indicated that after an extended period of remote work and reflection during lockdowns, employees developed new priorities that emphasized personal well-being. A 2022 global survey by PwC reported by the World Economic Forum (WEF) found that approximately one in five workers worldwide planned to quit their job in the coming year (WEF, 2022b; PwC 2022). Mid-career workers (30s and 40s) in particular switched jobs at high rates, often moving to roles with higher degrees of autonomy and flexibility or entering some form of self-employment.

By 2022, employers in many countries faced labor shortages in certain fields, a sharp reversal from the surplus of labor in 2020. For example, restaurants and hospitality businesses that reopened often struggled to rehire staff who had permanently moved on. Healthcare felt a severe pinch: after the strain of successive COVID waves, over 10.6 million health and social care workers in the United States quit their jobs between 2020 and early 2022, further contributing to ongoing staffing shortages (U.S. Bureau of Labor Statistics, 2022a, 2022b, 2022c). This mass exit of burned-out healthcare staff (mostly women) is sometimes called the "Great Resignation of women in health care" (Women in Global Health, 2022).

Perhaps the most visible transformation has been the normalization of remote work. Pre-pandemic, only a small fraction of jobs were done remotely. That changed within mere days and weeks in March 2020, when hundreds of millions of employees globally shifted to working from home due to lockdowns and travel restrictions. Companies rapidly adopted teleconferencing, cloud collaboration tools, and new management practices to accommodate distributed teams. By mid-2020, estimates suggest that over half of the workforce in high-income countries was working remotely at least part-time.

By 2023, remote and hybrid work remained widespread, though the trend gradually declined from the previous pandemic peaks. Globally, around 28% of employees worked remotely at least some of the time, up from roughly 20% in 2020—a dramatic shift from pre-pandemic norms (Sherif, 2024a, 2024b, 2024c, 2024d). In the United States, about 28–30% of workers continued to work from home at least one day a week, with only around 12–15% fully remote by 2024 (Aksoy et al., 2024; U.S. Bureau of Labor Statistics, 2023, 2024a, 2024b). Despite a push by some industry leaders for a return to the office, many companies adopted permanent hybrid policies, prompting employees to relocate away from urban centers and redefining where and how people work. However, this shift has remained deeply unequal: remote work is far more common among higher-educated, white-collar professionals, whereas most blue-collar and service roles cannot be performed remotely—widening labor market disparities.

As of 2024, global employment has broadly recovered, and even improved overall compared to pre-pandemic norms, but not uniformly. According to the ILO's projections, the global unemployment rate fell to 5.1% in 2023 and is projected to decline to 4.9% in 2024, remaining stable through 2025 (Reuters, 2024). This is below the 5.4% rate from 2019, though many countries remain below their pre-2020 employment trend lines. A new divide has emerged: higher-income countries have seen strong rebounds, while lower-income countries continue to struggle with depressed employment and stagnant wages. Informal employment is also rising again, as millions have returned to insecure, unprotected jobs out of necessity (Reuters, 2023a, 2023b).

While many labor markets have shown signs of recovery, the pace has been deeply uneven. Women, youth, hospitality workers, and low-wage earners—especially those in the informal economy—have experienced the most fragile and incomplete rebound. These disparities reinforce existing structural inequities,

Table 16.5 Global Unemployment Trends by Income Group and Gender, 2019–2024

Region/Group	*2019 (%)*	*2020 (%)*	*2021 (%)*	*2022 (%)*	*2023 (%)*	*2024 (proj.) (%)*
Global Average	5.40	6.60	6.20	5.30	5.10	4.9–5.2
High-Income Countries	4.80	7.30	6.20	5.00	4.50	4.3–4.5
Upper-Middle Income	5.20	6.40	6.10	5.70	5.30	5.1–5.3
Lower-Middle Income	5.40	6.60	6.30	6.00	5.50	5.3–5.5
Low-Income Countries	5.90	6.80	6.70	6.50	5.70	5.6–5.8
Women (Global)	5.60	7.40	7.80	6.20	5.70	5.4–5.6
Men (Global)	5.20	6.30	6.50	5.60	5.10	4.7–4.9

Sources: ILO (n.d., 2020, 2021a, 2021b, 2022, 2023, 2024), World Bank (n.d.), Reuters (2023a, 2023b, 2024).

Note: Unemployment figures reflect modeled estimates from the ILO and World Bank datasets. 2024 values are projections. Income tiers follow World Bank classification.

Table 16.6 Global Remote Work Adoption by Income Group and Gender (2020–2024)

Region/Group	*2020 (%)*	*2021 (%)*	*2022 (%)*	*2023 (%)*	*2024 (est.) (%)*
Global Average	20	25	26	28	25–30
High-Income Countries	30	32	33	35	30–35
Upper-Middle Income	18	20	22	24	20–25
Lower-Middle Income	10	12	14	15	12–18
Low-Income Countries	5	6	7	8	5–10
Women (Global)	–	–	–	22–28	20–25
Men (Global)	–	–	–	25–32	25–30

Sources: Aksoy et al. (2024), Sherif (2024a, 2024b, 2024c, 2024d), World Bank (n.d.).

Note: Estimates are based on aggregated international surveys and regional labor data. "Remote work" definitions vary by study (e.g., hybrid vs. fully remote).

particularly in regions lacking social protections. Informal workers—who constitute a majority of the workforce in many low- and middle-income countries—were among the most impacted. The ILO estimated that informal workers lost up to 60% of their income during the first wave of the pandemic. Many remain excluded from formal re-employment pathways. Without targeted efforts to support labor formalization, equitable wage growth, and workforce inclusion, the global recovery risks leaving millions behind, and further entrenching systemic vulnerabilities in the years to come.

Disrupted Education and Long-Term Learning Gaps

Education systems worldwide experienced the largest disruption in modern history due to COVID-19. Practically overnight, schools in nearly every country closed in 2020 to curb virus transmission—disrupting education for an entire generation of learners. The scale and duration of school closures were unprecedented—and so too are the consequences for learning and human capital development (Table 16.7).

At the peak of the crisis in April 2020, over 1.6 billion learners in more than 190 countries—94% of the world's student population—were out of school due to temporary closures (UNESCO, 2021a, 2021b). This figure indicates that virtually all schoolchildren were impacted in some way. Over 100 million teachers and school staff were also suddenly navigating the new realities of closed classrooms and distance teaching. The closures ranged from a few weeks in some countries to over a year in others. According to UNESCO, by one year into the pandemic (March 2021), half of all students worldwide were still experiencing full or partial school closures, and 29 countries had schools fully closed at that time (UNESCO, 2021a, 2021b).

With brick-and-mortar schools shut, education systems scrambled to provide remote learning infrastructure and curriculum. Solutions included online classes via videoconference, educational TV and radio broadcasts, printed learning packets, and mobile phone-based lessons. However, the capacity to deliver quality remote education varied enormously. High-income countries largely pivoted to online learning: teachers and students connected over Zoom or Google Meet, and tailored digital platforms were used at scale. In poorer regions, an underdeveloped digital infrastructure severely constrained access. An estimated 463 million children—at least one-third of the world's schoolchildren population—could not be reached by remote learning during school closures (UNICEF, 2020). This inaccessibility stemmed from a wide digital divide: two-thirds of children globally lack internet access at home (UNICEF & ITU, 2020), and even among those with connectivity, many had to share a single device with siblings or parents. As a result, remote learning primarily benefited better-off students, while millions of disadvantaged children had minimal to no formal instruction for prolonged periods.

Research now confirms that the pandemic caused major learning losses globally. Even in contexts where remote learning was offered, students absorbed significantly less than under in-person instruction. The World Bank, UNICEF, and UNESCO jointly reported that the share of children in low- and middle-income countries who are unable to read a simple text by age ten (a measure known as "learning poverty") jumped from 57% pre-pandemic to an estimated 70% in 2022 (World Bank, 2022). "As a result of the worst shock to education and learning in recorded history, learning poverty increased by a third," the report states. This means that millions more children are now unable to meet even basic literacy benchmarks by age ten—setting back global education progress by years.

The extent of learning loss correlates closely with the length of school closure and the quality of remote instruction. Latin America, which experienced some of the longest closures, saw particularly severe setbacks: modeling projected that learning poverty in Latin America and the Caribbean could reach 80%, up from approximately 50% pre-pandemic (World Bank, 2022). In South Asia, the figure rose to an estimated 78%, from a pre-pandemic level of around 60%. Sub-Saharan Africa saw a smaller increase in percentage terms but already had the world's highest baseline learning poverty rate, rising from around 86% to potentially over 89% in some areas (World Bank, 2022).

The World Bank has warned that this generation of students risks losing $21 trillion in lifetime earnings (in present value) due to pandemic-related learning deficits—up from earlier estimates of $17 trillion (World Bank, 2022). This staggering figure represents a cumulative global loss in future productivity, with implications for both individual well-being and ongoing national development.

Beyond academics, students's social and emotional development suffered. Children missed out on peer interaction, extracurricular activities, and the structure that schools provide. Education systems also play critical non-academic roles—such as providing nutrition (via school meals), access to health services, and protection from abuse. These functions were jeopardized when schools closed.

Educators and policymakers are now focused on learning recovery through remedial programs, extended instructional time, targeted tutoring, curriculum streamlining, and re-enrollment campaigns (Table 16.8). The success of these efforts has varied across countries, and many require sustained investment. Unfortunately, an analysis found that two-thirds of low-income countries cut their education budgets

Table 16.7 Educational Disruption and Learning Loss During COVID-19 (by Region)

Region	*Learners Affected (2020 Peak Disruption)*	*Remote Learning Access*	*Learning Poverty Increase*
Europe & Central Asia	213 million (98%)	Broad access (online and platforms)	Minimal/modest increases *(regionally varied)*
North America	96 million (95%)	High access (online)	Modest increases
East Asia & Pacific	325 million (90%)	Mixed; digital in urban, gaps in rural	Moderate increases *(regionally varied)*
South Asia	391 million (90%)	Limited access, especially rural	**+18 points** *(from 60% to 78%)*
Latin America & Caribbean	160 million (95%)	Major urban-rural divide	**+30 points** *(from 50% to 80%)*
Middle East & North Africa	110 million (89%)	Uneven; major gaps in war/conflict areas	Limited data *(increase assumed)*
Sub-Saharan Africa	250 million (80–85%)	Severe limitations	**+3 points** *(from 86% to 89%)*
Global	1.6 billion (94%)	463 million students lacked access	**+13 points** *(from 57% to 70%)*

Sources: World Bank (2022, 2023), UNESCO (2021a, 2021b, 2023a, 2023b), UNICEF (2020, 2021b); World Bank, UNESCO, & UNICEF (2022).

Note: "Learning poverty" is defined as the share of ten-year-olds unable to read and understand a simple sentence. Estimates reflect pre-pandemic baselines and projected 2022 values.

in 2020–2021 amid the broader economic downturn—just when more funding was needed most (UNESCO, 2021a, 2021b). While recovery is underway, the trajectories from region to region have been fragmented at best.

While some signs of rebound have emerged, bridging the post-pandemic education gap will require not just resources, but a sustained global commitment to equity, targeted recovery strategies, and long-term investment in resilient learning systems.

Trust, Institutions, and Public Sentiment After Crisis

The pandemic was not only a test of public health and economic systems but also a referendum on public trust in institutions. In times of crisis, people look to governments, health authorities, media, and international organizations for guidance and truthful information. COVID-19 presented an enormous challenge in this regard—one that, in many cases, institutions struggled to meet, leading to a volatile trajectory for public trust from 2019 to 2025 (Table 16.9).

When COVID-19 first struck, there was evidence of a short-lived "rally around the flag" effect and a palpable sense of unity among communities worldwide. In the early phase (spring 2020), many populations gave their governments the benefit of the doubt, hoping for decisive leadership and a quick resolution. In fact, the

Table 16.8 Educational Recovery and Response Trends (2024–2025)

Region	*Recovery Efforts*	*2025 Outlook*
Europe & Central Asia	Strong catch-up programs (tutoring, summer school)	Most countries near full recovery
North America	Investments in school-based mental health & tutoring	Progress steady; equity gaps remain
East Asia & Pacific	Targeted programs in some countries; uneven implementation	Moderate gains; urban areas rebounding faster
South Asia	Patchy recovery plans; NGO-supported in many areas	Partial recovery underway
Latin America & Caribbean	Regional emphasis on remedial education & re-enrollment	Learning levels improving, but below baseline
Middle East & North Africa	Conflict-affected areas lag; others piloting recovery tools	Recovery fragmented
Sub-Saharan Africa	Limited systemic recovery; community and donor-led efforts	Minimal rebound; high learning poverty persists

Sources: World Bank (2023), OECD (2024b), UNESCO (2023a, 2023b).

Note: This table summarizes early qualitative trends. Recovery progress varies widely by region, and consistent quantitative data remains limited, especially in low- and middle-income countries.

Edelman Trust Barometer found that "government was the most trusted institution as recently as May 2020, when the world sought leadership capable of tackling a global pandemic" (WEF, 2022a). However, as the pandemic dragged on, public trust in government responses plummeted in many countries. By January 2022, the same Edelman survey revealed that "government leaders are the least trusted" societal figures, and that only about four in ten people trusted their government to do what is right (WEF, 2022a).

Several factors contributed to the steep erosion of trust. Many governments were perceived as incompetent or inconsistent, with early missteps such as slow responses, lack of preparedness, inadequate PPE stockpiles, and confusing guidance on mask use undermining credibility. In places where leaders failed to transparently share COVID data or explain the rationale behind decisions, trust declined even further. This was especially apparent in the debate over the origins of SARS-CoV-2: the outright refusal by some officials to credibly entertain alternative outbreak scenarios signaled a lack of trust in the public's ability to engage with uncertainty. Though likely motivated by a desire to prevent panic or misinformation, these approaches backfired dramatically. As temporary restrictions extended into years, growing segments of the population became deeply resentful of government mandates, fueling protests, and the politicization of public health—an environment that opportunistic actors exploited to sow division and erode institutional trust. In countries where pandemic responses were seen as corrupt or disproportionately benefiting elites, trust deteriorated even further.

Table 16.9 Shifts in Public Trust Across Key Institutions During and After COVID-19

Institution/Sector	*Key Global Patterns (2020–2025)*
National Governments	• Trust peaked early in 2020 but fell sharply by 2022. • 39% global trust reported in 2023 (OECD). • Declines tied to confusion, delays, and perceived inequity.
Scientists/Health Experts	• Most trusted group early in the pandemic (87%). • Dropped to 73% by 2024, mostly among politicized groups. • Remain highly credible overall.
Traditional Media (e.g., news organizations)	• Faced backlash over inconsistent or politicized coverage. • Perceived bias fueled public skepticism and mistrust. • Confidence dropped further in 2022–2023.
Social Media Platforms	• Enabled fast info-sharing but also misinformation. • High trust linked to lower vaccine uptake and conspiracy content. • Usage remained high despite growing criticism.
Multilateral Organizations (e.g., WHO, UN)	• Trust split: 47% trust vs. 27% distrust (2020). • Criticized for slow response and political entanglements. • Struggled to coordinate global equity efforts.

Sources: Edelman Trust Institute (2023–2025); OECD (2023, 2024a); Kennedy & Tyson (2023); Tyson & Kennedy (2024); Tyson et al. (2025); Thornton (2022); Chen et al. (2023); Ferreira Caceres et al. (2022); Skafle et al. (2022); Zimmerman et. Al (2023); COVID-19 National Preparedness Collaborators (2022).

By late 2021 and 2022, trust in national governments was near record lows in many places. The OECD's 2023 survey found only ~39% of people on average trusted their national government (OECD, 2023, 2024a). This low trust is problematic beyond the pandemic, as it can impede compliance with any public policy and foster broader instability. A global analysis of 177 countries found that differences in infection and death rates were most strongly linked to levels of public trust, political polarization, and governance quality—not just GDP or healthcare system capacity (COVID-19 National Preparedness Collaborators, 2022). These findings further stress how institutional credibility and social cohesion were central to pandemic outcomes.

By contrast, scientists and healthcare professionals generally emerged as the most trusted voices during the pandemic. The Edelman survey reported that "scientists are the most trusted in society—trusted by 75% of people," far higher than any other group (WEF, 2022a). People placed considerable faith in doctors, nurses, and public health experts to guide them. However, even trust in science was not immune to polarization. A Pew study in 2023 found that in the United States, public trust in scientists and the benefits of science had declined compared to pre-pandemic levels, particularly among right-leaning or fringe political groups (Kennedy & Tyson, 2023). By 2025, this trend had persisted. Trust in scientists to act in the public's best interest dropped from 87% in early 2020 to 73% by late 2024, with the decline largely concentrated among conservative segments of the population (Tyson & Kennedy, 2024).

As discussed in Chapter 10 of the iceberg framework, the WHO warned early on of the rising tide of misinformation that accompanied the pandemic—what it called an "infodemic." Social media proved to be a double-edged sword: it helped disseminate health information quickly but also allowed rumors and falsehoods to spread like wildfire. Multiple studies have found that misinformation about COVID-19 vaccines circulated widely on these platforms, contributing to confusion and hesitancy (Ferreira Caceres et al., 2022; Skafle et al., 2022; Zimmerman et al. 2023). A study spanning 2020–2021 found that greater trust in social media correlated with lower vaccination rates and higher excess mortality, suggesting that people who relied on social media for information were more likely to believe misinformation and resist public health measures, despite overwhelming evidence of benefit outweighing risk (Chen et al., 2023). By 2024, over 40% of Americans said they were unsure what the current COVID-19 guidelines were, even five years into the pandemic, and 57% said false or misleading information had contributed significantly to the failures in the national response (Tyson et al., 2025).

COVID-19 also put multilateral organizations like the WHO in the spotlight. A global survey in 2020 indicated that about 47% of the world's population trusted the United Nations, including the WHO, while 27% expressed distrust. The pandemic likely strained that trust further, as global institutions struggled to maintain expert authority and legitimacy amid mounting geopolitical tensions and inconsistent national cooperation.

Eroded institutional trust has practical consequences for pandemic management and beyond. A *BMJ* study of 177 countries found that "trust in government and in other people was associated with lower COVID infection rates," strongly implying that greater social trust enabled more effective collective action and better health outcomes (Thornton, 2022).

Looking forward, rebuilding trust is a critical policy challenge. As of 2025, while the acute threat of the pandemic has largely waned, many societies are left with a trust hangover. A Pew survey from late 2024 found that only 40% of Americans believe the country would respond better to a future health emergency than it did to COVID-19. Another 43% expect the response would be about the same, and 16% think it would be worse. Confidence in the U.S. public health system remains modest, with just 61% saying it would do a good job in another crisis. In contrast, nearly 7 in 10 Americans said they believe their local community would respond well—possibly indicating greater faith in decentralized, community-based resilience over national institutions (Tyson et al., 2025). Our discussion of mental models in Chapter 11 of the iceberg framework highlights the importance of adaptive, locally tailored, community-based approaches to complement top-down interventions during emergencies. An Edelman 2023 analysis warns of a "vicious cycle of distrust" in many countries that could destabilize societies if not addressed (Edelman Trust Institute, 2023). Healing this will require honest institutional reflection and a sustained effort to engage the public in rebuilding credibility.

Conclusion

The COVID-19 pandemic has been a world-altering event, leaving lasting marks on nearly every facet of global society. Between 2019 and 2025, we witnessed sharp reversals in life expectancy, education, and mental health; sweeping changes in how we work and learn; and a significant erosion of public trust. While some trends have improved—such as rebounding life expectancy, job recovery, and school reopenings—others, like deepened learning gaps and institutional distrust, remain unresolved or have worsened.

These impacts have been profoundly uneven. Wealthier nations were better equipped to manage the crisis—though far from immune to failure—and how they choose to recover will shape outcomes far beyond their borders. In contrast, lower-income countries and marginalized communities often endured the harshest consequences, further widening global inequalities and complicating the path to recovery.

Above all, the pandemic exposed critical weaknesses in health systems, safety nets, and governance structures. But it also revealed the potential of human resilience, scientific innovation, and collective action. The challenge now is to ensure that the hard lessons of COVID-19 inform long-term decisions. The choices made in the pandemic's aftermath will determine not just national trajectories, but the shared future of global well-being.

References

Aksoy, C. G., Barrero, J. M., Bloom, N., Davis, S. J., Dolls, M., & Zarate, P. (2024, April). *Working from home in 2025: Five key facts*. Stanford Institute for Economic Policy Research. https://siepr.stanford.edu/publications/essay/working-home-2025-five-key-facts

Cancino, R. S., Su, Z., Mesa, R., Tomlinson, G. E., & Wang, J. (2020). The impact of COVID-19 on cancer screening: Challenges and opportunities. *JMIR Cancer*, *6*(2), e21697. https://doi.org/10.2196/21697

Centers for Disease Control and Prevention (CDC). (2022, October 25). *Global orphanhood associated with COVID-19*. CDC. https://archive.cdc.gov/www_cdc_gov/globalhealth/covid-19/orphanhood/index.html

Centers for Disease Control and Prevention (CDC). (2023, October 24). *Health workers face a mental health crisis*. CDC Vital Signs. https://www.cdc.gov/vitalsigns/health-worker-mental-health/index.html

Centers for Disease Control and Prevention (CDC). (2024a, August 6). CDC data show improvements in youth mental health but need for safer and more supportive schools. CDC Newsroom. https://www.cdc.gov/media/releases/2024/p0806-youth-mental-health.html

Centers for Disease Control and Prevention (CDC). (2024b, August 8). *Protecting the nation's mental health*. CDC Mental Health. https://www.cdc.gov/mental-health/about/what-cdc-is-doing.html

Chen, S. X., Ye, F. T., Cheng, K. L., Ng, J. C. K., Lam, B. C. P., Hui, B. P. H., Au, A. K. Y., Wu, W. C. H., Gu, D., & Zeng, Y. (2023). Social media trust predicts lower COVID-19 vaccination rates and higher excess mortality over 2 years. *PNAS Nexus*, *2*(10), pgad318. https://doi.org/10.1093/pnasnexus/pgad318

Coronado, F., Melvin, S. C., Bell, R. A., & Zhao, G. (2022). Global responses to prevent, manage, and control cardiovascular diseases. *Preventing Chronic Disease*, *19*, E76. https://doi.org/10.5888/pcd19.220347

COVID-19 Mental Disorders Collaborators (The Lancet). (2021). Global prevalence and burden of depressive and anxiety disorders in 204 countries and territories in 2020 due to the COVID-19 pandemic. *The Lancet*, *398*(10312), 1700–1712. https://doi.org/10.1016/S0140-6736(21)02143-7

COVID-19 National Preparedness Collaborators (The Lancet). (2022). Pandemic preparedness and COVID-19: An exploratory analysis of infection and fatality rates, and contextual factors associated with preparedness in 177 countries, from Jan 1, 2020, to Sept 30, 2021. *Lancet* (London, England), *399*(10334), 1489–1512. https://doi.org/10.1016/S0140-6736(22)00172-6

Edelman Trust Institute. (2023). *2023 Edelman Trust Barometer: Global report*. Edelman. https://www.edelman.com/trust/2023/trust-barometer

Edelman Trust Institute. (2024). *2024 Edelman Trust Barometer: Global report*. Edelman. https://www.edelman.com/trust/2024/trust-barometer

Edelman Trust Institute. (2025). *2025 Edelman Trust Barometer: Global report*. Edelman. https://www.edelman.com/trust/2025/trust-barometer

Ferreira Caceres, M. M., Sosa, J. P., Lawrence, J. A., Sestacovschi, C., Tidd-Johnson, A., Rasool, M. H. U., Gadamidi, V. K., Ozair, S., Pandav, K., Cuevas-Lou, C., Parrish, M., Rodriguez, I., & Fernandez, J. P. (2022). The impact of misinformation on the COVID-19 pandemic. *AIMS Public Health*, *9*(2), 262–277. https://doi.org/10.3934/publichealth.2022018

GBD 2019 Mental Disorders Collaborators (The Lancet) (2022). Global, regional, and national Burden of 12 mental disorders in 204 countries and territories, 1990–2019: A systematic analysis for the Global Burden of Disease Study 2019. *The Lancet. Psychiatry*, *9*(2), 137–150. https://doi.org/10.1016/S2215-0366(21)00395-3

GBD 2021 Europe Life Expectancy Collaborators (The Lancet) (2025). Changing life expectancy in European countries 1990–2021: A subanalysis of causes and risk factors from the Global Burden of Disease Study 2021. *The Lancet. Public Health*, *10*(3), e172–e188. https://doi.org/10.1016/S2468-2667(25)00009-X

Goodwin, R. D., Dierker, L. C., Wu, M., Galea, S., Hoven, C. W., & Weinberger, A. H. (2022). Trends in U.S. depression prevalence from 2015 to 2020: The widening treatment gap. *American Journal of Preventive Medicine*, *63*(5), 726–733. https://doi.org/10.1016/j.amepre.2022.05.014

Hillis, S., N'konzi, J. N., Msemburi, W., Cluver, L., Villaveces, A., Flaxman, S., & Unwin, H. J. T. (2022a). Orphanhood and caregiver loss among children based on new global excess COVID-19 death estimates. *JAMA Pediatrics*, *176*(11), 1145–1148. https://doi.org/10.1001/jamapediatrics.2022.3157

Hillis, S., Unwin, J., Cluver, L., Sherr, L., Villaveces, A., Flaxman, S., …, & Ibrahim, M. (2022b). *Children: The hidden pandemic – Orphanhood and caregiver loss based on excess COVID-19 death estimates*. Global Reference Group on Children Affected by COVID-19. https://stacks.cdc.gov/view/cdc/108199

Hillis, S. D., Unwin, H. J. T., Chen, Y., Cluver, L., Sherr, L., Goldman, P. S., Ratmann, O., Donnelly, C. A., Bhatt, S., Villaveces, A., Butchart, A., Bachman, G., Rawlings, L., Green, P., Nelson, C. A. 3rd, & Flaxman, S. (2021). Global minimum estimates of children affected by COVID-19-associated orphanhood and deaths of caregivers: A modelling study. *Lancet* (London, England), *398*(10298), 391–402. https://doi.org/10.1016/S0140-6736(21)01253-8

Huang, J., Hu, Y., & Wu, Y. et al (2025). Global burden of malaria before and after the COVID-19 pandemic based on the global burden of disease study 2021. *Scientific Reports*, *15*, 9113. https://doi.org/10.1038/s41598-025-93487-3

International Labour Organization ((ILO). (2020, June 30). *ILO Monitor: COVID-19 and the world of work* (5th ed.). https://www.ilo.org/sites/default/files/wcmsp5/groups/public/%40dgreports/%40dcomm/documents/briefingnote/wcms_749399.pdf

International Labour Organization (ILO). (n.d.). *ILOSTAT database: Labor market indicators*. https://ilostat.ilo.org/data/

International Labour Organization (ILO). (2021a, July 19). *Fewer women than men will regain employment during the COVID-19 crisis*. https://www.ilo.org/resource/news/fewer-women-men-will-regain-employment-during-covid-19-recovery-says-ilo

International Labour Organization (ILO). (2021b). *World employment and social outlook: Trends 2021*. https://www.ilo.org/publications/world-employment-and-social-outlook-trends-2021

International Labour Organization (ILO). (2022). *World employment and social outlook: Trends 2022*. https://www.ilo.org/publications/flagship-reports/world-employment-and-social-outlook-trends-2022

International Labour Organization (ILO). (2023). *World employment and social outlook: Trends 2023*. https://www.ilo.org/publications/flagship-reports/world-employment-and-social-outlook-trends-2023

International Labour Organization (ILO). (2024). *World employment and social outlook: Trends 2024*. https://www.ilo.org/publications/flagship-reports/world-employment-and-social-outlook-trends-2024

Jones, C. E., Danovaro-Holliday, M. C., & Mwinnyaa, G., & others. (2024). Routine vaccination coverage — Worldwide, 2023. *MMWR. Morbidity and Mortality Weekly Report, 73*(43), 978–984. https://doi.org/10.15585/mmwr.mm7343a4

Kearney, M. S., & Levine, P. B. (2022, April). *The US COVID-19 baby bust and rebound* (NBER Working Paper No. 30000). National Bureau of Economic Research. https://www.nber.org/papers/w30000

Kennedy, B., & Tyson, A. (Pew Research Center). (2023, November 14). *Americans' trust in scientists, positive views of science continue to decline: Among both democrats and republicans, trust in scientists is lower than before the pandemic*. Pew Research Center. https://www.pewresearch.org/science/2023/11/14/americans-trust-in-scientists-positive-views-of-science-continue-to-decline/

Kestel, D. (2022). *The state of mental health globally in the wake of the COVID-19 pandemic and progress on the WHO special initiative for mental health (2019–2023)*. United Nations Chronicle. https://www.un.org/en/un-chronicle/state-mental-health-globally-wake-covid-19-pandemic-and-progress-who-special-initiative

Msemburi, W., Karlinsky, A., & Knutson, V. et al (2023). The WHO estimates of excess mortality associated with the COVID-19 pandemic. *Nature*, *613*, 130–137. https://doi.org/10.1038/s41586-022-05522-2

National Alliance on Mental Illness (NAMI). (n.d.). *Mental health by the numbers*. https://www.nami.org/about-mental-illness/mental-health-by-the-numbers

Organisation for Economic Co-Operation and Development (OECD). (2023). *Government at a glance 2023*. OECD Publishing. https://www.oecd.org/en/publications/government-at-a-glance-2023_3d5c5d31-en.html

Organisation for Economic Co-Operation and Development (OECD). (2024a). *OECD survey on drivers of trust in public institutions – 2024 results: Building trust in a complex policy environment*. OECD Publishing. https://doi.org/10.1787/9a20554b-en

Organisation for Economic Co-Operation and Development (OECD). (2024b). *Education at a glance 2024: OECD indicators*. OECD Publishing. https://www.oecd.org/en/publications/education-at-a-glance-2024_c00cad36-en.html

Our World in Data. (2023). *Life expectancy is returning to pre-pandemic levels*. https://ourworldindata.org/data-insights/life-expectancy-is-returning-to-pre-pandemic-levels

Panchal, N., Saunders, H., Rudowitz, R., & Cox, C. (KFF). (2023, March 20). *The implications of COVID-19 for mental health and substance use*. KFF. https://www.kff.org/mental-health/issue-brief/the-implications-of-covid-19-for-mental-health-and-substance-use/

Pare, S. (2024, March 12). *COVID pandemic knocked 1.6 years off global life expectancy, study finds*. LiveScience. https://www.livescience.com/health/coronavirus/covid-pandemic-knocked-16-years-off-global-life-expectancy-study-finds

Patel, K., Robertson, E., Kwong, A. S. F., Griffith, G. J., Willan, K., Green, M. J., Di Gessa, G., Huggins, C. F., McElroy, E., Thompson, E. J., Maddock, J., Niedzwiedz, C. L.,

Henderson, M., Richards, M., Steptoe, A., Ploubidis, G. B., Moltrecht, B., Booth, C., Fitzsimons, E., Silverwood, R., …, & Katikireddi, S. V. (2022). Psychological distress before and during the COVID-19 pandemic among adults in the United Kingdom based on coordinated analyses of 11 longitudinal studies. *JAMA Network Open*, *5*(4), e227629. https://doi.org/10.1001/jamanetworkopen.2022.7629

PricewaterhouseCoopers (PwC). (2022). *Global workforce hopes and fears survey 2022*. https://www.pwc.com/gx/en/issues/workforce/hopes-and-fears-2022.html

Reuters. (2023a, January 16). *Global jobs growth will halve in challenging 2023: ILO*. https://www.reuters.com/markets/global-jobs-growth-will-halve-challenging-2023-ilo-2023-01-16/

Reuters. (2023b, May 31). *Low-income countries to be left behind without action on jobs: ILO*. https://www.reuters.com/world/low-income-countries-be-left-behind-without-action-jobs-ilo-2023-05-31/

Reuters. (2024, January 10). *Global unemployment seen rising modestly in 2024: UN labour body*. https://www.reuters.com/markets/global-unemployment-seen-rising-modestly-2024-un-labour-body-2024-01-10/

Roth, G. A., Mensah, G. A., Johnson, C. O., et al. (2020). Global burden of cardiovascular diseases and risk factors, 1990–2019: Update from the GBD 2019 study. *Journal of the American College of Cardiology*, *76*(25), 2982–3021. https://doi.org/10.1016/j.jacc.2020.11.010

Sapien Labs. (2025). *Mental state of the world in 2024*. https://mentalstateoftheworld.report/

Schöley, J., Aburto, J. M., Kashnitsky, I., et al. Life expectancy changes since COVID-19. *Nature Human Behaviour*, *6*, 1649–1659 (2022). https://doi.org/10.1038/s41562-022-01450-3

Sherif, A. (Statista). (2024a, December 11). *Struggles with working remotely worldwide from 2020 to 2023*. Statista. https://www.statista.com/statistics/1111316/biggest-struggles-to-remote-work/

Sherif, A. (Statista). (2024b, June 14). *Work from home: Remote & hybrid work – Statistics & facts*. Statista. https://www.statista.com/topics/6565/work-from-home-and-remote-work/

Sherif, A. (Statista). (2024c, November 12). *Percentage of employees who work from home all or most of the time worldwide from 2015 to 2023*. Statista. https://www.statista.com/statistics/1450450/employees-remote-work-share/

Sherif, A. (Statista). (2024d, February 27). *Percentage of employees who work fully or mostly remote worldwide in 2023, by industry*. Statista. https://www.statista.com/statistics/1451594/remote-work-share-by-industry-globally/

SingleCare Team. (2024). *Mental health statistics 2024*. https://www.singlecare.com/blog/news/mental-health-statistics/

SingleCare Team. (2025). *Mental health statistics 2025*. https://www.singlecare.com/blog/news/mental-health-statistics/

Skafle, I., Nordahl-Hansen, A., Quintana, D. S., Wynn, R., & Gabarron, E. (2022). Misinformation about COVID-19 vaccines on social media: Rapid review. *Journal of Medical Internet Research*, *24*(8), e37367. https://doi.org/10.2196/37367

Thornton, J. (2022). Covid-19: Trust in government and other people linked with lower infection rate and higher vaccination uptake. *BMJ* (Clinical research ed.), *376*, o292. https://doi.org/10.1136/bmj.o292

Tyson, A., & Kennedy, B. (Pew Research Center). (2024, November 14). *Public trust in scientists and views on their role in policymaking: Trust moves slightly higher but remains lower than before the pandemic*. Pew Research Center. https://www.pewresearch.org/science/2024/11/14/public-trust-in-scientists-and-views-on-their-role-in-policymaking/

Tyson, A., Lipka, M., & Deane, C. (Pew Research Center). (2025, February 12). *5 years later: America looks back at the impact of COVID-19—Most Americans say the pandemic drove the country apart*. Pew Research Center. https://www.pewresearch.org/politics/2025/02/12/5-years-later-america-looks-back-at-the-impact-of-covid-19/

UNESCO. (2021a, March 23). *One year into COVID-19 education disruption: Where do we stand?* https://www.unesco.org/en/articles/one-year-covid-19-education-disruption-where-do-we-stand

UNESCO. (2021b). *One year into COVID: Prioritizing education recovery to avoid a generational catastrophe [Programme and meeting document]*. https://unesdoc.unesco.org/ark:/48223/pf0000376984

UNESCO. (2023a). *Education: From COVID-19 school closures to recovery*. https://www.unesco.org/en/covid-19/education-response

UNESCO. (2023b). *Global education monitoring report 2023: Technology in education – A tool on whose terms?* UNESCO Publishing. https://unesdoc.unesco.org/ark:/48223/pf0000385723

UNICEF. (2020). *COVID-19: Are children able to continue learning during school closures? A global analysis of the potential reach of remote learning policies*. https://data.unicef.org/resources/remote-learning-reachability-factsheet/

UNICEF. (2021a, October 5). *Impact of COVID-19 on poor mental health in children and young people: Tip of the iceberg*. https://www.unicef.org/press-releases/impact-covid-19-poor-mental-health-children-and-young-people-tip-iceberg

UNICEF. (2021b). *The State of the World's Children 2021: On my mind – Promoting, protecting and caring for children's mental health*. https://www.unicef.org/reports/state-worlds-children-2021

UNICEF. (2021c, July 15). *COVID-19 pandemic leads to major backsliding on childhood vaccinations*. https://www.unicef.org/press-releases/covid-19-pandemic-leads-major-backsliding-childhood-vaccinations-new-who-unicef-data

UNICEF. (2024, April 6). *Aid cuts threaten fragile progress in ending maternal deaths, UN agencies warn*. https://www.unicef.org/press-releases/aid-cuts-threaten-fragile-progress-ending-maternal-deaths-un-agencies-warn

UNICEF & ITU. (2020). *How many children and young people have internet access at home?* https://www.unicef.org/reports/how-many-children-and-young-people-have-internet-access-home-2020

United Nations. (2022). *Global population growth and sustainable development*. https://www.un.org/development/desa/pd/sites/www.un.org.development.desa.pd/files/undesa_pd_2022_global_population_growth.pdf

United Nations Office on Drugs and Crime (UNODC). (2023). *Global study on homicide 2023*. https://www.unodc.org/documents/data-and-analysis/gsh/2023/Global_study_on_homicide_2023_web.pdf

U.S. Bureau of Labor Statistics. (2022a, June 23). *American Time Use Survey—2021 results*. https://www.bls.gov/news.release/archives/atus_06232022.pdf

U.S. Bureau of Labor Statistics. (2022b, March 9). *Job openings and labor turnover survey highlights: January 2022*. U.S. Department of Labor. https://www.bls.gov/news.release/archives/jolts_03092022.htm

U.S. Bureau of Labor Statistics. (2022c, November 16). *Empirical evidence for the "Great Resignation"*. Monthly Labor Review. https://www.bls.gov/opub/mlr/2022/article/empirical-evidence-for-the-great-resignation.htm

U.S. Bureau of Labor Statistics. (2023, June 22). *American time use survey—2022 results*. https://www.bls.gov/news.release/archives/atus_06222023.pdf

U.S. Bureau of Labor Statistics. (2024a, June 27). *American time use survey—2023 results*. https://www.bls.gov/news.release/pdf/atus.pdf

U.S. Bureau of Labor Statistics. (2024b, July 15). 35 percent of employed people did some or all of their work at home on days they worked in 2023. *The Economics Daily*. https://www.bls.gov/opub/ted/2024/35-percent-of-employed-people-did-some-or-all-of-their-work-at-home-on-days-they-worked-in-2023.htm

Vaduganathan, M., Mensah, G. A., Turco, J. V., et al (2022). The global burden of cardiovascular diseases and risk: A compass for future health. *Journal of the American College of Cardiology*, *80*(25), 2361–2371. https://doi.org/10.1016/j.jacc.2022.11.005

Villaveces, A., Chen, Y., Tucker, S., et al (2025). Orphanhood and caregiver death among children in the United States by all-cause mortality, 2000–2021. *Nature Medicine*, *31*, 672–683. https://doi.org/10.1038/s41591-024-03343-6

Women in Global Health (WGH). (2022). *The great resignation: Why women health workers are leaving*. https://womeningh.org/great-resignation/

World Bank. (n.d.). *World Development Indicators: Unemployment and labor force statistics*. https://databank.worldbank.org/source/world-development-indicators

World Bank. (2020a, June 8). *COVID-19 to plunge global economy into worst recession since World War II [Press release]*. https://www.worldbank.org/en/news/press-release/2020/06/08/covid-19-to-plunge-global-economy-into-worst-recession-since-world-war-ii

World Bank. (2020b, June). *Global economic prospects: Pandemic, recession—the global economy in crisis*. https://www.worldbank.org/en/publication/global-economic-prospects

World Bank. (2021a, January 11). *COVID-19 leaves a legacy of rising poverty and widening inequality*. https://blogs.worldbank.org/developmenttalk/covid-19-leaves-legacy-rising-poverty-and-widening-inequality

World Bank. (2021b, January 11). *Updated estimates of the impact of COVID-19 on global poverty: Turning the corner on the pandemic in 2021?* https://blogs.worldbank.org/opendata/updated-estimates-impact-covid-19-global-poverty-turning-corner-pandemic-2021

World Bank. (2022, June 23). *70% of 10-year-olds now in learning poverty, unable to read and understand a simple text [Press release]*. https://www.worldbank.org/en/news/press-release/2022/06/23/70-of-10-year-olds-now-in-learning-poverty-unable-to-read-and-understand-a-simple-text

World Bank. (2023). *Learning recovery to accelerate education outcomes: Guidance notes for policymakers*. https://www.worldbank.org/en/topic/education/publication/learning-recovery

World Bank, UNESCO, & UNICEF. (2022). *The state of global learning poverty: 2022 update*. https://www.worldbank.org/en/topic/education/publication/state-of-global-learning-poverty

World Economic Forum (WEF). (2022a, January 18). *Edelman Trust Barometer 2022: What you need to know*. https://www.weforum.org/stories/2022/01/edelman-trust-barometer-2022-report/

World Economic Forum (WEF). (2022b, June 24). *The Great Resignation is not over: A fifth of workers plan to quit in 2022*. https://www.weforum.org/stories/2022/06/the-great-resignation-is-not-over/

World Health Organization (WHO). (2022a, February 3). *Cancer services disrupted by up to 50% in all countries reporting, a deadly impact of COVID-19*. https://www.who.int/europe/news/item/03-02-2022-cancer-services-disrupted-by-up-to-50-in-all-countries-reporting-a-deadly-impact-of-covid-19

World Health Organization (WHO). (2022b, July 15). *COVID-19 pandemic fuels largest continued backslide in vaccinations in three decades*. https://www.who.int/news/item/15-07-2022-covid-19-pandemic-fuels-largest-continued-backslide-in-vaccinations-in-three-decades

World Health Organization (WHO). (2022c, March 2). *COVID-19 pandemic triggers 25% increase in prevalence of anxiety and depression worldwide*. https://www.who.int/news/item/02-03-2022-covid-19-pandemic-triggers-25-increase-in-prevalence-of-anxiety-and-depression-worldwide

World Health Organization (WHO). (2022d, October 27). *Global tuberculosis report 2022*. https://www.who.int/publications/i/item/9789240061729

World Health Organization (WHO). (2022e, October 27). *Tuberculosis deaths and disease increase during the COVID-19 pandemic*. https://www.who.int/news/item/27-10-2022-tuberculosis-deaths-and-disease-increase-during-the-covid-19-pandemic

World Health Organization (WHO). (2022f, December 8). *World malaria report 2022*. https://www.who.int/teams/global-malaria-programme/reports/world-malaria-report-2022

World Health Organization (WHO). (2023, August 29). *Opioid overdose*. https://www.who.int/news-room/fact-sheets/detail/opioid-overdose

World Health Organization (WHO). (2024, May 24). *COVID-19 eliminated a decade of progress in global level of life expectancy*. https://www.who.int/news/item/24-05-2024-covid-19-eliminated-a-decade-of-progress-in-global-level-of-life-expectancy

Zimmerman, T., Shiroma, K., Fleischmann, K. R., Xie, B., Jia, C., Verma, N., & Lee, M. K. (2023). Misinformation and COVID-19 vaccine hesitancy. *Vaccine*, *41*(1), 136–144. https://doi.org/10.1016/j.vaccine.2022.11.014

17 The Long COVID Conundrum

From Medical Mystery to Public Health Priority

Long COVID is a complex, long-lasting condition affecting a significant portion of those infected with the virus. It involves a wide range of symptoms—such as fatigue, brain fog, respiratory, and cardiovascular issues—driven by interconnected biological mechanisms. The condition disproportionately affects certain groups and poses ongoing challenges due to the lack of approved treatments, though multidisciplinary care is commonly used. With hundreds of millions affected globally and major economic costs, long COVID remains a pressing public health concern necessitating continued research, preventive measures, and coordinated care for the millions affected.

Introduction to Long COVID

Long COVID, also referred to as post-COVID-19 condition (PCC) or post-acute sequelae of SARS-CoV-2 infection (PASC), describes a constellation of symptoms that either persist or develop following the resolution of acute COVID-19 infection. These symptoms can involve multiple organ systems and often significantly impair daily functioning and quality of life. The WHO defines PCC as symptoms that begin within three months of initial COVID-19 infection and last for at least two months, in the absence of an alternative diagnosis (World Health Organization (WHO), 2025).

Although the majority of individuals recover from acute COVID-19, estimates of long COVID's prevalence vary significantly based on methodology, population studies, and definition criteria. A comprehensive 2025 meta-analysis examining 442 studies worldwide found a global pooled prevalence of 36% among COVID-19-positive individuals, with notable geographic variations: 35% in Asia, 39% in Europe, 30% in North America, and as high as 51% in South America (Hou et al., 2025). However, a more conservative estimate comes from a 2023 Scottish population cohort study which found that while 64.5% of participants reported at least one symptom 6 months after infection, so did 50.8% of matched participants who were never infected, suggesting the crude prevalence attributable to SARS-CoV-2 was closer to 6.6% after adjustment for confounders (Hastie et al., 2023). In the United States, a CDC survey from late 2024 found that approximately 8.4% of adults reported ever having had long COVID, with 3.6% reporting current symptoms and

DOI: 10.4324/9781003595564-22

2.3% experiencing activity-limiting long COVID (Vahratian et al., 2024). With widespread vaccination and the emergence of newer variants, the risk appears to have decreased compared to earlier pandemic waves, yet every additional infection continues to carry the potential for long-term health impacts.

Long COVID represents a priority challenge to global healthcare systems. Its multisystem nature, fluctuating symptoms, and variable presentations make it a complex condition to diagnose, manage, and study. The condition does not discriminate based on initial disease severity either, as individuals who experienced only mild acute symptoms can develop debilitating post-acute sequelae, though those with more severe initial illness face heightened risk (Ewing et al., 2025). What makes long COVID particularly challenging is its heterogeneity, both in symptoms and underlying mechanisms, requiring personalized approaches to treatment and management (Peluso & Deeks, 2024).

Symptoms and Clinical Presentations

The clinical presentation of long COVID is remarkably diverse, with over 200 symptoms documented in affected individuals (Table 17.1). These symptoms can differ significantly from person to person, with severity ranging from mild to incapacitating. Common symptoms include fatigue, muscle pain, shortness of breath, chest pain, cognitive dysfunction ("brain fog"), and post-exertional malaise, where symptoms worsen after physical or mental activity.

Fatigue stands out as one of the most pervasive and debilitating symptoms, often described as an overwhelming exhaustion that significantly interferes with daily activities. This is not ordinary tiredness that improves with rest but rather a profound energy depletion that can render simple tasks insurmountable. Accompanying this fatigue, many patients experience shortness of breath, even in the absence of exertion or observable lung damage on imaging studies. Persistent muscle

Table 17.1 Primary Long COVID Symptom Clusters and Estimated Prevalence

Symptom Cluster	*Common Symptoms*	*Prevalence (%)*
Fatigue/energy	Profound exhaustion, post-exertional malaise, unrefreshing sleep	**64–20**
Respiratory	Shortness of breath, cough, chest tightness	**44–20**
Cognitive	Brain fog, memory issues, concentration difficulties, word-finding problems	**35–16**
Cardiovascular	Palpitations, tachycardia, chest pain, POTS	**30–13**
Neurological	Headache, paresthesia, dizziness, dysautonomia	**22–16**
Psychological	Anxiety, depression, PTSD, sleep disturbances	**33–18**
Musculoskeletal	Myalgia, arthralgia, weakness	**20–9**
Sensory	Loss/distortion of smell or taste, vision changes, tinnitus	**29–3**

Note: Prevalence ranges compiled from multiple studies including Hou et al. (2025), Davis et al. (2023), Jangnin et al. (2024), Hou et al. (2025), DePace and Colombo (2022), Yan et al. (2025), Trott et al. (2022). Percentages vary based on study population, timing, and methodology.

and joint pain further compound mobility limitations, creating a cycle of reduced activity that can lead to deconditioning.

Cognitive impairment, colloquially known as "brain fog," manifests as difficulty concentrating, memory lapses, word-finding problems, and reduced executive function. These neurological symptoms can be particularly distressing for patients, affecting their ability to work, maintain relationships, and engage in previously enjoyed activities. Sleep disturbances are equally common, including insomnia, disrupted sleep patterns, and unrefreshing sleep, which further amplify fatigue and cognitive difficulties.

Many patients also experience cardiovascular symptoms, including palpitations, chest pain, and manifestations of autonomic dysfunction such as postural orthostatic tachycardia syndrome (POTS), where the heart rate increases abnormally upon standing. This dysautonomia can cause dizziness, fainting, and exercise intolerance. Psychological symptoms, including anxiety and depression, often accompany these physical manifestations, though it remains unclear whether these represent direct neuropsychiatric effects of the virus or secondary responses to chronic illness (Ewing et al., 2025).

What distinguishes long COVID from many other post-infectious syndromes is the fluctuating nature of these symptoms. Patients frequently report "good days and bad days," with unpredictable flare-ups that can be triggered by physical exertion, stress, or seemingly without cause. These patterns often resemble myalgic encephalomyelitis/chronic fatigue syndrome (ME/CFS), particularly in the hallmark symptom of post-exertional malaise, where even minimal activity leads to a disproportionate worsening of symptoms (Peluso & Deeks, 2024).

Beyond these immediate symptoms, long COVID is associated with increased risks of serious medical conditions, including stroke, cardiovascular disease, diabetes, and persistent mental health disorders. This heightened risk of comorbidities further complicates the clinical picture and emphasizes the need for comprehensive, long-term care approaches for affected individuals (Ewing et al., 2025).

The National Institutes of Health's RECOVER COVID Initiative has identified distinct symptom clusters that represent five different subtypes of long COVID: change of taste and smell (subtype 1), chronic cough (subtype 2), brain fog (subtype 3), palpitations (subtype 4), and post-exertional soreness, dizziness, and gastrointestinal symptoms (subtype 5). This subtyping approach could lead to more targeted clinical care and improve symptom management (Geng et al., 2025).

Pathophysiological Mechanisms of Long COVID

The pathophysiology underlying long COVID represents a complex interplay of multiple mechanisms rather than a single causative pathway (Table 17.2). Current research suggests several interdependent processes that contribute to the diverse manifestations of the condition (Davis et al., 2023).

According to a 2024 review in *Nature Medicine*, several mechanistic pathways are implicated in long COVID, including viral persistence, immune dysregulation, mitochondrial dysfunction, complement dysregulation, endothelial inflammation,

Table 17.2 Possible Pathophysiological Mechanisms of Long COVID

Mechanism	*Description*	*Clinical Implications*
Viral persistence	– Viral RNA/proteins in tissues – Possible viral reservoirs	– Chronic inflammation – Symptom recurrence
Immune dysregulation	– Elevated cytokines – Immune exhaustion – Autoantibodies	– Fatigue – Autoimmune-like symptoms
Endothelial dysfunction	– Vascular injury via ACE2 targeting – Microthrombi formation – Cytokine-induced endotheliitis	– Brain fog – Chest pain – Breathlessness
Mitochondrial dysfunction	– Impaired cellular energy production – Metabolic stress	– Exercise intolerance – Post-exertional malaise
Microbiome dysbiosis	– Gut flora disruption – Persistent inflammation	– GI symptoms – Systemic immune effects
Neuroinflammation	– CNS inflammation – Blood-brain barrier disruption – Microglial activation	– Cognitive dysfunction – Mood/sleep disturbances

Sources: Adapted from Al-Aly et al. (2024), Davis et al. (2023), Peluso and Deeks (2024), and Li et al. (2023).

Note: Mechanisms are interdependent and may contribute collectively to symptom presentation.

and microbiome dysbiosis (Al-Aly et al., 2024). With advancements in research during 2024–2025, scientists have made significant progress in understanding these mechanisms, though evidence on why persistent symptoms occur is still limited in some areas.

Viral persistence represents one of the most compelling theories. Evidence suggests that SARS-CoV-2 RNA and proteins can be identified in various tissues months after the initial infection, potentially serving as ongoing sources of antigenic stimulation. This persistence may explain why some patients continue to experience symptoms long after the acute phase has resolved. Studies have detected viral remnants in gut tissues, neural structures, and even adipose tissue, suggesting that the virus may establish reservoirs that evade complete clearance by the immune system (Li et al., 2023; Moser et al., 2023).

Immune dysregulation forms another critical component of long COVID pathophysiology. Patients with long COVID appear to have increased levels of cytokines compared to healthy controls, and these inflammatory mediators are associated with the persistence of symptoms. This significant increase in cytokines, especially interleukin 6 (IL-6), which can penetrate the blood-brain barrier, appears to alter neuronal functions and cause complications in the central nervous system. The dysregulated immune response may include sustained inflammation, immune cell exhaustion, and the development of autoantibodies that target the body's own tissues.

This autoimmune component might explain why some long COVID symptoms resemble known autoimmune conditions (Tziolos et al., 2023).

Microvascular and endothelial dysfunction also play important roles. In a study by Fogarty et al. (2021), patients recovering from COVID-19 showed elevated levels of biomarkers associated with blood vessel lining damage, including von Willebrand factor, factor VIII, and thrombomodulin, proteins involved in blood clotting and vascular health. Other studies have found elevated levels of endothelial cells in COVID-19 survivors, which were related to high cytokine levels, implying that endotheliitis can be the result of inflammation. The SARS-CoV-2 virus has a particular affinity for the ACE-2 receptors abundant on vascular endothelial cells, potentially causing widespread damage to the circulatory system. This endothelial injury can lead to microthrombi formation, impairing oxygen delivery and tissue perfusion. The resulting microvascular dysfunction may contribute to multi-organ symptoms, particularly in the brain, heart, and lungs (Pelle et al., 2022; Xu et al., 2023).

Mitochondrial dysfunction and metabolic reprogramming offer another explanatory framework, particularly for the profound fatigue experienced by many long COVID patients. Recent research in 2025 has identified the virus's impact on mitochondria, the energy powerhouses of cells, as a key factor in long COVID pathogenesis. The metabolic stress induced by viral infection, coupled with prolonged inflammation, can disrupt cellular energy production. This dysfunction is especially evident in immune cells and muscle tissue, potentially explaining the exercise intolerance and post-exertional malaise characteristic of the condition (Molnar et al., 2024).

Additionally, prevailing theories for underlying mechanisms include persisting viral reservoirs, sustained inflammation, host microbiome factors, persistent autoimmune responses, and endothelial dysfunction leading to blood clotting. The gut microbiome, which plays a crucial role in immune regulation, can be significantly altered by SARS-CoV-2 infection. These changes may persist long after the acute illness, potentially contributing to systemic inflammation and gastrointestinal symptoms (Zhang et al., 2023).

Neuroinflammation deserves special consideration given the prominence of neurological and psychiatric symptoms in long COVID. Central nervous system inflammation, accompanied by microglial activation and potential disruption of the blood-brain barrier, may explain persistent mood disorders, cognitive impairment, and sleep disturbances. Neuroimaging studies have demonstrated structural and functional changes in the brains of long COVID patients, particularly in regions involved in attention, memory, and emotional regulation (Al-Aly et al., 2024).

It's important to recognize that these mechanisms are not mutually exclusive but rather operate in concert, creating a complex landscape of dysfunction that manifests differently among individuals based on genetic predisposition, comorbidities, and environmental factors. The variability in long COVID presentations likely reflects this mechanistic heterogeneity, further emphasizing the need for personalized approaches to diagnosis and treatment.

Clinical Manifestations Across Organ Systems

The far-reaching impact of SARS-CoV-2 extends well beyond the respiratory system, affecting virtually every organ and physiological system in the body. Long COVID can manifest across a wide array of body systems (Table 17.3), reflecting the virus's unusual capacity to cause lingering symptoms and long-term complications through direct organ damage, immune dysregulation, and viral persistence, even in those who experienced only mild acute illness.

Table 17.3 Organ System Manifestations in Long COVID

Organ System	*Key Manifestations*	*Potential Mechanisms*
Neurological	– Cognitive dysfunction – Headache – Dysautonomia – Sleep disorders – Anosmia/dysgeusia	– Neuroinflammation – BBB disruption – Autoimmunity – Vagus nerve dysfunction
Cardiovascular	– Myocarditis – Palpitations – POTS – Chest pain – Increased MI/stroke risk	– Endothelial damage – Microthrombi – Direct viral cardiac injury – Inflammation
Respiratory	– Dyspnea (shortness of breath) – Cough – Reduced exercise capacity – Pulmonary fibrosis	– Ongoing inflammation – Microvascular damage – Fibrotic changes
Gastrointestinal	– Abdominal pain – Diarrhea – Nausea – Appetite changes	– Viral persistence in gut – Microbiome disruption – Enteric nervous system damage
Musculoskeletal	– Myalgia – Arthralgia – Weakness – Post-exertional malaise	– Inflammatory cytokines – Mitochondrial dysfunction – Autoimmunity
Reproductive	– Menstrual irregularities – Erectile dysfunction – Fertility concerns	– Vascular endothelial damage – Hormonal dysregulation – Immune effects
Renal	– Decreased GFR – Proteinuria – Electrolyte abnormalities	– Microvascular damage – Inflammation – Direct viral effect on ACE2
Dermatological	– Rashes – Urticaria – Hair loss – Chilblains	– Immune dysregulation – Microvascular changes – Mast cell activation

Note: Based on data from Al-Aly et al. (2024), Davis et al. (2023), Li et al. (2023), Peluso and Deeks (2024). BBB = blood-brain barrier; POTS = postural orthostatic tachycardia syndrome; GFR = glomerular filtration rate; MI = myocardial infarction; ACE2 = angiotensin-converting enzyme 2.

Neurological and Psychiatric Manifestations

The nervous system is frequently affected in long COVID, with neurological and psychiatric symptoms among the most commonly reported and debilitating. Cognitive deficits represent a significant burden for patients, encompassing memory loss, reduced executive function, and impaired attention. These cognitive changes can be profound enough to interfere with routine activities and employment. Structural changes in the brain have been documented via MRI up to six months post-infection, including gray matter loss and functional disruption in frontal, temporal, and occipital lobes. These findings suggest that COVID-19 may accelerate neurodegenerative processes, with concerning parallels noted between the pathological changes in COVID-19 and conditions such as Alzheimer's and Parkinson's diseases (Davis et al., 2023; Ewing et al., 2025; Li et al., 2023).

Psychiatric symptoms feature prominently in long COVID, with depression, anxiety, post-traumatic stress disorder, and insomnia widely reported. While some of these manifestations may represent psychological responses to chronic illness, neuroimaging and neurochemical studies suggest direct neuropsychiatric effects of the virus. The psychological burden is compounded by the unpredictable nature of symptoms and the often-inadequate recognition of long COVID in healthcare settings (Davis et al., 2023).

Dysautonomia, or autonomic nervous system dysfunction, emerges as a particularly troublesome aspect of long COVID, potentially involving the vagus nerve. This dysfunction can result in abnormal heart rate, blood pressure regulation, and digestive processes. A common manifestation is POTS, where patients experience rapid heart rate increases upon standing, accompanied by dizziness, weakness, and sometimes fainting. Ongoing inflammation and disruption of the blood-brain barrier, with viral invasion mechanisms, including vascular and olfactory pathways, may underlie many of these neurological manifestations (Davis et al., 2023; Ewing et al., 2025).

Cardiovascular Manifestations

Cardiovascular sequelae represent another prominent feature of long COVID. Patients face increased risks of myocardial infarction, heart failure, arrhythmias, and deep vein thrombosis, even those with mild initial infections. Cardiac inflammation has been well-documented, with cardiovascular MRI showing myocardial involvement in 60–78% of patients post-COVID, regardless of prior heart disease or illness severity. This inflammation can lead to scarring and potentially permanent damage to heart tissue (Ewing et al., 2025).

Persistent ischemic changes and an elevated incidence of stroke are concerning, with COVID-19 patients up to seven times more likely to experience stroke compared to those with influenza. The mechanisms behind these cardiovascular complications include direct viral infection of heart tissue, systemic inflammation affecting the heart, and endothelial damage leading to thrombotic events (Merkler et al., 2020). Additionally, SARS-CoV-2 infection of coronary vessels has been linked to inflammation and destabilization of atherosclerotic plaques, predisposing patients to acute cardiovascular events long after the initial infection has resolved (Ewing et al., 2025).

Respiratory Manifestations

Given that COVID-19 begins as a respiratory infection, it's unsurprising that the lungs remain a critical site of both acute and chronic symptoms. Chronic cough, breathlessness, and reduced pulmonary function persist in many patients, even without obvious imaging abnormalities. This discrepancy between symptoms and diagnostic findings often leads to dismissal of patients' complaints, despite their very real functional limitations.

Pulmonary fibrosis and long-term scarring are present in a subset of patients. This scarring reduces lung compliance, impairs gas exchange, and can lead to progressive respiratory decline. Even in patients without evident fibrosis, persistent inflammation and microvascular changes may contribute to ongoing respiratory symptoms and exercise limitation (Ewing et al., 2025).

Gastrointestinal Manifestations

The gastrointestinal system represents another significant target for long COVID, with persistent diarrhea, nausea, abdominal pain, and bloating reported by many patients. These symptoms likely reflect a combination of intestinal inflammation, dysbiosis, and possibly viral persistence in gut tissues. Studies have detected viral persistence in gut tissues and stool samples up to seven months post-infection, suggesting ongoing viral activity in the gastrointestinal tract (Davis et al., 2023).

The gut microbiome, crucial for immune regulation and neurological function, can be substantially altered by SARS-CoV-2 infection, potentially contributing to both gastrointestinal and systemic symptoms. A meta-analysis of nearly 300,000 patients showed gastrointestinal symptoms in 22% of those with long COVID, highlighting the significance of enteric involvement (Ewing et al., 2025).

Musculoskeletal Manifestations

Long COVID frequently affects the musculoskeletal system, with myalgias, joint pain, and fatigue often resembling fibromyalgia or chronic fatigue syndrome. These manifestations are particularly distressing for previously active individuals, who may find themselves unable to perform even basic physical activities without experiencing severe post-exertional malaise. The mechanisms underlying these symptoms likely include a combination of direct muscle inflammation, immune-mediated processes, and metabolic dysregulation affecting energy production in muscle tissues (Li et al., 2023).

Exercise intolerance and prolonged post-exertional malaise are common, especially in younger individuals and previously active patients. These features parallel those seen in ME/CFS, suggesting shared pathophysiological pathways (Li et al.,

2023). Some patients also develop autoimmune-like presentations, such as new-onset rheumatologic disorders or worsening of existing musculoskeletal conditions, further complicating the clinical picture (Tziolos et al., 2023).

Other System Manifestations

Beyond these major systems, long COVID affects virtually every aspect of human physiology. The reproductive system shows significant impacts in both sexes, with menstrual irregularities, fertility challenges, and hormonal disruptions in women, and erectile dysfunction, hypogonadism, and deteriorated sperm quality in men. Placental and fetal impacts, including increased risks of stillbirths, preeclampsia, and preterm births, have been documented due to the virus's ability to cross the placental barrier (Ewing et al., 2025).

Liver involvement, while less prominent than other organ systems, manifests as enzyme abnormalities and potential worsening of pre-existing liver diseases (Li et al., 2023). Renal complications include acute kidney injury during acute COVID-19, with persistent dysfunction reported in some long COVID patients, creating a risk of chronic kidney disease that requires long-term monitoring and intervention (Ewing et al., 2025).

Metabolic disruptions are increasingly recognized, with long COVID potentially impairing pancreatic function and contributing to incident diabetes, both type 1 and type 2. Insulin resistance and beta-cell dysfunction may result from direct viral attack on pancreatic tissue or from systemic inflammation affecting metabolic regulation (Ewing et al., 2025).

The breadth and depth of organ system involvement in long COVID stresses its nature as a true multisystem condition, requiring comprehensive evaluation and multidisciplinary management approaches. As our understanding of these manifestations continues to evolve, so too will our approaches to diagnosis, monitoring, and treatment of this complex condition.

Risk Factors and Predictors

Understanding who is most likely to develop long COVID has been a central focus of research efforts, yielding insights that are both scientifically valuable and clinically relevant. Several demographic, clinical, and viral factors have emerged as significant predictors of long COVID risk, though the complex interplay between these variables remains an area of active investigation (Table 17.4).

Sex and Gender Differences

Sex emerges as one of the most consistent predictors of long COVID risk, with women disproportionately affected, particularly by fatigue and cognitive symptoms. The global meta-analysis by Hou et al. (2025) identified female sex as one of the three strongest risk factors for long COVID, alongside being unvaccinated for COVID-19 and having pre-existing comorbidities.

Table 17.4 Risk Factors for Long COVID Development

Risk Factor	*Strength of Association*	*Likelihood of Long COVID*
Female sex	Strong	1.31–1.44× increased risk
Age	Moderate	Highest prevalence among 30–49 years
Severe acute COVID-19	Very strong	2.37× with hospitalization
Unvaccinated status	Strong	1.41× vs. any vaccination
Multiple reinfections	Very strong	2.14× with 2 infections 3.75× with ≥3 infections
Pre-existing conditions	Very strong	2.48× higher odds
Socioeconomic disadvantage	Moderate	Higher in lower-income countries (29.8 vs. 14.4%)
Race/ethnicity	Moderate	Black: 1.097×, Hispanic: 1.349× higher odds vs. White
Ancestry	Moderate	Arab/North African: highest at 36.1%
Variant	Moderate	Ancestral > Alpha > Delta/Omicron (in terms of long COVID risk)

Note: Compiled from multiple studies, including Shah et al. (2025), Adjaye-Gbewonyo et al. (2023), Tsampasian et al. (2023), Gao et al. (2022), Soares et al. (2024), Hermans et al. (2025), Jacobs et al. (2023b), Slawson (2023). Odds/hazard ratios vary across studies due to methodological differences, population characteristics, and adjustments for confounders. Risk factors often interact with each other, potentially amplifying or mitigating effects.

A comprehensive NIH-funded study from the RECOVER-Adult cohort, which followed over 12,000 participants across the United States, found that individuals assigned female at birth were significantly more likely to develop long COVID than males. After adjusting for demographic factors, comorbidities, and clinical characteristics, women were found to have a 31–44% increased risk of developing long COVID. This elevated risk was most evident in women between the ages of 40 and 54 (Shah et al., 2025).

Importantly, the relationship between female sex and long COVID appears influenced by age, menopausal status, and pregnancy. Among nonpregnant women in the 40–54 age group, the risk was even higher, while this association was not significant in women aged 18–39, suggesting a possible protective role of pregnancy or hormonal variation in younger women. Women with long COVID also reported higher frequencies of hallmark symptoms, particularly fatigue, brain fog, palpitations, dizziness, and post-exertional malaise (Shah et al., 2025).

These patterns suggest that sex-specific biological mechanisms, such as differences in immune response, inflammation, and hormonal regulation, may contribute to the increased vulnerability of women to post-COVID conditions. The findings parallel trends seen in other post-viral syndromes like ME/CFS and fibromyalgia, which also disproportionately affect women, highlighting the importance of considering sex and gender in both the diagnosis and management of long COVID (Shah et al., 2025).

Age-Related Factors

Age presents a more complex picture in relation to long COVID risk. While the highest prevalence is observed among adults aged 30–59, different age groups appear vulnerable to different aspects of the condition. An *Annals of Neurology* cross-sectional study investigated neurologic post-acute sequelae of SARS-CoV-2 infection (Neuro-PASC) in 200 post-hospitalized and 1,100 non-hospitalized adults, categorized by age. While older adults (65+) had more comorbidities and abnormal neurologic findings, younger (18–44) and middle-aged (45–64) individuals experienced a higher burden of Neuro-PASC symptoms, including fatigue, sleep disturbances, and cognitive dysfunction, which significantly impacted their quality of life (Choudhury et al., 2025).

Notably, the worst cognitive performance was seen in younger non-hospitalized patients, challenging early assumptions that long COVID predominantly affected older populations or those with severe acute illness. These findings highlight the profound public health and economic implications of Neuro-PASC, particularly as it disproportionately affects younger adults in their prime working years, potentially straining healthcare systems, worsening mental health, and hindering societal productivity and economic stability (Choudhury et al., 2025).

Racial, Ethnic, and Socioeconomic Disparities

Long COVID does not affect all populations equally, with significant disparities observed across racial, ethnic, and socioeconomic lines. A 2025 study published in *BMJ Global Health* examining participants across 14 nations found that 25.1% of patients reported symptoms of long COVID six months after symptomatic COVID-19 infection. The study revealed significant disparities: individuals in lower-middle-income countries reported long COVID symptoms at a rate of 29.8%, more than double the 14.4% rate observed in participants from high-income countries. Ethnic disparities were also pronounced—36.1% of participants of Arab or North African descent experienced long COVID symptoms, the highest among all ethnic groups studied. The authors concluded that "the burden to health and healthcare-related costs may fall disproportionately on countries with the least capacity to carry them" (Hermans et al., 2025).

These international findings align with racial and ethnic disparities observed in the United States. A study of over 62,000 COVID-19 patients in New York City found that Black and Hispanic individuals were more likely than white individuals to experience several long COVID-related symptoms and conditions. Among hospitalized patients, Black individuals were more likely to be newly diagnosed with diabetes and headaches compared to white patients. Hispanic patients also had higher rates of headaches and shortness of breath. Among non-hospitalized patients, Black individuals had elevated rates of pulmonary embolism and new-onset diabetes, while Hispanic individuals reported more frequent headaches and chest pain (Khullar et al., 2023).

These disparities likely reflect long-standing inequities in healthcare access, exposure risk, socioeconomic conditions, and systemic racism. Furthermore, racial and ethnic minorities are often underrepresented in clinical research, which may limit our understanding of how long COVID affects these groups and contribute to disparities in diagnosis and treatment.

Socioeconomic status intersects with these racial and ethnic factors as well, further shaping long COVID risk and outcomes. Limited access to healthcare and higher occupational exposure contribute to elevated risk among economically disadvantaged populations, according to a large, nationwide study conducted in Denmark published in *The Lancet Regional Health* that observed these interactions among migrant populations.

The study analyzed over 2.2 million confirmed COVID-19 cases between January 2020 and August 2022. Although the overall risk of long COVID diagnosis was not strongly associated with income or educational level within individual ethnic groups, migrants with low income were found to have a significantly higher risk of developing long COVID compared to low-income native Danes. This trend was especially evident among Eastern European, Southeast Asian, Middle Eastern, and North African migrants. For example, Southeast Asian migrants with low income were more than twice as likely to be diagnosed with long COVID than their Danish counterparts, and Eastern European and North African migrants also faced a substantially elevated risk (Mkoma et al., 2025).

Thus, occupational exposure emerged as a key contributor to long COVID risk. Migrant workers employed in sectors such as transportation, customer service, office administration, and education experienced higher rates of long COVID than Danish workers in the same industries. These jobs often involve public-facing duties, limited flexibility, and reduced access to paid sick leave, all factors that likely increase both exposure to infection and barriers to recovery (Mkoma et al., 2025).

These burdens, all tied to socioeconomic vulnerability, highlight the need for stronger workplace protections, equitable access to healthcare, and targeted policy interventions that address the specific challenges faced by economically disadvantaged labor groups.

Pre-Existing Health Conditions

Several pre-existing health conditions have been identified as significant predictors of long COVID risk. Large cohort studies, including the NIH RECOVER Initiative, have shown that obesity, chronic illnesses, psychiatric history, and autoimmune conditions all increase vulnerability to persistent post-COVID symptoms. These conditions may predispose individuals to more severe acute illness, dysregulated immune responses, or impaired recovery mechanisms. Psychological distress prior to infection, such as anxiety or depression, has also been linked to a substantially higher risk, sometimes even more strongly than physical health factors (Jacobs et al., 2023a).

The relationship between prior health status and long COVID risk points to the importance of preventive care and chronic disease management in reducing post-COVID complications. It also calls for targeted surveillance and early intervention in high-risk populations with multiple comorbidities.

Acute Illness Severity and Reinfection

The severity of initial COVID-19 illness and the occurrence of reinfections are key predictors of long COVID development. Individuals who required hospitalization or ICU care during the acute phase face a significantly increased risk of developing long-term complications across multiple organ systems, including pulmonary, neurological, and cardiovascular systems.

Reinfection adds further risk. A large cohort study published in *Nature Medicine*, which analyzed health records from over 5.8 million individuals, found a clear dose-response relationship: compared to those with a single infection, individuals with two infections had a 2.07 times higher risk of developing at least one post-acute sequela, while those with three or more infections had a 2.35 times higher risk. These risks persisted up to a year after reinfection, regardless of vaccination status (Bowe et al., 2022).

Reinfections also increased the risk of all-cause mortality and hospitalization and were associated with a higher burden of symptoms like fatigue, mental health issues, and organ dysfunction. These findings further emphasize the importance of preventing reinfection and managing severe cases to reduce the burden of long COVID, challenging the often believed notion that repeated COVID-19 infections become progressively milder or less consequential (Bowe et al., 2022).

Vaccination Status

Vaccination status has emerged as another critical factor influencing the risk of developing long COVID. While vaccination does not completely eliminate the risk of persistent symptoms following SARS-CoV-2 infection, accumulating evidence suggests that it provides a protective effect.

A large body of observational research, including several systematic reviews and meta-analyses, indicates that individuals who received any COVID-19 vaccination had a 22–29% lower risk of developing long COVID compared to unvaccinated individuals. When stratified by vaccine dosing, those who completed a primary course (typically two doses) experienced a 19% lower risk, while those who received booster vaccinations (≥3 doses) showed a 26% lower risk relative to unvaccinated peers. Importantly, booster doses also conferred a 23% additional risk reduction when compared to primary vaccination alone (Green et al., 2024). This protective effect of vaccination is further supported by the 2025 global meta-analysis by Hou et al. (2025), which identified being unvaccinated as one of the three strongest risk factors for developing long COVID.

The observed reduction in long COVID risk may be attributed to several mechanisms. Vaccination reduces the likelihood of severe acute infection, which itself is a key predictor of long COVID. Additionally, vaccine-induced immune responses may enhance viral clearance, limit viral persistence, and mitigate systemic inflammation—all factors implicated in the pathogenesis of prolonged symptoms (Peluso & Deeks, 2024).

However, vaccine efficacy varies by SARS-CoV-2 variant and time since vaccination. For instance, U.K. data showed that long COVID was 50% less common after Omicron BA.1 infection in double-vaccinated individuals compared to Delta infections, but this effect was less pronounced or absent in triple-vaccinated individuals across variant comparisons (Davis et al., 2023). Furthermore, booster vaccination does not uniformly improve outcomes for individuals already experiencing long COVID. A large international survey found that 57.9% of participants reported improvements in symptoms following vaccination, 17.9% reported deterioration, and the remainder experienced no change (Strain et al., 2022). Similarly, a systematic review published in *The Lancet eClinicalMedicine* found that 63% of studies showed vaccination improved ongoing symptoms of long COVID, while 36% reported small changes or worsening in some patients (Notarte et al., 2022).

Despite these nuances, the cumulative evidence supports the continued use of seasonal and booster COVID-19 vaccines—not only for preventing severe acute disease but also for mitigating the risk of chronic post-viral sequelae. These findings carry implications for public health policy and individual decision-making, especially in populations at heightened risk of long COVID.

Viral Variant

Since the emergence of COVID-19, some form of definitional long COVID has been reported across all major SARS-CoV-2 variants. While the core symptoms remain relatively consistent, including fatigue, cognitive dysfunction, and respiratory complaints, their severity, duration, and frequency have varied depending on the circulating variant, vaccination rates, and individual risk factors.

The ancestral strain and Alpha variant were associated with more prolonged, multisystem symptoms, including severe fatigue, dyspnea (loss of taste or smell), chest pain, palpitations, cognitive impairment, anosmia, and joint and muscle pain. These early variants typically produced symptoms lasting more than six months and affected multiple organ systems simultaneously (Spinicci et al., 2022).

The Delta variant, which circulated in mid- to late 2021, was characterized by more severe acute illness, leading to a higher risk of persistent symptoms (Du et al., 2022). The heightened severity of Delta infections contributed to a higher hospitalization rate and more cases of post-ICU syndrome. Notably, the protection offered by a single dose of mRNA vaccine was substantially lower against Delta. This marked the beginning of a trend where vaccine efficacy began to show signs of reduced performance against emerging variants (Lok et al., 2024).

With the emergence of Omicron and its subvariants, the clinical picture shifted somewhat. Although Omicron can still lead to long COVID, it has been associated with milder acute illness and a lower overall risk of developing long COVID (estimated at 20–50% reduction compared to Delta) (Antonelli et al., 2022). Interestingly, studies have reported that during the Omicron-dominant period, long COVID symptoms shifted away from cardiopulmonary and neuropsychiatric manifestations and more frequently involved gastrointestinal issues, metabolic disorders, and musculoskeletal symptoms compared to the pre-Omicron period (Lok et al., 2024). The reduced risk with Omicron likely reflected a combination of higher vaccination rates and the variant's inherently milder acute illness profile, though unvaccinated individuals and those experiencing reinfections remained at significant risk for long COVID (Padilla et al., 2024).

These evolving patterns add further importance to variant-specific insights to guide care and implement prevention strategies. As the virus continues to evolve, ongoing surveillance and research will be essential to understand how new variants might affect the long-term consequences of infection.

Global Prevalence of Long COVID

The global burden of long COVID represents one of the pandemic's most significant long-term public health challenges. According to a 2024 *Nature Medicine* review, the cumulative global incidence is around 400 million individuals, with an estimated annual economic impact of approximately $1 trillion, which is roughly equivalent to about 1% of the global economy (Al-Aly et al., 2024). However, prevalence estimates vary considerably across regions due to differences in case definitions, methodology, sampling approaches, follow-up duration, and whether study results are crude or adjusted for non-COVID control groups (Table 17.5). Most figures reflect symptoms lasting 4–12+ weeks in COVID-positive individuals, though criteria for attribution and severity differ. Due to this lack of a universally accepted, standardized diagnostic criteria for long COVID, any data regarding prevalence should be interpreted with caution and viewed directionally rather than definitively.

In the United States, where the CDC defines long COVID as persistent symptoms three months or more after initial infection, prevalence estimates range from

Table 17.5 Global Long COVID Prevalence by Region

Region	*Long COVID Prevalence by COVID-Positive (%)*	*Long COVID Prevalence by Total Population (%)*
Global	**54** (2021) **45** (2022) **36** (2025)	**5–6**
Asia	**40.9** (2022) **35** (2025)	**1.5–2**
Europe	**62.7** (2022) **39** (2025)	**6–7**
North America	**38.9** (2022) **30** (2025)	**3–4**
South America	**51** (2025)	**4–6**
Africa	**48.6** (2023) **42.1** (2025)	**1–2** (limited data)
Oceania	**18** (2025)	**1–1.5**

Note: Based on data from European Centre For Disease Prevention and Control (ECDC) (2022), Groff et al. (2021), O'Mahoney et al. (2023), Al-Aly et al. (2024), Hou et al. (2025), Di Gennaro et al. (2023), Frallonardo et al. (2023) and Alie et al. (2025). Prevalence among COVID-positive individuals reflects the proportion of infected individuals reporting persistent *symptoms at 4–12+ weeks post-infection. Prevalence by total population adjusts for overall infection rates and reflects the estimated burden across the general population.*

6 to 9% in the general population (Adjaye-Gbewonyo et al., 2023; Centers for Disease Control and Prevention (CDC), 2025; Vahratian et al., 2024). Recent CDC data indicates that while rates of new cases have decreased since the beginning of the pandemic, long COVID remains a serious public health concern as millions of U.S. adults and children have been affected (CDC, 2025). The NIH's RECOVER Initiative continues to gather data on prevalence, risk factors, and outcomes to inform national response strategies.

The United Kingdom has implemented robust long COVID surveillance through the Office for National Statistics (ONS), defining the condition as symptoms lasting more than four weeks after infection. Data from 2023 indicates that approximately 2.9% of the U.K. population (about 2 million people) reported ongoing symptoms consistent with long COVID, with fatigue, cognitive impairment, and breathlessness most commonly reported. This comprehensive population-based approach has provided valuable insights into the condition's community burden and natural history (Office for National Statistics (ONS), 2023).

In Canada, where the definition similarly emphasizes symptoms persisting beyond three months, self-reported data suggests approximately 1.4 million people have or had long COVID, with higher rates among women and individuals with comorbidities (Government of Canada, 2022). Australia estimates that 5–10% of confirmed COVID-19 cases develop persistent symptoms, focusing particularly on those lasting beyond 12 weeks (Australian Institute of Health and Welfare, 2022).

Asian countries have also documented significant long COVID burdens. In Japan, survey data during the Omicron-dominant period estimates that approximately 12% of individuals experienced symptoms lasting two months or longer (Iba et al., 2024). Data from South Korea estimated a prevalence of 19.7% among adults at three months after initial infection (Son et al., 2024).

In middle- and lower-income regions, data collection has been more challenging, but evidence suggests potentially higher burdens of long COVID. Studies in India report prevalence ranging from 29 to 46% for symptoms persisting for four or more weeks (Arjun et al., 2022; Singh et al., 2024). Brazil has documented rates up to 27% in infected healthcare workers, where over half reported three or more symptoms four weeks post-infection (Marra et al., 2023).

These global patterns reveal several important trends. First, while definitions and surveillance methods vary, long COVID affects a substantial minority of those infected with SARS-CoV-2 across all regions. Second, the burden appears disproportionately high in regions with limited healthcare resources and among disadvantaged populations, highlighting global health inequities. Third, prevalence estimates have generally declined since the pandemic's early phases, likely reflecting a combination of vaccination effects, variant evolution, improved treatments for acute disease, and increased population immunity.

The global prevalence data stresses the need for standardized definitions, improved surveillance systems, and coordinated international research efforts. As the pandemic continues its transition to endemicity, understanding and addressing the long-term burden of post-COVID conditions remains a critical global health priority that will shape healthcare for years to come.

Diagnosis, Treatment, and Management Strategies

The approach to long COVID diagnosis, treatment, and management requires a personalized, multidisciplinary framework that addresses both symptom relief and functional improvement. Given the condition's heterogeneity, no single diagnostic test or treatment regimen applies to all patients, necessitating tailored approaches based on predominant symptoms, organ system involvement, and individual circumstances. Different organizations use varying terminology and time frames to define and diagnose long COVID, which can complicate comparisons across studies and clinical settings (Table 17.6). Despite five years of research since the start of the pandemic, as of 2025, there is still no specific approved treatment for long COVID, though significant advances in understanding the condition have occurred (Del Carpio-Orantes, 2025).

Diagnostic Approaches

Currently, there is no single laboratory test that can determine if symptoms or conditions are due to long COVID, and a positive SARS-CoV-2 test is not required for diagnosis. Healthcare providers consider a diagnosis based on clinical evaluations, and results of routine blood tests, chest X-rays, and electrocardiograms may be normal in someone with long COVID. This reality often leads to diagnostic challenges and patient frustration, as objective findings may not align with subjective symptom burden (CDC, 2025).

Table 17.6 Time Frames for Long COVID Diagnosis Across Major Health Organizations

Organization	*Term Used*	*Time Frame for Diagnosis*
WHO (global)	*Post-COVID-19 condition*	Symptoms lasting ≥3 months post-infection
CDC (the United States)	*Long COVID/PASC*	Symptoms persisting ≥3 months after infection
NHS (the United Kingdom)	*Post-COVID syndrome/ long COVID*	Symptoms continuing ≥12 weeks after infection
ESCMID (Europe)	*Post-COVID-19 condition/long COVID*	Symptoms lasting ≥12 weeks after infection
NICE (the United Kingdom)	*Long COVID*	Symptoms lasting ≥4 weeks after infection
AUS DoH (Australia)	*PASC*	Symptoms lasting ≥3 months post-infection

Note: This table summarizes how major health authorities define long COVID based on the time elapsed since acute infection. While terminology and thresholds vary slightly, all definitions recognize prolonged symptom duration as a key criterion.

Adapted from World Health Organization (WHO) (2025), Centers for Diseases Control and Prevention (CDC) (2025), NHS (2023), Yelin et al. (2022), NICE (2020), and Australian Government Deaprtment of Health and Aged Care (2024). Some frameworks distinguish between ongoing symptoms (typically 4–12 weeks) and post-COVID syndrome (>12 weeks). Notably, many definitions do not require laboratory confirmation, acknowledging testing access limitations and symptom variability. WHO = World Health Organization; CDC = U.S. Centers for Disease Control and Prevention; NHS = United Kingdom National Health Service; ESCMID = European Society of Clinical Microbiology and Infectious Diseases; NICE = United Kingdom National Institute for Health and Care Excellence; AUS DoH = Australian Department of Health; PASC = Post-Acute Sequelae of SARS-CoV-2.

Diagnosis typically begins with a comprehensive history focusing on temporal relationship to COVID-19 infection, symptom patterns, exacerbating and alleviating factors, and functional impact. Physical examination may reveal findings such as orthostatic blood pressure changes, neurocognitive abnormalities, or cardiopulmonary signs, though many patients with significant symptoms have normal examinations (Yale Medicine, n.d.).

Laboratory investigations often include inflammatory markers (C-reactive protein, erythrocyte sedimentation rate), complete blood count, comprehensive metabolic panel, thyroid function, and cardiac enzymes. More specialized testing may be warranted based on specific symptoms, such as D-dimer for suspected coagulopathy, pulmonary function tests for respiratory complaints, or neuropsychological evaluation for cognitive symptoms. Advanced imaging, including cardiac MRI, chest CT, or brain MRI, may reveal objective abnormalities in some patients (Tsilingiris et al., 2023).

Importantly, diagnosis often requires excluding alternative explanations for symptoms, which necessitates a thorough evaluation rather than premature attribution to long COVID. Comorbid conditions can coexist with or mimic long COVID, complicating the diagnostic picture and requiring careful clinical judgment.

Treatment Approaches

Treatment of long COVID remains largely symptomatic and supportive, though evolving research continues to inform more targeted approaches. Symptom relief represents a cornerstone of management, with medications addressing specific complaints such as pain (nonsteroidal anti-inflammatory drugs, acetaminophen), anxiety (selective serotonin reuptake inhibitors, cognitive behavioral therapy), insomnia (sleep hygiene interventions, melatonin), and dysautonomia (increased fluid intake, compression garments, beta-blockers) (Providence, 2024).

Rehabilitation plays a crucial role in functional recovery, with physical therapy addressing deconditioning, breathing techniques, and gradual exercise tolerance. However, standard graded exercise approaches may worsen symptoms in patients with post-exertional malaise, necessitating energy conservation strategies and careful activity pacing instead. Occupational therapy provides valuable assistance with daily living activities, energy management, and workplace accommodations, while cognitive rehabilitation may help address memory, attention, and executive function deficits (Swarnakar & Yadav, 2022).

The multisystem nature of long COVID often requires specialist involvement from various disciplines. Cardiology consultation may be needed for palpitations, chest pain, or POTS symptoms; neurology for persistent headaches, paresthesias, or cognitive issues; pulmonology for breathlessness or chronic cough; psychiatry for mood disturbances; and rheumatology for joint pain or suspected autoimmune phenomena. This multidisciplinary approach allows for comprehensive evaluation and coordinated care plans but requires effective communication and coordination between providers to avoid fragmented or inefficient management (Yale Medicine, n.d.).

Self-management strategies empower patients to actively participate in their recovery. These include symptom tracking to identify patterns and triggers, pacing techniques to avoid post-exertional symptom exacerbation, dietary modifications to address gastrointestinal symptoms, stress reduction practices, and prioritization of restorative sleep. Environmental accommodations, such as workplace modifications, assistive devices, or schedule adjustments, can also significantly improve function and quality of life. These strategies align well with our discussion in Part 3 about implementing lifestyle medicine approaches that support long-term resilience, autonomy, and holistic recovery.

Emerging Therapeutic Approaches

As understanding of long COVID pathophysiology deepens, several promising therapeutic approaches are emerging, though most remain investigational (Table 17.7). The NIH has significantly expanded research funding, allocating $662 million over fiscal years 2025–2029 to support long COVID research, including clinical trials of potential treatments through the RECOVER-Treating Long COVID (RECOVER-TLC) program (National Institutes of Health (NIH), 2024).

Clinical trials have explored several treatment approaches with mixed results. Temelimab, a disease-modifying drug for multiple sclerosis, and BC007, designed to neutralize functional autoantibodies, both failed to demonstrate superiority over placebo in trials (GeNeuro, 2024). Extended treatment with nirmatrelvir/ritonavir (Paxlovid) has shown some promise in reducing long COVID symptoms in certain patients, though results remain inconsistent across studies (Cohen et al., 2025).

A promising treatment undergoing investigation is baricitinib, an FDA-approved immunomodulator for rheumatoid arthritis. The REVERSE-LC trial, a phase 3 multicenter study launched in 2025, is testing whether six months of baricitinib can improve neurocognitive and physical function in patients with long-term symptoms (Vanderbilt Health, 2025). The trial will enroll 550 patients who have had cognitive problems for at least six months after COVID-19 infection.

Other experimental approaches include the use of monoclonal antibodies, which showed promise in a small study reporting full recovery in some patients after being given Regeneron (Scheppke et al., 2024). Non-pharmacological interventions being studied include transcranial direct current stimulation for neuropsychiatric symptoms and repetitive transcranial magnetic stimulation (rTMS) for fatigue and brain fog (Lavretsky, 2025).

Yale New Haven Long COVID Multidisciplinary Care Center evaluates people experiencing long COVID symptoms and works closely with an array of specialists to find the best treatments for them. The Yale Center of Infection & Immunity is working to unravel disease pathogenesis of long COVID through multi-pronged approaches to biological analysis that will hopefully lead to insights useful for diagnosis and treatment (Yale School of Medicine, 2024).

Table 17.7 Current Treatment Approaches for Long COVID by Symptom Category

Symptom Category	*Standard Approaches*	*Emerging Treatments*	*Evidence Level*
Fatigue/PEM	– Pacing – Energy conservation – Nutritional support	– Low-dose naltrexone – Coenzyme Q10 – Nicotinamide adenine dinucleotide – RECOVER-ENERGIZE	*Limited RCTs; RECOVER trials*
Cognitive dysfunction	– Cognitive rehab – Sleep hygiene	– tDCS – Brain training – Neurostimulation devices – Modafinil – RECOVER-NEURO	*Early trials*
Respiratory symptoms	– Pulmonary rehab – Breathing exercises – Inhaled corticosteroids	– Antifibrotics (pirfenidone) – Hyperbaric oxygen – WEHI antiviral (preclinical)	*Small trials; preclinical*
Cardiovascular/ POTS	– Fluids and salt – Compression – Beta-blockers – Recumbent exercise	– Ivabradine – Gamunex-C intravenous immunoglobulin – RECOVER-AUTONOMIC	*RECOVER trials ongoing*
Immune dysregulation	– Antihistamines – Low-inflammatory diet – Mast cell stabilizers	– Baricitinib (SILC trial) – Intravenous immunoglobulin – Plasmapheresis	*Phase 2/3 trials*
Viral persistence	– Symptom-based care	– Antivirals (e.g., Paxlovid) – Metformin – RECOVER-VITAL	*Mixed trial results*
Psychological/ sleep	– CBT – SSRIs/SNRIs – Stress reduction	– Modafinil – Solriamfetol – RECOVER-SLEEP	*General use; trials ongoing*

Note: This table provides the summary of updated treatment pathways for long COVID as of 2025. Emerging therapies are under active investigation through the NIH RECOVER Initiative and other international studies.

Adapted from RECOVER (2024a, 2024b, 2024c, 2024d, 2024e), Bramante et al. (2024), Isman et al. (2024), Novak (2024), Bermudo-Peloche et al. (2025), Smith (2024), Swarnakar and Yadav (2022), Hadanny et al. (2024), Bader et al. (2025), Vanderbilt Health (2025), Halpern (2024), Del Carpio-Orantes (2025), España-Cueto et al. (2025), Lessene et al. (2025). PEM = post-exertional malaise; POTS = postural orthostatic tachycardia syndrome; CBT = cognitive behavioral therapy; tDCS = transcranial direct current stimulation; WEHI = Walter and Eliza Hall Institute of Medical Research; SILC = Schmidt Initiative for Long COVID.

Integrated Care Models

The most robust approach to long COVID management incorporates multiple complementary strategies. Effective symptom management combines medications and non-pharmacological approaches targeting specific symptoms while avoiding polypharmacy. Multidisciplinary care coordinates specialists relevant to the patient's symptom profile, ensuring comprehensive treatment planning. Patient education plays a crucial role, teaching pacing techniques, symptom recognition, and self-management strategies. Social support involves facilitating connections with support groups and addressing social determinants of health that may impact recovery.

Additionally, connecting eligible patients with clinical trials of emerging therapies offers access to potential new treatments while advancing scientific understanding of the condition. As we enter the fifth year since the pandemic's onset, long COVID management continues to evolve. While significant progress has been made in understanding the condition, approved treatments remain limited, highlighting the ongoing need for research and innovation in care approaches (RECOVER, n.d.).

Prognosis, Recovery, and Future Outlook

The trajectory of recovery from long COVID varies considerably among affected individuals, reflecting the condition's heterogeneous nature and multiple contributing factors. Understanding prognosis helps set realistic expectations, guide management approaches, and inform public health planning for long-term care needs.

While the observed outcomes vary widely, several factors appear to predict more favorable recovery trajectories. Milder acute illness severity is strongly associated with better recovery prospects, as patients who avoided hospitalization typically experience fewer long-term complications. Younger age generally correlates with more complete resolution of symptoms, with adolescents and young adults showing greater resilience than older populations. The absence of pre-existing conditions significantly improves recovery pathways, as comorbidities can complicate and prolong the healing process. Early symptom-directed intervention often proves beneficial, potentially preventing the progression to chronic symptoms when appropriate treatment is initiated promptly. Additionally, comprehensive multidisciplinary care that addresses the full spectrum of symptoms tends to yield better functional outcomes than fragmented or specialty-specific approaches.

Conversely, several risk factors predict prolonged or incomplete recovery. Severe acute COVID-19 requiring hospitalization frequently leads to more persistent sequelae, particularly among those who needed intensive care. The presence of multiple comorbidities complicates recovery, as pre-existing conditions can interact with and amplify long COVID manifestations. The development of organ damage during acute illness, such as myocarditis or pulmonary fibrosis, creates lasting functional impairments that may never fully resolve. Advanced age correlates with slower and less complete recovery, reflecting diminished physiological reserve and repair capacity. Female sex also appears to confer greater vulnerability to persistent symptoms. The specific symptom profile further influences recovery patterns, with respiratory symptoms generally improving more rapidly than neurological manifestations, which can persist for months or years.

Psychological adjustment represents an important aspect of recovery. Many patients experience frustration, anxiety, and grief related to persistent symptoms and functional limitations. Developing effective coping strategies, realistic expectations, and appropriate support systems can significantly impact quality of life even when physical symptoms persist. Healthcare providers play a crucial role in validating patients' experiences, providing compassionate care, and helping navigate the uncertainty inherent in long COVID recovery.

Reinfection remains a significant concern for those who have experienced long COVID. Evidence suggests that previous long COVID does not protect against developing similar or even more severe symptoms following subsequent SARS-CoV-2 infections. This vulnerability stresses the importance of continued prevention efforts, including vaccination, masking in high-risk settings, and other protective measures, particularly for those with a history of long COVID.

The concept of recovery itself warrants careful consideration in the context of long COVID. Rather than defining recovery solely as complete symptom resolution, many patients and clinicians have adopted more nuanced approaches focusing on functional improvement, adaptation, and quality of life. This perspective acknowledges that some individuals may not return to their pre-infection baseline but can nonetheless achieve meaningful improvements and develop effective management strategies for residual symptoms.

Long-term monitoring remains essential for all long COVID patients, even those experiencing apparent recovery. The condition's relapsing-remitting nature means symptoms may reappear after periods of improvement, and new complications may emerge over time. Regular follow-up allows for appropriate intervention, adjustment of management strategies, and monitoring for potential late-onset sequelae like cardiovascular or metabolic disorders associated with previous SARS-CoV-2 infection.

As our understanding of long COVID continues to evolve, so too will our ability to predict individual recovery trajectories and develop targeted interventions to promote healing. Ongoing research into biomarkers and risk factors may eventually enable more personalized prognostic assessments and treatment approaches, offering hope for improved outcomes even for those currently experiencing persistent symptoms. In this way, long COVID represents both a public health emergency and an opportunity to transform how we understand, research, and respond to complex, chronic conditions. Sustained investment, equitable care models, and inclusive research will be essential to mitigate its long-term impact and build a more resilient, patient-centered healthcare future.

References

Adjaye-Gbewonyo, D., Vahratian, A., Perrine, C. G., & Bertolli, J. (2023). *Long COVID in adults: United States, 2022*. NCHS Data Brief, no 480. National Center for Health Statistics. DOI: https://dx.doi.org/10.15620/cdc:132417

Al-Aly, Z., Davis, H., McCorkell, L., Soares, L., WulfHanson, S., Iwasaki, A., & Topol, E. J. (2024). Long COVID science, research and policy. *Nature Medicine*, *30*(8), 2148–2164. https://doi.org/10.1038/s41591024031736

Alie, M. S., Tesema, G. A., Abebe, G. F., & Girma, D. (2025). The prolonged health sequelae "of the COVID19 pandemic" in sub-Saharan Africa: A systematic review and meta-analysis. *Frontiers in Public Health*, *132025*. https://www.frontiersin.org/journals/publichealth/articles/10.3389/fpubh.2025.1415427

Antonelli, M., Pujol, J. C., Spector, T. D., Ourselin, S., & Steves, C. J. (2022). Risk of long COVID associated with delta versus omicron variants of SARSCoV2. *The Lancet*, *399*(10343), 2263–2264. https://doi.org/10.1016/S01406736(22)009412

Arjun, M. C., Singh, A. K., Pal, D., Das, K., G, A., Venkateshan, M., Mishra, B., Patro, B. K., Mohapatra, P. R., & Subba, S. H. (2022). Characteristics and predictors of long COVID among diagnosed cases of COVID19. *PLoS ONE*, *17*(12), e0278825. https://doi.org/10.1371/journal.pone.0278825

Australian Government Department of Health and Aged Care. (2024, February). *National Post-Acute Sequelae Of COVID-19 (PASC) Plan*. https://www.health.gov.au/sites/default/files/2024-02/national-post-acute-sequelae-of-covid-19-plan.pdf

Australian Institute of Health and Welfare. (2022). *Long COVID in Australia – A review of the literature, catalogue number PHE 318*. AIHW, Australian Government.

Bader, M., Calleja, D. J., Devine, S. M., Kuchel, N. W., Bernadine, L., Wu, X., Birkinshaw, R. W., Bhandari, R., Loi, K., Volpe, R., Khakham, Y., Au, A. E., Blackmore, T. R., Mackiewicz, L., Dayton, M., Schaefer, J., Scherer, L., Stock, A. T., Cooney, J. P., & Schoffer, K. (2025). A novel PLpro inhibitor improves outcomes in a preclinical model of long COVID. *Nature Communications*, *16*(1), 2900. https://doi.org/10.1038/s41467-025-57905-4

Bermudo-Peloche, G., Del Rio, B., Vicens-Zygmunt, V., Bordas-Martinez, J., Hernández, M., Valenzuela, C., Laporta, R., Rigual Bobillo, J., Portillo, K., Millán-Billi, P., Balcells, E., Badenes-Bonet, D., Bolivar, S., Rodríguez-Portal, J. A., López Ramirez, C., Tomás, L., Fernández de Roitegi, K., Sellarés, J., Castillo, D., González, J., …, & Molina-Molina, M. (2025). Pirfenidone in post-COVID-19 pulmonary fibrosis (FIBRO-COVID): A phase 2 randomised clinical trial. *The European Respiratory Journal*, *65*(4), 2402249. https://doi.org/10.1183/13993003.02249-2024

Bowe, B., Xie, Y., & AlAly, Z. (2022). Acute and postacute sequelae associated with SARSCoV2 reinfection. *Nature Medicine*, *28*(11), 2398–2405. https://doi.org/10.1038/s41591-022-02051-3

Bramante, C. T., Beckman, K. B., Mehta, T., Karger, A. B., Odde, D. J., Tignanelli, C. J., Buse, J. B., Johnson, D. M., Watson, R. H. B., Daniel, J. J., Liebovitz, D. M., Nicklas, J. M., Cohen, K., Puskarich, M. A., Belani, H. K., Siegel, L. K., Klatt, N. R., Anderson, B., Hartman, K. M., & Rao, V. (2024). Favorable antiviral effect of metformin on SARS-CoV-2 viral load in a randomized, placebo-controlled clinical trial of COVID-19. *Clinical Infectious Diseases*, *79*(2), 354–363. https://doi.org/10.1093/cid/ciae159

Centers for Disease Control and Prevention (CDC). (2025, February 3). *Long COVID basics*. CDC. https://www.cdc.gov/covid/long-term-effects/index.html

Choudhury, N. A., Mukherjee, S., Singer, T., Venkatesh, A., Perez Giraldo, G. S., Jimenez, M., Miller, J., Lopez, M., Hanson, B. A., Bawa, A. P., Batra, A., Liotta, E. M., & Koralnik, I. J. (2025). Neurologic manifestations of long COVID disproportionately affect young and Middle-Age adults. *Annals of Neurology*, *97*(2), 369–383. https://doi.org/10.1002/ana.27128

Cohen, A. K., Jaudon, T. W., Schurman, E. M., Kava, L., Vogel, J. M., HaasGodsil, J., Lewis, D., Crausman, S., Leslie, K., Bligh, S. C., Lizars, G., Davids, J., Sran, S., Peluso, M., & McCorkell, L. (2025). Impact of extended-course oral nirmatrelvir/ritonavir in established long COVID: A case series. *Communications Medicine*, *4*(1), 261. https://doi.org/10.1038/s43856-024-00668-8

Davis, H. E., McCorkell, L., Vogel, J. M., & Topol, E. J. (2023). Long COVID: Major findings, mechanisms and recommendations. *Nature Reviews Microbiology*, *21*(3), 133–146. https://doi.org/10.1038/s41579-022-00846-2

Del Carpio-Orantes, L. (2025). *Therapeutic updates on long COVID: Where things stand 5 years later*. IDSA. https://www.idsociety.org/science-speaks-blog/2025/therapeutic-updates-on-long-covid-where-things-stand-5-years-later/

DePace, N. L., & Colombo, J. (2022). Long-COVID syndrome and the cardiovascular system: A review of neurocardiologic effects on multiple systems. *Current Cardiology Reports*, *24*(11), 1711–1726. https://doi.org/10.1007/s11886-022-01786-2

Di Gennaro, F., Belati, A., Tulone, O., Diella, L., Fiore Bavaro, D., Bonica, R., Genna, V., Smith, L., Trott, M., Bruyere, O., Mirarchi, L., Cusumano, C., Dominguez, L. J., Saracino, A., Veronese, N., & Barbagallo, M. (2023). Incidence of long COVID-19 in people with previous SARS-Cov2 infection: A systematic review and meta-analysis of 120,970 patients. *Internal and Emergency Medicine*, *18*(5), 1573–1581. https://doi.org/10.1007/s11739-022-03164-w

Du, M., Ma, Y., Deng, J., Liu, M., & Liu, J. (2022). Comparison of long COVID19 caused by different SARSCoV2 strains: A systematic review and meta-analysis. *International Journal of Environmental Research and Public Health*, *19*(23). https://doi.org/10.3390/ijerph192316010

España-Cueto, S., Loste, C., Lladós, G., López, C., Santos, J. R., Dulsat, G., García, A., Carmezim, J., Carabia, J., Ancochea, Á, FernándezPrendres, C., MoralesIndiano, C., Quirant, B., MartínezCáceres, E., Sanchez, A., Parraga, I. G., Chamorro, A., Alba, S. J., Abad, E., & MuñozMoreno, J. A. (2025). Plasma exchange therapy for the post COVID19 condition: A phase II, double-blind, placebo-controlled, randomized trial. *Nature Communications*, *16*(1), 1929. https://doi.org/10.1038/s41467-025-57198-7

European Centre For Disease Prevention and Control (ECDC). (2022). *Prevalence of post COVID-19 condition symptoms: a systematic review and meta-analysis of cohort study data, stratified by recruitment setting Key facts*. https://www.ecdc.europa.eu/sites/default/files/documents/Prevalence-post-COVID-19-condition-symptoms.pdf

Ewing, A. G., Salamon, S., Pretorius, E., Joffe, D., Fox, G., Bilodeau, S., & Bar-Yam, Y. (2025). Review of organ damage from COVID and long COVID: A disease with a spectrum of pathology. *Medical Review*, *5*(1), 66–75. https://doi.org/10.1515/mr-2024-0030

Fogarty, H., Townsend, L., Morrin, H., Ahmad, A., Comerford, C., Karampini, E., Englert, H., Byrne, M., Bergin, C., O'Sullivan, J. M., Martin-Loeches, I., Nadarajan, P., Bannan, C., Mallon, P. W., Curley, G. F., Preston, R. J. S., Rehill, A. M., McGonagle, D., Ni Cheallaigh, C., Baker, R. I., … Irish COVID-19 Vasculopathy Study (iCVS) investigators (2021). Persistent endotheliopathy in the pathogenesis of long COVID syndrome. *Journal of Thrombosis and Haemostasis: JTH*, 19(10), 2546–2553. https://doi.org/10.1111/jth.15490

Frallonardo, L., Segala, F. V., Chhaganlal, Kajal, D., Yelshazly, M., Novara, R., Cotugno, S., Guido, G., Papagni, R., Colpani, A., Vito, D., Barbagallo, M., Madeddu, G., Babudieri, S., Lochoro, P., Ictho, J., Putoto, G., Veronese, N., Saracino, A., & Gennaro, D. (2023). Incidence and burden of long COVID in Africa: A systematic review and meta-analysis. *Scientific Reports*, *13*(1), 21482. https://doi.org/10.1038/s41598-023-48258-3

Gao, P., Liu, J., & Liu, M. (2022). Effect of COVID-19 vaccines on reducing the risk of long COVID in the real world: A systematic review and meta-analysis. *International Journal of Environmental Research and Public Health*, *19*(19), 12422. https://doi.org/10.3390/ijerph191912422

GeNeuro. (2024, June 28). *GeNeuro Announces Results of the GNC-501 study in post-Covid-19 syndrome*. https://geneuro.ch/wp-content/uploads/GeNeuro_GNC501-Results_28062024_EN-3.pdf

Geng, L. N., Erlandson, K. M., Hornig, M., Letts, R., Selvaggi, C., Ashktorab, H., Atieh, O., Bartram, L., Brim, H., Brosnahan, S. B., Brown, J., Castro, M., Charney, A., Chen, P., Deeks, S. G., Erdmann, N., Flaherman, V. J., Ghamloush, M. A., Goepfert, P., &

Goldman, J. D. (2025). 2024 update of the RECOVER-adult long COVID research index. *JAMA*, *333*(8), 694–700. https://doi.org/10.1001/jama.2024.24184

Government of Canada. (2022). *Post-COVID-19 condition in Canada: What we know, what we don't know, and a framework for action.* Science.gc.ca. https://science.gc.ca/site/science/en/office-chief-science-advisor/initiatives-covid-19/post-covid-19-condition-canada-what-we-know-what-we-dont-know-and-framework-action

Green, R., Marjenberg, Z., Gregory, Banerjee, A., Wisnivesky, J., Delaney, B. C., Peluso, M. J., Wynberg, E., & Abduljawad, S. (2024). The impact of vaccination on preventing long COVID in the Omicron era: A systematic review and meta-analysis. *MedRxiv*, 2024.11.19.24317487. https://doi.org/10.1101/2024.11.19.24317487

Groff, D., Sun, A., Ssentongo, A. E., Ba, D. M., Parsons, N., Poudel, G. R., Lekoubou, A., Oh, J. S., Ericson, J. E., Ssentongo, P., & Chinchilli, V. M. (2021). Short-term and long-term rates of postacute sequelae of SARS-CoV-2 infection: A systematic review. *JAMA Network Open*, *4*(10), e2128568–e2128568. https://doi.org/10.1001/jamanetworkopen.2021.28568

Hadanny, A., Zilberman-Itskovich, S., & Catalogna, M. *et al* (2024). Long term outcomes of hyperbaric oxygen therapy in post Covid condition: Longitudinal follow-up of a randomized controlled trial. *Scientific Reports*, *14*, 3604. https://doi.org/10.1038/s41598-024-53091-3

Halpern, L. (2024, November 23). *IVIG Demonstrates Effectiveness in Several Neuroimmune Conditions, Indicating Potential for Long COVID Treatment.* Pharmacy Times. https://www.pharmacytimes.com/view/ivig-demonstrates-effectiveness-in-several-neuroimmune-conditions-indicating-potential-for-long-covid-treatment

Hastie, C. E., Lowe, D. J., McAuley, A., Mills, N. L., Winter, A. J., Black, C., Scott, J. T., O'Donnell, C. A., Blane, D. N., Browne, S., Ibbotson, T. R., & Pell, J. P. (2023). True prevalence of long-COVID in a nationwide, population cohort study. *Nature Communications*, *14*(1), 7892. https://doi.org/10.1038/s4146702343661w

Hermans, L. E., Wasserman, S., Xu, L., & Eikelboom, J. (2025). Long COVID prevalence and risk factors in adults residing in middle- and high-income countries: Secondary analysis of the multinational anti-coronavirus therapies (ACT) trials. *BMJ Global Health*, *10*(4), e017126. https://doi.org/10.1136/bmjgh2024017126

Hou, Y., Gu, T., Ni, Z., Shi, X., Ranney, M. L., & Mukherjee, B. (2025). Global prevalence of long COVID, its subtypes and risk factors: An updated systematic review and meta-analysis. *MedRxiv*, 2025.01.01.24319384. https://doi.org/10.1101/2025.01.01.24319384

Iba, A., Hosozawa, M., Hori, M., Muto, Y., Muraki, I., Masuda, R., …, & Iso, H. (2024). Prevalence of and risk factors for Post–COVID-19 condition during omicron BA.5–Dominant wave, Japan. *Emerging Infectious Diseases*, *30*(7), 1380–1389. https://doi.org/10.3201/eid3007.231723

Isman, A., Nyquist, A., Strecker, B., Harinath, G., Lee, V., Zhang, X., & Zalzala, S. (2024). Low-dose naltrexone and NAD+ for the treatment of patients with persistent fatigue symptoms after COVID-19. *Brain, Behavior, & Immunity - Health*, *36*, 100733. https://doi.org/10.1016/j.bbih.2024.100733

Jacobs, E. T., Catalfamo, C. J., Colombo, P. M., Khan, S. M., Austhof, E., Cordova-Marks, F., Ernst, K. C., Farland, L. V., & Pogreba-Brown, K. (2023a). Pre-existing conditions associated with post-acute sequelae of COVID-19. *Journal of Autoimmunity*, *135*, 102991. https://doi.org/10.1016/j.jaut.2022.102991

Jacobs, M. M., Evans, E., & Ellis, C. (2023b). Racial, ethnic, and sex disparities in the incidence and cognitive symptomology of long COVID-19. *Journal of the National Medical Association*, *115*(2), 233–243. https://doi.org/10.1016/j.jnma.2023.01.016

Jangnin, R., Ritruangroj, W., Kittisupkajorn, S., Sukeiam, P., Inchai, J., Maneeton, B., Maneetorn, N., Chaiard, J., & Theerakittikul, T. (2024). Long-COVID prevalence and its association with health outcomes in the post-vaccine and antiviral-availability era. *Journal of Clinical Medicine*, *13*(5). https://doi.org/10.3390/jcm13051208

Khullar, D., Zhang, Y., Zang, C., Xu, Z., Wang, F., Weiner, M. G., Carton, T. W., Rothman, R. L., Block, J. P., & Kaushal, R. (2023). Racial/ethnic disparities in post-acute sequelae of SARS-CoV-2 infection in New York: An EHR-based cohort study from the RECOVER Program. *Journal of General Internal Medicine*, *38*(5), 1127–1136. https://doi.org/10.1007/s11606-022-07997-1

Lavretsky, H. (2025). *A pilot rTMS trial for neuropsychiatric symptoms of long-COVID a study on COVID-19 brain fog, fatigue, and transcranial magnetic stimulation*. UCH Clinical Trials; University of California Health. https://clinicaltrials.ucbraid.org/trial/NCT06586398

Lessene, G., Doerflinger, M., Komander, D., Devine, S., Bader, S., Calleja, D., Devine, S., Kuchel, N., Lu, B., Wu, X., Birkinshaw, R., Bhandari, R., Loi, K., Volpe, R., Khakham, Y., Au, A., Blackmore, D. T., Mackiewicz, L., Dayton, M., & Schäfer, J. (2025, April 9). *Tackling the "silent pandemic": Breakthrough study puts first long COVID treatment on horizon*. WEHI. https://www.wehi.edu.au/news/tackling-the-silent-pandemic/

Li, J., Zhou, Y., Ma, J., Zhang, Q., Shao, J., Liang, S., Yu, Y., Li, W., & Wang, C. (2023). The long-term health outcomes, pathophysiological mechanisms and multidisciplinary management of long COVID. *Signal Transduction and Targeted Therapy*, *8*(1), 416. https://doi.org/10.1038/s4139202301640z

Lok, L. S. C., Sarkar, S., & Lam, C. C. I., et al. (2024). Long COVID across SARS-CoV-2 variants: Clinical features, pathogenesis, and future directions. *MedComm – Future Medicine.*, *3*, e70004. https://doi.org/10.1002/mef2.70004

Marra, A. R., Sampaio, V. S., Ozahata, M. C., Lopes, R., Brito, A. F., Bragatte, M., …, & Rizzo, L. V. (2023). Risk factors for long coronavirus disease 2019 (long COVID) among healthcare personnel, Brazil, 2020–2022. *Infection Control & Hospital Epidemiology*, *44*(12), 1972–1978. https://doi.org/10.1017/ice.2023.95

Merkler, A. E., Parikh, N. S., Mir, S., Gupta, A., Kamel, H., Lin, E., Lantos, J., Schenck, E. J., Goyal, P., Bruce, S. S., Kahan, J., Lansdale, K. N., LeMoss, N. M., Murthy, S. B., Stieg, P. E., Fink, M. E., Iadecola, C., Segal, A. Z., & Cusick, M., Campion, T. R. Jr., Diaz, I., Zhang, C., & Navi, B. B. (2020). Risk of ischemic stroke in patients with coronavirus disease 2019 (COVID19) vs patients with influenza. *JAMA Neurology*, *77*(11), 1366–1372. https://doi.org/10.1001/jamaneurol.2020.2730

Mkoma, G. F., Goldschmidt, M. I., Petersen, J. H., Benfield, T., Cederström, A., Rostila, M., Agyemang, C., & Norredam, M. (2025). Socioeconomic disparities in long COVID diagnosis among ethnic minorities in Denmark. *Social Science & Medicine*, *372*, 117944. https://doi.org/10.1016/j.socscimed.2025.117944

Molnar, T., Lehoczki, A., Fekete, M., Varnai, R., Zavori, L., ErdoBonyar, S., Simon, D., Berki, T., Csecsei, P., & Ezer, E. (2024). Mitochondrial dysfunction in long COVID: Mechanisms, consequences, and potential therapeutic approaches. *GeroScience*, *46*(5), 5267–5286. https://doi.org/10.1007/s11357-024-01165-5

Moser, J., Emous, M., Heeringa, P., & RodenhuisZybert, I. A. (2023). Mechanisms and pathophysiology of SARSCoV2 infection of the adipose tissue. *Trends in Endocrinology & Metabolism*, *34*(11), 735–748. https://doi.org/10.1016/j.tem.2023.08.010

National Institutes of Health (NIH). (2024, December 12). *NIH adds funds to long COVID-19 research, advances work on new clinical trials*. National Institutes of Health (NIH). https://recovercovid.org/news/nih-adds-funds-long-covid-research-advances-work-new-clinical-trials

NHS. (2023). *Coronavirus» post-COVID syndrome (Long COVID)*. NHS England. https://www.england.nhs.uk/coronavirus/post-covid-syndrome-long-covid/

NICE. (2020, December 18). *Overview | COVID-19 rapid guideline: managing the long-term effects of COVID-19 | Guidance | NICE*. https://www.nice.org.uk/guidance/ng188

Notarte, K. I., Catahay, J. A., Velasco, J. V., Pastrana, A., Ver, A. T., Pangilinan, F. C., Peligro, P. J., Casimiro, M., Guerrero, J. J., Margarita, Ma., Lippi, G., Henry, B. M., & Fernández-de-las-Peñas, C. (2022). Impact of COVID19 vaccination on the risk of developing longCOVID and on existing longCOVID symptoms: A systematic review. *EClinicalMedicine*, *53*. https://doi.org/10.1016/j.eclinm.2022.101624

Novak, S. (2024, November 27). *New data: The most promising treatments for long COVID.* Medscape. https://www.medscape.com/viewarticle/new-data-most-promising-treatments-long-covid-2024a1000lm5

O'Mahoney, L. L., Routen, A., Gillies, C., Ekezie, W., Welford, A., Zhang, A., Karamchandani, U., SimmsWilliams, N., Cassambai, S., Ardavani, A., Wilkinson, T. J., Hawthorne, G., Curtis, F., Kingsnorth, A. P., Almaqhawi, A., Ward, T., Ayoubkhani, D., Banerjee, A., Calvert, M., & Shafran, R. (2023). The prevalence and long-term health effects of long Covid among hospitalised and nonhospitalised populations: A systematic review and meta-analysis. *EClinicalMedicine*, *55*. https://doi.org/10.1016/j.eclinm.2022.101762

Office for National Statistics (ONS). (2023, March 30). *Prevalence of ongoing symptoms following coronavirus (COVID-19) infection in the UK - Office for National Statistics.* ONS. https://www.ons.gov.uk/peoplepopulationandcommunity/healthandsocialcare/conditionsanddiseases/bulletins/prevalenceofongoingsymptomsfollowingcoronaviruscovid19infectionintheuk/30march2023#cite-this-statistical-bulletin

Padilla, S., Ledesma, C., García-Abellán, J., García, J. A., Fernández-González, M., de la Rica, A., Galiana, A., Gutiérrez, F., & Masiá, M. (2024). Long COVID across SARSCoV2 variants, lineages, and sub-lineages. *IScience*, *27*(4). https://doi.org/10.1016/j.isci.2024.109536

Pelle, M. C., Zaffina, I., Lucà, S., Forte, V., Trapanese, V., Melina, M., Giofrè, F., & Arturi, F. (2022). Endothelial dysfunction in COVID-19: Potential mechanisms and possible therapeutic options. *Life (Basel, Switzerland)*, *12*(10), 1605. https://doi.org/10.3390/life12101605

Peluso, M. J., & Deeks, S. G. (2024). Mechanisms of long COVID and the path toward therapeutics. *Cell*, *187*(20), 5500–5529. https://doi.org/10.1016/j.cell.2024.07.054

Providence. (2024, October 9). *The connection between dysautonomia and long COVID.* Providence. https://blog.providence.org/blog/the-connection-between-dysautonomia-and-long-covid

RECOVER. (n.d.). *About RECOVER | RECOVER COVID initiative*. RECOVER; National Institutes of Health. https://recovercovid.org/about

RECOVER. (2024a). *RECOVER clinical trials | AUTONOMIC*. RECOVER; National Institutes of Health. https://trials.recovercovid.org/autonomic

RECOVER. (2024b). *RECOVER clinical trials | ENERGIZE*. RECOVER; National Institutes of Health. https://trials.recovercovid.org/energize

RECOVER. (2024c). *RECOVER clinical trials | NEURO*. RECOVER; National Institutes of Health. https://trials.recovercovid.org/neuro

RECOVER. (2024d). *RECOVER clinical trials | VITAL*. RECOVER; National Institutes of Health. https://trials.recovercovid.org/vital

RECOVER. (2024e). *RECOVER: Researching COVID to enhance recovery*. RECOVER; National Institutes of Health. https://recovercovid.org/news/nih-open-long-covid-clinical-trials-study-sleep-disturbances-exercise-intolerance-and-post

Scheppke, K. A., Pepe, P. E., Jui, J., Crowe, R. P., Scheppke, E. K., Klimas, N. G., & Marty, A. M. (2024). Remission of severe forms of long COVID following monoclonal antibody (MCA) infusions: A report of signal index cases and call for targeted research. *The American Journal of Emergency Medicine*, *75*, 122–127. https://doi.org/10.1016/j.ajem.2023.09.051

Shah, D. P., Thaweethai, T., Karlson, E. W., Bonilla, H., Horne, B. D., Mullington, J. M., Wisnivesky, J. P., Hornig, M., Shinnick, D. J., Klein, J. D., Erdmann, N. B., Brosnahan, S. B., Lee-Iannotti, J. K., Metz, T. D., Maughan, C., Ofotokun, I., Reeder, H. T., Stiles, L. E., Shaukat, A., Hess, R., & RECOVER Consortium (2025). Sex differences in long COVID. *JAMA Network Open*, *8*(1), e2455430. https://doi.org/10.1001/jamanetworkopen.2024.55430

Singh, M. M., Sharma, H., & Bhatnagar, N., et al. (May 20, 2024) Burden of long COVID-19 in a cohort of recovered COVID-19 patients in Delhi, India. *Cureus*, *16*(5), e60652. https://doi.org/10.7759/cureus.60652

Slawson, D. C. (2023). Likelihood of long COVID varies by variant, sex, and vaccination status. *American Family Physician*, *107*(2), 199.

Smith, A. (2024, May 2). *U of M study finds metformin reduces COVID-19 viral load, viral rebound.* University of Minnesota. https://med.umn.edu/news/u-m-study-finds-metformin-reduces-covid-19-viral-load-viral-rebound

Soares, L., Assaf, G., McCorkell, L., Davis, H., Cohen, A., Moen, J., Shoemaker, L., Liu, L., Lewis, D., Robles, R., McWilliams, C., Lin, J., Akintonwa, T., Saravia, A., Wei, H., & Fitzgerald, M. (2024). *Long COVID and associated outcomes following COVID19 reinfections: Insights from an International PatientLed Survey.* https://doi.org/10.21203/rs.3.rs-4909082/v1

Son, H.-E., Hong, Y.-S., Lee, S., & Son, H. (2024). Prevalence, risk factors, and impact of long COVID among adults in South Korea. *Healthcare*, *12*(20), 2062. https://doi.org/10.3390/healthcare12202062

Spinicci, M., Graziani, L., Tilli, M., Nkurunziza, J., Vellere, I., Borchi, B., Mencarini, J., Campolmi, I., Gori, L., Giovannoni, L., Amato, C., Livi, L., Rasero, L., Fattirolli, F., Marcucci, R., Giusti, B., Olivotto, I., Tomassetti, S., Lavorini, F., & Maggi, L. (2022). Infection with SARSCoV2 variants is associated with different long COVID phenotypes. *Viruses*, *14*(11). https://doi.org/10.3390/v14112367

Strain, W. D., Sherwood, O., Banerjee, A., Van der Togt, V., Hishmeh, L., & Rossman, J. (2022). The impact of COVID vaccination on symptoms of long COVID: An international survey of people with lived experience of long COVID. *Vaccines*, *10*(5), 652. https://doi.org/10.3390/vaccines10050652

Swarnakar, R., & Yadav, S. L. (2022). Rehabilitation in long COVID-19: A mini-review. *World Journal of Methodology*, *12*(4), 235–245. https://doi.org/10.5662/wjm.v12.i4.235

Trott, M., Driscoll, R., & Pardhan, S. (2022). The prevalence of sensory changes in post-COVID syndrome: A systematic review and meta-analysis. *Frontiers in Medicine, 92022.* https://doi.org/10.3389/fmed.2022.980253

Tsampasian, V., Elghazaly, H., Chattopadhyay, R., Debski, M., Naing, Garg, P., Clark, A., Ntatsaki, E., & Vassiliou, V. S. (2023). Risk factors associated with post-COVID19 condition: A systematic review and meta-analysis. *JAMA Internal Medicine*, *183*(6), 566–580. https://doi.org/10.1001/jamainternmed.2023.0750

Tsilingiris, D., Vallianou, N. G., Karampela, I., Christodoulatos, G. S., Papavasileiou, G., Petropoulou, D., Magkos, F., & Dalamaga, M. (2023). Laboratory findings and biomarkers in long COVID: What do we know so far? Insights into epidemiology, pathogenesis, therapeutic perspectives and challenges. *International Journal of Molecular Sciences*, *24*(13), 10458. https://doi.org/10.3390/ijms241310458

Tziolos, N. R., Ioannou, P., Baliou, S., & Kofteridis, D. P. (2023). Long COVID-19 pathophysiology: What do we know so far? *Microorganisms*, *11*(10), 2458. https://doi.org/10.3390/microorganisms11102458

Vahratian, A., Saydah, S., Bertolli, J., Unger, E. R., & Gregory, C. O. (2024). Prevalence of post-COVID19 condition and activity-limiting post-COVID19 condition among adults. *JAMA Network Open*, *7*(12), e2451151. https://doi.org/10.1001/jamanetworkopen.2024.51151

Vanderbilt Health. (2025, January 27). *Discoveries in medicine – Treatment on trial to reverse long COVID effects*. Discoveries in Medicine; Vanderbilt Health. https://discoveries.vanderbilthealth.com/2025/01/treatment-on-trial-to-reverse-long-covid-effects/

World Health Organization (WHO). (2025, February 26). *Post COVID-19 condition (long COVID)*. WHO; World Health Organization: WHO. https://www.who.int/news-room/fact-sheets/detail/post-covid-19-condition-(long-covid)

Xu, S., Ilyas, I., & Weng, J. (2023). Endothelial dysfunction in COVID19: An overview of evidence, biomarkers, mechanisms and potential therapies. *Acta Pharmacologica Sinica, 44*(4), 695–709. https://doi.org/10.1038/s41401-022-00998-0

Yale Medicine. (n.d.). *Long COVID (post-COVID conditions, PCC)*. Yale Medicine. https://www.yalemedicine.org/conditions/long-covid-post-covid-conditions-pcc

Yale School of Medicine. (2024). *Center for infection & immunity*. Center for Infection & Immunity; Yale School of Medicine. https://medicine.yale.edu/cii/

Yan, D., Liu, Y., Chen, R., Zhou, L., Wang, C., Ada, M., Chen, X., Song, Q., & Qian, G. (2025). Follow-up of long COVID based on the definition of WHO: A multi-centre cross-sectional questionnaire-based study. *BMC Public Health, 25*(1), 1412. https://doi.org/10.1186/s12889-025-22671-x

Yelin, D., Moschopoulos, C. D., Margalit, I., GkraniaKlotsas, E., Landi, F., Stahl, J., & Yahav, D. (2022). ESCMID rapid guidelines for assessment and management of long COVID. *Clinical Microbiology and Infection, 28*(7), 955–972. https://doi.org/10.1016/j.cmi.2022.02.018

Zhang, F., Lau, R. I., Liu, Q., Su, Q., Francis, C., & Ng, S. C. (2023). Gut microbiota in COVID-19: Key microbial changes, potential mechanisms and clinical applications. *Nature Reviews Gastroenterology & Hepatology, 20*(5), 323–337. https://doi.org/10.1038/s41575-022-00698-4

18 Converging Disease Outbreaks

A Harbinger of Future Pandemics

The COVID-19 pandemic did more than introduce a single novel pathogen—it disrupted established viral ecosystems and set the stage for a new phenomenon: disease convergence. This section examines how pandemic-era mitigation measures reshaped viral dynamics, giving rise to what experts have dubbed the "tripledemic"—and more recently, the "quad-demic." These overlapping outbreaks are not coincidental but rather the interconnected consequences of prolonged behavioral and environmental shifts brought on by the pandemic.

COVID-19's Disruption of the Viral Ecosystem

Before the pandemic, respiratory viruses followed relatively predictable seasonal patterns (Figure 18.1). However, COVID-19 prevention measures—such as masking, social distancing, restricted public gatherings, and improved hygiene—suppressed not only SARS-CoV-2 but also influenza and respiratory syncytial virus (RSV). These mitigation efforts inadvertently created what researchers have called an "immunity debt" (Munro & House, 2024). Fewer people—especially

2020	2021	2022	2023	2024	2025
COVID	COVID	COVID	COVID	COVID	COVID
		FLU	FLU	FLU	FLU
		RSV	RSV	RSV	RSV
		MPOX	MPOX	MPOX	MPOX
				NOROVIRUS	NOROVIRUS

Figure 18.1 Resurgence of Multiple Infectious Diseases During the COVID-19 Period (2020–2025). Flu and RSV Saw Significant Resurgence from 2022 to 2025, Mpox from 2022 to 2024, and Norovirus from 2024 to 2025.

Source: Adapted from Buensalido (2023).

DOI: 10.4324/9781003595564-23

children—were exposed to common seasonal viruses during extended lockdowns and periods of reduced social contact. As a result, many never developed immunity to illnesses that had largely disappeared during the pandemic.

The First Tripledemic (2022–2023): Convergence of Respiratory Viruses

The term *tripledemic* gained traction in late 2022, as healthcare systems faced simultaneous surges of COVID-19, influenza, and RSV (Figure 18.2). Unlike previous years, when these viruses typically peaked at staggered intervals, they converged—overwhelming hospitals, particularly emergency departments (ED) and pediatric units (Wells, 2023).

Spatial-temporal analyses showed a shift in viral dynamics: compared to winter 2021, COVID-19 rates declined, while influenza and RSV infections rose sharply. These peaks occurred earlier than usual, defying established seasonal patterns. In several countries, flu hospitalizations peaked an average of 4.3 weeks earlier than pre-pandemic norms. RSV has become especially erratic, surfacing during spring, summer, or early fall in places like the United States, France, and Australia. These shifting patterns—sometimes varying even between regions of the same country—complicated both clinical preparedness and national public health forecasting (Lee et al., 2024).

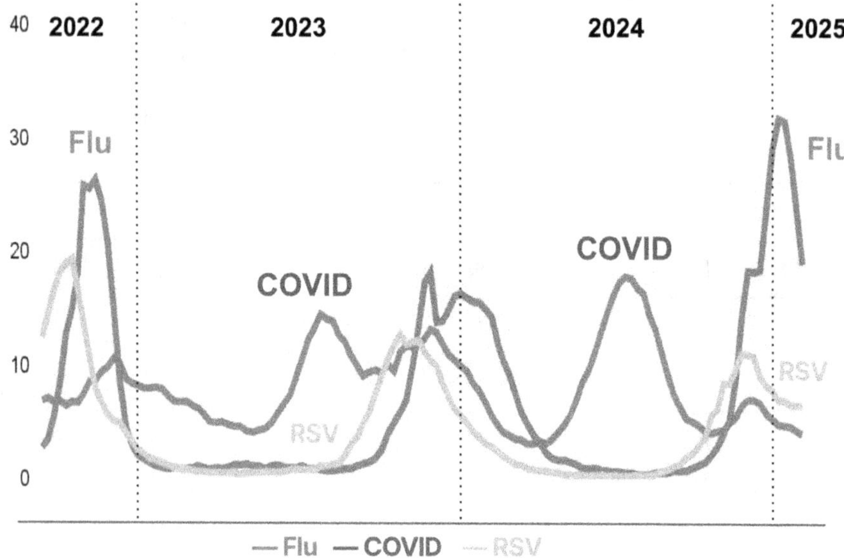

Figure 18.2 Test Positivity Rates for COVID-19, Influenza, and RSV in the United States (2022–2025). Flu and RSV Peaked During the Winters of 2022, 2023, and 2024.

Source: Adapted from CDC (2025b).

This convergence placed extraordinary strain on healthcare infrastructure. Pediatric hospitals were especially affected, with many children experiencing RSV for the first time. In Canada, RSV hospitalization rates for children doubled compared to the 2021–2022 season, and ICU admissions tripled compared to pre-pandemic years (Fitzpatrick et al., 2024).

Many hospitals operated at or beyond capacity with EDs facing long wait times and pediatric units converting overflow spaces to manage the influx of patients. While each virus was manageable on its own, their combined impact created a crisis that tested both healthcare resources and the endurance of frontline workers still recovering from earlier pandemic waves (McDonnell Busenbark, 2023).

The compounded burden of RSV, influenza, and COVID-19 pushed many healthcare systems close to their breaking point. These seasonal shifts have made it increasingly difficult to time vaccination campaigns or prepare for hospital surges, leading public health systems to adopt more flexible, real-time response strategies. By January 2023, however, the *tripledemic* began to fade as case numbers for all three viruses declined (Nirappil, 2023).

The Second Tripledemic (2023–2024): Countermeasures and Adaptive Responses

By the 2023–2024 respiratory season, healthcare systems had gained valuable experience managing concurrent viral outbreaks and began adopting a more proactive, coordinated approach. This shift was supported by new preventive tools—most notably nirsevimab, a long-acting monoclonal antibody that marked the first major breakthrough in RSV prevention in decades. Approved by the U.S. FDA in July 2023, nirsevimab provides extended protection for four to six months and is authorized for use in all healthy infants and children aged 8–19 months (Jones et al., 2023).

In parallel, three RSV vaccines were approved for use in adults: ABRYSVO (Pfizer), AREXVY (GSK), and mRESVIA (Moderna). ABRYSVO is indicated for adults aged 60 and older, as well as younger adults at increased risk, and is the only RSV vaccine approved for use during pregnancy to protect newborns through maternal immunization. AREXVY targets adults aged 60 and over and certain high-risk individuals aged 50–59 but is not recommended during pregnancy. mRESVIA is currently limited to adults 60 and older and is not intended for maternal use. The CDC recommends a single dose of any of the three RSV vaccines for all adults ages 75 and older and for adults ages 60–74 that are at increased risk for severe RSV (CDC, 2024).

Public health authorities also recalibrated vaccination campaigns in anticipation of continued viral convergence. The CDC emphasized timely and widespread uptake of both influenza and COVID-19 vaccines, while healthcare systems updated their surge protocols based on lessons from the previous winter. Despite these efforts, the *tripledemic* pattern persisted, albeit with reduced severity and altered timing. CDC surveillance indicated that while the overall disease burden was more manageable, the viral ecosystem remained unsettled. Increasingly, public health agencies began treating the three respiratory diseases not as isolated threats but as a combined seasonal challenge, prompting more integrated approaches to surveillance, prevention, and response. Hospitals mirrored this shift by implementing formal "*tripledemic* preparedness" measures, including cross-training staff to handle different respiratory infections, maintaining adaptable space for patient overflow, and developing clear triage protocols tailored to simultaneous surges (CDC, 2023).

The Mpox Outbreak (2022–2024): A Global Health Emergency

As healthcare systems were adapting to the ongoing *tripledemic* challenges, a separate and significant infectious disease threat emerged: the global outbreak of mpox (formerly known as monkeypox). Identified in May 2022, this marked a turning point, as the virus spread beyond its historically endemic regions in Africa to dozens of countries worldwide (WHO, 2022). As a result, the WHO declared mpox a Public Health Emergency of International Concern (PHEIC) on two separate occasions during this period.

The first declaration came on July 23, 2022, in response to its rapid global spread. By September 2022, more than 62,000 cases had been reported across 104 countries—including 97 that had not previously encountered mpox outbreaks. This declaration was lifted on May 11, 2023, following a sustained decline in cases (Haque et al., 2024; Ilic et al., 2022).

The second PHEIC was declared on August 14, 2024, amid a resurgence driven by the more virulent Clade Ib variant. Originating in the Democratic Republic of the Congo, this outbreak spread to neighboring countries—including Burundi, Kenya, Rwanda, and Uganda—and was notable for a higher case fatality rate and broader demographic impact (Michaud et al., 2024).

As of early 2025, the Clade Ib variant continues to circulate primarily in Central and Eastern Africa, with over 21,000 confirmed cases and more than 65 deaths reported globally since the resurgence began. While a number of countries—including the United States, China, Sweden, and Thailand—reported imported cases, there has been no evidence of sustained community transmission outside of Africa (CDC, 2025e).

Overall, the mpox outbreaks further highlighted the global need for stronger genomic surveillance, improved healthcare infrastructure in endemic regions, and more responsive international coordination. Occurring alongside the continued burden of respiratory virus surges, these emergencies placed additional strain on public health systems already stretched by overlapping crises.

The Third Tripledemic (2024–2025): The Quad-demic Emerges with Norovirus

In addition to the usual trio of respiratory viruses, a fourth pathogen surged into prominence: norovirus, a highly contagious gastrointestinal virus. Unlike COVID-19, influenza, and RSV—which primarily spread through droplet or airborne transmission—norovirus spreads via the fecal-oral route and causes severe vomiting and diarrhea. During the 2024–2025 season, outbreaks spiked to levels not seen since 2012, surpassing even pre-pandemic norms (Kee, 2025).

By early January 2025, ED visits across multiple regions circulated simultaneously. U.S. surveillance data reported peak test positivity rates of 18.6% for influenza, 11.4% for RSV, 6.6% for COVID-19, and 27.9% for norovirus (CDC, 2025a). The surge in norovirus cases was notable not only for its scale but also for its timing, which was concurrent with the peaks of the three major respiratory viruses. While winter increases in norovirus are typical, this level of overlap with respiratory outbreaks was considered highly atypical and deeply concerning to health experts.

The convergence of four active pathogens posed new challenges for diagnosis, treatment, and infection control. Clinicians reported a rise in co-infections, particularly among children, with some patients presenting with two or more infections simultaneously—an uncommon phenomenon prior to the pandemic. These co-infections were associated with more severe illness and higher rates of hospitalization (Xie et al., 2025).

The *quad-demic* also demanded a more layered infection control strategy. While respiratory viruses primarily spread through airborne droplets, norovirus transmits via contact with contaminated surfaces. As a result, healthcare facilities were forced to implement protocols addressing multiple transmission routes simultaneously—further straining resources and staff capacity.

The Norovirus Surge (2024–2025): Evolution of a Familiar Threat

The norovirus component of the quad-demic marked a striking return for a virus that had been largely dormant during the early years of the COVID-19 pandemic. Between 2020 and 2021, norovirus activity dropped sharply due to widespread mitigation measures. For example, Germany reported only 242 outbreaks from March 2020 to December 2022—a dramatic decline compared to pre-pandemic norms (Jacobsen et al., 2024). As restrictions eased in 2022 and 2023, norovirus gradually resumed its typical seasonal behavior. But the 2024–2025 season brought a massive resurgence.

In the United States, NoroSTAT-participating states recorded 2,407 norovirus outbreaks between August 2024 and April 2025—nearly double the 1,230 outbreaks reported during the same period the year before (CDC, 2025f). A similar trend occurred in the United Kingdom, which documented 308 outbreaks by week 7 of the 2024–2025 season—a 39% increase over the five-season average (UK Health Security Agency, 2025).

Several factors contributed to this resurgence. The emergence of new viral strains—especially the GII.17 variant, which accounted for roughly 70% of U.S. outbreaks between September and December 2024—was a key driver (CDC, 2025d). Population-level immunity had also waned due to reduced exposure during the pandemic years, leaving many more susceptible. The return of widespread in-person activities—such as dining out, travel, and large gatherings—further accelerated transmission across reconnected social networks.

This norovirus surge added yet another layer of strain to already burdened healthcare systems, particularly affecting young children, the elderly, and immunocompromised individuals. In response, the United Kingdom's National Health Service launched trials for the first-ever mRNA-based norovirus vaccine, developed by Moderna. The trial enrolled 2,500 participants—primarily older adults—with the goal of reducing hospital admissions during peak seasons (National Institute for Health and Care Research (NIHR), 2024).

The New Viral Equilibrium: Broader Implications for Public Health

By April 2025, signs of stabilization began to emerge. U.S. surveillance data showed that peak hospitalization rates for the 2024–2025 respiratory season reached 18.3 per 100,000—down from 21.0 the year before. Most notably, COVID-19 hospitalizations fell by nearly 50%, suggesting a slow shift toward a new viral equilibrium as population-level immunity continues to build (CDC, 2025c).

This evolving post-pandemic viral landscape reflects a complex interplay of factors. Despite the availability of effective preventive tools, vaccination uptake remains suboptimal in many regions, despite broad availability, and the viral ecosystem itself continues to shift, exemplified by the disappearance of the influenza B/Yamagata lineage—absent since March 2020—which prompted a transition to modified quadrivalent or trivalent flu vaccines for the 2024–2025 season (Gallagher, 2024).

The *tripledemic* and *quad-demic* years have reshaped how infectious diseases are tracked and managed. As respiratory virus seasons become increasingly asynchronous worldwide, global coordination has become more difficult. Outbreaks no longer align neatly between hemispheres, undermining traditional staggered preparedness models and reinforcing the need for more dynamic, real-time surveillance systems. A new paradigm—"viral ecosystem management"—has emerged, emphasizing that interventions aimed at one virus can ripple across others, requiring more holistic, systems-level strategies. Public messaging has also shifted to highlight the interconnected nature of viral threats, helping communities understand that preventive behaviors often guard against multiple illnesses at once.

The cascade of overlapping outbreaks between 2020 and 2025 has revealed deep vulnerabilities in public health infrastructure. These events foreshadow the urgent need for sustained investment in vaccine innovation, global surveillance networks, and resilient healthcare systems—especially in preparation for a future where concurrent outbreaks may become the norm rather than the exception. The lessons learned during this turbulent period—integrated monitoring, flexible surge capacity, and ecosystem thinking—provide a critical foundation as we confront the next wave of global health challenges: the rise of emerging and reemerging zoonotic threats, from pathogens both known and unknown.

References

Buensalido, J. A. L. (2023). Rhinovirus (RV) infection (common cold): Practice essentials, background, pathophysiology. *Medscape*. https://emedicine.medscape.com/article/227820-overview?form=fpf

CDC. (2023, October 6). *DSLR Friday update*. CDC. https://www.cdc.gov/readiness/media/pdfs/DSLR-Friday-Update_October-6_2023_508C.pdf

CDC. (2024, August 30). *RSV vaccine guidance for older adults*. CDC. https://www.cdc.gov/rsv/hcp/vaccine-clinical-guidance/older-adults.html

CDC. (2025a). *Interactive dashboard*. The National Respiratory and Enteric Virus Surveillance System (NREVSS); CDC. https://www.cdc.gov/nrevss/php/dashboard/index.html

CDC. (2025b). *Respiratory virus activity levels*. CDC. https://www.cdc.gov/respiratory-viruses/data/activity-levels.html#cdc_data_surveillance_section_5-wastewater-map

CDC. (2025c, February 19). *2024-2025 respiratory disease season outlook – February update*. CDC. https://www.cdc.gov/cfa-qualitative-assessments/php/data-research/season-outlook24-25-feb-update.html

CDC. (2025d, May 12). *CaliciNet data*. CDC. https://www.cdc.gov/norovirus/php/reporting/calicinet-data.html

CDC. (2025e, May 14). *Clade I Mpox outbreak originating in Central Africa*. CDC. https://www.cdc.gov/mpox/outbreaks/2023/index.html

CDC. (2025f, May 20). *NoroSTAT data*. CDC. https://www.cdc.gov/norovirus/php/reporting/norostat-data.html

Fitzpatrick, T., Buchan, S. A., Mahant, S., Fu, L., Kwong, J. C., Stukel, T. A., & Guttmann, A. (2024). Pediatric respiratory syncytial virus hospitalizations, 2017–2023. *JAMA Network Open*, *7*(6), e2416077–e2416077. https://doi.org/10.1001/jamanetworkopen.2024.16077

Gallagher, A. (2024, November 25). *Disappearance of B/Yamagata strain influences flu vaccine, public health decisions*. Pharmacy Times. https://www.pharmacytimes.com/view/disappearance-of-b-yamagata-strain-influences-flu-vaccine-public-health-decisions

Haque, M. A., Halder, A. S., Hossain, M. J., & Islam, M. R. (2024). Prediction of potential public health risk of the recent multicountry monkeypox outbreak: An update after the end declaration of global public health emergency. *Health Science Reports*, *7*(6), e2136. https://doi.org/10.1002/hsr2.2136

Ilic, I., ZivanovicMacuzic, I., & Ilić, M. (2022). Global outbreak of human monkeypox in 2022: Update of epidemiology. *Tropical Medicine and Infectious Disease*, *7*, 264. https://doi.org/10.3390/tropicalmed7100264

Jacobsen, S., Faber, M., Altmann, B., Marques, M., Bock, C. T., & Niendorf, S. (2024). Impact of the COVID-19 pandemic on norovirus circulation in Germany. *International Journal of Medical Microbiology*, *314*, 151600. https://doi.org/10.1016/j.ijmm.2024.151600

Jones, J. M., Fleming-Dutra, K. E., & Prill, M. M. et al (2023). Use of Nirsevimab for the prevention of respiratory syncytial virus disease among infants and young children: Recommendations of the advisory committee on immunization practices — United States, 2023. *MMWR Morbidity and Mortality Weekly Report*, *72*, 920–925. http://dx.doi.org/10.15585/mmwr.mm7234a4

Kee, C. (2025, January 3). *Norovirus 2025: How to stay safe as outbreaks surge In US*. TODAY. https://www.today.com/health/disease/norovirus-2025-rcna185976

Lee, W.-J., Tseng, H. K., Jacob, G., Tenrisau, D., & McGaff, C. (2024, May 9). *Where COVID has shifted flu and RSV seasons | Think Global Health*. Think Global Health. https://www.thinkglobalhealth.org/article/where-covid-has-shifted-flu-and-rsv-seasons

McDonnell Busenbark, M. (2023, July 24). *The problem of emergency department crowding*. Children's Hospital Association. https://www.childrenshospitals.org/news/childrens-hospitals-today/2023/07/the-problem-of-emergency-department-crowding

Michaud, J., Moss, K., & Kates, J. (2024, October 2). *The current international Mpox emergency and the U.S. role: An explainer | KFF*. KFF. https://www.kff.org/global-health-policy/issue-brief/the-current-international-mpox-emergency-and-the-u-s-role-an-explainer/

Munro, A., & House, T. (2024). Cycles of susceptibility: Immunity debt explains altered infectious disease dynamics post-pandemic. *Clinical Infectious Diseases*, *ciae493*. https://doi.org/10.1093/cid/ciae493

National Institute for Health and Care Research (NIHR). (2024, October 23). *UK's first norovirus mRNA vaccine trial launched*. NIHR. https://www.nihr.ac.uk/news/uks-first-norovirus-mrna-vaccine-trial-launched

Nirappil, F. (2023, January). Covid, flu, RSV declining in hospitals as "tripledemic" threat fades. *Washington Post*. https://www.washingtonpost.com/health/2023/01/22/covid-declining-flu-rsv-tripledemic/

UK Health Security Agency. (2025, February 27). *National norovirus and rotavirus report, week 9 report: Data to week 7 (data up to 16 February 2025)*. GOV.UK. https://www.gov.uk/government/statistics/national-norovirus-and-rotavirus-surveillance-reports-2024-to-2025-season/national-norovirus-and-rotavirus-report-week-9-report-data-to-week-7-data-up-to-16-february-2025

Wells, K. (2023, March 3). *A surge in sick children exposed a need for major changes to U.S. hospitals*. NPR. https://www.npr.org/sections/health-shots/2023/03/03/1160490089/a-surge-in-sick-children-exposed-a-need-for-major-changes-to-u-s-hospitals

WHO. (2022, May 29). *Multi-country monkeypox outbreak in non-endemic countries: Update*. WHO. https://www.who.int/emergencies/disease-outbreak-news/item/2022-DON388

Xie, J., Florin, T. A., Funk, A. L., Tancredi, D. J., Kuppermann, N., & Freedman, S. B. (2025). Respiratory viral co-infection in SARS-CoV-2-infected children during the early and late pandemic periods. *The Pediatric Infectious Disease Journal*, *44*(4). https://journals.lww.com/pidj/fulltext/2025/04000/respiratory_viral_co_infection_in.12.aspx

19 A Gathering Storm

The Rise of New Zoonotic Threats

While Chapter 18 examined how COVID-19 disrupted existing viral patterns and ushered in a new era of disease convergence, this section addresses a distinct but related threat: the accelerating emergence of entirely new zoonotic diseases, both known and unknown. The tripledemic and quad-demic represented a reshuffling of known pathogens, but zoonotic spillover events introduce novel viruses to which humans have no immunity—with SARS-CoV-2 being the most recent prominent example. The scale of this potential threat is grim: scientists estimate that 1.7 million undiscovered viruses exist in mammals and birds, with up to 850,000 potentially capable of infecting humans. As human activities increasingly encroach upon natural habitats and climate change alters ecological relationships, the barriers that once separated humans from these reservoirs of unknown pathogens are rapidly eroding.

Zoonotic Spillover Is Accelerating

Emerging infectious diseases are crossing from animals to humans at an unparalleled pace. Scientists estimate that over 60% of known human pathogens and approximately 75% of new or emerging infectious diseases are zoonotic in origin (World Health Organization (WHO), 2023). From HIV's jump from non-human primates to humans in the 20th century to the 21st-century outbreaks of SARS, Ebola, and COVID-19, spillover events have become disturbingly common. It is estimated that zoonoses cause about 1 billion infections and millions of deaths worldwide each year (WHO, 2020). This trend shows no sign of abating as factors like population growth, ecosystem disruption, and global travel create more opportunities for pathogens to spill over into human populations (Daszak et al., 2020).

Recent research confirms that spillover events are becoming more common and more widely dispersed geographically (Plowright et al., 2017). As shown in Table 19.1, the 21st century has already witnessed numerous major zoonotic spillover events, from Nipah virus to COVID-19 to newer strains of mpox. Each of these events has been linked to specific human activities that facilitate animal-to-human transmission.

Human disruption of natural ecosystems is a key driver behind many recent zoonotic outbreaks. As forests are cleared for agriculture, logging, mining, and

DOI: 10.4324/9781003595564-24

Table 19.1 Major Zoonotic Disease Spillovers of the 21st Century

Disease	*Year Identified*	*Reservoir/ Intermediate Host*	*Geographic Origin*	*Contributing Factors*
Nipah virus	1998	**Fruit bats → pigs**	Malaysia	*Deforestation; orchard farming*
SARS *(SARS-CoV-1)*	2002	**Horseshoe bats → civets**	Guangdong, China	*Wildlife markets; urban density*
H5N1 *(avian influenza)*	2003	**Wild birds → poultry**	Hong Kong/ China	*Poultry farming; live markets*
H1N1 *("Swine Flu")*	2009	**Pigs (avian/ swine/ human mix)**	Mexico	*Intensive pig farming; travel*
MERS	2012	**Bats → camels**	Arabian Peninsula	*Camel trade; close contact*
Ebola	2014	**Fruit bats (suspected)**	West Africa	*Bushmeat; forest encroachment*
Zika virus	2015	**Primates → mosquitoes**	Brazil (epidemic)	*Urban spread; climate shift*
COVID-19 *(SARS-CoV-2)*	2019	**Possibly bats → unknown**	Wuhan, China	*Wildlife trade; globalization*
Mpox *(new strain)*	2022	**Rodents, small mammals**	Democratic Republic of Congo	*Wildlife contact; global travel*

Sources: Data compiled from Centers for Disease Control and Prevention (CDC) (2025a), United Nations Environment Program (UNEP) and International Livestock Research Institution (2020).

urban expansion, wildlife that once lived deep in remote habitats is forced into closer contact with human communities and livestock. This loss of habitat and biodiversity increases human exposure to animal reservoirs of disease. For example, the Nipah virus emerged when deforestation and fires in Southeast Asia drove fruit bats into orchards near pig farms; the bats transmitted the virus to pigs, which then infected farmers (UNEP, 2020).

Climate and Globalization as Force Multipliers

Climate change and globalization act as force multipliers for zoonotic disease threats. Warming temperatures, shifting rainfall patterns, and more extreme weather events are reshaping the geographic range and seasonality of many diseases. Climate models project that over the next 50 years, rising temperatures will drive wildlife species to migrate to cooler areas, leading to over 15,000 new instances of viruses jumping between species that would not otherwise meet (Carlson et al., 2022).

The Lancet Countdown on health and climate change reported that the number of months suitable for malaria transmission in highland areas of the Americas and Africa has risen significantly since the 1950s as temperatures climbed (Romanello et al., 2022). Dengue fever, historically confined to the tropics, has expanded its range significantly; 2024 proved to be one of the worst years on record for dengue globally, with over 10 million cases reported across more than 175 countries (WHO, 2024b).

Climate change can also resurrect dormant microbial threats. In 2016, a heatwave melted Siberian permafrost and exposed decades-old anthrax spores from a reindeer carcass, causing an outbreak that killed a child and thousands of reindeer (Doucleff, 2016). As Table 19.2 illustrates, the geographic distribution of disease vectors is projected to shift significantly by 2050 due to climate influences.

Meanwhile, globalization has drastically shortened the path from local outbreak to global pandemic. In our hyperconnected world, a virus can spread from a remote village to major cities on all continents in as little as 36 hours (CDC, 2025b). The increased volume of human mobility—approximately 4.5 billion airline passenger-trips per year pre-pandemic—means even infections that emerge in isolated areas can quickly become global threats (CDC, 2025c).

Globalized trade also moves animals and goods in ways that propagate disease. The United States imports over 220 million live wild animals annually, many

Table 19.2 Expanding Disease Vector Ranges due to Climate Change

Disease/Vector	*Current Range (2025)*	*Projected Range (2050)*	*Key Climate Drivers*
Dengue (Aedes)	100+ countries, tropics, subtropics, some temperate	Southern United States, Southern Europe, highlands	Warmer temps; longer breeding seasons
Malaria (Anopheles)	African and Andean highlands (expanded season)	Higher elevations, Southern Europe	Warming increases mosquito and parasite survival
Lyme disease (Ticks)	Expanded 45% north in North America	Canada, Russia, Scandinavia	Milder winters; longer active seasons
West Nile (Culex)	The United States, Europe, parts of Asia and Canada	Higher latitudes and elevations	Heat and rainfall boost mosquito spread
Zika (Aedes)	Americas, Pacific, Asia, parts of Europe	Southern United States, Southern Europe	Urban heat islands; climate-driven expansion
Vibrio (bacteria)	Atlantic coasts, Baltic Sea	Arctic coastlines, longer seasonal windows	Ocean warming; salinity shifts
"Icebox" Pathogens	Siberian anthrax cases (2016), isolated risks	Dormant viruses may reemerge	Arctic permafrost thaw (2–4× global rate)

Sources: Data synthesized from Romanello et al. (2022), WHO (2022; 2024a), Chason et al. (2023), U.S. EPA (2025), United Nations Environment Program (UNEP) and International Livestock Research Institution (2020), Doucleff (2016), Baker-Austin et al. (2024), Shukla et al. (2019); Pörtner et al. (2022). Note: Range projections based on climate models assuming continued warming trends. Actual distribution depends on multiple factors beyond climate, including public health interventions, land-use changes, and adaptation measures.

with minimal health screening (Linder et al., 2023). Combined with increasing urbanization—nearly 60% of humanity now lives in cities—these factors create ideal conditions for rapid disease spread once a novel pathogen emerges (WHO, 2025b).

The Wildlife Trade and Agricultural Interfaces

The commercial wildlife trade and industrial agriculture create distinct but equally dangerous pathways for zoonotic spillover. Millions of live animals are shipped internationally each year for food, pets, fur, and traditional medicine, often with minimal health screening. This creates opportunities for exotic pathogens to jump to new hosts. The SARS coronavirus (SARS-CoV-1) likely spilled over via wildlife sold in a live animal market in 2003, illustrating the dangers of this trade (Wang et al., 2006).

Modern agricultural practices have also transformed in ways that elevate pandemic risks. Industrial livestock facilities concentrate billions of animals in dense, homogenous populations that create ideal conditions for pathogen evolution. The strain of influenza behind the 2009 "swine flu" pandemic emerged from pig farming operations that allowed avian, swine, and human flu viruses to reassort into a novel virus (Jilani et al., 2024).

Table 19.3 provides a comprehensive overview of zoonotic risk factors across various agricultural and wildlife trade practices, highlighting the specific pathogens associated with each sector and potential mitigation strategies.

The risks remain high today. The United States processed over 10 billion livestock animals in 2022, the largest number on record (Linder et al., 2023). Highly pathogenic avian influenza (H5N1) illustrates the ongoing danger—since 2021, a particular strain has caused the largest global avian influenza outbreak in decades, resulting in more than 280 million domestic birds dying or being culled worldwide (Weston, 2024).

In late 2022, an H5N1 outbreak on a mink farm in Spain provided evidence of mammal-to-mammal spread of this virus, raising concerns that H5N1 could acquire mutations for efficient human transmission (Peacock et al., 2025). Meanwhile, antimicrobial resistance continues to develop in agricultural settings, fostering drug-resistant bacteria that can infect humans—creating what health authorities have called a "silent pandemic" developing alongside more acute threats (Ahmed et al., 2024).

Preparing for Pathogen X

In the wake of COVID-19, global health authorities have fundamentally reimagined how they approach potential pandemic threats. The WHO's strategic watchlist of priority pathogens has evolved significantly, with the 2024 update representing a paradigm shift in global health preparedness strategy. While previous iterations focused on individual pathogens with known pandemic potential, the latest framework has elevated the concept of "Pathogen X" to a position of central importance.

Table 19.3 Zoonotic Risk Factors in Agricultural and Wildlife Trade Practices

Sector and Practice	*Pathogen Risks*	*Mitigation Strategies*
	Industrial Livestock Production	
Poultry farming	Avian influenza (H5N1, H7N9), *Salmonella*	Lower density, biosecurity, surveillance
Pig farming	Swine flu (H1N1), Nipah, cysticercosis	Biosecurity, reduced antibiotics, monitoring
Cattle feedlots	*Escherichia coli*, drug-resistant TB, prions, anthrax	Waste controls, vaccination, feed safety
	Wildlife Trade Practices	
Live wildlife markets	SARS, COVID-19, avian influenza	Regulation, sanitation, species separation
Exotic pet trade	Mpox, herpes B, *Salmonella*	Screening, quarantine, import limits
Bushmeat hunting	Ebola, HIV, simian viruses	Education, alternative proteins, hunting limits
Traditional medicine trade	Viral and bacterial pathogens	Regulation, synthetic substitutes
	Agricultural-Wildlife Interfaces	
Fruit plantations near forests	Nipah, Hendra viruses	Buffer zones, bat exclusion, crop screening
Irrigation/dam projects	Vector-borne diseases, leishmaniasis	Water controls, safe practices
Wildlife-livestock contact zones	Brucellosis, tuberculosis, Rift Valley fever	Fencing, vaccination, surveillance

Sources: Data synthesized from The Center for Food Security & Public Health (2021), CDC (2024a), Lin et al. (2023), and United Nations Environment Program (UNEP) and International Livestock Research Institution (2020).

Pathogen X represents the ultimate wildcard—an as-yet-unknown microbe with the potential to trigger a global pandemic. It is not a specific virus or bacterium but rather a conceptual placeholder for the next major disease threat that has not yet emerged or been identified. This shift in focus acknowledges an uncomfortable truth: despite our growing surveillance capabilities and scientific knowledge, the next pandemic could be caused by a pathogen we haven't yet discovered or recognized as dangerous (Coulson, 2024).

The WHO's 2024 watchlist, outlined in Table 19.4, represents this more comprehensive approach. Rather than focusing exclusively on individual pathogens, the framework adopts a family-focused strategy that acknowledges the potential for any viral family to produce the next pandemic threat. Scientists initially assessed 28 viral families and one core group of bacteria, totaling 1,652 pathogens, before identifying approximately 30 specific viral pathogens across multiple families that pose high risk of causing Public Health Emergencies of International Concern (PHEIC) (WHO, 2024d).

Central to this approach is the concept of "prototype pathogens"—carefully selected representatives from viral families with pandemic potential that serve

Table 19.4 WHO's 2024 Priority Pathogen Watchlist

Example Pathogens	*Associated Diseases*	*Pathogen Family*	*Transmission*
Lassa virus	Lassa fever	Arenaviridae	Rodents (*Mastomys*), bodily fluids
SARS-CoV-2, MERS-CoV	COVID-19, MERS	Coronaviridae	Droplets, close contact, animals
Ebola, Marburg	Viral hemorrhagic fevers	Filoviridae	Bodily fluids, animal exposure
Dengue, Zika, yellow fever	Dengue, Zika, yellow fever	Flaviviridae	Aedes mosquitoes
Sin Nombre, Seoul virus	Hantavirus syndromes	Orthohantavirus	Rodent excreta, aerosols
Influenza A variants (H1N1, H5N1, etc.)	Seasonal/pandemic flu	Orthomyxoviridae	Droplets, animal-to-human
Nipah, Hendra	Encephalitis, respiratory illness	Paramyxoviridae	Bats, contaminated food, animals
Monkeypox virus	Mpox	Poxviridae	Contact, droplets, fomites
Oropouche virus	Oropouche fever	Peribunyaviridae	Biting midges
Klebsiella, Shigella, Yersinia	Pneumonia, dysentery, plague	Enterobacteriaceae	Food/water, vectors, contact
Vibrio cholerae	Cholera	Vibrionaceae	Contaminated water/food
Pathogen X	*Unknown future pandemic*	*Conceptual*	*Unknown*

Sources: Data compiled from WHO Pathogens Prioritization (WHO, 2024d) and Ukoaka et al. (2024). Note: The 2024 WHO framework identified approximately 30 specific viral pathogens across multiple families as high risk for causing Public Health Emergencies of International Concern (PHEIC). This table presents key representatives from each family.

as research models. These prototypes are chosen based on their pathogenic significance, understood replication mechanisms, and availability of animal models (Ukoaka et al., 2024). By developing countermeasures for these prototype pathogens, scientists can create platforms adaptable to related threats—including potentially Pathogen X.

The elevation of Pathogen X in the WHO framework has practical implications for global health security. It drives investment in adaptable vaccine and drug development platforms that can be rapidly retooled for novel threats. It encourages the development of broad-spectrum antivirals that might work against entire viral families rather than specific pathogens. And perhaps most importantly, it pushes surveillance systems to look beyond known threats to detect unusual disease patterns that might signal the emergence of something new.

The real-world utility of this approach has already been demonstrated. When a new strain of mpox was detected in the Democratic Republic of Congo and declared a PHEIC in August 2024, response teams were able to leverage platforms developed for other poxviruses (PAHO, n.d.). Similarly, the H5N2 avian influenza confirmed in Mexico in May 2024, which spread throughout the United States in late 2024 and early 2025, benefited from surveillance and response mechanisms designed with the flexible Pathogen X framework in mind (WHO, 2024c).

The WHO has complemented this watchlist with the Preparedness and Resilience for Emerging Threats (PRET) Initiative to strengthen pandemic preparedness at national, regional, and global levels. This initiative explicitly addresses the challenge of Pathogen X by drawing on lessons from past epidemics—particularly those caused by respiratory pathogens, which pose ongoing global risks. They emphasize the importance of community involvement, cross-sector cooperation, and maintaining consistent, long-term efforts to avoid the common cycle of panic and neglect in public health emergencies (WHO, 2025a).

This focus on Pathogen X represents a humbling acknowledgment of the limits of scientific prediction. Despite sophisticated modeling and extensive cataloging of potential threats, the next pandemic could emerge from an unexpected source—perhaps a virus currently circulating undetected in wildlife, a known pathogen that acquires new properties through mutation, or even a virus released from melting permafrost due to climate change.

The challenge of Pathogen X stresses the importance of the broader zoonotic threat landscape described throughout this section. The same drivers that increase the risk of spillover from known high-risk pathogens—deforestation, wildlife trade, climate change, intensive agriculture—also elevate the chances of encountering an as-yet-unknown virus with pandemic potential. The concept reminds us that our focus cannot solely be on the threats we can name but must extend to strengthening the systems that protect us from those we cannot yet imagine.

Prevention over Reaction: Building Global Defense at the Source

The mounting evidence of zoonotic threat acceleration has catalyzed a shift in global health strategy: from reacting to outbreaks toward preventing them at their source. This approach is embodied in the One Health framework—the principle that human, animal, and environmental health are inseparable and must be addressed together (CDC, 2024b). Once largely theoretical, One Health has moved into practical implementation as agencies worldwide recognize that siloed approaches cannot adequately address interconnected threats.

In 2021, the World Health Organization (WHO), the Food and Agriculture Organization of the United Nations (FAO), the World Organisation for Animal Health (WOAH), and the United Nations Environment Programme (UNEP) launched a joint One Health action plan to integrate surveillance and control across sectors (World Organisation for Animal Health (WOAH), n.d.). This initiative brings together veterinarians, epidemiologists, wildlife biologists, climate scientists, and physicians to share data and coordinate efforts to detect emerging pathogens before they spread widely. The international Pandemic Fund established in 2022 has made

Table 19.5 Core Pillars of One Health for Pandemic Prevention

Domain	*Key Strategies*	*Challenges*
Human Health	– Early detection systems – Sanitation, vaccination, health access – Community risk and literacy education	– Fragile health systems – Misinformation – Resource disparities
Animal Health	– Wildlife trade regulation – Farm biosecurity – Disease surveillance in animals	– Enforcement gaps – Human-animal contact risks
Environmental Health	– Halt deforestation – Protect ecosystems – Address climate stressors	– Land-use conflict – Economic pressures – Climate disruption

Source: Adapted from Horefti (2023), One Health (2019), and United Nations Environment Program (UNEP) and International Livestock Research Institution (2020).

One Health a core focus, directing financing to low- and middle-income countries to strengthen veterinary and environmental health systems alongside public health (World Bank Group, 2025).

Table 19.5 outlines the core pillars of the One Health model for pandemic prevention, highlighting strategies and challenges across human health, animal health, and environmental health domains. These three interdependent domains form the foundation for a comprehensive approach to preventing zoonotic threat emergence.

Primary prevention at the source has gained emphasis as the most upstream strategy to stop future pandemics. Several critical preventive measures have emerged as priorities: halting deforestation to minimize wildlife-human pathogen exchange (Daszak et al., 2020); improving farm biosecurity and strengthening wildlife trade regulation (Linder et al., 2023); maintaining safe and appropriate guidelines for agricultural animals and emphasizing handwashing after animal contact (WHO, 2020); and addressing climate change to reduce ecosystem stress that drives disease spillovers (Romanello et al., 2022).

Table 19.6 presents cross-cutting strategies to operationalize the One Health approach, including integrated surveillance, community engagement, research and development, climate adaptation, and global governance mechanisms. These strategies represent the institutional, technological, and policy approaches needed to activate One Health at scale.

At the global governance level, momentum has built to solidify lessons from COVID-19 into binding commitments. The Pandemic Preparedness Accord negotiations aim to establish new rules for sharing data, samples, and resources during health emergencies (WHO, 2025c). This represents a crucial step toward ensuring coordinated responses and fortified capacities so that no country is left vulnerable when dangerous pathogens emerge.

By addressing the underlying drivers of risky human-animal contact and ecosystem disruption, while strengthening early detection and response capabilities,

Table 19.6 Cross-Cutting Strategies to Operationalize One Health

Domain	*Key Strategies*	*Challenges*
Integrated surveillance	– Cross-sector data sharing – Hotspot monitoring – Genomic tracking	– Siloed systems – Tech gaps – Privacy concerns
Community engagement	– Risk and literacy education – Livelihood support – Behavioral change programs	– Mistrust – Poverty – Cultural resistance
Research and development	– Broad-spectrum antivirals – Scalable vaccines – Predictive modeling	– High cost – IP barriers – Weak incentives
Climate adaptation	– Climate-resilient health systems – Vector control – Forecasting tools	– Funding gaps – Adaptation complexity
Global governance	– Pandemic accord – Coordinated response – Sustainable prevention funding	– Political will – Global equity divides

Sources: Adapted from United Nations Environment Program (UNEP) and International Livestock Research Institution (2020), One Health (2019), and Horefti (2023).

we can reduce the likelihood of future pandemics or, at minimum, contain them before they spread globally. The world is awakening to the reality that we must live with biological threats, but we are not helpless against them. Science, surveillance, and solidarity offer powerful tools to navigate the gathering storm of zoonotic threats.

References

Ahmed, S. K., Hussein, S., Qurbani, K., Ibrahim, R. H., Fareeq, A., Mahmood, K. A., & Mohamed, M. G. (2024). Antimicrobial resistance: Impacts, challenges, and future prospects. *Journal of Medicine, Surgery, and Public Health, 2*, 100081. https://doi.org/10.1016/j.glmedi.2024.100081

Baker-Austin, C., Lake, I., Archer, E., Hartnell, R., Trinanes, J., & Martinez-Urtaza, J. (2024). Stemming the rising tide of Vibrio disease. *The Lancet. Planetary Health, 8*(7), e515–e520. https://doi.org/10.1016/S2542-5196(24)00124-4

Carlson, C. J., Albery, G. F., Merow, C., Trisos, C. H., Zipfel, C. M., Eskew, E. A., Olival, K. J., Ross, N., & Bansal, S. (2022). Climate change increases cross-species viral transmission risk. *Nature, 607*(7919), 555–562. https://doi.org/10.1038/s41586-022-04788-w

Centers for Disease Control and Prevention (CDC). (2024a, May 20). *About bovine tuberculosis in humans*. CDC. https://www.cdc.gov/tb/about/m-bovis.html

Centers for Disease Control and Prevention (CDC). (2024b, October 30). *About One Health*. CDC. https://www.cdc.gov/one-health/about/index.html

Centers for Disease Control and Prevention (CDC). (2025a). *CDC current outbreak list*. Centers for Disease Control and Prevention. https://www.cdc.gov/outbreaks/index.html

Centers for Disease Control and Prevention (CDC). (2025b, January 15). *2024 global outbreak responses*. CDC. https://www.cdc.gov/global-health/annual-report-2024/outbreaks.html

Centers for Disease Control and Prevention (CDC). (2025c, April 23). *Air travel*. CDC. https://www.cdc.gov/yellow-book/hcp/travel-air-sea/air-travel.html

The Center for Food Security and Public Health (CFSPH). (2021). *Zoonotic Disease Prevention and Biosecurity Resources*. Iowa State University, College of Veterinary Medicine. https://www.cfsph.iastate.edu/zoonoses/

Chason, R., Crowe, K., Muyskens, J., & Chikwendiu, J. (2023, October 23). *Where malaria is spreading*. Washington Post. https://www.washingtonpost.com/climate-environment/interactive/2023/malaria-disease-spread-climate-change-warming/

Coulson, M. (2024, February 15). *Defining Disease X*. Johns Hopkins Bloomberg School of Public Health. https://publichealth.jhu.edu/2024/what-is-disease-x

Daszak, P., Amuasi, J., das Neves, C. G., Hayman, D., Kuiken, T., Roche, B., Zambrana-Torrelio, C., Buss, P., Dundarova, H., Feferholtz, Y., Foldvari, G., Igbinosa, E., Junglen, S., Liu, Q., Suzan, G., Uhart, M., Wannous, C., Woolaston, K., Mosig Reidl, P., O'Brien, K., Pascual, U., Stoett, P., Li, H., & Ngo, H. T. (2020) Workshop Report on Biodiversity and Pandemics of the Intergovernmental Platform on Biodiversity and Ecosystem Services. IPBES Secretariat. Bonn, Germany. https://doi.org/10.5281/zenodo.4147317

Doucleff, M. (2016, August 3). *Anthrax outbreak in Russia thought to be result of thawing permafrost*. Npr.org. https://www.npr.org/sections/goatsandsoda/2016/08/03/488400947/anthrax-outbreak-in-russia-thought-to-be-result-of-thawing-permafrost

Horefti, E. (2023). The importance of the One Health concept in combating zoonoses. *Pathogens (Basel, Switzerland)*, *12*(8), 977. https://doi.org/10.3390/pathogens12080977

Jilani, T. N., Jamil, R. T., & Siddiqui, A. H. (2024, March 4). *H1N1 influenza (Swine Flu)*. NIH; StatPearls Publishing. https://www.ncbi.nlm.nih.gov/books/NBK513241/

Lin, C. N., Okabayashi, T., Tummaruk, P., & Ooi, P. T. (2023). Editorial: Zoonotic diseases among pigs. *Frontiers in Veterinary Science*, *9*, 1122679. https://doi.org/10.3389/fvets.2022.1122679

Linder, A., McCarthy, V. W., Green, C., Nadzam, B., Jamieson, D., & Stilt, K. (2023). *Animal markets and zoonotic disease in the United States*. Brooks Institute for Animal Rights Law & Policy Program; Harvard Law School. https://animal.law.harvard.edu/wp-content/uploads/Animal-Markets-and-Zoonotic-Disease-in-the-United-States.pdf

One Health. (2019). *Taking a multisectoral One Health approach: A tripartite guide to addressing zoonotic diseases in countries*. World Health Organization (WHO), Food and Agriculture Organization of the United Nations (FAO) and World Organisation for Animal Health (WOAH).

Pan American Health Organization (PAHO). (n.d.). *Mpox outbreak*. PAHO; WHO. https://www.paho.org/en/mpox

Peacock, T. P., Moncla, L., Dudas, G., VanInsberghe, D., Sukhova, K., Lloyd-Smith, J. O., Worobey, M., Lowen, A. C., & Nelson, M. I. (2025). The global H5N1 influenza panzootic in mammals. *Nature*, 637(8045), 304–313. https://doi.org/10.1038/s41586-024-08054-z

Plowright, R. K., Parrish, C. R., McCallum, H., Hudson, P. J., Ko, A. I., Graham, A. L., & LloydSmith, J. O. (2017). Pathways to zoonotic spillover. *Nature Reviews Microbiology*, *15*(8), 502–510. https://doi.org/10.1038/nrmicro.2017.45

Pörtner, H.-O., Roberts, D. C., Tignor, M., Poloczanska, E. S., Mintenbeck, K., Alegría, A., Craig, M., Langsdorf, S., Löschke, S., Möller, V., Okem, A., & Rama, B. (eds.) (2022). *Climate Change 2022: Impacts, Adaptation, and Vulnerability*. Contribution of Working Group II to the Sixth Assessment Report of the Intergovernmental Panel on Climate Change. IPCC. Cambridge University Press, Cambridge, UK and New York, NY, USA, p. 3056. doi:10.1017/9781009325844.

Romanello, M., Napoli, D., Drummond, P., Green, C., Kennard, H., Lampard, P., Scamman, D., Arnell, N., AyebKarlsson, S., Ford, L. B., Belesova, K., Bowen, K., Cai, W.,

Callaghan, M., CampbellLendrum, D., Chambers, J., Dalin, C., Dasandi, N., Dasgupta, S., & van Daalen, K. R. (2022). The 2022 report of the *Lancet* countdown on health and climate change: Health at the mercy of fossil fuels. *The Lancet*, *400*(10363), 1619–1654. https://doi.org/10.1016/S01406736(22)015409

Shukla, P. R., Skea, J., Calvo Buendia, E., Masson-Delmotte, V., Pörtner, H.-O., Roberts, D. C., Zhai, P., Slade, R., Connors, S., van Diemen, R., Ferrat, M., Haughey, E., Luz, S., Neogi, S., Pathak, M., Petzold, J., Portugal Pereira, J., Vyas, P., Huntley, E., Kissick, K., Belkacemi, M., & Malley, J. (eds.) (2019). Climate Change and Land: An IPCC Special Report on Climate Change, Desertification, Land Degradation, Sustainable Land Management, Food Security, and Greenhouse Gas Fluxes in Terrestrial Ecosystems. In press.

Ukoaka, B. M., Odunayo, F. R., Rahmat, A. B., Ngozi, A. L., Shalom, C. C., & Bassey, E. E. (2024). Updated WHO list of emerging pathogens for a potential future pandemic: Implications for public health and global preparedness. *Infectious Medicine*, *32*(4), 463–477. https://doi.org/10.53854/liim-3204-5

United Nations Environment Programme (UNEP) and International Livestock Research Institute (2020). *Preventing the next pandemic: Zoonotic diseases and how to break the chain of transmission*. https://www.unep.org/resources/report/preventing-future-zoonotic-disease-outbreaks-protecting-environment-animals-and

US Environmental Protection Agency (EPA). (2025, February). *Climate change indicators: Lyme disease*. US EPA. https://www.epa.gov/climate-indicators/climate-change-indicators-lyme-disease

Wang, L. F., Shi, Z., Zhang, S., Field, H., Daszak, P., & Eaton, B. T. (2006). Review of bats and SARS. *Emerging Infectious Diseases*, *12*(12), 1834–1840. https://doi.org/10.3201/eid1212.060401

Weston, P. (2024, September 4). *Forgotten epidemic: With over 280 million birds dead how is the avian flu outbreak evolving?* The Guardian. https://www.theguardian.com/environment/article/2024/sep/04/forgotten-epidemic-with-over-280-million-birds-dead-how-is-the-avian-flu-outbreak-evolving

World Bank Group. (2025). *Health emergencies*. World Bank. https://www.worldbank.org/en/topic/pandemics

World Health Organization. (2020, July 29). *Zoonoses*. World Health Organization. https://www.who.int/news-room/fact-sheets/detail/zoonoses

World Health Organization (WHO). (2022, December 8). *Zika virus*. WHO. https://www.who.int/news-room/fact-sheets/detail/zika-virus

World Health Organization (WHO). (2023). *Zoonotic disease: Emerging public health threats in the region*. WHO EMRO; WHO. https://www.emro.who.int/about-who/rc61/zoonotic-diseases.html

World Health Organization (WHO). (2024a, April 23). *Dengue and severe dengue*. WHO. https://www.who.int/news-room/fact-sheets/detail/dengue-and-severe-dengue

World Health Organization (WHO). (2024b, May 30). *Dengue – Global situation*. WHO. https://www.who.int/emergencies/disease-outbreak-news/item/2024-DON518

World Health Organization (WHO). (2024c, June 5). *Human infection caused by avian Influenza A (H5N2) – Mexico*. WHO. https://www.who.int/emergencies/disease-outbreak-news/item/2024-DON520

World Health Organization (WHO). (2024d). Pathogens prioritization a scientific framework for epidemic and pandemic research preparedness. In *WHO*. WHO. https://cdn.who.int/media/docs/default-source/consultation-rdb/prioritization-pathogens-v6final.pdf

World Health Organization (WHO). (2025a). *Call to action on respiratory pathogen pandemic planning*. World Health Organization. https://iris.who.int/bitstream/handle/10665/380524/9789240084650-eng.pdf?sequence=1

World Health Organization (WHO). (2025b, March 25). *Urban health*. WHO. https://www.who.int/news-room/fact-sheets/detail/urban-health

World Health Organization (WHO). (2025c, May 20). *World Health Assembly adopts historic pandemic agreement to make the world more equitable and safer from future pandemics*. WHO. https://www.who.int/news/item/20-05-2025-world-health-assembly-adopts-historic-pandemic-agreement-to-make-the-world-more-equitable-and-safer-from-future-pandemics

World Organisation for Animal Health (WOAH). (n.d.). *One Health.* WOAH – World Organisation for Animal Health. https://www.woah.org/en/what-we-do/global-initiatives/one-health/

20 From Iceberg to Lighthouse

A Final Reflection

The Iceberg Revisited: From Visible Events to Hidden Drivers

Five years after the emergence of SARS-CoV-2, we find ourselves at a critical juncture for reflection. The pandemic that once seemed an abstract threat on distant shores transformed with stunning speed into a global catastrophe that fundamentally altered our world. As we've traced the journey from those first alarming reports in Wuhan to today's evolved understanding, the Iceberg Theory has provided us an invaluable framework for comprehending not just what happened, but why events unfolded as they did (Table 20.1).

Events

Like the ill-fated Titanic confronting what appeared to be a manageable obstacle while failing to foresee the deadly mass beneath the surface, our global community encountered COVID-19 with a dangerous misreading of the true threat. The visible events—rising case counts, health system strain, policy decisions, and scientific breakthroughs—commanded our attention, but these represented merely the tip of a much larger and more complex reality.

Trends / Patterns

Beneath these observable manifestations, patterns emerged that proved decisive in shaping the pandemic's trajectory. The virus's remarkable evolutionary capacity produced increasingly transmissible and immune-evasive variants from Alpha to Omicron and beyond. Transmission dynamics revealed how geography, seasonality, and human behavior combined to create distinct infection waves across the globe that proliferated and re-manifested anew. Vaccines demonstrated changing effectiveness against these evolving threats, while testing, surveillance, and treatment approaches underwent their own reactive evolution in real time.

Systemic Structures

Deeper still lay the systemic structures that either supported or hindered effective response. Healthcare systems, despite theoretical preparedness, often collapsed

DOI: 10.4324/9781003595564-25

Table 20.1 The COVID-19 Iceberg: A Framework for Understanding the Pandemic

Iceberg Layer	*Examples and Dynamics*	*Key Takeaway*
1. Events (Surface)	• Case surges • Overwhelmed ICUs • Lockdowns and mandates • Social and economic disruption	These dramatic signals were visible but reactive symptoms—not root causes.
2. Trends/ patterns	• Variant evolution • Seasonal and geographic waves • Booster and new vaccine cycles • Shifting testing and tracking strategies	Recurring dynamics that hinted at deeper feedback loops and adaptation challenges.
3. Structures	• Health system capacity • Global supply chains • Vaccine access and equity • Communication infrastructures	Pre-existing institutional architecture shaped not just one country—but how global health governance functions.
4. Mental models	• Cognitive biases • Cultural values • Risk perception • Institutional trust	Mental models determined how leaders acted, how societies complied, how systems responded, and how behaviors manifested.

under prolonged duress and strain. Supply chains revealed critical vulnerabilities, particularly in the production and distribution of vaccines, treatments, and protective equipment. Communication networks alternately informed and confused populations struggling to navigate the uncertainties of the crisis. Economic systems demonstrated both remarkable adaptability and troubling disparities in how burdens were distributed.

Mental Models / Behaviors

But at the deepest level—the true foundation of the iceberg—lay something more fundamental: the mental models through which we understand and respond to crisis itself. Individual cognitive frameworks determined how people processed risk and uncertainty. Cultural perspectives shaped whether populations viewed crisis response through collective or individualistic lenses. Institutional trust influenced whether public health guidance was embraced or rejected. And our psychological responses to fear and extended crisis ultimately determined whether protective behaviors could be sustained over time.

The Seven Unknowns Revisited: A Path Forward

The seven critical unknowns we identified in the introduction—the virus's origin, true mortality figures, evolutionary capacity, immunity dynamics, long COVID's nature, actual infection rates, and viral ecosystem disruption—served as portals into understanding the pandemic's deeper dimensions. In the following analysis, we examine these questions through the iceberg model to illuminate strategic directions for the future.

What Is the True Origin of SARS-CoV-2?

Despite years of investigation, the origin remains uncertain—whether zoonotic spillover or lab-based incident. This uncertainty fueled geopolitical tension and public mistrust.

Future Direction:

i Establish a permanent, independent global pathogen origins observatory, free from political influence, backed by the WHO and a coalition of transparent scientific bodies.
ii Standardize biosafety protocols globally with real-time audits and data sharing between labs and governments.
iii Foster science diplomacy, creating international agreements that protect pandemic investigations from political interference.

Insight: Global science must be uncoupled from national interest when investigating zoonotic threats.

How Many People Truly Died from COVID-19?

Excess mortality estimates suggest that actual deaths were two to three times higher than official reports, revealing fragile, inconsistent data systems.

Future Direction:

i Develop automated, real-time mortality and morbidity tracking using digital death registries, AI-assisted reporting, and standardized metrics across nations.
ii Integrate excess mortality modeling as a standing public health function—not only during pandemics.
iii Promote radical transparency in health data to build trust and enable swift action.

Insight: Truth in numbers is not optional; it's the foundation of global health equity and response.

Why Does the Virus Mutate so Rapidly?

SARS-CoV-2 demonstrated extraordinary genetic agility, outpacing public health strategies and vaccine updates.

Future Direction:

i Shift from strain-specific to universal, pan-coronavirus vaccines, leveraging platforms like mRNA, self-amplifying RNA, and nanoparticle delivery.
ii Expand global genomic surveillance networks, especially in low-resource settings, to ensure equitable early detection.
iii Link vaccine R&D pipelines to real-time variant evolution using AI modeling.

Insight: Vaccine innovation must match viral speed—not in reaction, but in anticipation.

How Long Does Immunity Last, and How Should Vaccination Evolve?

Immunity proved transient; antibody levels dropped within months, while cellular immunity remained more durable. This disrupted traditional vaccination schedules.

Future Direction:

i Move toward personalized vaccine regimens, guided by immune profiling and infection history.
ii Develop immunity dashboards for population-level monitoring—just as weather is forecasted, so should immune risk.
iii Invest in long-acting vaccine technologies and mucosal (e.g., nasal) delivery methods for broader, longer protection.

Insight: Vaccine strategies must treat the immune system as dynamic, not static.

What Is Long COVID, and What Are Its Long-Term Consequences?

Long COVID became a hidden pandemic—millions developed lingering symptoms with unclear mechanisms, ranging from fatigue to cognitive dysfunction.

Future Direction:

i Create dedicated long COVID centers integrating rehabilitation, neurology, cardiology, and mental health.
ii Launch longitudinal cohorts and biobanks to study post-viral syndromes beyond COVID.
iii Acknowledge and integrate post-infectious chronic disease care into national health systems.

Insight: A virus's impact does not end with viral clearance. Chronicity must be planned for, not ignored.

What Was the Actual Infection Rate Globally?

Testing limitations and asymptomatic spread masked the true extent—many waves were underestimated, affecting models and public health responses.

Future Direction:

i Institutionalize wastewater surveillance, seroprevalence studies, and digital symptom tracking as core public health infrastructure.
ii Use smart population sampling powered by AI to dynamically adjust for underreporting.
iii Build real-time dashboards of community-level viral presence, combining multiple data streams.

Insight: Surveillance must shift from reactive case counting to proactive environmental sensing.

Why Did Influenza and RSV Vanish, Then Return with a Vengeance?

During COVID's peak, flu and RSV nearly disappeared—then returned off-season and more severe, highlighting complex viral interactions.

Future Direction:

i Develop a multi-virus surveillance platform, incorporating flu, RSV, COVID, and other emerging pathogens.
ii Study viral interference and immune imprinting across various pathogens.
iii Prepare hospitals with season-agnostic surge readiness plans that consider all major infectious threats.

Insight: Respiratory pathogens interact in complex ecological systems. Our interventions must account for viral interference and ecosystem effects.

Collectively these unknowns reveal both our shortcomings and our opportunities. Beneath the visible failures lie pathways to lasting resilience—if we commit to thinking systemically, acting globally, and responding structurally.

From Darkness to Light: A Lighthouse on the Horizon

What have we learned from peering beneath the surface? Most fundamentally, those technical solutions alone cannot address the full scope of complex crises. Countries with sophisticated medical infrastructure but fragmented social trust often fared worse than those with more modest resources but coherent leadership and public cohesion. We've seen how institutional trust represents the bedrock of effective crisis response, how cultural context shapes the reception of health measures, and how psychological resilience determines a population's capacity to adapt to prolonged emergency.

The pandemic exposed how deeply our fates are intertwined. No nation controlled its destiny alone, as supply chains, variant emergence, and information flows transcended borders. The disproportionate impact on vulnerable populations revealed that equity isn't just a moral imperative, but a practical necessity for effective global pandemic control.

Perhaps most importantly, we've learned that preparation must extend beyond infrastructure and protocols to address the deeper psychological and social dimensions of crisis response. Building population-wide literacy around uncertainty, risk assessment, and collaborative action will prove as crucial as stockpiling ventilators or developing new vaccine platforms.

While COVID-19 may have receded into historical memory for the vast majority, the conditions that allowed it to wreak such havoc with expediency continue to intensify more than ever. These driving forces make future pandemics not merely possible, but inevitable.

Now, at this five-year milestone, we stand before a profound truth: the light we've gained through immense sacrifice must illuminate not just our understanding of the past, but our creation of the future. This book began with an iceberg; let us end it with a lighthouse. We have descended through the layers of the pandemic iceberg, from its visible peaks to its darkest depths. Yet this journey of understanding serves no purpose if we resurface unchanged.

The question before us now is not whether we have comprehended the crisis, but whether we have the courage to be transformed by it—to remake our systems,

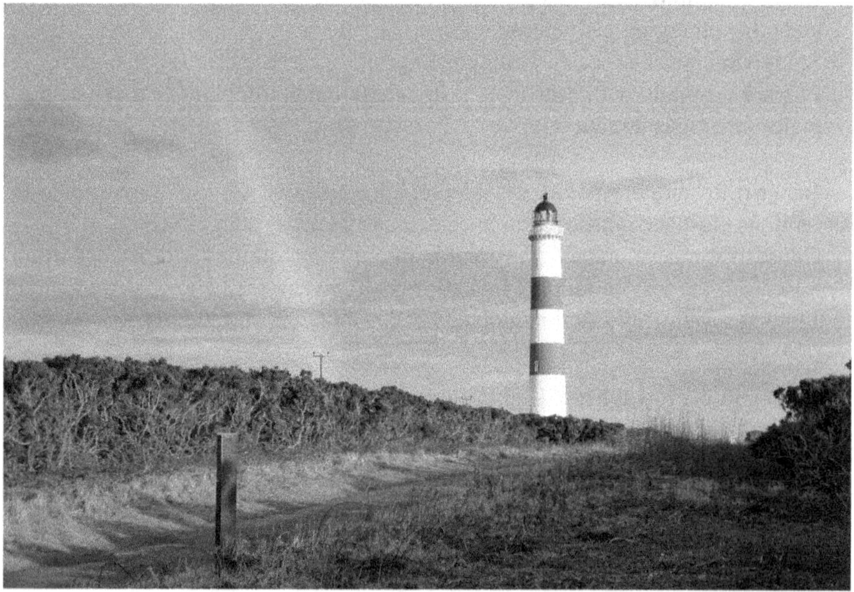

Figure 20.1 Lighthouse.

to recalibrate our institutions, and to reimagine our shared future in this light where there was only shadow before. The next pandemic awaits, not as a distant possibility, but as an evolutionary certainty. And when it arrives, it will test not our fleeting memory of COVID-19, but the wisdom we extracted from its devastating passage through our world.

The lighthouse asks us not to forget, but to illuminate. Not to retreat, but to navigate. The next crisis will come, but with what we have learned, we can meet it not as casualties of chance, but as designers of resilience.

Index

Note: Page references in *italics* denote figures and in **bold** tables.

1918 influenza pandemic 12, 49; and COVID-19 pandemic 24–31; evolution of respiratory protection 26–27; mortality patterns and demographic impact 24–26, *25*, **26**; non-pharmaceutical interventions 26; pathogen identification and characterization 28; personal hygiene 27; public health interventions **27**; public health leadership and communication 29–30; vaccine development 28–29; *see also* pandemics

ABRYSVO 357
acute illness severity and reinfection 338, 346
Adaptive COVID-19 Treatment Trial (ACTT-1) 259
adaptive models 209–210
adequate hydration 281–282
adequate vitamin intake 280–281, **280–281**
age-related factors 336
aging 273–275, *274*; and immune challenges of COVID-19 273–274, *274*; social and healthcare marginalization 275; vulnerability 273–274, *274*
Agley, J. 215
agricultural interfaces 366, **367**
Airhihenbuwa, C. O. 193
Alpha variant 83, 87–88
American College of Sports Medicine (ACSM) 283
American Rescue Plan 150
Ancestral Wave 86–87
anchoring bias 179
Andriani, L. 186
Annals of Behavioral Medicine 289
antiviral strategies 107–109, **108**; hydroxychloroquine 107, 158; molnupiravir 260; nirmatrelvir-ritonavir (Paxlovid) 107–109; remdesivir 107
Antonine Plague 19–20
AREXVY 357
AstraZeneca 138, 157, 260
Australia: contact tracing **251**; empathetic communication 207; lockdowns 131–132; vaccine hoarding 145; WBE 103
availability heuristic 178–179

balanced diets 275, 279; impact on COVID-19 outcomes 279, **279**; as potential protective factor against COVID-19 278–282
Balmis, Francisco Javier 35
bamlanivimab 260
baricitinib 109, 344
Basabe, N. 193
bias: anchoring 179; cognitive 174, **175**, 181–183, **183**; confirmation 177–178; normalcy 177, 182; optimism 176–177, 182; worst-case 179–180
biological pathway: immune system 288; stress 288
Black Death 7, 11–12, 22, 49; early quarantine measures 20; overview 17; as plague 20–21; scientific breakthroughs in study of 18–19; scientific milestones **21**; Venice 20
BMC Public Health 215, 270
Brazil 131; *Auxílio Emergencial* program 154; *Bolsa Família* program 154; household and business support measures **151**
British Journal of Sports Medicine 283–284

Canada: RSV hospitalization 357; universal public healthcare system 130; vaccine hoarding 145, **146**; WBE 103
cardiovascular manifestations 332–333
CARES Act 149
casirivimab/imdevimab (REGEN-COV) 111
Centers for Disease Control and Prevention (CDC) 156, 196, 199, 211, 237, 239, 269
Child Tax Credit 150
China: Belt and Road Initiative 145; healthcare worker burnout 136; household and business support measures **151**; human-to-human transmission 61; interventions in 70; SARS-CoV-2 virus 13, 28, 41, 60; stimulus measures 153; vaccine exports 145; "zero-COVID" strategy 129–130
chronic diseases 269–270; and excessive alcohol consumption 293; impact of the pandemic 269–270; vulnerability 269–270
Circadian vaccination timing: age-specific timing considerations 286, **287**; midday administration effectiveness 286
Clade Ib variant 358
Clark, E. 199
climate as force multipliers 364–366, **365**
Clinical Infectious Diseases 272
clinical manifestations across organ systems **331**, 331–334
clinical presentations, long COVID **327**, 327–328
Coalition for Epidemic Preparedness Innovations (CEPI) 143
cognitive biases 174, **175**; across cultures 181–183, **183**; *see also* bias
cold chain crisis 140–142, **142**
collective mental models 184–194
communication breakdowns: infodemic 159; pandemic communication 156–157; public health communication 160–162; vaccine hesitancy and public trust 157–158; *see also* public trust
confirmation bias 177–178
confusion to mandates 237
"Conspiracy Belief" model 212, **213**, 214–216
conspiracy theories and mental models 214–216
contact tracing/quarantine policies 249–252; Australia **251**; de-prioritization of 250; digital 130; fatigue and focused response 250; Germany **251**; global approaches to 250–251; lessons learned 251–252; rapid scaling/uneven implementation 250; of select regions **251**; South Korea 137, **251**; Taiwan 130, **251**; United Kingdom **251**; United States 250; voluntary and situational practices 250
convergence: disease outbreaks 355–360; of respiratory viruses 356–357
coronavirus family 41–42; challenges of COVID-19 45–46; lessons from outbreaks 44–45; similarities and differences 43–44
Corta el Contagio ("Cut the Transmission") campaign 264
COVID-19 iceberg *see* iceberg
COVID-19 pandemic 13, 22, 44–45; and 1918 influenza pandemic 24–31; age vulnerability 273–274, *274*; antiviral therapies for **108**; applying pandemic wisdom to 52–53; cases confirmed 2020 to 2025 *1*; demographic impact 24–26, *25*, **26**; demographic shifts 303–305; disrupted education and long-term learning gaps 313–315, **315**, **316**; disruption of viral ecosystem 355–356; and drug use 294–295; evolution of respiratory protection 26–27; and excessive alcohol consumption 293–294; exercise helps combat 283–284; global economic responses 154–156; global impacts of 303; global vaccination coverage *4*; hospitalizations in United States *6*; Iceberg Theory 62–63; immune challenges of 273–274, *274*; immunodeficiency and 272–273; impact of stress on 289; indirect health outcomes **306**, 306–308; and institutions 315–318, **317**; landscape 14–15; life expectancy 303–305; Mediterranean diet and 282; mental health fallout 308–310, **309**; mortality patterns 24–26, *25*, **26**, **306**, 306–308; non-pharmaceutical interventions 26; overview 1–7; *vs.* past pandemics 53–54; pathogen identification and characterization 28; personal hygiene 27; policy interventions during 148–156; potential protective factor against 278–282; public health interventions **27**; public

health leadership and communication 29–30; public sentiment after crisis 315–318, **317**; reported deaths from 2020 to 2025 *2*; scientific milestones **21**; severity linked to obesity 271–272; six-dimensional analysis 303; sleep and 286, **287**; *vs.* smallpox **36**, 36–38; smallpox management lesson for 38; social connections and 291–292; socioeconomic interventions during 148–156; surveillance 101–103, **102**, **104**; timeline of **66**; tobacco use and 292–293; trajectory 81–112; treatment evolution 106–112; and trust 315–318, **317**; uneven global impact 92–93; vaccine development 28–29; workforce transformation 310–313, **312**, **313**
COVID-19 treatments: chronological timeline 257–262; clinical implementation 261; early discoveries and treatment development 259; late 2020 260; monoclonal antibody therapies 260; regulatory transitions and innovation 261–262; rise of variants and oral antivirals 260–261
COVID-19 vaccination rates 262–264; economic factors and vaccine hesitancy 263; exploration of global 262–264; Nicaragua and vaccine inequity 263–264; vaccination rates by income 262–263; vaccination rates by region 262, **262**
COVID-19 vaccines: manufacturer, origin, type, and initial efficacy of **258–259**; types available globally 257
COVID-19 Vaccines Global Access program (COVAX) 141, 144, 148, 263; financial model 144; initiative 157; and vaccine equity 143–144
crisis temporality 209–210
cultural mental models: in pandemic response **192**; of prolonged crisis 204–205
culture: cognitive biases across 181–183, **183**; "loose" 182; "tight" 183
Cyprian Plague 19–20

Daly, M. 204, 209
Defense Production Act (DPA) 139
de Lorme, Charles 19
Delta variants 2, 83, 88; vaccine initial effectiveness 93–94
demographic shifts 303–305
diagnosis: diagnostic approaches 342–343; long COVID conundrum **342**, 342–346, **345**
Diamond Princess cruise ship 61, 67
dietary foundations of immune health 279–282
Digestive and Liver Disease 294
disease outbreaks, converging 355–360
disrupted education 313–315, **315**, **316**
Dolinski, D. 176
drug use and COVID-19 294–295

Ebola outbreak 50–51
economic disruption, and COVID-19 pandemic 72–75, **73**
emergency use authorizations (EUA) 107
Emergent BioSolutions 138
emerging therapeutic approaches 344–345
epistemic bubbles 178
ethnic disparities 336–337
Evusheld 260, 261
excessive alcohol consumption and COVID-19 293–294
exercise: combating COVID-19 283–284; effects on human body 283; strengthening body's defenses against infection 283–285
Eyam 20

Farhadi, A. 198
Fauci, Anthony 29
fear and uncertainty responses 210–221
fear-based messaging 216–218
first tripledemic (2022–2023) 356–357
first wave of COVID-19 pandemic 65–67
Fleming, Alexander 18
flexible skepticism 181
Fogarty, H. 330
Food and Agriculture Organization of the United Nations (FAO) 369
France 71, 100, 130, 140, 152, 356; *France Relance* industrial recovery plan 152; household and business support measures **151**; partial unemployment scheme *(Chômage Partiel)* 152
Freud, Sigmund 62
future outlook, and long COVID 346–347
future pandemics 355–360

gastrointestinal manifestations 333
genomic sequencing 24, 52, 105

Germany 130, 139, 359; contact tracing **251**; cultural approaches to uncertainty 190; health institutes 198; household and business support measures **151**; *Kurzarbeit* program 152; normalcy bias 182; Robert Koch Institute (RKI) 207; TRIPS waiver 139–140
Ghebreyesus, Tedros Adhanom 67
GISAID initiative 101
Giuntella, O. 205–206
Global Alliance for Vaccines and Immunization (GAVI) 143
Global Dashboard for Vaccine Equity 146
global genomic surveillance 103–105
global health equity 147–148
global health security (GHS) Index 132
globalization 365–366; as force multipliers 364–366, **365**
global prevalence of long COVID **340**, 340–341
Global South 140, 147–148
global vaccine equity 143–144; *see also* vaccine manufacturing
governance responses, to COVID-19 pandemic 69–72
Great Depression 72, 310
GSK 261, 357
Guterres, António 147

H1N1 influenza pandemic (2009) 50, 185
Haffkine, Waldemar 18
hand hygiene policies 240–242; continued emphasis with evolving guidance 242; foundational public health message 241; global hand hygiene policies 242; lessons learned 242; reduced focus/targeted use 242; as routine practice 242; of select regions **243**; in United States (2020–2025) 241–242
Haug, N. 196
health: behaviors 278–296; impacts and COVID-19 outcomes of substance use **295**; and loneliness 290–291; risks and consequences during pandemic 292–296; and social isolation 290–291
Health Belief Model (Rosenstock) 176
healthcare systems: and COVID-19 pandemic 67–69; ICU system **68**
healthcare systems resilience 129–137; healthcare workforce burnout **134**, 134–136; ICU capacity 137
healthcare workforce: burnout **134**, 134–136; capacity 134–136; factors associated with increased burnout risk **136**
health systems preparedness 129–137; Africa 131; Asia 129–130; Europe 130; North America 130; Oceania 131–132; preparedness paradox 132–134, **133**; South America 131
Hemingway, Ernest 62
highly pathogenic avian influenza (H5N1) 366
high-quality protein 280
high-risk factors 269–275; aging 273–275, *274*; chronic diseases 269–270; immunodeficiency 272–273; obesity 270–272
historical pandemics 49–50; *see also* pandemics
HIV/AIDS pandemic 13, 131, 272
hospital-based immune therapies **110**
human body: and adequate hydration 281–282; defenses against infection 283–285; effects of exercise on 283
human negligence: and COVID-19 60–62; and pandemics 60–62
hydroxychloroquine 107, 158

Iceberg Theory 60, *65*, 375–381; 90% submerged principle 60; application 62; COVID-19 pandemic 62–63; events 375, **376**; framework for understanding the pandemic **376**; mental models/behaviors 376, **376**; origins 62; systemic structures 375–376, **376**; Titanic analogy 59; trends/patterns 375, **376**; from visible events to hidden drivers 375–376; *see also* systems thinking
immune system: sleep and 285–286; stress and 288
immunity: dietary foundations of immune health 279–282; immune strength 285–287
immunodeficiency challenges 272–273
immunomodulation 109–110
implicit and explicit temporality in crisis 202
India 14, 18, 35, 71, 83, 88, 91; *Atmanirbhar Bharat Abhiyan* 154; Delta variant 260; *Emergency Credit Line Guarantee Scheme* 154; household and business support measures **151**; initial COVID-19 data collection 198; multi-faceted response 154; TRIPS waiver initiative 139; vaccine exports 144

indirect health outcomes **306**, 306–308
individual mental models 174–184; anchoring bias 179; availability heuristic 178–179; cognitive biases 174, **175**; confirmation bias 177–178; individual differences 174–176; interactive cognitive biases 180; normalcy bias 177; optimism bias 176–177; worst-case bias 179–180
"The Inequality Virus" 155
influenza 5, 25; H1N1 28; and healthcare systems 356
"Information Avoidance" approach 212, **213**, 217
information processing models **213**
institutional memory: 1918 influenza pandemic 30–31; COVID-19 pandemic 30–31
institutional mental models: adaptive models **201**; frameworks of trust and authority 194–201, **195**; rigid models **201**
institutions: after crisis 315–318, **317**; construction and modulation of temporal urgency 207–208
integrated care models 345–346
intellectual property: global vaccine 139–140; *vs.* public health responsibility 139–140
interactive cognitive biases 180
interactive mental models 208–209
interagency mental models of coordination 197
International Labour Organization (ILO) 310, 313

Japan 61, 66, 130, 133, 189–190, 204; collective societies 182; conservative fiscal approach 153; cultural approaches to uncertainty 190; cultural mask-wearing norms 183; cultural principles of giri and wa 185; employment protection schemes 187; household and business support measures **151**; social harmony 184–186; *Special Cash Payments* program 152; "tight" culture 183; voluntary compliance 240
Jenner, Edward 35
Johnson & Johnson 138–139
Johnson-Laird, P. N. 174
Journal of Adolescent Health 293
The Journal of Clinical Investigation 286
Journal of the American Medical Association (JAMA) 283
Justinian Plague 13

Kaasa, A. 186
Keys, Ancel 282
Kim, J. H. 208–209

labor market protection strategies 150–152
Lahooti, M. 198
The Lancet 289, 308
Lancet Commission 155
The Lancet Countdown 364
The Lancet eClinicalMedicine 339
The Lancet Regional Health 337
life expectancy 303–305
lifestyle: balanced diets 278–282; exercise 283–285; as a shield 278–296; sleep and circadian rhythms 285–287; social connections 290–292; stress management 287–290; substance use 292–296
lighthouse 375–381, *380*
Liu, Y. 188
Li Wenliang 61, 66
lockdown policies 245–247; during 2023–2025 246; global lockdown policies 246; lessons learned 247; localized restrictions and reopenings 246; post-Omicron shift 246; of select regions **247**; in United States (2020–2025) 246–247; widespread and disorganized lockdowns 246
loneliness, health impacts of 290–291
long COVID 5, 112, 326–347; acute illness severity and reinfection 338; age-related factors 336; cardiovascular manifestations 332–333; clinical manifestations across organ systems **331**, 331–334; diagnosis **342**, 342–346, **345**; diagnostic approaches 342–343; future outlook 346–347; gastrointestinal manifestations 333; global prevalence of **340**, 340–341; integrated care models 345–346; introduction to 326–327; management strategies **342**, 342–346, **345**; musculoskeletal manifestations 333–334; neurological/psychiatric manifestations 332; pathophysiological mechanisms of 328–330, **329**; pre-existing health conditions 337; prognosis 346–347; racial, ethnic, and socioeconomic

disparities 336–337; recovery 346–347; respiratory manifestations 333; risk factors and predictors 334–340, **335**; sex and gender differences 334–335; symptoms and clinical presentations **327**, 327–328; system manifestations 334; therapeutic approaches 344–345; treatment **342**, 342–346, **345**; treatment approaches 343–344; vaccination status 338–339; viral variant 339–340
long-term complications 111–112
long-term learning gaps 313–315, **315**, **316**

Maaravi, Y. 185, 191
management strategies, and long COVID **342**, 342–346, **345**
masking policies and evolution 237–238; from confusion to mandates 237; global masking approaches 238; lessons learned 238; Omicron and decentralized approach 238; seasonal and situational use 238; of select regions **239**; in the United States 237–238; vaccine rollout and policy shifts 238
McNeill, William 19
Mediterranean diet 282
mental health: fallout 308–310, **309**; nurturing during challenging times 287–290
mental models *174*; of adaptation and normalcy 205–206; of authority and expertise 188–190; of collective identity and social harmony 184–186; of crisis duration and endurance 202–204; of data and evidence 198; formation and individual differences 174–176; as foundations for public health response 193–194; as foundations of institutional response 199–201; individual 174–184; of individual autonomy and personal rights 186–188; of information processing during crisis 212–214; of institutional authority and legitimacy 196–197; of institutional endurance and trust 206–207; of public communication 198–199; within public health institutions 194–196; of risk and uncertainty 190–192; of stability and change 177; of threat and information 210–221; through cognitive biases 174; of truth and knowledge 177–178; updating and adaptation 180–181
mental resilience 218–221
MERS-CoV virus 41–42, **42**, 52, 185; *vs.* SARS-CoV-2 virus 43–44
Mexico 130; conservative fiscal response 154; household and business support measures **151**
misinformation 158–159; and conspiracies **160**; management 53
Moderna 138, 141
molnupiravir 260
Mompesson, William 20
Morgan, M. G. 174
mortality patterns **306**, 306–308
mpox outbreak (2022–2024) 358
mRESVIA (Moderna) 357
mRNA vaccines 2–3; constraints 138; IP barriers 140; temperature-controlled supply chains 140–141, 144; vaccinia capping enzyme 138
multidimensional impact of fear 210–211
musculoskeletal manifestations 333–334

nanoSTING 261
National Center for Drug Abuse Statistics 294
National Institutes of Health (NIH) 259; RECOVER COVID Initiative 328, 335, 337, 341
Nature 270
Nature Human Behaviour 289
Nature Medicine 328, 338, 340
neuroinflammation 330
neurological and psychiatric manifestations 332
new viral equilibrium 360
New York Stock Exchange 72
New Zealand 131, 133, 191, 199–200; communication strategy 137; empathetic communication 207; leadership 191; public communication strategies 72
next-generation vaccine development: nasal vaccine delivery systems (nanoSTING) 261; pan-coronavirus candidates 261–262; Project NextGen initiatives 262
Nicaragua: case study 263–264; success in overcoming vaccine inequity 263–264
nirmatrelvir-ritonavir (Paxlovid) 107–109
non-pharmaceutical interventions (NPIs) 189, 237–252; contact tracing and quarantine 249–252; hand hygiene 240–242; lockdown policies 245–247; masking 237–238; school and business closures 242–245; social distancing 238–240; travel bans 247–249

normalcy bias 177, 182
norovirus surge 358–360
Novavax 96, 141
nutrition 279–282
NWSS (National Wastewater Surveillance System) 103; *see also* wastewater-based epidemiology (WBE)

obesity 270–272; COVID-19 severity linked to 271–272; impact of the pandemic 270–271; as pandemic amplifier 270–272
Omicron variants 2, 83–84, 89; and decentralized approach 238; monoclonal antibodies 111; vaccine initial effectiveness 94
One Health framework 369–370, **370**; core pillars for pandemic prevention **370**; cross-cutting strategies to operationalize **371**; *see also* World Health Organization (WHO)
Operation Warp Speed 130
optimism bias 176–177, 182

Pan-American Health Organization 263
pandemic preparedness *see* health systems preparedness
pandemic resilience 278–296
pandemic response: health systems resilience and preparedness 129–137; and institutions 128–162; and systems 128–162
pandemics: comparison **12**; health risks and consequences during 292–296; historical 49–50, **51**; and human negligence 60–62; management through history 19–21; past *vs.* COVID-19 pandemic 53–54; preparing for future 31; role of religious communities during 19–20; vulnerable groups in 269–275
pathogen identification and characterization: 1918 influenza pandemic 28; COVID-19 pandemic 28
Pathogen X 366–369, **368**
pathophysiological mechanisms of long COVID 328–330, **329**
Paxlovid 260–261
Paycheck Protection Program (PPP) 149–150
PCR testing and diagnostics 44, 100, **102**
personal hygiene: 1918 influenza pandemic 27; COVID-19 pandemic 27
personal protective equipment (PPE) 44, 68–69, 71, 135, 316
Perspectives in Psychological Science 290
Peru 131
Pfizer 260, 357
Pfizer-BioNTech 140, 141, 144
physical activity: and COVID-19 outcomes **284**; immunoregulatory effects of 283; reduced motivation for 271; regular 283–284
Pierce, M. 208
"Plagues and Peoples" (McNeill) 19
Plandemic documentary 159
PNAS Nexus 271
Post-Acute Sequelae of SARS-CoV-2 (PASC) *see* long COVID
pre-existing health conditions 337
prognosis, and long COVID 346–347
Project NextGen initiatives 262
Protection Motivation Theory (Rogers) 176
"prototype pathogens" 367–368
Psychological Bulletin 288
psychological stress 288–289
"psychology of uncertainty" 220
public health: broader implications for 360; building preparedness resilience 136–137; communication 160–162; interventions **27**; measures and COVID-19 pandemic 69–72; new viral equilibrium 360; responsibility *vs.* intellectual property 139–140
Public Health Emergency of International Concern (PHEIC) 156
public health leadership and communication: 1918 influenza pandemic 29–30; COVID-19 pandemic 29–30
public sentiment after crisis 315–318, **317**
public trust: and misinformation 158–159; and vaccine hesitancy 157–158; *see also* communication breakdowns

quad-demic emerges with norovirus 358–359

racial disparities 336–337
Rajkumar, R. P. 187
RECOVERY trial 259
Redfield, Robert 156
REGEN-COV (casirivimab and imdevimab) 260
remdesivir 107, **108**, 109, 259
respiratory manifestations 333
respiratory viruses 356–357

REVERSE-LC trial 344
ring vaccination 35, 37
risk factors/predictors, and long COVID 334–340, **335**
Robinson, E. 204, 209
Ros, M. 193
Royal Philanthropic Vaccine Expedition 35
RSV seasonal infections 5; hospitalizations in the United States *7*
RSV vaccines (Arexvy; Abrysvo; mRESVIA) 357
Russia: Sputnik V vaccine 145; vaccine diplomacy 145
Rwanda 131, 358

SARS-CoV-2 virus 1, 13, 21, 41–42, **42**, 45–46, 158, 185, 260; Alpha variant 83; Delta variant 83; epidemiological trends by **87**; eradication challenge 37; evolution of 82–86, **85**, 99–106; immunity landscapes 91–92; initial phase 82–83; *vs.* MERS-CoV virus 43–44; mutation and adaptation 4; Omicron variant 83–84; origin of 4; regional and seasonal transmission patterns of **90**; regional variation 91–92; seasonal and environmental patterns 89–91, **90**; testing challenges 99–100; testing technologies 100–101; transmission dynamics 86–93; urban dynamics 91–92; vaccine-induced immunity 5
Schatz, Albert 18
school and business closures 242–245; closure no longer a strategy 244; global approaches to 244; gradual reopening with caution 244; lessons learned 244; Omicron and return to normal operations 244; of select regions **245**; in United States 243–244; widespread closures 243–244
Science 196, 216
“Scientific Consensus” model 212
Scientific Reports 197
seasonal and situational use 238
second tripledemic (2023–2024) 357–358
Serum Institute of India (SII) 139
seven critical unknowns 376–379; actual infection rate globally 379; immunity 378; influenza and RSV 379; long COVID and long-term consequences 378; mortality estimates 377; true origin of SARS-CoV-2 377; virus mutation 377–378
sex and gender differences 334–335
Simond, Paul-Louis 14, 18
Sinopharm 145
Sinovac 145
six pillars of lifestyle medicine: balanced diet 278–282; physical activity/exercise 271, 283–284, **284**; sleep and Circadian rhythms 285–287; social connections 290–292; stress management 287–290; substance use patterns 292–296
sleep: and Circadian rhythms 285–287; and COVID-19 286, **287**; and COVID-19 outcomes **287**; and immune system 285–286
smallpox 12–13; *vs.* COVID-19 **36**, 36–38; eradication 35–36, 50; historical perspective 34–35; Intensified Smallpox Eradication Program 35; management lesson for COVID-19 38; ring vaccination 35, 37
social and healthcare marginalization 275
social connections: and COVID-19 291–292; health impacts of loneliness 290–291; health impacts of social isolation 290–291; importance of 290; relationships and overall well-being 290–292
social distancing policy 238–240; easing and reinstating with variants 239–240; global social distancing strategies 240; lessons learned 240; as recommendation, not rule 240; shift toward personal responsibility 240; strict nationwide recommendations 239; in the United States 239–240
social distancing strategies: 6-foot rule implementation and evolution 72; "15 Days to Slow the Spread" campaign 239; regional variation patterns 91–92; of select regions **241**
social isolation 290–291
“Social Media–Dependent” model 212
societal disruption, and COVID-19 pandemic 72–75, **73**
socioeconomic disparities 336–337
South Africa 131; *COVID-19 Social Relief of Distress* 154; household and business support measures **151**

South Korea 61, 66–67, 71–72, 185–187, 189–190, 200, 240; actions taken during pandemic 133–134; digital contact tracing systems 130; drive-through testing centers 130; early pandemic testing 99–100; economic and public health approaches 152; *Emergency Disaster Relief Payment* program 152; extensive contact tracing efforts 137; health authorities 196; household and business support measures **151**; mental models 181; technological innovation 136–137; technology-driven response 153
Spanish Influenza *see* 1918 influenza pandemic
specialized interventions 110–111
Sputnik V vaccine 145
Stanley, Thomas 20
stimulus programs 149–150
Strategic National Stockpile (SNS) 133; *see also* health systems preparedness; personal protective equipment (PPE); supply chains
Streptomycin 18–19
stress and immune system 288
stress management: biological pathway 288; and COVID-19 outcomes 289; global surge in psychological stress 288–289; nurturing mental health during challenging times 287–290; stress and immune system 288
structural inequities 149–150
substance use: drug use 294–295; excessive alcohol consumption 293–294; health impacts and COVID-19 outcomes of **295**; health risks and consequences during pandemic 292–296; tobacco use 292–293
supply chains: building resilient 142–143; cold chain crisis 140–142, **142**; temperature-controlled 140–141
supportive care 110–111
systems thinking 53, 59, 62, *63*; *see also* Iceberg Theory

Taiwan 191; contact tracing 130, **251**; digital surveillance tools 130; healthcare workforce management 135–136; household and business support measures **151**; *Triple Stimulus Voucher* program 153
temporal disorientation and uncertainty 206
temporal mental models: processing extended crisis and adaptation 201–210; and responses across COVID-19 pandemic **203**
Third Plague Pandemic 14
third tripledemic (2024–2025) 358–359
Titanic analogy 59
tobacco use and COVID-19 292–293
"Toxic Wild West Syndrome" 187
travel ban policies 247–249; global approaches to 248; lessons learned 249; normalization of travel 248; of select regions **249**; strict and expanding bans 248; transition to risk mitigation 248; in United States 248; variant-driven adjustments 248
treatment: approaches 343–344; long COVID conundrum **342**, 342–346, **345**
treatment timeline evolution 3, 257–262; clinical implementation 261; early discoveries and treatment development 259; monoclonal antibody therapies 260; regulatory transitions and innovation 261–262; rise of variants and oral antivirals 260–261
TRIPS Agreement 139
trust after crisis 315–318, **317**
Tuttle, Thomas 29

UNESCO 74, 313–314
UNICEF 141, 211, 264, 307, 314
United Kingdom (U.K.): contact tracing **251**; *Coronavirus Job Retention Scheme* 151; COVAX 144; Furlough scheme 150–151; hospitalization trends 88; Household Longitudinal Study 207–208; NHS system strain 130; preparedness paradox 132–133; *Self-Employment Income Support Scheme* 151; vaccine hoarding 145–146
United Nations Environment Programme (UNEP) 369
United Nations Office on Drugs and Crime 294
United States: burnout rate 135; contact tracing and quarantine policies in 250; COVAX 144; fragmented federal response 130; hand hygiene policies 241–242; healthcare worker burnout 136; hospitalizations in *6*; human-to-human transmission 61; individualism 182; individual liberty 188; intensive care units, stress on 88; large-scale

lockdowns 61; lockdown policies in 246–247; "loose" culture 182; masking policies in 237–238; mental models 204; optimism bias 182; political ideology 178; political polarization impacts 246; PPP implementation issues 149–150; public communication strategies 72; RSV seasonal infections 7; school and business closures in 243–244; social distancing policy 239–240; social distancing policy in 239–240; stimulus packages 149–150; structural inequities 149–150; testing capacity 100; Toxic Wild West Syndrome 187; travel ban policies in 248; vaccine hoarding 145
UN's State of the World's Children 2021 report 309

vaccination status 338–339
vaccine: diplomacy 144–145; efficacy and immunity 93–99; global disparities 97–99, **98**; hoarding 145–147, **146**, **147**; initial effectiveness 93–94, **94**; platform diversity 95–96, **96**; real-world effectiveness 96–97; rollout and policy shifts 238; and treatments 257–264
vaccine development: 1918 influenza pandemic 28–29; COVID-19 pandemic 28–29
vaccine hesitancy 3, 144, 157, 159, 188, 192, 216, 263–264
vaccine inequity 263–264
vaccine manufacturing: building resilient supply systems 142–143; cold chain crisis 140–142, **142**; global struggles of 137–139; mRNA vaccines constraints 138; Serum Institute of India 139; traditional vaccine challenges 138–139; *see also* global vaccine equity
vaccine nationalism 37, 143–144, 146, 148
Van Bavel, J. J. 175, 178, 200
Venice 20; Black Death 20
viral variant 339–340
VISION Network 97
vulnerable groups 269–275

Waksman, Selman 18–19
Wang, Y. 188
wastewater-based epidemiology (WBE) 103
well-being: importance of relationships for overall 290–292; individual 185, 314; mental 219, 275, 296, 310; personal 185, 311; physical 275, 290; psychological 176, 289; social 291
wildlife trade 366, **367**
workforce transformation 310–313, **312**, **313**
World Bank 106, 154–155, 311, 314
World Economic Forum (WEF) 311
World Health Organization (WHO) 11, 61, 198, 200, 217, 259, 260, 261, 308, 310, 369; 2024 priority pathogen watchlist **368**; infodemic 159; mRNA Technology Transfer Hub 140; Preparedness and Resilience for Emerging Threats (PRET) Initiative 369; Public Health Emergency of International Concern (PHEIC) 156; vaccine equity framework 148
World Organisation for Animal Health (WOAH) 369
World Trade Organization (WTO) 139–140
World War II 311
worst-case bias 179–180

Xiao, Y. 215

Yersin, Alexandre 14, 18
Yersinia pestis 11, 14, 18, 20–21

Zika virus outbreak 52
zoonotic spillover events 363–364, **364**
zoonotic threats: building global defense at the source 369–371, **370**, **371**; climate as force multipliers 364–366, **365**; globalization as force multipliers 364–366, **365**; Pathogen X 366–369, **368**; prevention over reaction 369–371, **370**, **371**; rise of new 363–371; wildlife trade and agricultural interfaces 366, **367**; zoonotic spillover events 363–364, **364**

For Product Safety Concerns and Information please contact our EU representative GPSR@taylorandfrancis.com
Taylor & Francis Verlag GmbH, Kaufingerstraße 24, 80331 München, Germany

www.ingramcontent.com/pod-product-compliance
Lightning Source LLC
Chambersburg PA
CBHW052117230326
41598CB00079B/3775

* 9 7 8 1 0 3 2 9 8 3 8 0 6 *